2015 ChiroCode DeskBook

23RD ANNUAL EDITION

A Practice Management

B Insurance and Reimbursement

C Medicare Guidelines

D Documentation Guidelines

E Claims and Appeals

F Compliance and Audit Protection

G Diagnosis Codes

H Procedure Codes

I Supply Codes

ChiroCode INSTITUTE

To activate your ChiroCode DeskBook online tools go to ChiroCode.com/onlinetools. Click on "Activate" then enter your online activation code below:

Write your user name and password here for quick access.
User: _____
Password: _____

LJ213

Copyright Notice and Disclaimer

Published and copyrighted © by ChiroCode®, Inc. 1993-2015 All rights reserved.

No part of this publication may be reproduced, distributed or transmitted in any form or by any means including photocopying, recording, or other electronic or mechanical methods, without the prior written permission of the publisher, except in the case of brief quotations embodied in critical reviews and certain other noncommercial uses permitted by copyright law. Online content for this DeskBook is licensed for a single-user only. For permission, please email all queries to ChiroCode, Inc. at operations@ChiroCode.com.

This publication is distributed with the understanding that the publisher is not engaged in rendering legal or accounting or medical services. If legal advice or other expert assistance is required, the services of a competent professional person should be sought.

ChiroCode Institute assumes no liability for data contained or not contained herein. It does not directly nor indirectly practice law or give legal opinions. It assumes no responsibility for the consequences attributable to or related to any use or interpretation of any information or views contained in or not contained in this publication. Absolute accuracy cannot be guaranteed. Neither ChiroCode Institute nor the American Chiropractic Association (ACA) are responsible for informing the purchaser of any updates.

The inclusion of hyperlinked information and additional content on the American Chiropractic Association website is independent of ChiroCode Institute and does not constitute an endorsement of that content.

ChiroCode® DeskBook is a registered trademark of ChiroCode, Inc.

CPT copyright 2014 American Medical Association. All rights reserved.

Current Procedural Terminology (CPT) codes and descriptions are copyright 2014 American Medical Association (AMA). All Rights Reserved. Fee schedules, relative value units, conversion factors and/or related components are not assigned by the AMA, are not part of CPT, and the AMA is not recommending their use. The AMA does not directly or indirectly practice medicine or dispense medical services. The AMA assumes no liability for data contained or not contained herein. CPT is a registered trademark of the American Medical Association.

Visit ChiroCode.com for more information.

Printed in the U.S.A.

ChiroCode, Inc.
62 East 300 North
Spanish Fork, UT 84660 USA

Phone (801) 528-6876 Fax (602) 997-9755

ChiroCode.com

ISBN: 978-0-9913390-2-0

2015 ChiroCode DeskBook
CONTENTS

INTRODUCTION
- Welcome ... v
- What's New for 2015 ... vi
- Acknowledgments ... viii
- Endorsements ... ix
- ChiroCode DeskBook Online Tools ... xii
- Additional Tools and Resources ... xiii
- ACA Code of Ethics ... xiv
- Legend to Using Resource Icons ... xvi

A – PRACTICE MANAGEMENT
1. Starting and Maintaining a Thriving Practice ... A - 3
2. Compliance Considerations ... A - 9
3. Office Equipment and Software ... A - 13
4. Business Financial Standards ... A - 17
5. Supportive and Productive Staff ... A - 25

B – INSURANCE AND REIMBURSEMENT
1. Understanding Insurance Reimbursement ... B - 3
2. Types of Insurance Plans ... B - 21
3. Establishing Fees ... B - 39

C – MEDICARE GUIDELINES
1. Understanding Medicare ... C - 3
2. Medicare Coverage ... C - 15
3. Medicare Fees ... C - 30
4. Medicare Appeals ... C - 36
5. Physician Quality Reporting System ... C - 44

D – DOCUMENTATION GUIDELINES
1. The Documentation Challenge ... D - 3
2. Record Keeping ... D - 7
3. Assessment Visits ... D - 18
4. Treatment Visits ... D - 28
5. Treatment Plans and Assessments ... D - 33

E – CLAIMS AND APPEALS
1. Claims Processing ... E - 3
2. 1500 Claim Form ... E - 11
3. Guidelines for Unpaid Claims ... E - 37
4. ERISA Appeals ... E - 47

F – COMPLIANCE AND AUDIT PROTECTION

1. The Need for Compliance .... F - 3
2. HIPAA Compliance .... F - 14
3. Medicare Compliance .... F - 30
4. OIG Compliance Program Guidance .... F - 35
5. Audit Protection .... F - 45

G – DIAGNOSIS CODES

1. Diagnosis Coding .... G - 3
2. Commonly Used ICD-9-CM Diagnosis Codes (Anatomic List) .... G - 12
3. Commonly Used ICD-10-CM Diagnosis Codes (Anatomic List) ..... G - 21
4. Numeric ICD-9-CM (Tabular) List .... G - 33
5. Alphabetic List (ICD-9-CM) .... G - 111

H – PROCEDURE CODES

1. Procedure Coding .... H - 3
2. Commonly Used Codes .... H - 11
3. Evaluation and Management .... H - 21
4. CPT Procedures
   a. Evaluation and Management Codes .... H - 35
   b. Surgery Codes .... H - 48
   c. Diagnostic Imaging Codes .... H - 52
   d. Laboratory Codes .... H - 62
   e. Medicine Codes (Chiropractic Manipulation and Therapies) ... H - 64
   f. Category III Codes .... H - 90
5. HCPCS Procedure Codes .... H - 92
6. Procedure Modifiers .... H - 97
7. Clinical Examples .... H - 112
8. Alphabetic List .... H - 128

I – SUPPLY CODES

1. Supply Coding .... I - 3
2. Commonly Used Supply Codes .... I - 7
3. HCPCS Supply Codes .... I - 8
4. HCPCS Supply Modifiers .... I - 31
5. Alphabetic List .... I - 34

REFERENCE PAGES

ACA Template Letters
Glossary
Frequently Asked Questions
ChiroCode DeskBook Index

Welcome

Welcome to this 2015 *ChiroCode DeskBook*–23rd Annual Edition–with *ChiroCode Online Tools* and *Resources*. The *ChiroCode DeskBook* is the original insurance reimbursement manual for chiropractic. In our continued pursuit of excellence, this edition has been completely revised in order to make it easier to follow and understand. This is truly a unique annual compilation of reimbursement essentials from authoritative sources, with commentary. For twenty-three years, the *ChiroCode DeskBook* has provided excellence in helping thousands of offices to be more profitable and successful. Comments like these are typical of satisfied subscribers: "It's nice to have a non-political coding and reimbursement book," "It's my Bible for getting paid," and, "Once again, you guys have the answer."

Our Commitment is to providing excellence in reimbursement information.

Our Mission is to lead the Chiropractic profession through the reimbursement process to achieve financial success through quality products, services, education, and consulting. We encourage and support appropriate reimbursement, ethical and compliant documentation and reporting of diagnoses, procedures, and supplies with appropriate and effective appeals when claims are denied.

Our Pledge is to help your practice survive and thrive with greater assurance through an accurate knowledge of current codes, clean claims, thorough and complete documentation, effective appeals for denied claims, refund demands, and compliance.

Universal Use We are honored by the widespread acceptance and use of this annual publication. It was initially developed as a factual and comprehensive reimbursement resource for doctors and has since grown to include much more than just reimbursement. Additionally, many payers, consultants, attorneys, colleges, boards, and other professionals have discovered it to be a valuable reference and reimbursement guide.

Support We encourage you to take advantage of our ChiroCode Alerts, which are sent by email. These alerts include the latest industry and coding news, *ChiroCode DeskBook* updates, notifications of *ChiroCode Webinars*, current *Quick Questions*, coding and reimbursement tips, and more. To register, go to: ChiroCode.com/register. Your information privacy is assured—it is never shared with others.

Feedback Your opinions and suggestions are welcome and appreciated. With your feedback we continue to improve year after year. Please send your comments and suggestions to support@chirocode.com.

Thank you for your confidence and trust.

LaMont J. Leavitt, President/CEO

What's New for 2015

At the ChiroCode Institute, we understand that the ever increasing post-payment reviews, audits, and demands on time are making it more difficult to keep up with all the challenges of running a successful chiropractic practice. In light of these challenges, the *ChiroCode DeskBook* has been updated and revised once again to make it easy for you to find needed information quickly and efficiently. Expanded online resources, flowcharts, checklists, chapter objectives, and outlines are just some of the helpful things in this edition.

Resources

To help providers find the resources in the book (webinars, training, articles and more), we've simplified the process. By numbering the resources, it makes it much easier to find an online reference or a specific document in our vast library of information. If you see a resource listed in the book, simply go to ChiroCode.com/deskbook-resources and look for the number. You can also do a search for the page and immediately go to the one you need.

Another benefit to this new approach is that resource pages on specific topics will also be continuously updated throughout the year with additional content as it becomes available. For example, if there's a new webinar on the EHR program, it will show up on the Documentation Resources page.

Practice Management

This section was updated and includes new segments or information on the impact of Health Reform Shared Savings Programs, malpractice insurance, cyber insurance, advantages and disadvantages of outsourcing in your practice as well as the impact of social media and the use of cell phones.

Insurance and Reimbursement

Understanding the impact of health reform is now more important than ever. This section has been updated with the essential information that your clinic needs. Additionally, the segment on Personal Injury has been completely revised for 2015.

Medicare Guidelines

This section of the *ChiroCode DeskBook* has new segments on "Accountable Care Organizations (ACOs)/Shared Savings Programs" and the Medicare Overpayment process. Additional tips and alerts have been added to the segment on ABNs. The updated "Medicare Part B Appeals Process" flowchart is also very helpful.

Documentation Guidelines

The Federal EHR program has had some significant changes that may impact provider payments in the coming years. This revised section addresses those issues and also includes a new segment titled "Common Errors" which can assist providers in performing an internal audit on their documentation. Several new tips have been added and some explanations clarified to make this section even more user-friendly.

Claims and Appeals

Claims processing guidelines are frequently updated and so Chapter 2 of this section has been updated to include the most current Medicare and NUCC instructions. Additionally, Chapter 3 includes a new segment on processing payer overpayments (voluntary refunds). It includes a generic form which can be used by providers when a payer does not have a specific form to use. The chapter on ERISA has been updated with important information on the impact of self-funded insurance plans.

Compliance and Audit Protection

Compliance is a constantly evolving area of importance for healthcare providers. As such, this section has been udpated with current information to assist providers in maintaining an active and effective compliance plan. Updated information on mobile devices and Windows operating systems provide further compliance guidance.

We have also included information on virtual cards and how this growing trend can significantly impact your practice.

Codes for Diagnoses, Procedures and Supplies

Current HIPAA-approved code excerpts for chiropractic services and supplies are found in the three sections: Diagnosis Codes, Procedure Codes, and Supply Codes. New codes for 2015 are indicated with the "●" symbol, and revised codes are shown with a "▲" symbol.

In *Section H-Procedure Codes*, Chapters 2 and 3 have been completely revised. Chapter 2 is built around an easy to follow Commonly Used Codes format and Chapter 3 contains a comprehensive breakdown on how to best select the proper Evaluation and Management codes.

Acknowledgments

Development of this annual edition requires extensive review and input. The contributions over many years from numerous chiropractic physicians, assistants, consultants and attorneys have made this book possible. Their efforts and professional input are sincerely appreciated but they are too numerous to list here. Special thanks also goes to all of the hardworking ChiroCode Institute support staff.

Senior editors:

> Brandy Brimhall, CPC CMCO CPCO CCCPC, ChiroCode Director of Education
>
> Evan Gwilliam, DC MBS BS CPC CCPC NCICS CCCPC CPC-I MCS-P CPMA, ChiroCode Vice President
>
> Raquel Shumway, ChiroCode Editorial Staff
>
> Wyn Staheli, ChiroCode Chief Content Officer
>
> Michael Bo Vocu, CCCPC, ChiroCode Editorial Staff

Other reviewers and contributors for this edition:

> David D. Berky, Find-A-Code, Chief Product Officer
>
> Ray Foxworth, DC FICC MCS-P, ChiroHealthUSA President
>
> Mario Fucinari, DC CCSP DAAPM MCS-P, AskMario.com
>
> Tom Grant Jr., DC, Grant Professional Strategies
>
> Alan M. Immerman, DC, Arizona Chiropractic Society President
>
> LaMont Leavitt, ChiroCode CEO
>
> Ron Short, DC CPC MCS-P, ChiroMedicare
>
> Jared Staheli, ChiroCode Editorial Staff
>
> Aimee Wilcox, MA CCS-P, Find-A-Code, Director of Education

Appreciative acknowledgement is expressed to the American Chiropractic Association's Insurance Relations Department as well as the Coding, Payment Policy and Medicare Committees for their invaluable input. Their contributions have been instrumental in making this the best coding manual within the chiropractic industry.

In Memoriam - We are pleased to rededicate this 23rd annual edition to a man who lived to help others, **D Henry Leavitt**. His vision and service to the industry have made ChiroCode what it is today.

ACA ENDORSEMENT

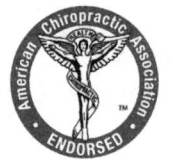

The goal of the *ChiroCode DeskBook* is to standardize coding and billing practices to aid proper reimbursement. This is the third year that the American Chiropractic Association (ACA) has given its endorsement to the *ChiroCode DeskBook* which involves detailed collaboration to produce timely and accurate information for the profession. ACA members and the entire chiropractic profession can expect the same quality information they have had access to for years and have come to trust from both organizations.

The U.S. health care system is in transition, making coding and billing more complex than ever before. The ACA is pleased to work with ChiroCode, and its well-established product, to give providers a comprehensive reference text to help navigate the often confusing myriad regulations that clinics must follow to be in compliance. Doctors face ongoing challenges with audits, changing payer policies, network limitations, state laws, and a changing coding landscape. Proper coding and documentation have never been more important, not only for accuracy, but to help doctors bill properly.

Having a comprehensive tool that is updated annually is a must for every chiropractic practice. Clinics can have confidence in the DeskBook because it comes from two trusted names within the profession.

Anthony Hamm, DC
ACA President

Leo Bronston, DC
Chairman, ACA Coding Committee

At the time of printing, the American Chiropractic Association (ACA) reviewed the 2015 *ChiroCode DeskBook* and endorses its content unless otherwise specified. The ACA's endorsement is exclusive to the 2015 *ChiroCode DeskBook*. **The endorsement does not extend to hyperlinked information, additional content on ChiroCode Institute's website, or other ChiroCode Institute products and services.** The ACA's endorsement of ChiroCode Institute's content is done so with the understanding that the ACA is not engaged in rendering legal, accounting, medical, practice management, coding or other professional services, and may not be held liable for any use or misuse of the content. The ACA's endorsement should not be construed as offering clinical advice and does not substitute for medical decision making, both of which are the responsibility of the treating physician.

ACA HIPAA Disclaimer

ACA recognizes that, as a federal regulation, HIPAA is complex. Providers should take care not only to be in compliance, but to assure they observe state laws and regulations which may provide similar protections/requirements. The information offered by ACA is provided as helpful tips and providers are encouraged to seek the counsel of a qualified healthcare law attorney licensed in their state for further guidance. To view the ACA's information on HIPAA, please go to ACAtoday.org/hipaa.

ACA Medicare Section/OIG Portion Disclaimer

At the time of printing, the federal government had not yet released its changes for 2015. Every effort was made to update the information in the 2015 *DeskBook* with information available at the time of review. Ongoing updates on CMS-related topics will be posted on the ACA website at ACAtoday.org/Medicare and through its articles and publications.

ACA Documentation Section Disclaimer

The American Chiropractic Association has developed a comprehensive Clinical Documentation Manual (3rd edition) apart from the *ChiroCode DeskBook*. The ChiroCode Documentation section refers to the ACA Clinical Documentation Manual (3rd edition), where appropriate, for additional examples and clarification which illustrate ACA's current and official policies and opinions regarding Documentation.

ACA Time of Service (TOS) Disclaimer

The ACA does not officially recommend that doctors of chiropractic use TOS discounts. This is due to the possibility of violating state and/or federal law. Before implementing a TOS discount, doctors of chiropractic should consult with a health care law attorney.

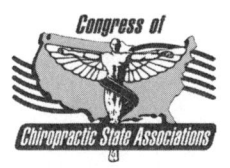

Dear Colleague:

The Board of Directors of the Congress of Chiropractic State Associations (COCSA) enthusiastically supports the annual *ChiroCode DeskBook*.

We believe this book belongs in the office of every Doctor of Chiropractic, particularly those who deal with third party payers such as Medicare, health insurers, automobile insurance companies and others who pay for chiropractic services. It is essential for any chiropractic office to ensure that their services are properly coded and billed.

This annual *ChiroCode DeskBook* assists Doctors of Chiropractic in becoming more successful. It allows the doctor to properly identify, accurately describe and report diagnoses, procedures, and supplies. It provides the tools needed to determine appropriate fees for reimbursement, to pursue proper payment and make effective appeals when denied. In addition to helping doctors understand coding, reimbursement, and compliance issues, this book also includes tips and other information that will enrich the chiropractic profession and make your practice more successful.

COCSA is proud of its association of many years with the ChiroCode Institute. They have given back so much to our chiropractic profession. We are pleased to support the annual *ChiroCode Deskbook* and believe you will find it to be an indispensable tool for your practice.

Dr. John LaMonica
President, Congress of Chiropractic State Associations

CHIROCODE DESKBOOK ONLINE TOOLS

ChiroCode DeskBook Online Tools are available to all *2015 ChiroCode DeskBook* subscribers at ChiroCode.com/onlinetools. The tutorial on the following pages will help you better understand the online tools.

Sign-in

If you purchased your *ChiroCode DeskBook* online from ChiroCode Institute's online store, you may use the same sign-in information to access your online tools. Otherwise, create a new account and follow the instructions to activate your book.

Online Tools

ChiroCode DeskBook Online Tools include:

- Online Resources
- ChiroCode Fee Calculator
- Medicare Fee Calculator for Chiropractic Codes

Online Resources

If you have ever had trouble finding that one form or report, you will love this new tool. Easily access all the resources in the book which may be referenced by either number or name. This includes the downloadable forms, the complete line-by-line instructions for the 1500 claim form and much more.

ChiroCode Fee Calculator

Calculate fees for all the codes in your *ChiroCode DeskBook* based on the Medicare fee schedule for any zip code entered. You will also be able to calculate two additional fee columns based on percentages of Medicare. Common percentages are 150% and 200%.

Medicare Fee Calculator for Chiropractic Codes

Calculate your Medicare fees including the Allowed Amount and Limiting Charge for your geographic area. This tool only calculates fees for the three Chiropractic codes that Medicare reimburses.

Additional Tools and Resources

Visit 🖱 ChiroCode.com/store to become a ChiroCode Premium member.

ChiroCode Premium Membership

ChiroCode Premium Membership includes:

- **Map-A-Code:** The Map-A-Code ICD-10 Crosswalk tool uses General Equivalence Mappings (GEMs) to map codes from ICD-9-CM to ICD-10-CM. Be sure to take advantage of the valuable and helpful 'page view" feature which allows you to see a page of codes all at once and aids in the coding decision process.
- **ChiroCode Webinars on Demand:** Hundreds of informative webinars are available, on a wide variety of useful topics to Chiropractic offices.
- **Email Coding Support:** Quickly get the answers you need by simply sending an email to ChiroCode Institute.
- **ChiroCode KnowledgeBase:** Hundreds of articles are available in this vast KnowledgeBase, in a searchable online format, with more articles added each month.
- **Discounts:** Take advantage of special discounts on many items available for purchase at 🖱 ChiroCode.com/store.
- **CCCPC Certification Practice Test:** Find out if you have the skills to become a ChiroCode Certified Chiropractic Professional Coder.

American Chiropractic Association (ACA) Membership

Visit 🖱 ACAtoday.org to read more about the ACA's mission and to become an ACA member.

ACA provides legislative and insurance advocacy, public relations, and educational opportunities for doctors of chiropractic for the advancement of the profession. Here are a few of the many benefits of ACA membership:

- New patients through Find a Doctor—ACA's online directory
- Coding and insurance questions answered for doctors of chiropractic
- Practice management and marketing tools
- Updates on issues affecting the profession, such as health care reform, electronic health records, integrative care, and more
- Guidance on coding, which includes helpful resources on ICD-10 and documentation of preventive services

ACA Code of Ethics

Preamble

This Code of Ethics is based upon the acknowledgement that the social contract dictates the profession's responsibilities to the patient, the public, and the profession; and upholds the fundamental principle that the paramount purpose of the chiropractic doctor's professional services shall be to benefit the patient.

    I. Doctors of chiropractic should adhere to a commitment to the highest standards of excellence and should attend to their patients in accordance with established best practices.

    II. Doctors of chiropractic should maintain the highest standards of professional and personal conduct, and should comply with all governmental jurisdictional rules and regulations.

    III. Doctor-patient relationships should be built on mutual respect, trust and cooperation. In keeping with these principles, doctors of chiropractic shall demonstrate absolute honesty with regard to the patient's condition when communicating with the patient and/or representatives of the patient. Doctors of chiropractic shall not mislead patients into false or unjustified expectations of favorable results of treatment. In communications with a patient and/or representatives of a patient, doctors of chiropractic should never misrepresent their education, credentials, professional qualification or scope of clinical ability.

    IV. Doctors of chiropractic should preserve and protect the patient's confidential information, except as the patient directs or consents, or the law requires otherwise.

    V. Doctors of chiropractic should employ their best good faith efforts to provide information and facilitate understanding to enable the patient to make an informed choice in regard to proposed chiropractic treatment. The patient should make his or her own determination on such treatment.

    VI. The doctor-patient relationship requires the doctor of chiropractic to exercise utmost care that he or she will do nothing to exploit the trust and dependency of the patient. Sexual misconduct is a form of behavior that adversely affects the public welfare and harms patients individually and collectively. Sexual misconduct exploits the doctor-patient relationship and is a violation of the public trust.

    VII. Doctors of chiropractic should willingly consult and seek the talents of other health care professionals when such consultation would benefit their patients or when their patients express a desire for such consultation.

    VIII. Doctors of chiropractic should never neglect nor abandon a patient. Due notice should be afforded to the patient and/or representatives of the patient when care will be withdrawn so that appropriate alternatives for continuity of care may be arranged.

    IX. With the exception of emergencies, doctors of chiropractic are free to choose the patients they will serve, just as patients are free to choose who will provide healthcare services for them. However, decisions as to who will be served should not be based on race, religion, ethnicity, nationality, creed, gender, handicap or sexual preference.

    X. Doctors of chiropractic should conduct themselves as members of a learned profession and as members of the greater healthcare community dedicated to the promotion of health, the prevention of illness and the alleviation of suffering. As such, doctors of chiropractic should collaborate and cooperate with other health care professionals to protect and enhance the health of the public with the goals of reducing morbidity, increasing functional capacity, increasing the longevity of the U.S. population and reducing health care costs.

XI. Doctors of chiropractic should exercise utmost care that advertising is truthful and accurate in representing the doctor's professional qualifications and degree of competence. Advertising should not exploit the vulnerability of patients, should not be misleading and should conform to all governmental jurisdictional rules and regulations in connection with professional advertising.

XII. As professions are self-regulating bodies, doctors of chiropractic shall protect the public and the profession by reporting incidents of unprofessional, illegal, incompetent and unethical acts to appropriate authorities and organizations and should stand ready to testify in courts of law and in administrative hearings.

XIII. Doctors of chiropractic have an obligation to the profession to endeavor to assure that their behavior does not give the appearance of professional impropriety. Any actions which may benefit the practitioner to the detriment of the profession must be avoided so as to not erode the public trust.

XIV. Doctors of chiropractic should recognize their obligation to help others acquire knowledge and skill in the practice of the profession. They should maintain the highest standards of scholarship, education and training in the accurate and full dissemination of information and ideas.

Legend for Using Resource Icons

ChiroCode DeskBook This icon indicates that there are other locations in the *ChiroCode Deskbook* which also have information on this subject and/or a more in-depth look at a concept.

Resource This icon directs the reader to a variety of resources. This can include links to online articles, websites, webinars and other helpful information from many sources which provides more in-depth information on a particular topic. This ensures that the most current and up-to-date information is available to our subscribers. See ChiroCode.com/deskbook-resources

Note: Webinars on Demand are now part of the resources. The complete webinar archive is available to ChiroCode Premium Members (you must be logged in to review them). See ChiroCode.com/webinars

Checklist This icon is used to point out items that need to be "checked off." These are things that your office needs to review and include in your office policies and procedures where applicable.

ChiroCode DeskBook Online Tools This icon represents resources that are available to those who have purchased and registered the current version of the *ChiroCode DeskBook*. These include tools such as the *ChiroCode Fee Calculator*. Go to ChiroCode.com/onlinetools.

Internet resource This icon is used to indicate that there are resources available on the internet for this topic.

ChiroCode Store This icon indicates helpful resources which may be purchased from the ChiroCode Store. Go to ChiroCode.com/store.

2015 ChiroCode® DeskBook | ChiroCode.com

1. Starting and Maintaining a Thriving Practice
Page A-3

2. Compliance Considerations
Page A-9

3. Office Equipment and Software
Page A-13

4. Business Financial Standards
Page A-17

5. Supportive and Productive Staff
Page A-25

PRACTICE MANAGEMENT

A

PRACTICE MANAGEMENT

OBJECTIVES

Practice Management is a very broad subject. There are many excellent seminars, books, and magazines which are devoted entirely to helping healthcare providers.

The purpose of this section is to not only assist providers who are just beginning to start their own practice, but also to outline some important concepts that currently practicing chiropractors need to be aware of in order to maintain a thriving practice. These are only guidelines and should be used as a starting point for a practice update. In some situations, it is advisable to obtain help from accountants or attorneys as the case may be.

Please note that billing codes and other important details for reimbursement and compliance are included in other sections of this book.

OUTLINE

1. Starting and Maintaining a Thriving Practice *A-3*
   - Introduction to Practice Management *A-3*
   - Business Basics *A-4*
   - Other Considerations *A-5*
   - Review *A-8*

2. Compliance Considerations *A-9*
   - Government Compliance Programs *A-9*
   - Professional Licensing *A-10*
   - Insurance *A-11*
   - Review *A-12*

3. Office Equipment and Software *A-13*
   - Equipment: Lease vs Purchase *A-13*
   - Selecting Software *A-15*
   - Review *A-16*

4. Business Financial Standards *A-17*
   - Financial Considerations *A-17*
   - Marketing Your Practice *A-20*
   - Review *A-24*

5. Supportive and Productive Staff *A-25*
   - Finding the Right People *A-25*
   - Training Staff *A-28*
   - Review *A-34*

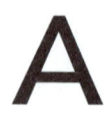

1. Starting and Maintaining a Thriving Practice

INTRODUCTION TO PRACTICE MANAGEMENT

Why become a doctor of chiropractic? Every provider has their own unique answer. Very few of them will include something like, "I wanted to be responsible for payroll taxes and understand OSHA regulations." Rather, most will answer that being a chiropractor is about helping the patient and making a difference in someone's life. It is a higher calling and sense of purpose that drives men and women to become doctors, or even support staff. The bottom line is that there must be a paycheck and there must be a business to provide that pay. This section serves two purposes:

1. Assist new doctors with understanding the business considerations of running a chiropractic practice, and
2. Assist seasoned doctors with guidelines and tips to brush up on important business matters.

The success of your practice depends on knowing and understanding current laws, regulations and policies. If you do not meet these requirements, you may not have a business to help people. This is why it is important to take time, on a regular basis, to assess how your business can improve from a business standpoint.

Your practice can not thrive without understanding and applying the following concepts which are taught throughout this *ChiroCode DeskBook*:

- Business requirements at the federal, state, and local level;
- Professional requirements such as licensing, training, and education;
- Financial standards for running an office and generating income;
- Marketing to attract new clients;
- Billing standards which are in full compliance to keep the income stream steady;
- Supportive people all working to help the practice succeed.

This section is hardly exhaustive, as there are volumes of information available on each of the topics included herein. Instead, important topics to evaluate are discussed and guidance is given on where to look for further resources. Make this your beginning point for a practice review.

See Resource 100 for additional information.

Business Basics

An excellent resource for your practice is the government's Small Business Association (SBA) website. Their "10 Steps for Starting a Business" is a thorough review for all practices, whether they are just getting started or they have been around for years and are well established.

The ten basic steps are:

1. Write a Business Plan
2. Business Assistance and Training
3. Choose a Business Location
4. Finance Your Business
5. Determine the Legal Structure of Your Business
6. Register a Business Name
7. Get a Tax Identification Number
8. Register for State and Local Taxes
9. Obtain Business Licenses and Permit
10. Understand Employer Responsibilities

See Resource 101 for more about these steps and links to a wealth of information for small business owners.

Not all these steps are in exact order. For instance, you can't obtain financing for your company unless you have registered the business structure and obtained a Taxpayer Identification Number (TIN). Banks rarely lend money to anyone without a solid business plan. The exception to this is if you obtain a private source of financing, such as from friends, family, or yourself.

If you need to ask someone questions, the SBA personnel can be helpful. The SBA also contracts with local business professionals to provide assistance to other small business professionals. You will find these contacts under their "Get Local Assistance" section.

State and Local Requirements

Next, review state and local government information for business owners. Become familiar with applicable laws surrounding starting and running a business in your location. If you're going to hire employees, then you will need to become familiar with your state's employment laws. Don't forget to review tax laws. Tax laws will be the biggest factor in deciding what kind of business structure you are going to use. You'll need the answers to these important questions:

- Does your state collect income tax, sales taxes, use taxes, or other miscellaneous taxes like personal property?
- Are you required to carry specific insurances such as workers compensation, general liability, or professional liability?
- Will you be required to provide specific benefits to your employees such as health insurance?
- What are the reporting requirements?

It is not feasible to include guidelines for every state in this book because the differences between states are often much bigger than you may realize. For this reason, if you are expanding your practice to another state, do not assume that things will work the same in the new state. Chances are that they will be quite dissimilar.

Do not forget to review your county and city business information to determine if there are other taxes and regulations which are applicable to your business. Counties and cities are the entities that issue business licenses and are in charge of other local services such as water and power. They also regulate where you may place your business. Pay close attention to zoning laws.

Professional Assistance

Most government entities assume that small businesses will be doing all the work on their own. For this reason, they don't offer much information about outsourcing certain tasks such as payroll to other companies. Be aware that managerial tasks such as payroll, human resources, accounting, and taxes can take up much of your time if you do them on your own. Outsourcing these tasks may help you save time, headaches, and money. A negative aspect to using these services is that you lose some control, and possibly some security. You are dependent upon them doing their job correctly. Research these businesses thoroughly to make sure they are reputable. Make sure your contract with them holds them responsible for any errors they make. HIPAA Covered Entities must have a signed Business Associate Agreement with them as well.

> See *Section F–Compliance and Audit Protection* for more about HIPAA Requirements.

> Business Associate Agreements are included in *Complete & Easy HIPAA Compliance* (Resource 116).

Location

One major decision that will have the most impact on your new chiropractic office is where it will be located. Remember the three "L's" of real estate: location, location, location. Your practice should be easy to find, and accessibility and parking should be prime considerations because many of your patients will have injuries which make parking difficult. Find out if there are any ordinances or zoning restrictions that might affect your location. Be sure that you leave room for growth. See the segment "Marketing Your Practice" in Chapter 4 of this section for more about location considerations.

This leads us to the ever difficult question of Owning versus Leasing.

OTHER CONSIDERATIONS

Office Space: Own vs Lease

Many business people like the autonomy and possible equity that arises from owning a building. However, 98 percent of all commercial, retail, and office space is for lease, not for sale, according to Franchise Update Media Group. Additionally, most properties that are available for purchase tend to be in less desirable locations. If you leave a leased space and decide to build or own in another location which is in close proximity to your old location, keep in mind that the previous landlord may fill the space you left behind with another chiropractor which could potentially lead to increased competition. Also, owners may need to become the plumber, painter, and electrician, etc., which can be a real burden. On the other hand, an owner can sell a practice, but retain the property, thereby creating a stream of income that can continue into retirement.

Move-in Costs

No matter where you set up your business, you need to factor in the cost of outfitting your location to do business. Computers, desks, tables, equipment, lighting, chairs, office supplies, websites, email, and cleaning services all have costs associated with them. These are the unexpected costs that tend to swamp a start-up business because they were never considered and factored into the pricing of products and services.

Solo or Group Practice?

Beyond an understanding of the basic business principles, providers should consider whether they desire to establish their practice as a solo practice or a group practice. They should also remember that anytime they decide to move or change locations, there are additional problems and costs associated with doing so.

Group Practice Options

Many providers like the autonomy of being an entrepreneur and having a solo practice. However, there are some other types of practices to consider: Multi-DC or Multi-Disciplinary Practices. If you are considering one of these options, it is wise to consult with a healthcare attorney to ensure that these unique situations are set up correctly in accordance with all applicable state and Federal regulations.

Multi-DC Clinics

There are some distinct advantages when more than one chiropractor is part of a practice; for example, shared expenses, shared ancillary staff, increased capacity to grow, sharing of emergency calls and increased flexibility in vacation time. However, there are some disadvantages such as having fewer patients per doctor. The following are some important points to consider:

- Whose NPI gets used in box 24? Whose NPI is in box 33?
- Who is considered the primary caregiver for the patient?
- What happens if the providers split, i.e. they decide to no longer practice together?
- What happens to the patient? What happens to the office?

These types of decisions need to be addressed and documented at the beginning of the relationship, not at the end. Consult with a good lawyer to ensure that all these issues are properly addressed.

Multi-Disciplinary Practice

A Multi-Disciplinary Practice (MDP) is simply a practice where at least two healthcare professionals of more than one specialty practice in the same location. These types of arrangements are also known as a Multi-Disciplinary Clinic or Center (MDC). Usually these specialties are MD/DO and a chiropractor; however, the possibilities are limitless. This concept has been used successfully for cancer treatment for some time. The patient benefits from having all their care in one place with this coordinated care plan between different specialties.

Providers benefit in a variety of ways. With an MDP, there is one less HIPAA administrative burden. When it comes to HIPAA rules regarding PHI, all healthcare providers within the MDP are considered to be one entity (so long as they are employees and not private contractors) and thus no additional authorized releases of PHI are required for them to communicate internally. Also, these types of clinics allow the business owners to share expenses and reduce or limit liability because there are checks and balances in place.

As part of these necessary checks and balances, pay particular attention to ensuring that improved clinical outcome is the basis for treatment and that necessary precautions are taken to avoid Stark Law self-referral violations. However, there are other important checks and balances to consider. As such, the ACA has established an official public policy regarding MDPs. If you are considering this type of practice, it would be wise to check their website for important information regarding this subject.

There are some disadvantages which should also be considered. When merging different disciplines, all parties need to be flexible and willing to view treatment options from the other provider's point of view. All providers need to be more concerned with patient outcome than about who is "in charge." Also, some DC's have found that they merely become a part-time appendage to the medicine machine. Like any good relationship, there will be an adjustment period as each learns to work in a cooperative manner for the greater good.

- See Resource 117 for additional information and resources.
- Go to ACAtoday.org/policy (Resource 118) for additional information on the ACA's public policy page.
- See *Section F–Compliance and Audit Protection* for more information about HIPAA authorizations, self-referral laws and other regulations.

Health Reform Shared Savings Programs

Accountable Care Organizations (ACOs) and Patient Centered Medical Homes (PCMHs) are patient care and reimbursement management models which focus on cost savings and improving patient healthcare outcomes through better coordination of care. Payment is often based on how well these goals are met. For these reasons, these models have received renewed attention due to the passage of the Patient Protection and Affordable Care Act (PPACA.) Like MDPs, these organizations bring together healthcare professionals and organizations which perform a variety of services in order to provide patient-centered care. Unlike MDPs, these types of programs usually must meet strict regulatory and accreditation requirements in order to be reimbursed by insurers.

- Go to ChiroCode.com/hcr or ACAtoday.org/HCR for more information about these new shared savings programs.

Other Helpful Tips

Here are some other helpful tips and ideas to consider for your practice:

- Don't pay for employment posters. Most if not all can be obtained for free from your state's department of labor.
- Have financial checks and balances in place. A leading cause of small business failure is embezzlement by an employee, partner, or relative.
- Keep your business receipts and statements. You will need them in case you are audited. To save space, scan them into a protected computer that is backed up.
- Don't accept sales phone calls at face value. Pretend they are calling your home and asking for your personal information. Businesses are scammed every day by telemarketers. Ask for their website and tell them that you will review their information carefully before making a purchase decision.

Last, But Not Least

Regularly evaluate your business practices. Set aside time to attend workshops, read magazines and look for ways to make your business even better. Always keep in mind the value of your time. Providers should not spend their time with basic managerial tasks when they could be seeing patients. Delegate as much as possible. This is where an excellent chiropractic assistant (CA) or office manager is essential.

Prioritize

In conclusion, every aspect of a practice is important. Patient care comes first. Coding and billing must be completed accurately and in a timely manner. Continuing education for the practitioners is necessary for licensure. Bills have to be paid and bank accounts balanced. Floors need to be swept and linens laundered. It all has to get done, and sometimes it may not be entirely clear which comes first. Picking priorities is an individual practice decision, but there are some guiding principles:

- Look to minimize risk.
- Look to maximize opportunity.
- If something can make money, think about it.
- If something can save money, think about it.
- If something can make money and save money, and is thoroughly scrutinized from a legal perspective to account for local, state, and federal regulations, do it right away.

In the case of your own practice, there may be some problem areas that need to be addressed immediately. Often, these situations are actually the consequence of some simple action not tended to according to a set procedure in a timely manner, likely because no procedure had been established. Remember that what you can do about something before it becomes a crisis can usually be done with little money and small pieces of time.

- Create your "Daily Policies and Procedures Manual" as found on page A-29.
- Create your "Compliance Manual" as found in *Section F-Compliance and Audit Protection.*
- It is recommended that practices hold regular staff meetings and training sessions to minimize risk and increase efficiencies. See page A-28 for more information.

Review: Starting and Maintaining a Thriving Practice

- What are the "10 Steps for Starting a Business" according to the Small Business Association? *A-4*
- Which law will play the biggest factor in deciding what kind of business structure to use? *A-4*
- What are the pros and cons of outsourcing some of your business tasks, such as payroll, HR, accounting and taxes? *A-5*
- What are the three "L's" of real estate? *A-5*
- What are two types of group practices which may be considered? *A-6*

2. Compliance Considerations

There are many different aspects to compliance that must be carefully considered in order to operate a safe and effective practice. There are government compliance programs, such as HIPAA, as well as professional licensing and business operational insurance requirements.

GOVERNMENT COMPLIANCE PROGRAMS

Providers must be aware of both state and federal compliance programs, and meet their requirements or risk fines and penalties, which can include severe monetary fines and/or imprisonment. These government programs include:

- **HIPAA**

    See *Section F–Compliance and Audit Protection* for more information about this program.

    See *Complete & Easy HIPAA Compliance* for complete HIPAA guidelines, including forms and training materials. (Resource 116)

- **OIG/Medicare**

    See *Section F–Compliance and Audit Protection* for more about OIG compliance.

    See *Section C–Medicare* for more information about Medicare compliance.

- **OSHA**

    The Occupational Safety and Health Administration (OSHA) sets the federal standards for employee health and safety. Their standards do not apply to patient safety.

    Employee safety standards, as required by OSHA, are an area of practice management that is often overlooked because of the common misperception that OSHA only applies to industrial workplaces. If you have employees, you must have an OSHA Compliance Program for each office of your practice.

    See *Section F–Compliance and Audit Protection* for more information about this compliance program.

- **CLIA**

    The Clinical Laboratory Improvement Amendments are the laboratory testing quality standards for healthcare providers. A number of simple tests and screens exist which use just a drop of blood, such as a blood sugar test for diabetes. Pay close attention to the scope of practice laws in your state regarding these tests. If such testing is within your state's scope, you should be aware and comply with the requirements of CLIA.

For a chiropractor to be able to draw blood, conduct dip-stick urinalisys or other waived tests, a "certificate of waiver" is required and it must be within your state scope of practice.

See Resource 103 for more information about the CLIA program.

Professional Licensing

Professional licensing is not only needed for doctors of chiropratic, other staff members could also benefit from maintaining professional licensure. For example, a certified coder has additional training which can help keep the number of denied claims at a minimum. Everyone in the office benefits from annually renewing licenses which require Continuing Education Units (CEUs) as part of the renewal process.

Go to ChiroCode.com/certification to learn how to become a ChiroCode Certified Chiropractic Professional Coder CCCPC™ (Resource 119).

See Resource 120 for additional information on professional licensing.

Chiropractic Licensing

The current academic requirements to become a doctor of chiropractic include two to four years of undergraduate work (prerequisites) and four years at a chiropractic college. Many states require a bachelor's degree and it is anticipated that this will become the standard in the future.

The National Board of Chiropractic Examiners (NBCE) is responsible for administering the exams that demonstrate proficiency for doctors of chiropractic. There are three written exams and one practical exam which are administered twice a year. There are also exams for specialties such as physiotherapy and acupuncture.

Although the NBCE administers the national exams, actual licensing takes place at the state level. Many states also require providers to pass state level board exams. These exams often focus on state laws regarding scope of practice. Be aware that some states may also require other board exams in addition to standard chiropractic care. For example, the Oregon Board of Chiropractic Examiners requires additional testing on obstetrics, proctology, and minor surgery.

Continuing Education Units (CEUs)

Most regulatory agencies and professional organizations require licensed or certified individuals to continue to develop their skills throughout their career. This is accomplished by attending courses or reading material to demonstrate that they are keeping up with developments in their field. States regulate the licensing of chiropractic physicians and dictate what is required to maintain licensure. Typically, they require doctors to earn continuing education units (or CEUs). Courses must be approved by the state licensing board and reported at regular intervals which are determined by the state.

Other Professional Licensing

Some states require licensing for chiropractic assistants (CAs), massage therapists (LMTs) and limited x-ray operators (LXMOs). The purpose is to ensure some level of proficiency when the physician delegates procedures to be performed on patients. The requirements for these types of licenses vary from state to state. In an effort to create uniform training and licensure requirements for CAs, the Federation of Chiropractic Licensing Boards (FCLB) recently implemented a national certification program.

Additionally, billing staff may find it useful to obtain coding certification. It is not a requirement, but certification can be helpful to ensure that claims are submitted as accurately as possible. Including special certified coder credentials on an appeal indicates to the reviewer that they are working with someone who is knowledgeable in the field. Though not required by any regulatory agency, ChiroCode suggests that staff consider earning the ChiroCode Certified Chiropractic Professional Coder (CCCPC) certification. This greatly decreases the likelihood of billing errors.

INSURANCE

This segment covers business insurance that every healthcare office should have. Insurance is one of those things that is often overlooked or forgotten, unless there is an incident or problem. It is easy to remember malpractice insurance because most third-party payers have minimum malpractice requirements. However, other types of business related insurance should also be considered.

See Resource 121 for additional information on business insurance.

Malpractice Insurance

While it may seem obvious that malpractice insurance is something you should have, there are several factors to take into consideration when determining the amount of coverage needed. First, review any state or contract requirements. When enrolling as a provider for an insurance carrier, pay particular attention to their required malpractice limits, as they may vary. Keep in mind that in the event of a lawsuit, higher limits may help your defense. A reputable business advisor can ensure that your limits meet your specific needs.

In addition to policy limits, there are other factors to consider. When choosing an insurance provider, don't base your decision solely on price. Keep in mind that other helpful benefits may be available, such as legal defense assistance or hot lines which can quickly address your questions Get quotes from more than one company and compare all differences carefully.

Another key factor to consider when selecting malpractice insurance is "claims made" versus "occurrence" coverage. "Claims made" covers events that occur and are reported during the time period of the policy. "Occurrence" covers events which occur during the policy term, which means that incidents are covered even after the policy holder no longer pays for coverage. For this reason, an occurence policy is usually more expensive than a claims made policy during the initial years of policy ownership.

And finally, it is important to consider the insurance company's financial stability, experience and knowledge of the chiropractic profession. Be sure you fully understand the coverage provided and the extent of their obligations to defend your practice should the need arise. For example, will you be reimbursed for lost wages while in court?

Other Insurance

Beyond legal protection, your business should also have adequate coverage for other potential losses, such as building damage or data breaches. Be aware that you can be over-covered, as well as under-covered, when it comes to this type of insurance.

Consider the following types of insurance which may be of additional benefit to your practice:

- **Property insurance** is for losses of building fixtures and equipment.

- **Business owners policy (BOP)** typically includes property insurance, general liability insurance, product liability insurance and business interruption insurance. Many chiropractic offices are small and as such, disruptions to business can create a heavy financial strain.
- **Disability insurance** is designed to provide supplementary income in the event of an illness or accident that prevents the insured from working. Choose a short and/or long term disability plan which may be purchased as a group, individual or supplemental policy. When looking for a policy, remember that a group policy may be more affordable than individual coverage.
- **Workers' Compensation insurance** provides coverage for employees who become ill, injured or die as the result of a work-related situation. Most states require all businesses to carry some form of workers' compensation insurance. Required coverage is determined by state law and can include medical care, rehabilitation costs, lost wages as well as death and/or disability benefits. Even if your state does not require this type of coverage, you may wish to consider this additional protection.
- **Cyber insurance** (also known as data breach insurance or cyber liability insurance) covers the unauthorized use of, or unauthorized access to, electronic data or software within your network or business. It can help cover the costs incurred after a data breach, including a HIPAA breach. Depending on the policy selected, it can include coverage for investigation costs, notification to individuals affected, litigation costs, federal/state fines, or even income losses resulting from damage to electronic data. Carefully review policies to determine exact coverage.

> **Tip:** What about medical records in the event of a disaster? As part of your HIPAA compliance plan, every office needs to have an official HIPAA Disaster Plan which should be accessible to all employees.
>
> See *Section F–Compliance and Audit Protection* for HIPAA Disaster Plan information.

Review: Compliance Considerations

- Which four government compliance programs have requirements that providers must meet to avoid the risk of fines and penalties? *A-9*
- Who in a Chiropractic practice could benefit from maintaining professional licensure? *A-10*
- What should be considered when choosing a malpractice insurance? *A-11*

3. Office Equipment and Software

Every office needs to have the necessary equipment to assist the provider in treating patients. This also includes equipment and/or software to properly document and efficiently file claims for each patient encounter. Providers need to consider the pros and cons of leasing, purchasing, or outsourcing required equipment. They must also select software and services that will help their practice maintain profitability with minimal headaches and hassles.

Equipment: Lease, Purchase, or Outsource?

This is one of the most commonly asked questions with major financial implications for any business. The answer depends on your situation. If you have limited capital or equipment that must be upgraded often, leasing or outsourcing can be a good option. Purchasing equipment can be a better option for established businesses or for equipment with a long usable life. These are only general guidelines and the decision should be made on a case-by-case basis. Here's a look at these options.

> **Beware of Manufacturing Coding Advice:** Manufacturers often give incorrect coding advice when it comes to equipment or supplies they are selling. Do not take their advice at face value. If there are any concerns, please contact ChiroCode Institute, ACA if you are an ACA member, or your professional association.

Leasing Equipment

Leasing business equipment and tools preserves capital in the short term and provides flexibility, but it often costs more in the long run.

Advantages

- **Less initial expense.** When a practice is new, cost can be THE deciding factor. Equipment leases usually do not have a large down payment which helps with cash-flow.
- **Tax deductible.** Lease payments can usually be deducted as business expenses on your tax return.
- **Flexible terms.** Leases are generally more flexible than loans for buying equipment. It makes it a good option for those with bad credit or those who need to negotiate a longer payment plan to lower business costs.
- **Easier to upgrade equipment.** Items such as computers tend to be quickly outdated, which shifts the costs to the lessor instead of the leasee. This leaves you free to lease newer, higher end items later, when cash-flow has improved.

Disadvantages

- **Higher overall cost.** With interest rates included as part of the cost, leasing is almost always more expensive than other purchasing options. Consult a financial advisor to determine if this is the best option for you.
- **You don't own the equipment.** You don't build equity, and if the item is not obsolete, this can be a financial loss.
- **Obligation to pay for entire lease term.** Even if you stop using the equipment, you are locked into the lease payments for the entire term. Pay close attention to clauses for loss or early termination fees which can be quite costly.

Purchasing Equipment

Ownership and tax breaks make buying business equipment appealing, but high initial costs mean this option isn't for everyone.

Advantages

- **Ownership.** This is an advantage on items which have a long life such as patient tables. The costs are lower in the long-run.
- **Tax incentives and possibility of depreciation deductions.** Consult with an accountant to carefully review applicable tax laws, such as I.R.S. Section 179, for any equipment that is being considered for purchase. If full purchase deductions are not available, depreciation deductions may apply.

Disadvantages

- **Higher initial expense.** Sometimes purchasing costs are high enough that making a cash purchase does not make financial sense. Loans often have up to a 20% down payment which may also be prohibitive.
- **Getting stuck with old equipment.** When it comes to high-tech purchases, ownership is not always the best financial decision because of a very low re-sale value.

Outsourcing Services

Outsourcing is another viable alternative to a lease or purchase which can often meet the needs of healthcare providers, especially new doctors. It is simply a contract with another business to perform services that are not available at your location. It is commonly utilized for laboratory or imaging services.

> **HIPAA Reminder**: If you outsource services for **treatment**, no Business Associate Agreement (BAA) is required. However, a BAA is required if you outsource other services which are NOT for treatment, payment or certain specified healthcare operations.

When choosing this option, it is important to pay close attention to referral laws to avoid allegations of fraud. Also keep in mind that providers participating in shared savings or other managed care programs should refer patients to facilities which are also participating in that same plan.

See *Section F–Compliance and Audit Protection* for more about referral laws and HIPAA requirements regarding BAAs.

Advantages

- **No initial expense.** No financial outlays are required. This is a powerful driving factor for new healthcare providers. It may make more financial sense to outsource radiology services to a local imaging facility or another provider's office than to try and do everything in-house. Although the revenue for taking and reading the films goes to the imaging center, your facility can avoid all the costs and liability risks of creating an x-ray suite and maintaining equipment.

- **Decreased liability.** Some types of services, such as radiology, can increase your liability. Malpractice claims could be filed for incorrectly interpreting an xray. Outsourcing can reduce (but not eliminate) this risk because another expert will have rendered an opinion regarding the image. In addition, it may not be necessary to add radiology services as part of your malpractice coverage.

- **No equipment upgrades or maintenance fees.** Technology is rapidly expanding which can necessitate a potentially costly equipment upgrade. For example, more advanced digital imaging technology can be more expensive than a standard xray machine. Outsourcing can allow providers to take advantage of the latest technologies without a financial burden.

Disadvantages

- **No tax incentives or benefits.** Unlike other options, which can reduce a provider's tax liability, outsourcing has no tax benefits.

- **Inconvenience.** Will the delay in imaging and lab results impact the patient's treatment plan? Will your patients feel frustrated if they have to go to another facility?

Summary

When deciding whether to buy, lease or outsource a particular piece of equipment or service, figuring out the the approximate net cost is an important task. Consider both tax breaks and resale value to determine which option is more cost-effective. Keep in mind that according to the IRS, major software purchases (including EHR systems) may be classified as a corporate asset, and therefore the cost must be depreciated according to IRS guidelines. It is good to consult with an accountant on these matters.

SELECTING SOFTWARE

There are many excellent software programs on the market for chiropractic offices. They range from full service practice management systems, to standalone EHR packages, to single function tasks like scheduling. Remember, software is not a one size fits all product. Here are a few basic tips and guidelines to use when selecting software:

- Carefully evaluate any programs that you are considering to ensure that they meet HIPAA privacy and security standards before doing a trial run. HIPAA compliance is a Meaningful Use (MU) requirement for EHRs.

    Windows XP Alert: As of April 8, 2014, Windows XP is no longer HIPAA compliant. It is recommended that providers update their computer operating systems as soon as possible.

    Go to ChiroCode.com/windows-xp-hipaa or ACAtoday.org/HIPAA for detailed information about this important change.

- **Always** try out a software program before you buy. Try more than one. Software can be a very personal thing–what one person likes, another may not.

- Evaluate the features and determine if the additional costs to purchase and train is worth the price. It might not be.
- Compare basic features versus deluxe ones; such as digitized x-rays or online automated scheduling. Sometimes it may be more cost effective to purchase small programs which perform one task; such as a standalone program versus an entire practice management system.
- Software customization is vital. No software will arrive **exactly** as you want, or need, it to be. The notion of being "out of the box" ready to meet your individual practice needs can be misleading, and will likely lead to disappointment. This is why it is important to be able to **easily** configure and customize new software.
- ICD-10 readiness – Ask the software vendor the following questions:
    - Is the software ICD-10-CM ready? If not, when will it be updated? It is important to obtain an exact implementation date, preferably in writing, from the vendor rather than a vague response.
    - Do I need to pay for an upgrade?
    - Will there be any training or assistance provided? If so, is there an additional cost for these services?
    - Will the software have a built in crosswalk? If so, is it based only on GEMs?
    - Will the software be able to report both ICD-9 and ICD-10 codes (also known as "dual processing" or "dual coding") if necessary?
    - When will the program be ready to test?

See *Section D–Documentation* for more about electronic health records software.

Go to ChiroCode.com to search for the latest articles and webinars on ICD-10 implementation (Resource 123), business software, EHR and more.

Review: Office Equipment and Software

- Why should you avoid getting coding advice from an equipment manufacturer? *A-13*
- What are the differences between leasing, owning, and outsourcing office equipment? *A-13 to A-15*
- What are four of the six basic tips to consider when choosing a software package? *A-15-A-16*

4. Business Financial Standards

Financial Considerations

There are many important financial considerations for your business. Revenue is **not** based on the work that was done. Rather, income is based on the ability of the business to be paid by the patient or a third-party payer. Thus, financial considerations are closely tied to the Reimbursement Life Cycle, which is explained in *Section B–Insurance and Reimbursement*.

This section covers the following five topics:

- Setting Fees
- Evergreen Contracts
- Patient Financial Responsibility
- Outsourcing/Billing Agencies
- Collections

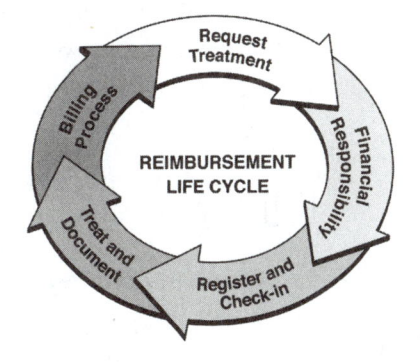

See *Section B–Insurance and Reimbursement* for more about the Reimbursement Life Cycle and how it impacts your office.

See Resource 124 for the latest articles and webinars on financial standards.

Setting Fees

There are numerous questions surrounding the subject of setting fees. How much should you charge? Can you discount your fees? What arrangements need special consideration in contracts? In reality, your office should have only one fee schedule. The only appropriate exceptions are time of service discounts, economic hardships (which must be clearly defined), and contractual obligations. That's it–otherwise, you could be alleged to have dual-fee schedules.

See Chapter 3–Fees of *Section B–Insurance and Reimbursement* for more about setting fees. See the segment "Other Fee Schedules" for more information about how to appropriately discount your fees.

See Resource 110 for additional comments, resources, networks, and opinions on discounts.

> **ACA Time of Service (TOS) Disclaimer:** The ACA does not officially recommend that doctors of chiropractic use TOS discounts. This is due to the possibility of violating state and/or federal law. Before implementing a TOS discount, doctors of chiropractic should consult with a health care law attorney.

Evergreen Contracts

Evergreen contracts are those agreements between the provider and the insurance company which automatically renew, usually on an annual basis. The nice thing about these types of contracts is that they automatically renew year after year, which means that you save significant time and effort every single year. Renewals or re-credentialing can take quite a bit of time when you have more than one contract. Like having your bills paid automatically every month, you know that you don't miss a deadline and have to pay those dreaded late fees.

However, there are some problems to consider. In some cases, providers found that changes in their contract not only decreased their fees, but also removed their right to appeal. They were unaware of this change because their contract was on auto-renewal.

> **Tip:** Review non-contract payments and fee schedules. Recently, a provider discovered that they were being paid the PPO rate for three years and they were not a contracted provider. Significant revenue was lost because they were writing it off when they were not obligated to do so.

Patient Financial Responsibilities

There are many considerations when it comes to establishing the patient financial responsibilities. It is important to have written policies explaining fees and payment policies. This protects the practice should there be charges or allegations of fraud.

Here are some important questions to ask:

- What type of claim will this be?
- What payment options are available to the patient?
- What policies do we need to have in place?

> See *Section B–Insurance and Reimbursement* for in depth coverage of how to establish financial responsibility.

Federal Truth in Lending Act

The Federal Truth in Lending Act was created in response to fraudulent creditor activities. Technically speaking, medical providers extend credit when they do not receive full payment at the time that services are rendered. This puts the burden on the provider to ensure that the patient understands late fee charges, re-billing fees, or interest rates which may be charged on balances due. Patient financial agreements must clearly specify these things in order to comply with this law.

> See *Section B–Insurance and Reimbursement* for in depth coverage of how to establish financial responsibility.

Outsourcing/Billing Agencies

The decision to outsource billing is a difficult one. You must weigh the need for control, compliance, and sensitivity to patient situations against the cost effectiveness of sending this work to be done elsewhere. Outsourcing is not for everyone. It may not make sense if you have a qualified employee who is capable of doing the billing and coding work themselves, and they have the time to do it. Keep your goals and compliance issues in mind whichever route you decide to pursue.

If you decide to outsource, consider the following:

- Carefully review contracts to determine how this arrangement will affect billing, collections, denials and appeals. What rights does the agency have and what rights does the provider retain?
- All HIPAA Compliance requirements must be met. Business Associate Agreements must be properly executed and updated to meet the new Omnibus Final Rule requirements.

> See *Section F–Compliance and Audit Protection* for more about Breach requirements, Business Associate Agreements and other important HIPAA Privacy and Security considerations when it comes to outsourcing.

Collections

Effective collection procedures must be part of the daily office routine. Every office should have a clearly defined, written Accounts Receivable policy which outlines the processes which must happen before an account is sent to a collection agency. Bad collection policies reflect poorly on the company financial statements because the longer a bill goes unpaid, the greater the overhead collection costs and the greater the risk of non-payment. If a solid internal collections process is established, it will reduce the need to seek outside help. Your collection policy should be clearly documented in your "Daily Policies and Procedures Manual" (see page A-29 for more information). The following is a very basic outline for a policy:

- After 30 days, send a "Reminder Letter," where the tone is friendly, especially if their insurance payment has just been received.
- After 45 days, send a "Second Reminder Letter" where the tone is more stern.
- After 60 days, send a "Third Reminder Letter" which includes a threat to send their account to a collection agency.
- After 90 days, send a "Collection Notice" informing the patient that their account has been sent to a collection agency.

If the patient's financial responsibility is clearly established at the beginning of their treatment, and co-pays and deductibles are paid immediately, then sending the account to collections should be a rare event. See "Ways to Avoid Collections" on the following page.

Collection Agencies

Outside third party collection agencies can be an effective means of collecting past due accounts. When considering a collection agency, ask the following questions:

- Are they HIPAA Compliant? This should be your primary concern because of increased fines and penalties. Business Associate Agreements should be executed to comply with HIPAA requirements.
- How long have they been in business? If they are new to the industry, their collection rates may be low because of lack of experience. Get references from other healthcare providers in your area. Having them local is helpful for both the patient as well as your office.

Overseas Billing Caution

To cut costs, many companies have outsourced their billing overseas. Recently, one provider had PHI stolen by someone employed by that overseas billing company. The provider was fined under HIPAA rules, but the billing company has not paid the fine, even though the contract stated they were responsible for HIPAA breaches.

- Do they have flexible business hours in which clients can conveniently reach them? Do they have a toll-free number? These things make it easier for collections to take place.
- Do they have an attorney on staff? Having legal counsel readily available can be beneficial for legal proceedings or when collection letters are needed.
- What are their collection fees? Some are higher than others. Keep in mind the adage that you get what you pay for.

If collection agencies are unsuccessful, there are some last resort options such as small claims courts, or seeking advice from an attorney. Small claims court is less costly than hiring an attorney and is not as time consuming as a full legal case. As such, it can be a viable alternative collection method for healthcare providers. Each state has a dollar limit on disputed claims, so contact the small claims court in your jurisdiction. Legal counsel is not required for small claims court; however, they may be able to give advice on more complex questions.

Ways to Avoid Collections

The following tips should help you avoid the need for collections services.

- Do verification of coverage before the patient arrives-you will know deductibles at that point.

    See *Section B–Insurance and Reimbursement* for more about verification of coverage.

- Don't wait. Collect co-pays immediately. However, some **preventive** services may not have a co-pay, so be careful. Consider having multiple payment options (i.e. cash, check, or charge) to make it more convenient for patients to pay.
- Establish financial agreements up front! Patients should be notified of their co-pay and patient portion amounts so that they know what fees they are responsible for when they come in.
- Consider taking payments by phone or via other methods such as web based portals.
- If a patient has elected to make payments on an outstanding balance, consider using an auto-debit service. The patient provides debit card information once, and agrees to a regular withdrawal at even intervals. It may be easier for a patient to fulfill their payment obligations with this type of arrangement.

    See *Section B–Insurance and Reimbursement* for more information about Financial Responsibility.

Marketing Your Practice

Marketing your practice requires addressing and reviewing the following:

- Location
- Advertising
- Joining panels
- Networking
- Medicare restrictions
- Practice management seminars or groups.

Location

When considering a location for your practice, be sure to look for an area which has a very high patient-to-doctor ratio. This ensures a large potential market just waiting for chiropractic care. Most communities already have a chiropractic office, so consider your target market and competition. Will you market to old or young, white collar or blue collar workers, etc? Where are the other chiropractic offices? These demographics can often be obtained from the local chamber of commerce.

Another necessary consideration is deciding whether to locate your practice in either a downtown or a suburban area. If you locate in the downtown area, your busiest time may be during the lunch hour, so having a long lunch break would be out of the question. Suburban areas tend to be busiest at the end of the day, and your practice may need to remain open until 7:00 or 8:00 in the evening in order to best serve clients.

Also, remember that areas of greater income tend to be over-crowded with healthcare providers; so don't overlook the possible opportunity of a higher number of potential clients in less affluent areas. If there are no other chiropractic offices in the area, you have less competition. In lower income areas where transportation might be an issue, make it easy for your patients to get to your office by choosing a location near public transportation.

> **Tip:** Location can also determine whether you participate with Medicare or other insurance plans. If you are in an area with a high elderly population, it will be in your best interest to be a Medicare provider. If your location is near a major manufacturer or mining company, you may want to consider participation as a Plan Provider.

Advertising

Advertising can be very helpful in driving customers to your practice. However, it is an area in which healthcare providers need to exercise caution. Advertising itself is not the problem, it is what is included in the ad or marketing materials that gets providers into trouble. Be aware of state laws and federal kick-back laws to avoid legal problems. Your state licensing board will have detailed information regarding state requirements for advertising.

> **Alert:** Ads cannot offer to waive insurance co-pays or deductibles–that is considered fraud.

In today's market, putting an ad in the newspaper or listing your practice in the yellow pages seems to have a minimal effect on increasing your clientele. While these methods may work for older populations, younger people may be reached more effectively through social media and other on-line resources for advertising. Many clinics are beginning to turn to social media like Facebook and pay-per-click advertising. You may wish to consult with an expert for advice on using these more modern marketing mediums. Also consider contacting professional associations for information and guidelines.

Social Media

Social media such as Facebook and Twitter are increasingly being used as marketing tools which have the added benefit of minimal costs. However, providers need to be very careful about what is posted on these types of platforms in order to avoid HIPAA violations as well as violations of federal and state laws. With so many connections between individuals, it is not difficult for someone to deduce an individual's Protected Health Information (PHI) from shared data which can lead to a HIPAA violation. A social media policy should be part of your official Policies and

Procedures Manual. As part of this policy, employees should be trained regarding acceptable uses of social media within the practice.

> See Resources 111 and 112 for additional information on the use of social media.

> See *Section F–Compliance and Audit Protection* for more about federal laws regarding gift giving and marketing. Also, review HIPAA marketing rules and PHI requirements to avoid violations when using social media.

Joining Panels

For providers seeking to expand their practice, joining an insurance panel of preferred providers can be an effective way to open more doors. However, some doctors who are new to an area may find their options limited by a small number of insurance carriers that are widely utilized in a particular region. Unless they can get on those panels, there are fewer patient options for them.

Carefully evaluate this option. If you are already overwhelmed and don't need any more patients, then do not join a panel simply to have your name on one more list. Insurance panels offer more patients in exchange for reduced reimbursement rates, so in some cases, this can be a losing proposition. It is wise to carefully evaluate the numbers and consider your individual business needs before signing any contracts.

> See *Section B–Insurance and Reimbursement* for more information including pros and cons regarding insurance panels.

> ACA members, see ACAtoday.org/contracts to review the article, "Adequately Review your Contract."

Networking

Another helpful marketing tool is networking. There are many national and local business networking groups available for providers to join (i.e. MGMA, BNI, Chamber of Commerce or Rotary Club). Most meet on a regular basis and business owners or managers are given opportunities to introduce their business to other businesses. These organizations enjoy a synergistic relationship in which they are all working to enhance their business by working with others. If you don't want to join one of these organizations, create your own networking group by inviting half a dozen business people out to lunch.

Medicare Restrictions

Exercise caution when advertising. In particular, pay close attention to OIG Special Advisory Bulletin, Offering Gifts and Other Inducements, August 2002. This advisory outlines what is acceptable and what is a violation of law.

You may **not** do the following:

- Waive Medicare co-insurance or deductibles.
- Offer incentives to Medicare patients for referrals.
- Offer free visits on birthdays.
- Offer flat fees for initial services (like $49 exam and X-rays).

> See Resource 113 to read the complete OIG advisory.

Practice Management Groups

Practice management groups and consultants for chiropractors are widely available. Many offer seminars and in-house consultations which aim to teach everything discussed here and more. Some charge a flat monthly fee, some have contracts, and some even take a percentage of your collections.

Please exercise caution when deciding to use such a service. Some are skilled at helping to fill in practice management gaps and can help increase your revenue stream and solve problem areas in your office. However, be aware that there are firms which can be very costly and yield little in the way of results. Here are some important questions to ask:

- Are they promising too much? If it sounds too good to be true, it might be.
- Do they have a proven track record? Can you speak to their customers? Are there reliable testimonials, not just scripted ones? Speaking to real customers lets you know more about the company.
- Talk to other providers to see which services they use and if they are satisfied with the results.
- What guarantees do they offer? If they offer a money-back guarantee, this is usually a good indication that they stand behind their work.
- Are they using strong salesmanship or scare tactics? If they do, step back and ask more questions.
- Are their recommendations ethical? Some firms have suggested coding and billing practices that are less than ethical. Compare their recommendations to the guidelines in this book. If it sounds questionable, you may want to take a closer look before signing up.

Working With Payers

Third party payers are quite often the lifeblood of most practices. According to the NBCE's Practice Analysis of Chiropractic 2010, 75% of the income in a typical healthcare practice depends upon third party payers. The trade off is the need for staff that have the expertise to handle everything. These staff members need to be tenacious and friendly and have the ability to carefully and appropriately follow up with all claims not paid correctly. Sometimes that involves going through an appeals process.

> **Tip:** Even though payers provide contact information on the back of the patient's insurance card, those toll-free numbers are not always helpful. Once you find someone that is helpful at that office, try to save their extension, direct line, or fax number so that you don't have to wade through phone menus the next time.

- See *Section B–Insurance and Reimbursement* for more about working with non-Medicare third-party payers.

- See *Section C–Medicare* for more about working with this government program.

- See *Section E–Claims and Appeals* for more about both submitting and appealing claims.

Go to ChiroCode.com and search on "Marketing" or "Third Party Payers" for the latest articles and webinars.

Review: Business Financial Standards

- Which questions should you know the answer to when writing your policy for patient responsibilities? *A-18*
- What considerations are most important when choosing a collection agency? *A-19*
- When is the right time to verify your patient's insurance coverage? *A-20*
- What questions should you answer to help find your target market? *A-20 to A-21*
- Which business networking groups are available to join? *A-22*
- What are some important questions to ask when choosing a practice management group? *A-23*

5. Supportive and Productive Staff

Finding the Right People

Chiropractic is a unique profession and it requires unique people. A front desk person needs to be friendly and professional. A biller needs to be both assertive and courteous at the same time. An associate doctor needs to appear confident, but not aloof. How do you find the right people for the right position? How do you keep them? How much do you pay them?

A great chiropractic assistant (CA) or office manager is invaluable. Keep in mind that turnover for these types of positions is normal for a healthcare business. However, the right kinds of incentives can make a big difference. Some business advisors suggest that monetary incentives are not as powerful as recognition, or bonus time off.

Additionally, businesses need to be aware of local, state and federal laws regarding employees, including hiring and firing. Be aware of union laws, medical leave requirements, mandated posters, OSHA and much more.

See Resource 125 for the latest articles and webinars on staffing.

Hiring and Firing

In hiring and firing employees, please consult applicable federal and state laws for specific do's and don'ts. It is also helpful to attend human resources workshops and/or seminars. Review the information located at the United States Department of Labor, and your state's division of labor. Here you will find information concerning regulations on wages, safety, unions, Family Medical Leave Act (FMLA), discrimination, and much more.

Go to www.dol.gov for information from the U.S. Department of Labor.

Exclusions Database

All potential applicants (as well as current staff members) must be screened against the OIG website for providers that are in their "Exclusions" database. You cannot hire or employ **anyone** on that list! Recently, a home health agency was heavily fined because they had employed staff members on the exclusions list. Even though there was no evidence of wrong-doing, and all claims were correctly billed, they still were fined.

Always check your applicants' eligibility for healthcare positions. Go to exclusions.oig.hhs.gov to search for excluded individuals.

Help Wanted Ads

Help wanted ads should be honest yet distinctive. Honesty is important because you don't want to hire someone and then have to refill the position again when the applicant is disillusioned because the job is nothing like the listing. Being distinctive is important because your ad needs to stand out from other potentially similar listings for the same position. What makes your office unique? Why would they want to be there?

Clearly defining job requirements or special skills helps eliminate unqualified applicants from the beginning. A good job description also helps screen applicants. If the pay is a range, then say so. If it is a salary with no room for negotiation, then say so. Be careful to avoid illegal items like age or race (see "Hiring Tips" below).

Precise application instructions are helpful for applicants and reduce extra office burdens. For instance, if you do not wish to have people "drop by," then specify that resumes should only be faxed, mailed, or emailed.

When it comes to listing or placing your ad, local newspapers are a good place, but don't forget to include your ad in trade magazines and other online job listing sites. A potential applicant may want to move to a new location if they see a job that really catches their eye.

Interviewing

Hopefully the help wanted ad(s) has yielded many potential candidates for the position. Carefully review their resumes and cover letters. Check their references to see if they may legally work and if they can, determine if they are on the Federal Exclusions Database (see the "State and Federal Requirements" segment on the following page).

When you have narrowed down your list of applicants, you may wish to do a telephone interview first. This demonstrates their telephone skills which is important to many positions in a chiropractic office. It also helps to weed out applicants that do not "fit" your organization before a formal face-to-face takes place.

During the interview process, whether in person or over the telephone, all questions must be focused on skills, work experience, behaviors and other job related information. Be careful to avoid questions that are illegal to ask during an interview. Avoid the following subjects:

Hiring Tips

- **Don't make the final decision alone.** Get feedback from others in the office. It is also good to include a few other office staff (no more than 3 people though) in the final interview process.
- **Trust your instincts.** If an applicant seems to have all the requirements, but something doesn't "feel" right about the person, pay attention. Better to be safe than sorry.
- **Hire for the long term.** Training an employee can be more costly than you realize. Look for candidates whose previous employment history shows commitment and professional growth. A series of short-term jobs often indicates that this individual will not stay long enough to re-coup your training costs.
- **Be consistent.** Your entire hiring process should be standardized and even included in your office policies and procedures manual. Be sure to include testing, interviews, and background and reference checks as part of that process.
- **Test Applicants.** Consider having applicants take a test to see if they are a good "fit" for your office. Tests such as the "Wonderlic" test or a personality profile can be helpful to identify which traits or attributes match the position.

- Age
- Race, ethnicity, or color
- Gender or sex (including gender identity or sexual orientation)
- Country of national origin or birth place
- Religion
- Disability
- Marital or family status or pregnancy

If they ask a question such as, "Would I be required to work on (a specific religious holiday)?", it is appropriate to answer their question, but do not pursue the subject further.

There are many different ways to conduct an interview. Just don't forget to follow all state and federal laws during this process.

State and Federal Requirements

There are two laws that are sometimes forgotten during this process. If you use a third-party payroll company, be sure to ask about:

1. The *Personal Responsibility and Work Opportunity Reconciliation Act of 1996 (PRWORA)* which requires employers to report new hire information to their state Office of Child Support Enforcement (OCSE). This information must be reported within 20 days of hiring a new employee.

2. The *Illegal Immigration Reform and Immigrant Responsibility Act (IIRIRA)*, which requires the Social Security Administration (SSA) and U.S. Citizenship and Immigration Services (USCIS), to initiate an employment verification program. Many states require the use of E-Verify for all new hires. Be aware of your state requirements.

   Go to dhs.gov/e-verify for access to the E-Verify system.

Firing

Firing is one of the least enjoyable aspects of practice management. As such, it is common to wait too long to fire an employee. If it is clear that they are not meeting job requirements and proper warnings have taken place, do not hesitate to fire them. It is better for everyone involved. However, understand that there are both legal and ethical issues that must be carefully considered. Except in cases where immediate dismissal is necessary, proper steps must be taken when firing an employee.

The way that firing is handled sends a message to the rest of the office—it can be either positive or negative. It is not the firing itself that creates problems in a business, it is "how" they were fired. Keep in mind that privacy rights prevent disclosure of the exact termination reasons. However, informing remaining employees that someone has been fired for violations of company policy can be a good reminder for everyone to go back and review company policies.

All employees should clearly understand what actions are considered grounds for termination. Include this information in an employee handbook, if you have one, or simply include it in your "Daily Policies and Procedures Manual." For example, your HIPAA Compliance Manual should include signed statements by staff in which they state that they understand that specific HIPAA violations result in immediate termination.

In cases of "underperforming," it is wise to document warnings and training sessions where you as the employer tried to "coach" them into a higher level of performance. If it is still clear that they are underperforming, you may suggest that they voluntarily quit, but be aware that quitting has an effect on unemployment benefits. Also be aware of differences in state laws regarding termination. In cases where fraud or HIPAA violations exist, it may be necessary to hire an attorney.

Finally, do not forget to do the following things:

- Include a letter clearly stating non-biased reasons for termination in the employee's file.
- Conduct a termination (or exit) interview and complete an Employee Exit Checklist. Some items on this list, such as changing passwords, might need to be done before the interview in order to protect company and patient information.
- Company property should be returned at this time. Physical property such as keys or computers need to be turned in. It may be necessary to change locks, depending on the reasons for termination.

See *Complete & Easy HIPAA Compliance* (Resource 116) for Employee Exit Checklists.

TRAINING STAFF

Training staff members is an integral part of an effective practice. Everyone needs reminders, especially when laws, rules and regulations are always changing. Also, as part of an effective HIPAA compliance plan, staff members are required to have "regular" training which is documented in the business compliance manuals. Newly hired employees need to be immediately trained regarding your HIPAA policies.

Federal and state requirements are just the beginning. Providers must also train staff on making a good first impression, either over the phone or when the patient walks in the door.

Remember that change is not always easy and we all tend to resist changing our routines. As such, keep these tips in mind:

- Provide encouragement at every opportunity. Daily support keeps the process moving forward.
- Give and receive criticisms carefully. Be polite and constructive.
- Immediately correct and address problems. If you wait, you send the message that it is not important.
- Focus on a hands-on, here-and-now approach.
- Improvement requires effort and effort requires enthusiasm. Reward those demonstrating a willingness to change.

Another helpful training tip is to have weekly staff meetings. This enables problems to be resolved quickly. A typical weekly meeting agenda might look like this:

1. Review minutes from last week
2. Share successes
3. Review statistics
4. Training/role play
5. Discuss progress on last week's projects
6. Discuss problems and potential solutions
7. Make assignments for next week's projects

Finally, it is important to remember that all these necessary tasks must happen efficiently and consistently. This results in additional time and cost savings for the practice. There are entire seminars and books which focus on only this one subject. Therefore, use these ideas as a review or starting point and then refer to other resources as needed.

Daily Policies and Procedures Manual

One way to avoid inefficiencies (and thus lost revenue) is to create your own office "Daily Policies and Procedures Manual." This manual enables everyone in the office to understand what needs to be done and how it needs to be done. Should someone be absent from the office, anyone on the staff, including the doctor, can go to this manual and know how to perform specific tasks. For example, suppose that the office manager gets a flat tire on the way to work. The doctor is there, but doesn't know how to take the phones off the answering service. If the manual is readily available, it is easy to go to the manual and look up the procedure.

The following subjects are typically included in this type of manual:

- **Telephone** procedures, including automated phone service, how to answer voicemail, how to put on hold, etc.
- **Employee-patient** procedures/standards including appointment scheduling and how to handle problem patients.
- **Mail** tasks, including incoming and outgoing correspondence standards, how to handle records requests, etc.
- **Medical records** tasks, including general filing, record processing and maintenance, archiving, etc.
- **Follow up tasks:** Tickler filing, patient reminders and follow-up procedures.
- **Housekeeping** tasks such as how to service equipment, inventory control, supply storage, ordering and purchasing, etc.
- **Managerial** tasks such as bookkeeping requirements.
- **Payment** tasks such as fee schedule(s), payment portals, accounts receivables/payables, billing and collecting, banking/deposits, etc.
- **Reporting** tasks including monthly cash flow, taxes, and performance reports.
- **Special circumstances,** such as referrals, or OSHA spills.
- **FAQ** section for answers to common or typical problems and situations.

This may seem like a lot to undertake, but it does not have to happen all at once. In fact, there may already be notes or "cheat sheets" here and there on workstations around the office regarding many of these items. Start by compiling this information into one place. Sample daily policies and procedures manuals on the internet can help guide this process.

> **Alert:** Be sure that the manual includes important and relevant federal/state requirements such as HIPAA standards for communicating with patients and releasing medical information.

Communications and First Impressions

Communicating well and making a patient feel comfortable and confident are important to building an effective and profitable practice. A potential client may decide they do not want to come into an office because they didn't like how the person answered the phone. They may decide not to return if they feel less than comfortable in the office. Because it is less expensive to keep a customer than to try and find new ones, this section focuses on some things that can be done to improve the patient experience.

All of the following are types of communications that could happen in a healthcare setting. Although some of these items are less common, like web-based posts, they are methods of communication and each should be carefully evaluated and considered when communicating with patents. Some forms of communication fall under HIPAA regulations.

- Face-to-face
- Telephone
- Fax
- Emails
- Paging (electronic or overhead)
- Instant messaging or text messaging
- Videoconferencing
- Web-based posts or blogs.

No matter what type of communication is being used, some of the same basic standards apply:

- Keep in mind HIPAA privacy and security.
- Be polite and professional.
- Respond promptly.
- Listen and give feedback.

First Impressions

What is the first thing that your patient sees when they walk in the door? What do they think when they are setting up their appointment? All these first impressions are important to the success of the practice. As a beginning point, walk around the office and ask these questions as if you are a new patient:

- Does the office appear organized?
- Is the patient waiting area clean and uncluttered?
- Is the atmosphere calm and inviting?
- How long is the wait time?
- Are the magazines in the waiting area interesting and current?
- Are the exam rooms comfortable - not too warm, not too cold?
- If there is music, is it calming?

Now, with new eyes, take steps to ensure that the best first impression is made. It can also be helpful to attend additional training or even enlist the help of family or friends to come in and act as if they are a new patient.

The Illusion of Communication

George Bernard Shaw said, "The single biggest problem with communication is the illusion that it has been achieved." To ensure good communication, always verify and re-state.

Telephone Skills and Duties

Telephone skills are highly important to establishing good first and second impressions. It is easy to tell if the person on the other end of the phone is smiling or not. Basic skills such as "Smile when you answer the phone and be pleasant, yet professional" should be emphasized.

Also, other phone duties should be documented in the "Daily Policies and Procedures Manual." Consider including guidelines such as these:

- **Hold times.** If you leave someone on hold for more than 90 seconds, check in with them and offer to either allow them to continue to hold or take a message and call them back promptly.
- **Call back and reminder calls.** Respond quickly to patient phone messages. They are your priority. Appointment reminder calls should happen daily before 3 pm.
- **Handling cranky/upset patients.** Remain calm. Do not raise your voice. Actively listen, then ask questions. Take a deep breath and count to 10 if necessary before responding. Sometimes all they need is to feel that someone is listening. If you are unsure about how to help them, do not be afraid to say "I need to research that problem. When is a good time to call you back?" Keep in mind that people may come across as being more unpleasant when they are in pain. Don't take it personally.
- **Personal calls.** Patients are the number one priority. For this reason, avoid making personal calls during regular hours. Making long distance or toll calls for personal reasons are not permitted.
- **Cell phones.** A personal cell phone is a distraction in the workplace and should not be accessed during work hours. Use only during breaks or in case of a true emergency.

> **Note**: There are cell phone policy templates available on the internet which may be used as a guide to establish your office policy. If your business owns the cell phone, be sure to include information on the appropriate uses and prohibitions on cell phones while driving. Include any laws and regulations specific to your state.

- **Handling solicitors.** It is office policy to never purchase anything over the telephone. Explain this policy to the caller and suggest that they send written materials for the doctor to review.
- **Working with attorneys.** It is office policy that attorney phone calls are a priority. If the doctor is unable to take the call quickly, look at the schedule and suggest some times that the doctor could return the call. If the matter is patient related, remember that privacy rules prevent you from either confirming or denying any information unless there is an appropriate release on file which allows you to consult with that attorney.

Keeping checklists near the phone with little reminders like "Smile - Breathe - Ask Questions - Listen - Write Down Specifics" can also be very helpful to ensure that good first impressions are not forgotten.

> **Tip:** Create a script and role play with staff members in weekly meetings. What items need to be communicated during a phone call? Practice makes perfect.

Handling Mail and Correspondence

Most offices receive large amounts of mail on a daily basis. Some items are considered high priority, such as checks and requests from third-party payers. Others fall into the "junk" mail category. Regardless of the amount of mail received, it is important that staff be well-trained on what is expected. Consider including the following items in the "Daily Policies and Procedures Manual":

- **Mail marked "personal."** Never open any mail marked "Personal." Set aside for the addressee.
- **Sorting mail.** Mail should be sorted by the following priority:
    1. Telegrams, registered letters, special deliveries, and express/overnight mail should be taken care of immediately.
    2. Checks should be sorted together.
    3. Other first-class mail.
    4. Newsletters.
    5. Third-class mail.
    6. Journals, magazines, and catalogs are the lowest priority.
- **Checks.** Insurance checks and patient checks go to the "Payments" folder. Keep insurance checks together with explanation of benefits (EOBs) or remittance advice notices (RAs) until they are entered into the accounting system.

Appointment Scheduling

The process of appointment scheduling can be unique for each provider. Overbooking can create frustration for both the patient and the provider. Underbooking can create cash flow problems. Your policy should be based upon the following considerations:

- How many days do you wish to be open for patient care per week? Do you want to designate times or days for marketing, networking, documentation, or golfing?
- How do you prefer to work? For example, do you prefer to only see new patients in the morning?
- How long do you typically spend on an established patient visit?

The answers to these questions then dictate the appointment schedule. For example, if you want two new patients per day, create two set time slots for new patients (i.e. 10 am and 3 pm). Instruct staff to never schedule regular patients during this time, unless it is an emergency. If no new patients are there when the time comes, that leaves an hour to dedicate to neglected tasks such as marketing.

> **Tip:** If a typical established patient visit takes ten minutes, consider "cluster booking" two patients at each 15 minute interval. One usually arrives a few minutes late, and the other a few minutes early.

In order to control the schedule, staff should be trained to always offer two choices. Would you like Monday or Tuesday? Morning or afternoon? Three or four o'clock? This drives patients into time slots you designate, but allows them to still feel like they have choices.

> **Alert:** Auditors are now routinely examining appointment books and/or daily schedules to look for discrepancies. Could you have seen that many patients in one day? Did your schedule properly allocate for level 4 and 5 E/M services? Is your scheduling software capable of making adjustments before end of day closeout to fix these unique cases?

Compliance/HIPAA/Breach

Federal and state laws and regulations should be part of any discussion on communications. It is very important that all staff members fully understand HIPAA privacy, security, and breach protocols. All these should be carefully documented in your HIPAA Compliance Manual. Everyone needs to be reminded and have ongoing training regarding these regulations. Through regular training, they will feel confident that they will be able to handle themselves in pressure situations such as a breach. They also get reminders about avoiding potential privacy violations.

See *Section F–Compliance and Audit Protection* for more about these programs.

Chiropractic Assistant (CA)

Generally speaking, a chiropractic assistant is someone who assists the chiropractor in their daily responsibilities of running a chiropractic office. Their responsibilities are extremely varied and can include all of the following:

- **Front desk tasks.** Greeting patients, answering phones, scheduling appointments, collecting payments, and managing patient flow.
- **Medical assistant tasks.** Giving patients the appropriate medical history and insurance forms to complete, acting as the doctor/patient liaison, therapy application, recording patient medical and treatment information, and patient education.
- **Coding and billing tasks.** These include collections, and responding to audits and requests for records.
- **Managerial tasks.** These can include performing the functions of the HIPAA Compliance Officer, human resources manager, marketing and advertising director.
- **Miscellaneous tasks.** Maintaining patient records, filing, ordering supplies, janitorial duties, and information technologies (fixing computers and equipment).

As mentioned previously, the Federation of Chiropractic Licensing Boards has recently instituted a Certified Chiropractic Clinical Assistant program. Although individual states may not have implemented this program yet, this program offers consistency in the education, training, and testing of CAs. Regardless of whether this position is filled by someone with certification or training, be aware of individual state scope of practice laws when it comes to patient treatment. Some procedures may only be supervised or administered by a board licensed professional.

Traditionally, there have not been formal education requirements for this position; however, this is changing. As more and more state scope of practice laws are requiring certification of chiropractic assistants – especially when it comes to patient treatment – some schools and chiropractic associations are beginning to offer formal CA education. Certification aside, it is extremely important that you understand scope of practice laws in order to know exactly what a CA can and cannot do in your state.

Independent Contractor (IC)

Generally speaking, an independent contractor (IC) is someone who leases space within the office. The space can be fully supplied (including staff, equipment and supplies) or only partially supplied depending on the needs of both parties. However, the key is "independent" as determined by financial and behavioral control and the relationship of the parties involved. The Internal Revenue Service has specific rules which determine if the arrangement is a true independent contractor status or if they are really an employee merely labeled as a contractor for the convenience of the employer.

Both parties can benefit from a truly independent agreement. The "hosting" office gets an additional boost with a built in locum tenens, a colleague for collaboration and financial support. The IC enjoys minimal start up costs, the benefits of an established location and the freedom to set their own hours.

Here are some important considerations for this type of arrangement:

- **Detailed Contract:** Responsibilities and duties for each party need to be clearly defined. For example, how will "walk ins" be distributed and how will collections be handled? Be aware of IRS regulations and ensure that a proper "independent" relationship is established. It would be wise to consult with an attorney to ensure that all state regulations are met.

    Note: the independent contractor must maintain proper licensure (see page A-10).

- **Business Associate Agreements:** Because of the independent nature of the agreement, a separate Business Associate Agreement should also be executed by both parties and included in their HIPAA Compliance Manuals.

- **Billing Protocols:** As a truly independent contractor, they must have their own NPI and bill with their NPI.

    Contact your payers and find out their billing policies regarding locum tenens/substitute doctors. If the IC is licensed in your state and your payers have no objection to substitute coverage, then claims may include the Q5 or Q6 modifier if required by the payer. Be sure to have the independent contractor's NPI on the line items and the practice NPI as the billing entity.

See Resource 114 for additional information.

See *Section F–Compliance and Audit Protection* for more about HIPAA Compliance with business associates.

Sample Business Associate Agreements are included with the *Complete & Easy HIPAA Compliance – Third Edition* (Resource 116).

- Go to ACAtoday.org/HIPAA for a "To Do" Checklist for Covered Entities & Business Associates-For Compliance with 2013 Regulations.
- Go to ACAtoday.org/content_css.cfm?CID=4314 (Resource 115) for additional information on idependent contractors.

Review: Supportive and Productive Staff
- What is an "Exclusions" database and where do you find it? *A-25*
- What information are you required to report within 20 days of hiring a new employee? *A-27*
- Which state requirements must be met when hiring new employees? *A-27*
- What steps can be taken to protect your practice when firing an employee? *A-27 to A-28*
- What is included in a "Daily Policies and Procedures Manual"? *A-29*
- How long is too long for your patient to hold on the telephone? *A-31*
- How can balancing a schedule be achieved? *A-32*
- What should be documented in your HIPAA Compliance Manual? *A-33*

1. Understanding Insurance Reimbursement
Page B-3

2. Types of Insurance Plans
Page B-21

3. Establishing Fees
Page B-39

B INSURANCE AND REIMBURSEMENT

INSURANCE AND REIMBURSEMENT

OBJECTIVES

The Reimbursement Life Cycle is the lifeblood of a chiropractic office. Here we introduce the five components of this cycle which begins with a request for treatment and ends with billing standards and protocols. This section covers the basics of this process such as the welcome process, establishing financial responsibility, understanding the different requirements of different types of insurance and the proper setting of fees. Other components of this Reimbursement Life Cycle such as Documentation are covered in other sections of the book.

Throughout this book, these different components are taught in order to help the reader understand what needs to be done to achieve the final desired result – payment or reimbursement which is not later taken away.

OUTLINE

1. Understanding Insurance Reimbursement *B-3*
   - Overview of Insurance Reimbursement *B-3*
   - The Reimbursement Life Cycle *B-5*
   - Review *B-20*

2. Types of Insurance Plans *B-21*
   - Traditional Insurance (Individual or Group Health Plans) *B-21*
   - Managed Care (HMO, PPO, etc.) *B-23*
   - Consumer Driven Plans *B-25*
   - No-Insurance and the Cash Practice *B-26*
   - Personal Injury *B-28*
   - Workers' Compensation *B-32*
   - Government Programs *B-35*
   - Federal Employee Plans *B-37*
   - Review *B-38*

3. Establishing Fees *B-39*
   - About Fees and Fee Schedules *B-39*
   - Fee Schedule Methodologies *B-40*
   - Dollar Conversion Factors *B-43*
   - ChiroCode Fee Calculations *B-44*
   - Other Fee Schedules *B-45*
   - Review *B-48*

1. Understanding Insurance Reimbursement

Billing and reimbursement issues are a critical component of your practice and therefore a thorough understanding is essential. The only way to ensure appropriate reimbursement (and keep it) is by knowing how to submit clean claims to payers with all the essential information.

Reimbursement is cyclic in nature and has a life of its own. In this section, we refer to this complex process as the Reimbursement Life Cycle. In order to appreciate the complexities of this process and see the "big picture," the Reimbursement Life Cycle image will be referred to throughout this book (see page B-5). This enables you to see how each section relates to this cycle and how the entire reimbursement process works.

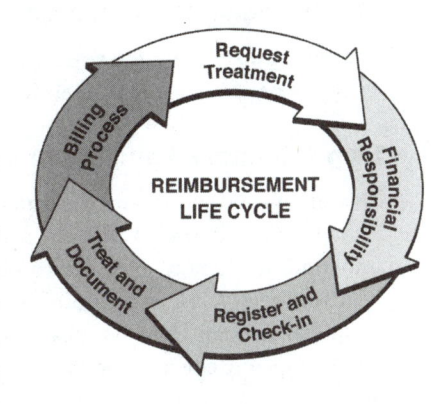

Concerns about avoiding false claims and allegations of fraud, along with expanding rules, regulations and the associated paperwork required, can make this process challenging but not impossible. This section teaches the concepts necessary for proper claims submission which leads to prompt and appropriate reimbursement.

OVERVIEW OF INSURANCE REIMBURSEMENT

Whether you do your own billing, use an outside billing service, or have your patients submit their own claims, you need to understand and follow the proper coding, billing and documentation protocols. It is the provider's responsibility to gather and submit the required information for reimbursement. This process of gathering and submitting information for reimbursement is what we refer to as the Reimbursement Life Cycle.

The five parts of the Reimbursement Life Cycle are:

1. Request for Treatment
2. Establish Patient Financial Responsibility
3. Registration Process
4. Treatment and Documentation
5. Billing Process

Step 1. Request for Treatment

All patient visits begin with the patient requesting care. The reason for the visit is referred to as the Chief Complaint (CC). Their visit and the associated documentation are related to this problem. During this phase, it is important to establish good communication between the patient and the office.

Step 2. Establish Patient Financial Responsibility

Financial responsibility (insurance, cash, etc) should be established as soon as possible, preferably before the patient comes in for the first visit. Both provider and patient need to understand who is responsible for payment of services. The patient needs to understand what they are responsible for versus what the insurance plan or company will or will not pay.

The section on Financial Responsibility (see page B-10) explains how different types of "coverage" should be handled and verified. This includes cash, health insurance, personal injury, and workers compensation.

Step 3. Registration Process

The registration step is the patient check-in process. This section covers what needs to happen when the patient arrives for their initial visit.

Step 4. Treatment and Documentation

This step includes not only the actual treatment of the patient, but it also includes other important processes such as the checkout process and the documentation of the visit. It is very important that treatment centers around the patient's CC. If you perform services **not** directly related to the CC (such as those conditions without subjective complaints but that have been identified through objective measures) be sure to thoroughly document the clinical correlation and therapeutic effect of the care.

The patient should be treated in accordance with appropriate practice parameters and protocols. At the conclusion of the treatment, either the patient needs to have an appropriate fee slip (superbill) to take to the front desk for checkout, or your EHR software must transfer the information there automatically. Part of the checkout process needs to include collecting the coinsurance and deductibles, if this did not happen during the registration process.

Step 5. Billing Process

The final step of the Reimbursement Process is the Billing Process. This includes completing and submitting the claim form, following up on the claim and appealing when necessary, understanding the EOBs and reviewing payments carefully. It is important to realize that in today's environment of denials, post-payment reviews and audits, receiving payment is NOT the end of the reimbursement cycle.

Impact of Healthcare Reform (HCR)

Traditional insurance and reimbursement models are changing due to the influence of HCR. Because HCR delivery and payment models are based on quality of patient care and cost-effective delivery, there may be variations to the Reimbursement Lifecycle steps as outlined in this section of the *ChiroCode DeskBook*.

See ChiroCode.com/HCR and ACAtoday.org/HCR for a more thorough review of the impact of healthcare reform on chiropractic care.

The Reimbursement Life Cycle

Step 1. Request for Treatment

The request for treatment most often begins with a phone call and the scheduling of an appointment. If this is a new patient, this is an excellent time to address your office policies regarding payment, scheduling and cancellations. The remainder of this section explains important information for new patients. If this is an established patient, most of this section is not necessarily applicable unless any pertinent office policies have changed since their last visit.

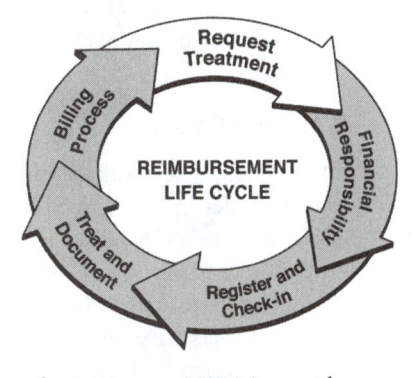

> See *Section F–Compliance and Audit Protection* for important HIPAA considerations regarding appointment reminders.

Before the Patient Arrives

When a patient calls to schedule an appointment, important office policies should be discussed with them. Briefly explain your office policies such as patient payment, insurance and cancellation policies as well as collect any insurance coverage information for verification. Let the patients know that you would like to assist them by contacting their insurance company for coverage details prior to their scheduled visit. This will help avoid confusion or delays during their initial visit. Also, request that patients have all of your office's required documents (assignments, releases, etc.) signed by the appropriate parties. See the "Welcome Packet" segment on the next page for more information about these requirements.

Explaining payment policies to your patients ahead of time will help reduce and eliminate confusion and anxiety. An easy transition is to simply ask the patient, *"Would you like to know about our fee and payment policy?"* With their consent, you have made for a comfortable transition to a discussion about financial responsibilities.

> See Chapter 3–Establishing Fees in this *Insurance and Reimbursement* section for more information on fee structures.

Sample Pre-Arrival Voice Script

When making the appointment, this voice script could be useful.

1. *"Please arrive 20 minutes before your scheduled appointment. This time is necessary to complete the required forms and paperwork before the doctor or therapist sees you. We have a special Welcome Packet which includes these forms which you may complete before coming in. It will save you some time."* [Then suggest either mailing, emailing or having them download the forms].
2. *"Would you like to know our payment policy? [pause] Payment is expected at the time of service, if the insurance billing has not been pre-approved. As a courtesy to you, we will supply the necessary information for your insurance carrier to process and consider for payment. However, your patient portion is due at the time of your visit, before leaving the office. We accept personal checks, cash, or credit card."*
3. *"Please bring your insurance card. We would like to make a copy of it for our records."*
4. *"If you have any questions, please call our office. Thank you."*

Note that in this process you have established your policy and terms. When this information is communicated by telephone, it may be helpful to also mail the written policies, along with a patient information packet which should include any health history forms that need to be completed.

Welcome Packet

There are many forms that need to be completed before a patient is seen. As suggested above, some providers mail a welcome packet to patients so they can fill out these forms before they arrive. Sometimes there isn't enough time between that initial call and the time of the patient visit in order to have those forms mailed. If this is the case, either email the required forms, or tell the patient to arrive 20 minutes early in order to complete them before the doctor sees them. Some providers have found it useful to have their welcome packet available on their practice website for downloading.

Your welcome packet should include the following:

- Welcome Letter
- Patient Financial Responsibility Letter
- Patient Information Form
- Medical and Health History Forms
- Informed Consent Form
- HIPAA Privacy Policy and Acknowledgement
- Financial Hardship Policy and Application (optional—only for cases of financial hardship; includes instructions for completing this application form)

Note: Although not included in what is given to the patient, the "Verification of Insurance Coverage" form should be started at this point (see page B-12).

WELCOME LETTER

The Welcome Letter should be sent to all new patients. Be sure to print on high quality paper on office letterhead and the tone of the letter should be warm, friendly and inviting. During this introduction phase, it is best to customize the letter for the patient instead of printing a generic form that just says "Dear Patient." This establishes the fact that the doctor sees them as an individual, not just another number.

Be sure to change the wording to fit your office tone and style. The ChiroCode example is only a starting point. For example, consider the following phrases:

- "eager to serve you and your family"
- "pleasure to welcome you to our practice"
- "extend a warm welcome to you and your family"
- "greatly anticipate meeting you"

See Resource 140 for a full-size version of this form, with instructions.

PATIENT FINANCIAL RESPONSIBILITY LETTER

Patient financial responsibility is a major source of problems in the billing process. Some practices have found that a letter outlining specific details about how the insurance process works reduces these problems by clearly outlining the insurance company's portion, as well as the portion for which the patient is personally responsible.

> See Resource 141 for a full-size version of this form, with instructions.

> See Step 2. Patient Financial Responsibility (page B-10) for more information about Informed Consent for Non-covered services.

Alert: Insurance Coverage Communication: When communicating with patients about "insurance coverage," do not use the word "insurance" alone. Instead, use "insurance-portion." This clarifies the true meaning for both the sender and listener as an effective checkmate to the false perception that "insurance" means total coverage. Always using both words together helps alleviate misunderstandings, and avoid frustration.

PATIENT INFORMATION FORM

The Patient Information form provides the basic information necessary for all types of practices. However, since it lacks specific questions regarding insurance information, it is better suited for a cash practice. It may be modified for use in all practices as long as proper insurance information is obtained.

> See Resource 142 for a full-size version of this form, with instructions.

> See Step 2. Establish Financial Responsibility (page B-10) for more about obtaining insurance verification. Now is a good time to start verifying insurance coverage—before the patient arrives.

See the legend for using resource icons on page *xvi*.

Insurance Information Form

The Insurance Information form provides the basic necessary information for insurance billing. Identifying the insurance type is critical for proper billing and appeals. The "Employer Sponsored" column is for ERISA appeals. The "My Authorization" portion allows you to use "signature on file" on all future claims. The "My Financial Responsibility" clarifies the patient portion.

> See Resource 143 for a full-size version of this form, with instructions.

Medical History and Health History Forms

The Medical History and Health History are very important documents for the initial patient visit. Most patients dislike filling out forms when they arrive and sometimes they do not bring all the necessary information with them. By completing this form before they arrive, not only do they save both the practice and themselves some time, the doctor also has the necessary information to meet documentation requirements for Review of Systems and Health History.

MEDICAL AND HEALTH HISTORY FORMS

> See Resource 144 for a full-size version of this form, with instructions.

> See *Section D–Documentation* for more about documentation requirements.

INFORMED CONSENT AGREEMENT FOR TREATMENT

For appropriate risk management, every office needs to have a signed Informed Consent Agreement prior to treatment. Consult with your legal counsel and your malpractice insurance carrier for specific forms they may recommend for your office (e.g., decompression therapy, pediatrics, etc.). Here is a basic and general consent form for those who have none.

> See Resource 145 for a full-size version of this form, with instructions.

Sample: *Informed Consent for Chiropractic Treatment*

HIPAA PRIVACY POLICY FORM AND ACKNOWLEDGEMENT

HIPAA requires patients to receive a notice of the provider's (clinic's) privacy practices. Their individual medical record needs to contain their signed acknowledgement that they have received this notice and reviewed its contents. Such a statement is included on the sample Patient Information Form, however the actual notice is not included in this section.

The requirements for this Notice of Privacy Practices have changed due to the January 2013 HIPAA Omnibus Rule. All patients need to be notified that their rights have changed.

> See *Section F–Compliance and Audit Protection* for more about HIPAA requirements including the Omnibus Rule changes.

> For detailed information about HIPAA requirements and all necessary forms which have been updated for Omnibus Rule requirements, see *Complete & Easy HIPAA Compliance* (Resource 116).

> Go to ACAtoday.org/HIPAA for additional information by the ACA about protecting patient privacy.

FINANCIAL HARDSHIP POLICY AND APPLICATION (OPTIONAL)

This is an optional form for use when the patient appears to have a problem financially where they would be unable to meet their co-pays or deductibles. This form is necessary and must be included in their chart if you intend to waive all or part of their co-pay (patient portion) or deductible. Caution is advised when implementing hardship waivers. They should be used only in cases where hardship is clearly indicated and properly documented. If not done correctly, waiving deductibles or co-pays could violate several federal laws. Waivers and reductions for co-pays, co-insurances, and deductibles should not be routine and should not be advertised in any way. See page B-46 for additional information.

Sample: *Financial Hardship Policy and Application*

See "Financial Hardship Policy" in Chapter 4. Fees of this *Insurance and Reimbursement* section for more about the proper use of hardship discounts.

See Resource 146 for a full-size version of this form, with instructions.

Step 2. Establish Patient Financial Responsibility

Establishing patient financial responsibility is not just about patient portion versus insurance payments. It is about eliminating surprises and establishing better communication between provider and patient about who pays for what. When it comes to chiropractic care, it could also be about personal injury or workers compensation. It is up to the provider to obtain the necessary information for proper billing to third-party payers as well as the patient.

The Insurance Information Form (see page B-8) is an excellent tool for assisting in this process. Used in conjunction with the Verification of Insurance Coverage Form (see page B-12), these tools establish the necessary financial requirements during the Check Out process.

See the "Patient Financial Responsibility Letter" on page B-7 for additional information.

See Resource 149 for additional information.

Informed Financial Consent Policy

The Informed Financial Consent Policy is the proper way to eliminate surprises and help the patient understand what their insurance may or may not cover. It should be used for non-covered or elective services, or at the beginning of a treatment plan. If you know that a service or item will not be covered, it is crucial to have an official written policy and to have the patient sign the necessary required forms. For a patient, this policy is sometimes referred to as an "estimate."

ESTIMATE OF MEDICAL FEES

For a third-party payer, using an estimate may be insufficient. Some payers have their own specific forms that must be used. For example, CMS has their own form called the Advanced Beneficiary Notice (ABN) which must be used to inform Medicare beneficiaries of the patient's financial responsibility when services may be denied/non-covered.

See *Section C–Medicare* for more about the ABN form and how to use it properly.

See Resource 147 for a full-size version of this form, with instructions.

Cash/No Insurance

Even if your practice does not accept any insurance, financial policies need to be clearly documented. Your "Patient Financial Policy" letter should clearly outline what payment options are available.

- See Chapter 2–Types of Insurance Plans in this *Insurance and Reimbursement* section for more information about Cash/No Insurance options.

- See Chapter 3–Fees in this *Insurance and Reimbursement* section for more information about discounts.

Personal Injury

Personal injury is for accidents such as auto, home or non work related business. Providers should be careful to gather all details of the incident including both personal injury and medical insurance coverage details.

See the "Personal Injury" segment on page B-28 for more information.

Workers' Compensation

This is for work related illness or injuries on the job where the employer pays for insurance which covers medical costs incurred, and replaces lost wages. Fees are based on their own specific fee schedule and vary by state.

See Chapter 2 in this *Insurance and Reimbursement* section for more about Workers' Compensation.

Health Insurance

Health insurance coverage is based on a payer's health benefit plan and is typically based on the concept of medically necessary services. There are several different types of health insurance and each one needs to be handled in accordance with their specific protocols. At this point in the visit, it is important to obtain copies of insurance cards and contact the company to verify coverage. Obtain necessary pre-authorizations or referrals prior to the initial visit.

Alert: If the patient's spouse or parents have an additional insurance plan, there could be multiple insurance coverage for the patient. It is very important to correctly determine which is the

Alert - *cont.*

primary insurance and which is secondary. The "birthday rule" can be helpful in establishing the proper coverage. Generally, when both spouses have insurance coverage, the husband's insurance plan is the primary for him, and the wife's insurance plan is the primary for her. For dependents, the primary insurance company is determined by the insured's birthdate, which is referred to as the "birthday rule." The primary insured is the person whose birthdate (month and day) comes earliest in the year. For example, if the father's birthday is September 20 and the mother's birthday is February 5, the mother's insurance would be the primary plan for their dependents since her birthday is earlier. The year of birth is not applicable.

- See *Section C–Medicare* for specifics on Medicare Coverage.
- See Chapter 2–Types of Insurance in this *Insurance and Reimbursement* section for more about these different types of insurance.

VERIFICATION OF INSURANCE COVERAGE FORM

If you will be billing insurance, coverage should be verified and all necessary pre-authorizations for treatment should be obtained. When you contact the insurer for coverage information, record the necessary insurance information using a "Verification of Insurance Coverage" form. This will help you to verify coverage for that individual. If they are enrolled in a particular insurance plan, it might require that the provider be a part of their panel for full coverage. Additional information on patient insurance coverage is found later in this section.

Alert: The new marketplace plans available through Health Insurance Exchanges (HIE) can complicate the verification process. Even though you may be an in-network provider for a specific carrier, this does **not** mean that you are an in-network provider for that same carrier for insurance plans purchased through an insurance exchange.

Only offices which are compliant with all HIPAA regulations can verify coverage *electronically* with health plans that have the information available. If your office is **not** HIPAA compliant, you may only verify insurance coverage by telephone or by regular mail (but not email). There may be other related information obtained about coverage during this verification process. Record it on this form.

- See Resource 148 for a full-size version of this form, with instructions.
- ACA members, go to ACAtoday.org/resourcecenter for a comprehensive Verification of Coverage form.

Sample: *Verification of Insurance Coverage*

Pre-authorization

Some payers may require pre-authorizations for certain types of services or for pre-approval of a specified number of visits. In some cases, you may need to have an official referral number before treatment begins. Pre-authorizations are commonly utilized in managed care situations.

Note: For some health plans, there may be situations in which additional benefits could be granted to patients who meet specific criteria. In such cases, it is important to document the clinical necessity for treatment beyond their usual limits. Your diagnosis should reflect the improvement or changes in your patient's condition as the case progresses. Be aware of individual payer policies.

See *Section D–Documentation* for more about record keeping standards.

Office Policies - Patient Information

Every office needs a standard written policy regarding the patient information/data which should be obtained. Employees need to be responsible for obtaining current and correct data. They should also understand that claims with missing or inaccurate patient information are delayed or denied. Some policy examples are:

- Information for the subscriber(s) of the insurance coverage should also be obtained.
- A photocopy of both front and back of the patient's health plan identification card should be kept on file and updated when the policy renews.

See *Section D–Documentation* for suggestions on organizing your patient records.

Step 3. Registration Process

Step 3 of the Insurance Reimbursement Life Cycle covers the patient arrival, check in and intake process. During this step, it is important to obtain patient demographics, verify insurance, obtain informed consent and financial responsibility forms, and take care of HIPAA Privacy requirements. Established patient registration is much simpler than that of a new patient.

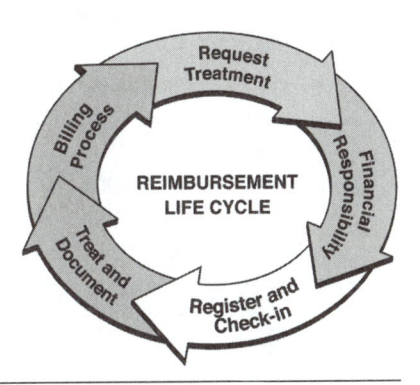

Tip: Co-pays and deductible amounts should have been established during the insurance verification process. It is helpful to have these amounts noted on the superbill/charge sheet before the patient encounter takes place.

Alert: Be aware of HIPAA regulations during this registration process. Simple sign-in sheets are fine, but the reason for the visit cannot be included. See Resource 151 for more information.

New Patient Initial Visit

When the patient arrives, it is important to ensure that all forms are properly completed and signed. If they have not already completed the forms in the Welcome Packet, give them time to fill them out. Pay particular attention to the following:

- Make copies of their insurance cards, both front and back and include it in their patient record.
- Validate the information on the insurance card with another valid form of identification such as a drivers license, to avoid security problems like patient misrepresentation and possible health care fraud. It is not necessary to copy the drivers license, just look at the name and address to ensure that the patient is who they claim to be. In fact, some states prohibit copying a drivers license, so be aware of your state law if you wish to make a copy.

- Referrals and/or pre-authorizations should have been obtained before the patient arrived. If not, call immediately to verify coverage.
- Make sure that all of the forms in the Welcome Packet are properly completed.
- Obtain signed copies of other forms, such as the Release of Information or liens, where applicable.

Established Patient Subsequent Visits

One common problem in a medical office is not catching changes in demographic or insurance information when an established patient arrives for a visit. Be sure to ask the patient if anything has changed since their last visit. This could also be done by phone prior to the appointment. Verify the following:

- **Patient information/demographics** such as address, phone or employment.
- **Insurance plan change or coverage.** Remember that coverage can change, and the patient may not know about it or remember to tell you. Periodically ask, and document any changes using the Insurance Verification form.
- **Health history.** If there have been significant changes, it might be beneficial to do an updated form if it has been some time since the patient was last in the office. Otherwise, be sure to remind the patient to tell the provider of these changes so they are part of the medical record.
- **Pain assessment.** After a specified number of days or visits, an updated pain assessment is required by most insurance companies. This is best done before the patient sees the provider.

> **Reminder:** Diagnoses are dynamic, not static. As necessary, your documentation/diagnosis should reflect the improvement or changes in your patient's condition as the case progresses. See the Documentation section in this book for more help with documentation.

> **Alert:** Medicare will pay for treatment as long as all documentation criteria are met and the treatment is documented as medically necessary.

Step 4. Treatment and Documentation

This step is the core of the patient encounter and drives the remainder of the Reimbursement Life Cycle. There are several tasks that need to happen beyond the actual treatment of the patient.

Document the Visit

As stated throughout this book, proper documentation of the visit is essential to payment. By properly following documentation protocol, you will appropriately capture the procedures and diagnoses which are required for billing. Your SOAP notes will be your supporting evidence. These notes show which systems were examined and which areas were treated. If there is any question when it comes time to bill, your billing specialist will need these records to ensure proper billing takes place.

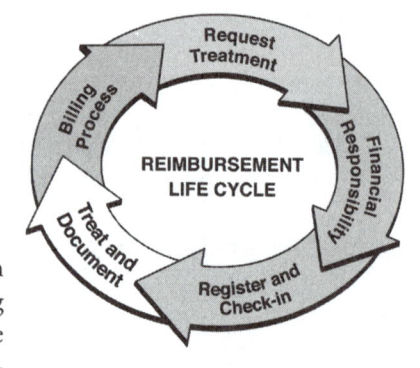

See *Section D–Documentation* for more about record keeping standards.

Clinical Documentation Manual by the ACA includes detailed documentation information (Resource 151).

Create a Treatment Plan

The treatment plan must be fully documented and be part of the patient record. This is one of the most forgotten components of documentation and one of the most highly scrutinized areas by auditors. Additionally, it is also advisable to send written instructions of this plan home with the patient or caregiver. It is very easy for them to forget details about what they need to do when at home and before the next visit.

See *Section D–Documentation* for more about treatment plan standards.

Complete Fee Slip

Using a superbill is one way of providing all the necessary information for billing on one form. Superbills are also known as care tickets, charge-slips, or encounter forms. No matter what they are called, their purpose is to simplify both the check-out and coding processes. It makes it easier for the provider to let the billing staff know what codes to use and it can also make it easier to give the patient what they need.

If you have a computerized system, it is recommended that the items on your form be coordinated with the sequence in which data is entered in your computer. This will save time, frustration, and reduce the possibility of data entry errors.

> **Alert:** Be aware that some automated billing systems review the documentation and select the billing codes based on internal EHR settings. Auditors have found that in many cases, these systems often up-code to a higher billing level when they should not. If you have one of these systems, always review the selected code and make sure that you have justification for the code selected. You must be able to either approve or disapprove what the computer has chosen before it is billed. Understand what you are billing for, as you have ultimate responsibility for what is submitted for reimbursement. Also, your documentation must support what is being billed.

Checkout Process

This is the final step in which the patient takes the super-bill to the front desk. At this time, it is important to not only schedule the next visit, but, even more importantly, to collect payment of the patient portion. The best time to collect the patient portion is when the benefit of the service is fresh in their minds and fully appreciated. You should collect payment before they leave the office, if it was not collected during the check-in process.

Step 5. Billing Process

Overhead costs for billing and administration can be up to 30% of the fees. For this reason, some providers have chosen to either switch to a cash practice or else outsource their billing to an agency. Regardless of who does the work, the billing process has its own work flow. The Billing Process Flowchart in Figure 2.1 outlines how this process can work.

See *Section A-Practice Management* for more information about Outsourcing and Billing Agencies.

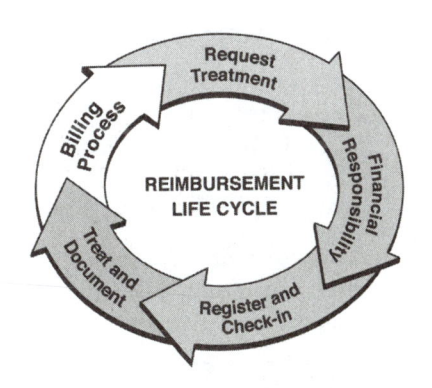

REIMBURSEMENT LIFE CYCLE: Request Treatment → Financial Responsibility → Register and Check-in → Treat and Document → Billing Process

Fighting to Keep Your Money

This should be the end of the claims cycle, but there is one more thing to consider: post-payment problems such as audits, refund demands, and take-backs.

Payment Concerns

As with all businesses, receipts, and collections are an integral part of staying in business. Insurance payers can be slow and the collection equation could become a central issue for your office. The best way to avoid collection problems is to avoid the pitfalls that create potential problems.

> See Chapter 4–Business Financial Standards in *Section A–Practice Management* for more information.

Prompt Filing

Both patients and insurance payers respond better to timely requests for payment. When insurance is involved, claims should be submitted promptly. Payers reject claims that exceed their claim filing time limits (usually 180 or 365 days, but some payers have shorter time frames). Know your payer policies regarding timely submission of claims and their deadlines.

- See *Section E–Claims and Appeals* for more about claims submission.
- See Chapter 3–Guidelines for Unpaid Claims in *Section E–Claims and Appeals*.
- See also Chapter 5–Audit Protection in *Section F–Compliance and Audit Protection* for more information.

Billing Managed Care

Managed care programs often have specific billing requirements. Obtain billing manuals and instructions directly from the carrier. Specific policies for referrals and coverage, along with claims submission requirements, are outlined within their billing manuals. Follow their guidelines carefully.

> **Note:** Routinely reevaluate the costs of membership and payment benefits related to provider participation with all plans. These programs could be costing more than they benefit the practice. When calculating costs, include the cost of increased provider time and administrative costs incurred in dealing with managed care controls.

Benefit Notices and Payment Reports

Once you receive a check from an insurance payer, that does NOT mean that you are done. Carefully review their attached benefit notices to ensure that the appropriate payment has been received. The following information explains some of these notices and what you can expect.

EXPLANATION OF BENEFITS

An Explanation of Benefits (EOB) is the explanation that accompanies either Medicare or private carrier disbursement or denial of healthcare benefits. This document is the key to knowing what was paid or not paid and why. Knowing how to read an EOB will help a practice collect proper reimbursement. There are terms used on EOBs, such as, "applied to deductible," "usual and customary," "patient co-pay," "allowable," etc., which make it easier to determine what the patient is responsible for paying. Becoming familiar with these terms will allow you to process payments in a more efficient manner.

REMITTANCE ADVICE

A Remittance Advice (RA) is similar to an EOB, in the manner that it is a notice of payments and adjustments sent to providers, billers, and suppliers. After a claim has been received and processed, a third party payer produces the RA, which may serve as a companion to a claim payment or as an explanation when there is no payment. The RA explains the reimbursement decisions including the reasons for payments, adjustments, or denials.

The codes listed on the RA help the provider identify any additional action that may be necessary. For example, some RA codes may indicate a need to resubmit a claim with corrected information, while others may indicate whether the payment decision can be appealed.

It is very important that the RA be thoroughly reviewed. The RA features valid codes and specific values that make up the claim payment. There are seven general types of adjustments:

- Denied Claim
- Zero Payment
- Partial Payment
- Reduced Payment
- Penalty Applied
- Additional Payment
- Supplemental Payment

> If your claim has not been paid correctly, then you **must** follow the appeals procedures and protocols for that payer. See *Section E-Claims and Appeals* for more information.

MEDICARE SUMMARY NOTICE

The Medicare Summary Notice (MSN) is a summary of all charges that providers and suppliers billed to Medicare over a 90-day period that is sent to the beneficiary. The MSN lists the details of the services received, Medicare payments and the patient portion or the amount a beneficiary may be billed for by the providers or suppliers. The MSN is mailed when claims are processed. Beneficiaries/patients should check this notice to be sure all the services, medical supplies, or equipment that providers billed to Medicare were actually received.

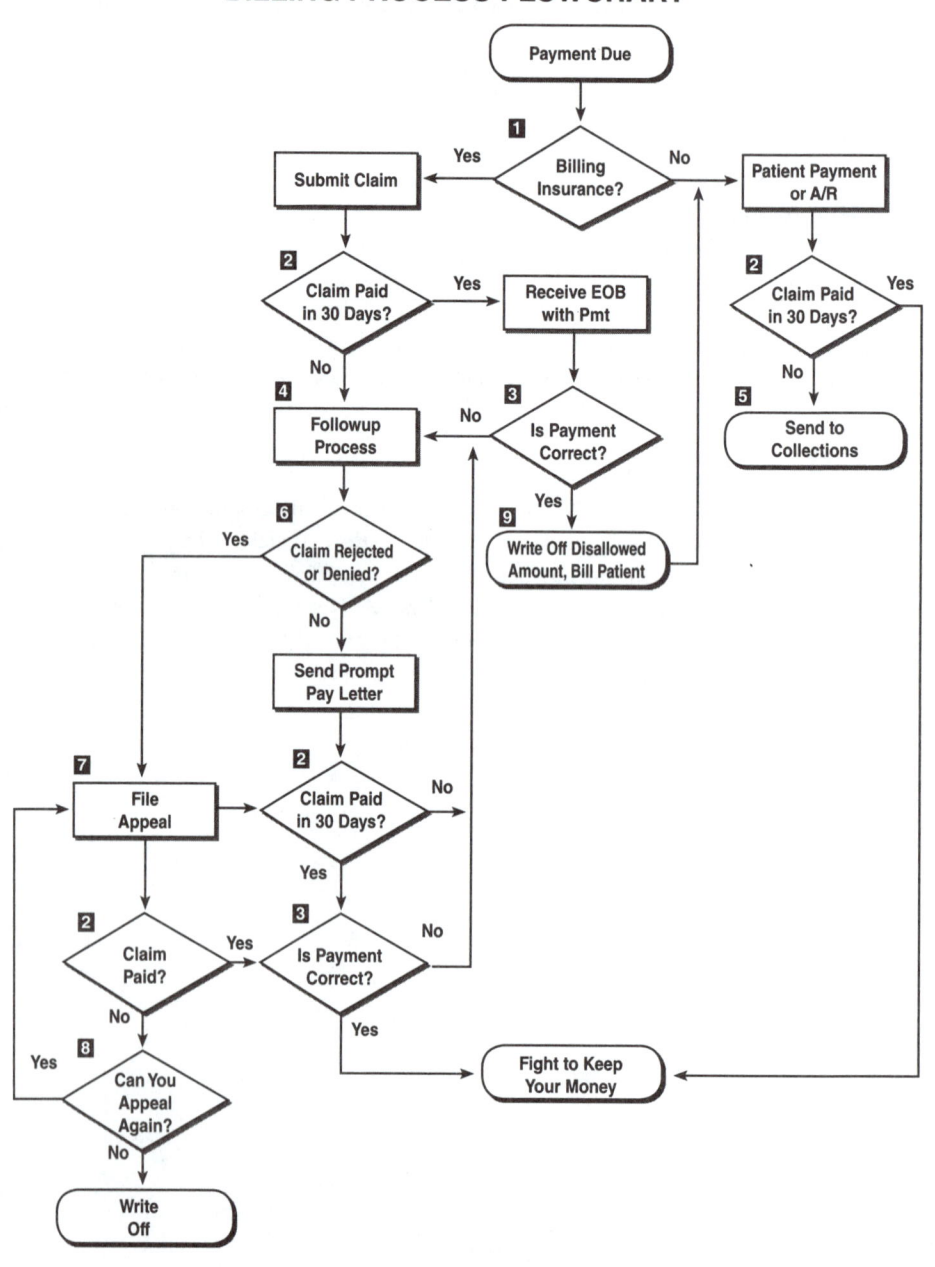

Billing Process Flowchart

The Billing Process Flowchart (see Figure 2.1) helps outline the decision process for maintaining an effective billing process. This is only a suggested work plan and is used for demonstration purposes to illustrate areas which may need more attention in your practice's policies and procedures. All billing begins with a service being completed and a payment is due. It doesn't end with the payment though. Often it is necessary to fight to keep that reimbursement.

FIGURE 2.1
Billing Process Flowchart

BILLING PROCESS FLOWCHART

```
                                    Payment Due
                                         │
                                        [1]
                          Yes          Billing          No
              ┌────────────────────── Insurance? ──────────────────────┐
              ▼                                                         ▼
        Submit Claim                                          Patient Payment
              │                                                   or A/R
             [2]                                                     │
              ▼                                                     [2]
        Claim Paid        Yes      Receive EOB                  Claim Paid       Yes
        in 30 Days? ──────────────► with Pmt                   in 30 Days? ──────┐
              │                         │                          │             │
             No                        [3]                         No            │
             [4]                        ▼              No         [5]            │
         Followup ◄──────────── Is Payment ──────────►        Send to            │
         Process                  Correct?                    Collections        │
              │                        │                                         │
             [6]                      Yes                                        │
              ▼                       [9]                                        │
   Yes   Claim Rejected       Write Off Disallowed                               │
  ┌───── or Denied?            Amount, Bill Patient                              │
  │           │                                                                  │
  │          No                                                                  │
  │           ▼                                                                  │
  │     Send Prompt                                                              │
  │     Pay Letter                                                               │
  │           │                                                                  │
  │          [2]                                                                 │
  │           ▼             No                                                   │
  │      Claim Paid ──────────────┐                                              │
  │      in 30 Days?              │                                              │
  │           │                   │                                              │
  │          Yes                  │                                              │
  │          [7]                 [3]                                             │
  ▼    File              Yes  Is Payment      No                                 │
  Appeal ◄───────────── Correct? ──────────┐                                     │
    ▲        [2]            │              │                                     │
    │         ▼            Yes             │                                     │
    │     Claim                            │                                     │
    │     Paid?                            │                                     │
    │         │                            │                                     │
    │        No                            ▼                                     │
  Yes       [8]                     Fight to Keep ◄────────────────────────────┘
  ┌──── Can You                     Your Money
  │     Appeal
  │     Again?
  │         │
  │        No
  │         ▼
  │      Write
  │       Off
```

Flowchart Notes

1. **BILLING INSURANCE?**
   - If you are billing insurance, you will need to submit a claim. This can be either electronic or paper. Remember, the cleaner the claim, the faster payment will be received.
   - If you are NOT billing insurance, implement an effective accounts receivable procedure.

2. **IS THE CLAIM PAID? IS IT PAID IN 30 DAYS?**
   - Unpaid claims must be reviewed at least every 30 days, more if there is a known problem that is being addressed with the payer.
   - If payment has been received, carefully compare the EOB against the submitted claim to ensure that payments are correct.

3. **IS PAYMENT CORRECT?**
   - If the payment is correct, then hopefully all is done and there are no post-payment reviews or audits to worry about. If the patient portion has not been collected, be sure to write off any disallowed amounts (if you are a contracted provider) and the bill the patient for the remaining balance.
   - If the payment is not correct, policies need to be in place to follow a specific procedure for both over-payments and under-payments. Over-payments will need to be paid back to the insurance company quickly to avoid allegations of fraud. Under-payments will need to reviewed and may need to be appealed.

4. **FOLLOWUP PROCESS**
   - Every office needs an established Follow up procedure. See "Claim Followup Procedures" in Chapter 3–Guidelines for Unpaid Claims in *Section E–Claims and Appeals* for more information.

5. **SEND TO COLLECTIONS**
   - The decision to send an account to collections should not be an emotional decision. It should be clearly outlined in your office Policies and Procedures.

6. **IS CLAIM REJECTED OR DENIED?**
   - If the claim has been rejected or denied, begin the claims appeals process. See *Section E–Claims and Appeals* for more about the steps that need to be taken.
   - If the claim is unpaid after 30 days and has not been rejected, then see the segment "Prompt Pay Laws" in Chapter 3–Guidelines for Unpaid Claims in *Section E–Claims and Appeals* for more about one possible option to encourage payment.

7. **FILE APPEAL**
   - If the claim has been rejected or denied, begin the claims appeals process. See *Section E–Claims and Appeals* for more about the specific steps which should be taken.

8. **CAN YOU APPEAL AGAIN?**
    - Most payers have a limit on the appeals process, so follow individual payer guidelines carefully. If you have exhausted your appeal options with the payer, consider external appeals, complaint to DOI, and notifying ACA or your state association.

        If these additional options are unsuccessful, then it may be necessary to write off the balance. In limited cases, you may be able to collect from the patient. Be aware of individual payer policies about "balance billing."

        See *Section E–Claims and Appeals* for more information about appeal options.

9. **WRITE OFF DISALLOWED AMOUNT, BILL PATIENT**
    - Once the claim has been adjudicated and an Explanation of Benefits (EOB) has been received, the disallowed amounts (if required by contract or law) should be deducted from the patient account to accurately reflect their "patient portion." Only bill the patient the amount which you are legally allowed to bill. Do not write off patient co-payments or deductibles unless the patient has an approved Financial Hardship Application (see page B-47).

Review: Understanding Insurance Reimbursement

- What are the five parts of the Reimbursement Life Cycle? *B-4*
- When should a discussion of practice policies take place with a new patient? *B-5*
- Which seven items should be included in a welcome packet? *B-6*
- What is the "insurance portion," and why is it important? *B-7*
- Whose responsibility is it to provide the necessary billing information to third-party payers? *B-10*
- How can the "Birthday rule" be helpful in establishing the proper coverage? *B-11*
- Which documentation component is one of the most forgotten, and one that is scrutinized by auditors? *B-15*
- How does it benefit you to know how to read an EOB? *B-16*

2. Types of Insurance Plans

This chapter explains the different types of insurance plans that a chiropractic office may encounter. It is important to understand that there are a variety of insurance plans, each designed to meet the demands of consumers. These range from traditional fee-for-service health plans to managed care plans. Types of insurance administered by federal and state government include Medicare, Medicaid, Workers' Compensation, etc., each of which serves a different purpose.

Although most payers use the universal 1500 Health Insurance Claim Form form, also referred to as the 1500 claim form, for paper claims, or the 837 format (5010) for electronic claims, some payers may have additional requirements or forms. Be aware of these differences.

- See *Section C–Medicare* for more information on Medicare.
- See *Section E–Claims and Appeals* for more about claims submission requirements and help with managing denials and appeals.

TRADITIONAL INSURANCE (INDIVIDUAL OR GROUP HEALTH PLANS)

Traditional indemnity plans or fee-for-service plans are purchased by individuals or groups. These plans review claims for payment after the service is rendered. These plans are becoming less common as people switch to Managed Care Organizations (MCOs) in an effort to save money. To help control the cost of medical care, traditional plans are increasingly adopting ideas from managed care plans, such as utilization review and prior authorization.

Healthcare Reform Entities Are NOT Insurance Plans

Led by provisions in the Affordable Care Act, three types of patient care and payment models do not adhere to traditional insurance protocols. Accountable Care Organizations (ACOs), Patient Centered Medical Homes (PCMHs) and Patient Centered Healthcare Homes (PCHCHs) are designed to improve the quality of patient care while simultaneously decreasing costs. As such, they are not fee-for-service insurance plans. Providers need to be aware of how these new entities function and become involved in this changing healthcare environment.

- See ChiroCode.com/hcr and ACAtoday.org/HCR for a more thorough review of the impact of healthcare reform on chiropractic care.

With indemnity health coverage, the patient could use the service of any doctor or any other medical service provider. Either the patient or the provider forwards the bill to the insurer who reimburses the medical costs based on an established formula or fee schedule.

The formula for most indemnity policies begins with the "usual and customary charge" reserved for covered medical service. The insurance firm pays a percentage (typically 80%) of these costs, after the patient has paid for services up to the deductible amount of the policy. The patient is responsible for the remaining 20%, plus any charges in excess of the usual and customary charges.

Annual and Lifetime Limits

Beginning January 1, 2014, the Patient Protection and Affordable Care Act (PPACA) changed the rules regarding annual and lifetime limits. Insurance companies can no longer set lifetime limits on "essential health benefits" as long as the patient is enrolled in that plan. Even though there are no longer lifetime limits on essential health benefits, there can be a yearly limit of $2 million.

Once medical costs reach a given amount in a calendar year, the customary costs for the benefits covered would be met in full by the insurance firm, and the insured does not pay the coinsurance any longer. This concept is called an "out-of-pocket maximum."

Keep in mind that currently existing plans, which have not undergone substantial changes, are "grandfathered," and will not be covered under these new rules.

See Resource 152 for additional information.

PPACA Essential Health Benefits (EHBs)

PPACA establishes the federal minimum standards for required health plan benefits. For 2014 and 2015, states have the flexibility to determine their own benchmarks for plans sold in the exchanges, and for small group and individual markets. HHS plans to reevaluate this policy for plans sold in 2016 and beyond. According to the National Conference of State Legislatures, most states mandate coverage for services provided by doctors of chiropractic, however, be aware of state specific EHB differences.

See Resource 153 for additional information.

The following are the required federal essential health benefits categories for all health plans offered in the individual and small group markets, both inside and outside the Health Insurance Marketplace:

- Ambulatory patient services
- Emergency services
- Hospitalization
- Maternity and newborn care
- Mental health and substance use disorder services, including behavioral health treatment

---

Federal vs State Minimum Standards

The Patient Protection and Affordable Care Act (PPACA) is a federal statute which includes federal standards for essential health benefits. States can enact their own minimum standards which may be more stringent, but they must, at the a minimum, meet the requirements of PPACA. It is important for all providers to be aware of their own state's statutes and regulations in addition to the federal requirements.

- Prescription drugs
- Rehabilitative and habilitative services and devices
- Laboratory services
- Preventive and wellness services and chronic disease management
- Pediatric services, including oral and vision care

Appeals

All payers have an appeals process if all or part of your claim is denied; however, these processes are not standardized throughout the industry. For example, Medicare has their own specific appeal guidelines which are different than the process required for employer sponsored plans which are governed by ERISA.

See *Section E–Claims and Appeals* for more information about appeals, including ERISA appeals.

Sickness vs. Wellness and Coverage

Figure 2.2, the Health Stability Scale for Insurance Coverage (on the following page), illustrates important coverage differences between **Sickness and Accident Insurance** (falsely called health insurance) and **Health Assurance** (also known as wellness).

When a patient is stable, many third party payers use the phrase, "Maximum Medical Improvement." This is generally a false and confusing statement. What most sickness and accident insurance payers are really attempting to express is: "The patient is now stable and/or symptom free, and thus beyond the contracted sickness and accident insurance benefits." In auto accident insurance cases it usually means: "The patient is now back to their pre-accident health condition, and the insurance contract does not provide for any benefits beyond this status."

Sickness and Accident Insurance contracts are all different, but they share a common goal: to make payments for treatment to correct a problem and return the patient to a stable condition. Rarely will they cover supportive care (to keep stable), preventive care (immunizations and screenings), or promote wellness. However, some are now beginning to cover screening services in an effort to reduce expenditures by catching diseases before they become costly.

Remember that Sickness and Accident Insurance is not "Health and Wellness Assurance" (see Figure 2.2). Communicating what it really is avoids confusion.

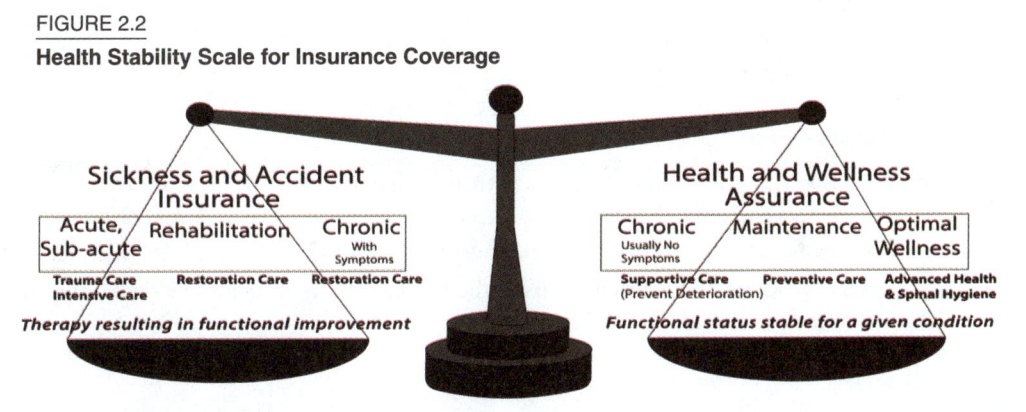

FIGURE 2.2
Health Stability Scale for Insurance Coverage

Sickness and Accident Insurance
- Acute, Sub-acute — Trauma Care, Intensive Care
- Rehabilitation — Restoration Care
- Chronic With Symptoms — Restoration Care

Therapy resulting in functional improvement

Health and Wellness Assurance
- Chronic Usually No Symptoms — Supportive Care (Prevent Deterioration)
- Maintenance — Preventive Care
- Optimal Wellness — Advanced Health & Spinal Hygiene

Functional status stable for a given condition

Managed Care (HMO, PPO, etc.)

Managed care was created as a way to contain costs and maintain quality care standards. Broadly speaking, managed care is any health care delivery system in which a party other than the physician or the patient influences the type of health care delivered. Although this broad definition may include indemnity insurance, which limits benefits using various methods based on cost and utilization, such a system is not truly managed. Limitations of benefits serve to limit non-selective access. A managed care system may limit benefits to its customers, and actively manage those limitations. A managed care system also actively manages both the medical and financial aspects of a patient's care.

Defining managed care is difficult because it is an evolving concept made up of disparate organizations. The sharp distinctions that once existed between different types of plans have clouded as these plans have adopted features that make some of their characteristics indistinguishable from each other. Managed Care Organizations (MCO) are also known as Health Maintenance Organizations (HMO). The characteristics most common to these plans include:

- Arrangements with selected providers who furnish a package of services to enrollees.
- Explicit criteria for selection of providers.
- Quality assurance, utilization review, and outcome measures.
- Incentives (financial or program coverage).
- Penalties to enrollees who do not use selected providers.
- Provider risk-sharing arrangements.
- Management by providers to ensure that enrollees or members receive appropriate care from the most cost-efficient mix of providers.

To Participate or Not Participate

Reimbursement from these plans often requires that you as a provider be on their panel, or network of "preferred" providers. Sometimes this is known as "participating." If you are not on their panel, ask if the patient's plan has an "out-of-network" or "opt-out" benefit. The "out-of-network" percentage of coverage may be lower than if you were participating; however, if you were participating, you would be required to accept their fee schedule and you would **not** be allowed to bill the patient for charges above the contracted amounts for covered benefits (called "balance billing").

Also check their list of covered and non-covered diagnosis and service codes. Managed care systems typically will either not cover or will limit coverage for particular diagnosis codes or procedures.

Learn as much as you can about the MCO before signing up. What is their financial status? What is their reputation for paying bills? How stable is their contract with the employer? Know your local market. Is the company under pressure to compete? If they have potential problems, signing up might not be a good option. If an MCO goes bankrupt (and they do), your only recourse may be to hire a lawyer and go to court.

Advantages of Participating

- *Increased Clientele*: Patient requests to their insurance carrier for the name of a provider in their area could be referred to you. This is free "marketing" for you. Check to see how many providers are currently on their panel for your area.
- *Direct Payment*: Payment comes from the HMO directly to the provider, without the risk of the patient not forwarding it to you.

Disadvantages of Participating

- *Panel Costs:* Quite often, there are costs associated with becoming part of a panel. Ask what those costs are, along with their anticipated referral rate. The amount of "participating fees" for their referral rate might not be worth the effort. It may be less expensive to run your own marketing campaign.
- *Lower Fees:* By participating, you agree to accept their "allowable" amount and only bill the patient for the applicable patient portion or "co-pay" and/or deductible. Ask what the allowable amounts are up front to avoid any unpleasant surprises. Some have very low fee schedules.
- *Higher Overhead Costs:* There could be additional overhead costs in administering other plans in your office. For example, you would need to maintain separate fee schedules and/or write off disallowed amounts. Be aware of any additional overhead expenses.

CONSUMER DRIVEN PLANS

This section covers Consumer Directed Healthcare Plans (CDHP), no insurance or cash, and medical discount plans for those who are uninsured or under-insured.

See Resource 154 for additional information.

Consumer Directed Healthcare Plans (CDHP)

In the late 1990s, Consumer Directed Healthcare Plans (CDHPs) were developed as a way to shift the control of healthcare dollars from the insurance companies to the patient (consumer). The goal of these types of plans is to allow the patient to take a more active role in their own health and healthcare decisions in an effort to control costs. The Patient Protection and Affordable Care Act (PPACA) has fueled the growth of CDHPs.

According to a 2014 survey, 57% of employers surveyed are implementing or expanding CDHPs and 32% of that 57% have a CDHP as the only healthcare option for their employees. Another survey reported that by 2016, 78% of large employers (those with more than 5,000 employees) are very likely to offer a CDHP to their employees. As employers seek to find cost effective solutions to the new healthcare requirements, CDHPs seem to be the best option available. In fact, only 4 percent of employees work for firms which offer traditional insurance plans. This phenomenal growth trend is expected to continue. For these reasons, providers need to understand how these plans work. The following section explains several different CDHP options.

Affordable Care Act Limited Provisions

The Affordable Care Act treats self-funded health benefit plans differently than fully insured plans. There are fewer regulations under the PPACA for self-funded plans and the new trend for employers appears to be moving towards the self-funded option. These differences make it essential for providers to verify coverage and plan information.

See Chapter 4–ERISA Appeals in *Section E–Claims and Appeals* for important information on self-funded plans.

Consumer Driven Health Care Options

Here is a summary of major consumer driven health insurance options:

- **Health Savings Accounts (HSA).** These accounts are similar to the former Archer Medical Savings Accounts in that they permit eligible individuals to save and pay for health care expenses on a tax-free basis. HSA patients are empowered to spend their own dollars. Funds are held in a tax-exempt trust or custodial account with a qualified HSA trustee who pays or reimburses qualified health care expenses. To qualify for an HSA, there must be a high deductible health plan (HDHP).

- **Medicare Medical Savings Accounts (MSA).** This consumer-driven option for Medicare beneficiaries is a huge boon for beneficiaries because it eliminates the need for MediGap coverage and costs, provides a way of paying for Medicare non-covered services, limits out-of-pocket exposure, and offers the opportunity to save-up for future expenses.

- **Health Reimbursement Arrangement (HRA).** In these employer-sponsored health plans, the employee/patient has control of their funds. Plans can vary, and if specifically allowed, these personally controlled reserve funds can roll over from year to year and continue to grow. The result of which is a diminished need for major medical insurance and associated controls by others.

- **Voluntary Employee Benefit Associations (VEBA).** VEBA is a classification by law that permits employees within a geographic area to band together for a common good. For example, school teachers in the state of Washington organized themselves. As a result, a majority of the healthcare reserves are controlled by each member for their account within the VEBA, but only a minority of the funds are needed for outside catastrophic insurance.

- **Multiple Employer Welfare Arrangements (MEWA).** MEWA is a type of plan, established by ERISA and regulated by the PPACA, in which two or more unrelated employers, including those who are self-employed, may establish a health benefit plan. This can be done through an insurance plan or some other type of funding.

  In concept, MEWAs are designed to give small employers access to low cost health coverage on terms similar to those available to large employers.

Impact of CDHP on Patients and Practitioners

The era of benefit rationing by third party payers will diminish as more patients control their funds. The providers of primary care and chiropractic services who give patients the best value-based care for dollars spent will be the most successful practitioners in the future. Providers will need to become more familiar with patient centered health care models, such as Patient Centered Medical Homes (PCMHs) and Accountable Care Organizations (ACOs) as regulations and guidelines under health care reform and quality improvement are implemented.

Herein is hope for healthcare costs for America and the chiropractic industry. This consumer controlled model is rapidly expanding. As individuals assume personal responsibility for their health, they become empowered. With that empowerment, the Thomas A. Edison vision can also be realized: *"The doctor of the future will dispense no medicine, but interest his patients in the care of the human frame and the cause and prevention of disease."*

See Resource 156 for more information.

No-Insurance and the Cash Practice

A growing number of chiropractic offices offer some form of a cash practice. Many health care providers are frustrated with inadequate reimbursement and excessive administrative requirements. If you're a doctor who desires to practice without third-party interference, while also getting a fair market value for your services, a no–insurance practice could be for you. This can be a positive business and financial decision. It provides an alternative to the labor-intensive health insurance reimbursement process. Physicians and their patients can both benefit from this type of arrangement.

The benefits of having a no-insurance program or cash practice with payment in full at the time of service by cash, check, or credit card are:

- Hassle-free health care
- Elimination of administrative and other overhead costs
- Less paperwork
- No insurance forms or bills to send
- No referral approval or authorization
- Lower fees to patients

The risks of a cash practice include having fewer patients initially, having false illusions that quality is not important, and being the possible target of unfair fee allegations by third-party payers.

All who pay at the time of service should get the same benefit, whether they have insurance or no insurance. A patient sees a doctor for a non-catastrophic reason and the patient pays in full before leaving—it's just that simple!

See Chapter 3–Fees for more information about discounting fee schedules.

See Resource 154 for additional information.

Alert: If you have a "cash practice", you are still subject to rules regarding Medicare beneficiaries. See *Section C-Medicare* for more information.

Healthcare Discount Programs

Healthcare discount programs, also known as medical discount programs, are **not** medical insurance. Rather, they are member programs where a fee is paid in order to be part of the "group" who qualifies for discounted services. In many states, these types of programs are regulated, so be sure that any plan you are considering joining is approved in your state.

Benefits

There are many patients that are either uninsured or under-insured. Legal discount programs can help doctors enjoy the benefit of offering a discount (other than Time of Service) to patients that are part of their network of paid subscribers. Those plans which utilize the network concept and are approved and registered in your state can help to fill in those gaps. It has been compared to being in a PPO for your cash and underinsured patients. Some plans require you to accept discounts prescribed by the plan. Other plans may allow you to set your own level of discounts.

Unlike the Time of Service discount which must be paid in full at the time of service, some of these plans allow the patient to benefit from lower fees which can be paid over time.

Look Before You Leap

Not all healthcare discount programs are the same. The Federal Trade Commission (FTC) is warning consumers to carefully evaluate these programs. Providers need to exercise caution as well, as some programs are not as wonderful as they claim. Carefully review contracts, minimum requirements and exercise due diligence in evaluating these plans and any applicable state laws and regulations. In some cases, these programs have not really benefited the patient or provider.

For these reasons, the American Chiropractic Association has issued an official policy regarding healthcare discount programs. In addition to warning about state regulations, this policy also includes the following warnings:

- Heed caution using a discount program in conjunction with, or in lieu of, a patient's Medicare benefits.
- Caution should also be observed when using a discount program in conjunction with, or in lieu of, third party payers and managed care organizations.
- Providers should completely review contracts and investigate the policies in place for renewal and cancellation of membership by patients and participation by providers to determine their rights under the contract.

- See Resource 110 to view additional comments, resources, networks, and opinions on discounts.
- See Resource 383 for information by the FTC regarding discount plans.

> **ACA Time of Service (TOS) Disclaimer:** The ACA does not officially recommend that doctors of chiropractic use TOS discounts. This is due to the possibility of violating state and/or federal law. Before implementing a TOS discount, doctors of chiropractic should consult with a health care law attorney.

Personal Injury

Personal injury claims are handled differently than health insurance claims. Situations involving "personal injury" (PI) in a chiropractic setting *usually* involve medical conditions arising from three main accident scenarios:

- Motor vehicle involvement
- Accidents occurring in and around a home, which may include automobile related injuries occurring at a residence
- Accidents occurring on a business-site not related to work

See the "Workers' Compensation" segment later in this chapter for information about on-the-job injuries.

In each of these accident scenarios, there are potentially several different sources of payment: fault-based insurance coverages (e.g., liability, uninsured motorist coverage); no-fault coverages (e.g., medical payments benefits, personal injury protection); and attorneys.

If these sources are limited or exhausted, then health insurance could be a source. Additionally, patient payments could include cash, Health Savings Plans/Flex Spending and Medical Cafeteria Plans.

This personal injury segment provides a general explanation of what is involved in personal injury cases. State laws regarding personal injury claims vary from state to state. Therefore it is crucial for healthcare providers to understand their own state requirements.

See Resource 159 for additional information on personal injury cases.

Sources of Medical Expense Recovery for Personal Injury Care

This section contains a non-exhaustive list of commonly used sources for medical expense recovery. Each state has a specific standard, which may or may not use any of these described sources. You should consult with your state association for a list of applicable sources. If any of these or similar types of medical benefits coverages are not available, then you might consider reimbursement by cash or medical expense financing.

If Personal Injury benefits are exhausted or not available, this should be noted in the patient record along with supporting documentation. In this situation, if standard health insurance or another type of coverage is available, then the patient may elect to have reimbursement requests for continued care submitted to their health insurance carrier. DO NOT bill both the PI carrier and health insurance carrier simultaneously. Be aware of individual state laws which may specify which carrier is to be billed first.

All verbal communication should be thoroughly documented. Due to limitations and rules of coverage with PI insurances, providers should make communication with the PI carrier a priority from the very beginning of care and as the patient progresses.

- **Liability.** Liability insurance covers general damages caused by the negligence or fault of an insured. In many states, general damages include compensation for pain and suffering, subject to certain minimum monetary thresholds, before legal action is taken to recover those claims.

    Liability coverage is not just limited to automobile policies. Homeowner's policies and select business policies often carry liability coverage that can serve as a source of medical expense payment when accidents occur in these settings.

- **Uninsured Motorist (UM) Coverage.** UM coverage is a medical expense recovery option utilized when the uninsured (at-fault) driver has no insurance. UM coverage is virtually identical to liability insurance, the primary difference being that it only becomes available when there are no liability policies for the patient to pursue (e.g., the patient was injured by a hit-and-run driver or the at-fault vehicle was not insured).

- **Underinsured Motorist (UIM) Coverage.** UIM benefits were designed to help cover an insured driver or passenger who has been injured by an underinsured and/or at-fault (in applicable states) motorist whose medical benefits **coverage is inadequate** to compensate the insured's losses. Generally speaking, this means that the injured party (driver or passenger) makes a medical benefits claim against the automobile insurance policy (UIM) of the driver in whose vehicle they occupied at the time of the accident (often their own insurance), if they obtain policy limits from the underinsured and/or at-fault (in applicable states) carrier and their loss exceeds those limits. In the case of an injured passenger, that passenger may also make a claim against their own PIP/MedPay and UIM policies. Because individual state laws may vary from this general statement, it is important to check your state laws regarding the application of liability claims benefits.

- **Medical Benefits Payments ("MedPay").** In many states, MedPay is optional. Insurance companies can choose to offer it or not. MedPay is limited only to medical expenses. It is also limited to the amount of medical benefits purchased by the insured. In the case of automobile insurance, MedPay "follows" both the insured and the car, i.e., it covers the insured regardless of what vehicle the insured was occupying at the time of the accident. It also provides medical benefits coverage for all occupants in the insured vehicle at the time of the accident.

See the legend for using resource icons on page *xvi*.

MedPay is not just limited to automobile policies. Homeowners and businesses may carry MedPay as well. Usually, filing claims against MedPay coverage does not result in a rate increase to the insured.

- **Personal Injury Protection (PIP).** PIP is very similar to MedPay. One key difference between PIP and MedPay lies in the fact that PIP commonly covers lost wages and lost services in addition to medical expenses (the carrier's total liability, however, will not exceed the set amount of benefits purchased by the insured). Another key difference lies in the fact that, whereas MedPay is usually optional, PIP may either be optional, required-unless-waived-in-writing, or mandated (such as in "no-fault" states), depending on state law. In cases where PIP is mandated, state law may designate it as primary (must be billed first) to any liability coverage that may be available.

- **Motorcycles.** Injuries from motorcycle accidents may not be covered in some states the same as motor vehicles. In many states, motorcycle medical benefits coverage is optional, a commonly overlooked exclusion.

- **Pedestrian/Bicycle.** Pedestrian vs. motor vehicle, or bicyclist vs. motor vehicle collision injuries are also seen in a chiropractic office. In some states, medical payments for injured pedestrians and cyclists are often covered under the motor vehicle MedPay or PIP automobile insurance benefits, regardless of who's at fault. Sometimes injured cyclists are covered the same as pedestrians; in other states and municipalities they are considered as vehicles and subject to its motor vehicle laws, rules or regulations. It would be prudent to learn your state laws and the benefits or limitations on this subject.

- **Plaintiff Attorneys.** The function of plaintiff attorneys (representing the patient) in personal injury cases is to protect the rights of the injured and maximize a fair recovery for their injuries, such as current and future treatment expenses. This is accomplished in a variety of ways, including, but not limited to liability and UM/UIM coverage for any type of damages recognized by law, including losses such as pain and suffering. When the patient is represented by an attorney, doctors of chiropractic are commonly asked not to seek payment directly from the at-fault insurance coverage, or to send office notes, narrative reports, lists of charges, or other information which might potentially jeopardize the patient's legal case. When the case is resolved, the task of the doctor of chiropractic is to obtain payment from the attorney out of any proceeds received by the attorney. Liens or Letters of Protection are legal tools to help in that recovery.

- **Letter of Protection or Liens.** Patients may enter into agreements with their doctors at the beginning of treatment in order to have their services paid at the conclusion of the case from the proceeds of a settlement or verdict. They may use several varieties of these methods, including "letters of protection (LOP)" or a "lien." Some doctors prepare LOPs or liens

---

The Difference between Liens and Assignment

Assignment is transferring rights to a third party. Whereas a lien is a legal claim against funds for payment of a debt or an amount owed for services rendered. Some personal injury cases have been overturned when assignment was used. Because state requirements can vary, it would be wise to consult with a local health care attorney to determine which is most appropriate for your office.

See ChiroCode.com/pi-resources (Resource 159) for help and information on personal injury cases.

themselves, while others request that the patient's attorney prepare the LOPs or liens indicating that the plaintiff attorneys will protect them for outstanding medical bills. Use caution and logic. The plaintiff attorneys' primary obligation is to represent and look out for the patient's interest, not the doctor's.

See Resource 160 for a full-size version of this form, with instructions.

"No-Fault" States

A minority of states have enacted No-Fault automobile insurance laws within their jurisdictions. No-Fault laws usually entail the following requirements or principles:

- Mandatory PIP coverage.
- Primacy of PIP coverage to liability (i.e., liability becomes secondary to PIP).
- Monetary or verbal medical expense thresholds which must be met before the patient has a right to seek a legal solution against a liability carrier.

Coding and Billing

For Personal Injury, use the standard code sets for procedures (CPT) and diagnoses (ICD). It is also important to use the "E" codes in the *Diagnoses* section of this book to specify the external cause of the injury (see the auto accident codes in the E810-E819 series). Carriers usually accept claims submitted on a 1500 claim form. Verify specific coding and billing requirements with the personal injury insurance carrier.

Attorneys may request office notes and charges accompanied by a narrative report. If your clinic is currently not using an EHR system, it is generally a good practice to have typed and or transcribed notes for personal injury cases due to the possibility of health related information being needed for legal reasons or for referral to another provider who may be collaborating on the case. Before preparing a long narrative, confirm that this is what is being requested. Often, attorneys will be satisfied with a brief summary describing the status of the patient at the conclusion of care. Don't forget to maintain HIPAA Privacy standards by obtaining the proper authorization from your patient prior to releasing any records or reports.

A HIPAA authorization for release of PHI is included with the *HIPAA Compliance* publication (see Resource 116).

See Chapter 2–HIPAA Compliance in *Section F-Compliance and Audit Protection* for additional information on HIPAA.

Claims adjusters enter the information from the claim form and the patient charts into their computers. Their software program (such as Colossus, Mitchell Medical, etc.) then evaluates your claim. A check is then authorized for their approved procedures. It is important to review their payment reports to identify any portion of your services that are denied or bundled. In some cases a corrected statement could resolve a problem. In other cases an appeal could be necessary to require them to follow accepted national guidelines (e.g. CPT, NCCI edits, etc.). Ultimately, when an account is not paid in full, the final resolution may require a legal solution against the insurance carrier.

Personal Liability Compensation

Liability for Personal Injury incidents goes beyond physician services which help restore patients to their pre-accident condition. When an insurance company is assessing liability, many factors related to the collision/accident need to be considered. This includes conditions not necessarily related to chiropractic care (i.e. abrasions, cuts, contusions, fractures, etc.) as well as work time loss, pain and suffering. These conditions, known as "value drivers," are considered when the computer software determines a settlement offer. The dollar range for the "settlement offer" is then conveyed to the claims adjuster. Therefore, when a doctor of chiropractic is the first physician to see the patient, it is critically important that every aspect of these types of visible and non-visible injuries be documented in the physician's report, even though another provider may be treating the other injuries. Common auto injuries, such as lacerations, may not be treated by the chiropractic physician, but they may delay treatment as the doctor waits for them to heal before he can perform manipulations in the affected areas.

Fee Schedules for Personal Injury

Each payer will have their own fee schedules; however, some state legislatures have mandated Personal Injury Protection or MedPay fee schedules. It is important to note that state laws can vary.

Conclusion

When you accept a PI patient, you are accepting a responsibility to properly manage and/or coordinate care for these acute traumatic care injury cases. This means not only providing care that the patient may need for an optimal recovery, but also to administrate each individual case as may be required by other involved parties (PI carrier, attorney, etc) and your local law. Because PI claims are handled differently than regular medical claims and PI laws vary from state to state, it is imperative to understand these differences.

Close communication with patients, personal injury carriers and attorneys (as may be necessary under certain circumstances) is essential. This ensures that necessary claim information is collected and also helps avoid misunderstanding or oversights regarding claims submission and payment.

Monitoring personal injury claims on a frequent and regular basis with personal injury carriers and/or attorneys (where applicable) is a measure of efficiency and protection for both the patient and the provider. Also, collecting the proper letter of protection or lien is a protective measure which can help the practice avoid potential reimbursement complications. Documenting your practice's personal injury claims procedure in your Policies and Procedures manual helps to ensure a smooth and seamless process.

See Resource 159 for additional help and information on handling personal injury cases.

Workers' Compensation (WC)

There are three possible scenarios regarding workers' compensation: the patient is covered by a WC carrier located in your own state, the patient is covered by a WC carrier located in another state, or the patient is covered by Federal Workers' Compensation. The following information pertains to state based workers' compensation claims. However, please note that Federal Workers' Compensation has very specific requirements. Please see "Federal Workers' Compensation" under "Government Programs" on page B-36.

Work-Related Illness or Injury

Employers pay the cost of the Workers' Compensation program. This program covers all medical costs incurred, and replaces wages lost as a result of a work related illness or injury. In addition, many states cover rehabilitation and retraining for the worker. Workers' Compensation is administered by each state. While many rules are similar, some states have regulations and guidelines that are unique. It is best to contact your workers' compensation board to ascertain which forms, requirements or reporting methods to use.

According to the U.S. Chamber of Commerce there are six basic objectives in Workers' Compensation law:

- Provide sure, prompt, and reasonable income and medical benefits to work accident victims, or income benefits to their dependents regardless of fault.
- Provide a single remedy and reduce court delays, costs, and workloads arising out of personal-injury litigation.
- Relieve public and private charities of financial drains, incident to uncompensated industrial accidents.
- Eliminate payment of fees to lawyers and witnesses as well as time-consuming trials and appeals.
- Encourage maximum employer interest in safety and rehabilitation through an appropriate experience-rating mechanism.
- Promote frank study of causes of accidents (rather than concealment of fault), reducing preventable accidents and human suffering.

Verification of Coverage

Proper verification of insurance coverage is the safest, smartest way to insure maximum reimbursement on all claims submitted. Sometimes it comes down to having a knowledge of what questions to ask. Some of the important items to verify include:

- **Employer:** Correct name, address, phone/fax number and contact person.
- **Payer:** Most states have many payers who write Workers' Compensation coverage. A few states (e.g., Nevada) require insurance through a state run agency. Others allow for self-insured coverage if the employee meets specified guidelines.
- **Date and time of injury or illness:** These items may affect the acceptance of the claim by the payer.
- **Description of how the accident or illness occurred:** This will help to verify the liability of the Workers' Compensation payer. This information will also help to provide a causal link between the work activity and the injury or illness.

When a patient comes to your office alleging a work-related injury, your first communication should be with the employer to ascertain the following information:

- Verify that the employer is familiar with the accident and the patient's injury.
- The employer's report of the accident/injury has been filed with the insurance carrier.
- The name of the Industrial Insurance carrier.
- The employer's Workers' Compensation policy number.

Once you are satisfied with the information from the employer, call the Workers' Compensation carrier and ask the following:

- Is the employer's Workers' Compensation policy still in force?
- Where should the claim be sent?

Proper billing and documentation can be very important in wrapping up the details of a claim.

- Charge only those fees allowable by the state in which you practice. Many states have guidelines for fees that are allowable.
- Code the diagnosis(es) most appropriate to the patient's condition. Like Medicare, carriers often have a list of allowable diagnosis codes. It is a good idea to verify coverage exclusions and requirements by checking the carrier's website.

> **Alert**: There are times when a patient is referred to your office with a specific diagnosis already assigned to their workers compensation case/claim. Obtain this information from the referring provider. Using a different diagnosis code can result in the claim being denied.

- Send copies of your complete chart notes, whenever required or requested, in addition to any applicable reports or forms required by your state.

If these reports and claims are sent and are within the guidelines set forth by the Industrial Commission, you should have no problem obtaining reimbursement.

First Report of Injury

States require a First Report of Injury to be completed. Whether the physician and/or the employer completes this report will vary by state. Currently, each state has their own unique form which needs to be used and the required elements to be reported may also vary. Additionally, many states are encouraging the use of electronic filing instead of paper claims.

The International Association of Industrial Accident Boards and Commissions (IAIABC) is currently working with the American National Standards Institute (ANSI) and other governmental agencies (e.g., Occupational Safety and Health Administration (OSHA)) to standardize the Physicians First Report of Injury form. Hopefully, this will simplify this process in the future.

Loss of Work Time

Communication with the employer and insurance company is very important. After the examination has been completed and it becomes apparent that there will be a loss of time from work, contact the employer and payer and inform them of the physician's findings. Indicate the estimated time off from work, treatment plan, and the necessity for any outside testing. Specific time frames for loss of work time vary by state. Refer to your state Workers' Compensation Board for applicable time frames.

State Guidelines and Fee Schedules

Medical care accounts for a large portion of the total cost of Workers' Compensation. Most states have initiated guidelines for controlling the medical dollars spent. These measures include adoption of fee schedules (state specific and/or the RBRVS), managed care mandates, choice of physician, pre-authorization for specific procedures and guidelines for frequency of care.

It is important for the provider to be familiar with the Workers' Compensation reimbursement guidelines for the state in which they practice. Nearly every state prohibits billing the patient for any or all services unless the claim has been denied.

As with most payers, Workers' Compensation payers may require pre-authorization for elective services. The procedures include diagnostic and therapeutic services such as CT, MRI, MRA, physical therapy, non-emergent surgical procedures and inpatient hospital care. It may be necessary to submit medical necessity documentation for peer review. Orthotics, prosthetics, and durable medical equipment may also need to be pre-authorized.

Some states govern the choice of provider to help control medical costs. States with managed care usually require the employee to use a designated physician or group. Some states with more stringent fee schedules may allow the patient to choose a physician. Other states may even limit the number of physician changes the patient may initiate.

When a clean claim is submitted, reimbursement is usually received in a timely manner. It is important to submit all required documentation with the initial billing. It may be necessary to provide explanations for unique circumstances and procedures.

If the claim is denied, determining the cause will help in submitting an appropriate appeal. Was the claim processed within state guidelines? Is the entire claim denied? Was pre-approval obtained prior to circumstances?

At times the payer may request an "independent medical evaluation." This is usually a medical opinion based upon records and evaluation of the patient to render an unbiased statement regarding the patient's condition and treatment plan. Most payers and providers negotiate a fee for this service unless a fee is specified in state guidelines.

The Workers' Compensation patient may also require the completion of an "impairment rating." Most states use the AMA's *Guide to the Evaluation of Permanent Impairment* rating (there are several versions, the most current is the 6th edition.) Some states modify the AMA's guide and others have their own specific criteria. This permanent impairment rating calculates a financial compensation for loss of function, body part, or other conditions that prohibit return to pre-injury status.

The medical disability evaluation code 99455 is reported when the treating physician completes the disability forms. When a non-treating physician completes the evaluation and necessary forms, code 99456 is used.

At times the physician may be asked to give a deposition or appear in court. Code 99075 for medical testimony is used to report that physician service. Fees should be agreed upon before the testimony or deposition is given. Billing should be directed to the requesting attorney.

Because the rules governing Workers' Compensation vary from state to state, there may be discrepancies regarding patients who are injured out of their home state or who move after an injury. Contacting the payer and determining the liability prior to service will save time, frustration and money. If the patient leaves the state governing the care of the claim, the laws protecting the patient may not be applicable.

See Resource 161 for additional information about impairment rating guide options.

GOVERNMENT PROGRAMS

The Department of Health and Human Services (HHS) oversees all government health care programs. They are administered by various agencies such as the Centers for Medicare & Medicaid Services (CMS), the Veterans Administration (VA) and even on the state level. This section gives a brief overview of these government services.

See *Section C–Medicare* for information about the Medicare program.

See Resource 162 for additional information.

Federal Workers' Compensation

For all injuries that are work related, Federal employees are entitled to those services and supplies which are recommended by a physician which are likely to cure, give relief, reduce the degree or period of disability, or aid in lessening the amount of monthly compensation. Preventive care is not a covered benefit.

In accordance with the Federal Workers' Compensation Act (FECA), chiropractic services are reimbursed only for subluxations. The following statement is from the American Chiropractic Association:

> "The services of chiropractors may be reimbursed only for treatment consisting of manual manipulation of the spine to correct a subluxation as demonstrated by x-ray to exist. The term 'subluxation' is defined as an incomplete dislocation, off-centering, misalignment, fixation, or abnormal spacing of the vertebrae anatomically which must be demonstrable on any x-ray film to individuals trained in the reading of x-rays. Chiropractors may interpret their own x-rays, and if a subluxation is diagnosed, OWCP [Office of Workers' Compensation Programs] will accept the chiropractor's assessment of any disability caused by it. Because doctors of chiropractic are considered physicians under the FECA, it is permissible for a patient to choose a doctor of chiropractic as his/her treating physician."

Note: To be paid for treating federal employees by the Federal Employees Workers Compensation Act (FECA), you must enroll with their bill consolidation contractor (ACS).

Go to ACAtoday.org/fep (Resource 163) for more detailed information by the American Chiropractic Association, including important billing information.

Military and Veterans

Military programs are offered through the Department of Defense (DOD) and the Department of Veterans Affairs (VA). The Department of Defense covers active duty service members and retirees from all branches of the military and their families. The Department of Veterans Affairs covers veterans and their eligible family members. Each program has different eligibility criteria and a variety of benefits packages.

Go to ACAtoday.org/pdf/government/VAFact2013.pdf (Resource 164) for a fact sheet about veteran's services.

TRICARE

TRICARE is the managed care program administered by the Department of Defense for active duty military, active duty service families, retirees and their families, and other beneficiaries. Chiropractic care is only available to active duty service members at specially designated facilities. There are only a limited number of facilities. If your office is near a military facility, and you qualify, this could be a unique opportunity for your practice.

⚙ See Resource 165 for more information.

CHAMPUS and CHAMPVA

The Civilian Health and Medical Program of the Uniformed Services (CHAMPUS) and the Civilian Health and Medical Program of the Veteran Services (CHAMPVA) are not health insurance programs, but they do make payment for health benefits provided through certain affiliations with the Uniformed Services and the Veterans Administration. Similar to the Medicare program, the physician agrees to accept the charge determination as payment in full and the patient is responsible for any deductible, coinsurance and non-covered services.

Only recently has the availability of chiropractic care improved as a result of recommendations issued by a congressionally-mandated advisory committee. Previously, no doctors of chiropractic served on the staff of any VA treatment facilities and "referrals" to those in private practice were severely limited. However, that is no longer the case. Eligible beneficiaries now have access to a doctor of chiropractic at numerous major VA treatment facilities within the U.S. The American Chiropractic Association (ACA) continues to work with Congress and the Department of Veterans Affairs to ensure that every eligible veteran has access to the essential services provided by doctors of chiropractic. Those who are interested in positions or contracts should contact their nearest VA office.

Patient-Centered Community Care

The VA Patient-Centered Community Care (VAPCCC or VAPC3) is a Veterans Health Administration (VHA) program created to provide eligible Veterans access to specialized services, which can include chiropractic care. PC3 contracts have been awarded to HealthNet and TriWest to provide care when the local VA is unable to readily provide those needed services.

EmpowerChiro has been awarded an exclusive agreement to provide chiropractic services for 28 states through TriWest. At the time of publication, HealthNet did not include chiropractic services.

⚙ See Resource 166 and 167 for more information.

Medicaid

Medicaid programs are available to anyone unable to afford private health insurance or unable to meet the requirements for Medicare benefits. The federal government and state governments cooperate in financing each Medicaid program. Each state decides which Medicaid health services will be provided and how they will be administered. There are distinct differences between the way Medicare and Medicaid programs are administered. Staff members involved with reimbursement must educate themselves regarding their own state's Medicaid policies. Interested doctors of chiropractic should contact their state health departments for detailed information on this program.

Approximately thirty states offer some form of coverage of chiropractic services. Some through traditional fee-for-service arrangements and others through managed care programs. Most plans limit coverage to subluxation only. Your local state health department can provide more specific information about Medicaid chiropractic benefits in your area.

Even though PPACA expanded Medicaid coverage in many states, because chiropractic services are an optional benefit, it remains to be seen how coverage will ultimately be affected.

Federal Employee Plans

By law, Federal Employees are entitled to both workers' compensation benefits for work-related injuries and the Federal Employees Health Benefits (FEHB) program. These programs have caused some problems for chiropractic in the past because providers mistakenly bill the same as they would any other program like Medicare. Also, some Federal agencies seem to be unaware that chiropractic services **are** covered. This section helps to clarify some of these issues.

Federal Employees Health Benefits (FEHB) Program

The Federal Employees Health Benefits (FEHB) Program is a system of "managed competition" through which employee health benefits are provided to civilian government employees and annuitants of the United States government. Workers pay one-third of the cost of insurance; the government pays the other two-thirds.

The FEHB program, which is administered by the United States Office of Personnel Management (OPM), allows some insurance companies, employee associations, and labor unions to market health insurance plans to governmental employees.

Review: Types of Insurance Plans

- What is the difference between Sickness/Accident Insurance and Health Assurance? *B-23*
- What are the factors in determining whether to be a participating or non-participating provider? *B-24*
- What are five consumer-driven health care options? *B-25 to B-26*
- What advantages does a cash practice offer? *B-27*
- Which covers lost wages, MediPay or PIP? *B-29*
- How do you obtain verification of coverage on a Workers' Compensation claim? Do they require preauthorization? *B-33*

3. Establishing Fees

About Fees and Fee Schedules

The establishment of appropriate fees for services is one of the greatest challenges in health care. The old concept—that you charge a fair amount based on your own costs and expected return on your investment—has given way to government controls and insurance mandates.

One of the most challenging tasks in a medical practice is to arrive at a fair and equitable fee that also meets all the requirements of the insurance industry. The objective of this section is to assist providers in having a better understanding of how fees are evaluated and established. This section includes tools and worksheets to help you calculate proper fees.

The most important thing to remember when setting fee schedules, is that you only have one standard fee schedule. This concept may seem odd considering the number of payer contracts your office may have; however, you must set one fee for each procedure code and that is your set fee. Period. Once you set your fee, that fee is only changed in the following situations:

- Contractual obligations with third-party payers such as insurance companies or medical discount plans (see page B-27).
- Prompt Pay/Time of Service (TOS) discounts (see page B-47).
- Financial Hardship Discounts (see page B-47).

Always bill your standard amount on submitted claims for reimbursement—**not** the contracted amount—unless your contract specifically states that your claim must only show the contracted amount. This is important for the following reasons:

1. Do you really want to get paid less? What if you have the wrong amount in your system and you are getting paid far less than you should? It has happened to many providers.
2. Do you want to lower national fee perceptions? When claims data is used to set UCR limits, claims which have contracted amounts instead of the real value for the service will cause the averages to lower over time. See "Usual, Customary and Reasonable (UCR)" below for more about keeping national fees realistic.

See *Section C–Medicare* for information about billing and fees for Medicare.

See Resource 170 for your Medicare Fee Calculations.

See Resource 171 for additional information and resources.

Price Fixing Warning

It is **illegal** for providers/physicians to discuss fees with each other and agree upon **dollar conversion factors** or **fees**. To do so is price fixing, and a violation of federal anti-trust laws.

Fortunately, there is information readily available in the public domain such as www.fairhealth.org. These resources, along with the *ChiroCode Medicare Fee Calculator for Chiropractic Codes* (Resource 170), can and should be studied to better understand the market forces affecting fees. Many payers will disclose their fee schedules when asked (when asking, it is appropriate to limit your request to only the codes relevant to your practice).

With knowledge, providers can make better informed decisions regarding their personalized fee schedule. Fees should be reviewed annually.

Fee Schedule Methodologies

There are two methodologies used to determine fees. The first is the "usual, customary, and reasonable" (UCR) which is based on billed charges. The second method is the RBRVS system which is based on the actual value of the work, practice expense, and malpractice expense of the procedures/services.

Usual, Customary, and Reasonable (UCR)

"Usual, customary, and reasonable" (UCR) refers to the base amount that third-party payers generally use to determine how much will be paid for services that are reimbursed under a health insurance plan. This amount is determined based on a review of the prevailing charges made by peer physicians for a particular health service within a specific geographical area. Typically, fee surveys are done by publishers and/or researchers through questionnaires for practitioners. Respondents report the fees which they are currently charging.

The UCR amount is generally set at different percentiles (e.g., 50th, 70th, 90th, etc.) which are mathematical formulas based by a comparison of all submitted fees by providers and establishing fee ranges. Think of the "bell curve" where results tend to group in the center - the very center of this curve would be 50%. When they say they pay 70% of the UCR, they mean that their "approved" fee is what 70% of the providers charge in that region and would be a higher payment than one who uses a 50th percentile. When a payer reduces a fee by using a UCR schedule it is important to know which percentage level they are using.

Federal law does not regulate how UCR reimbursements are calculated; however, the Centers for Medicare and Medicaid Services (CMS) provides general guidelines that the insurance carriers must follow. Ultimately, the insurance company has flexibility when setting the maximum reimbursement fee.

It is important to understand that when you create your fee schedule, you are contributing to the data pool used by payers in their fee schedules. You should **never** set your UCR fees to the contracted rates of your payers. Doing so will result in a continued reduction in fees. You need to keep your UCR rates at a fair and marketable rate and accept the reduction from your in-network payers until equitable fees come around once more.

Proponents of this method feel that it provides more meaningful and accurate data than the UCR method used by insurance companies, because the database is not being polluted with inaccurate information (e.g., a provider submits fees that are mandated under contract in which fees are arbitrary and low).

Tip: Do not confuse UCR percentiles with the patient portion. If you are **not** a contracted provider with a specific payer, and if that plan covers 80 percent of UCR charges, then the patient is responsible for both the remaining 20 percent, and for the difference between what is charged by the provider and what the plan considers UCR.

UCR Example

Typically, 70 percent of providers in your geographic area charge $100 for a particular service. ABC Insurance uses the 70th percentile to set their UCR at $100 for that service. John Smith has met his deductible for ABC Insurance and comes in for that service. You are an out-of-network provider and you bill ABC Insurance $110 for that service. ABC Insurance pays $80 based on their UCR and the 80 percent of the covered service. John Smith is responsible for the $30 balance ($20 coinsurance and $10 for the amount over ABC Insurance's UCR).

If you were an in-network provider, you would need to discount the patient's bill by $10 to meet the contracted UCR amount.

Relative Value Units

Use of the UCR as the standard for fees has been replaced with a more rational approach. Since 1994 nearly all payers have moved to the Resource-Based Relative Value Units (RVUs) methodology. The RVU system is composed of two parts:

1. **Resource-Based Relative Value Unit (RVU):** An intrinsic value of one procedure or service as it relates to another. It is a mathematical expression, not a dollar amount.

    Example:

99212	Office or other outpatient services, established patient, level 2	1.17
99213	Office or other outpatient services, established patient, level 3	1.97

2. **Dollar Conversion Factor (DCF):** A dollar amount, which when multiplied by the RVU converts the RVU into a fee.

    Example:

Code	RVU		DCF		Fee
99212	1.17	x	$35.82	=	$41.91
99213	1.97	x	$35.82	=	$70.57

Relative Value Units (RVUs) have become the foundation for fee calculations in health care. RVUs are the result of a 10-year study by the American Medical Association (AMA) and the Centers for Medicare & Medicaid Services (CMS) and were meant to establish parity in fees between specialties. On January 1, 1992, the Resource-Based Relative Value Scale (RBRVS) became the official CMS payment methodology for physician services provided to Medicare patients. Medicare's reimbursement approach was based on a research study by the Harvard University School of Public Health.

The intention of RBRVS was to establish a consistent and rational basis for assessing the resources that go into providing any physician service. Under RBRVS, RVUs are based on the human resources and other costs associated with the delivery of a specific procedure or service. For every procedure or service (as defined by current CPT and come HCPCS codes), the RBRVS defines the **physician's work, practice expense,** and **malpractice insurance** costs. A percentage multiplier then adjusts them for variations in expenses between geographic areas. Finally, a dollar conversion factor, based on a provider's or payer's financial objectives, is applied to yield a dollar-based fee schedule.

Although RBRVS is used as the foundation of the Medicare Fee Schedule, the methodology should not be equated with Medicare, nor should it be associated with perceived deficiencies in the development and implementation of Medicare payment policies. In fact, the Physician Payment Review Commission noted in its 1994 annual report to Congress: "As more payers adopt the RBRVS based fee schedule, it may be especially desirable for changes in health plans' conversion factors to reflect only their competitive and financial situations, and not be confused by shifts in Medicare payment policies that they do not share."

RBRVS has affected nearly every physician practicing in the United States today. Generally, evaluation and management services have experienced increases in allowed charges, while allowed charges for procedure-oriented services have decreased.

Payers and providers are choosing RBRVS as their basis for determining appropriate reimbursement for physician services. Whether addressing physician pricing, contracting, strategic and financial planning or productivity, RBRVS has become the most credible method available to fairly evaluate pricing and compensation for physicians/providers.

RVUs are not perfect and not every code has an RVU. However, they do represent a high degree of integrity. It is the most widely used payment system with providers and carriers. All other payment methodologies can be compared to it as a standard.

RBRVS Components

The three RVU components in the RBRVS methodology are:

1. Physician work
2. Practice expense
3. Malpractice expense

For each component, there is a Geographic Practice Cost Index (GPCI) for each specific geographic area. The relative costs of the physician work, practice expenses, and malpractice insurance in an area is compared to the national average for each component, and is adjusted accordingly with a GPCI. After the RVU is adjusted, it is multiplied by a **national** dollar conversion factor (CF).

In summary, the general formula for calculating RVUs for a given service in a geographic area can be expressed as:

(RVU physician work   x   GPCI for physician work)
+ (RVU practice expense   x   GPCI for practice expense)
+ (RVU malpractice   x   GPCI for malpractice expense)

= Total RVU

- **Relative Value Units (RVU) for Physician Work (PW):** Approximately 7,500 codes represent services included in the physician fee schedule. The initial physician work RVU was implemented into the CMS Medicare Fee Schedule in January 1992, and is updated every five years (2002, 2007, 2012, 2017, etc.).

- **Relative Value Units (RVU) for Practice Expense (PE):** The Balanced Budget Act (BBA) of 1997 mandated that the Practice Expense component be updated every five years.

    As part of this five year review of the Practice Expense (PE), CMS has made available the supporting data regarding the various subcomponents of the RVU for the PE (e.g., Direct Expenses such as equipment and supplies, and Indirect Office Expenses for overhead costs such as rent, phones, support staff, etc.).

    In 2010, CMS began a 4-year transition to a new methodology for determining PE RVUs using the updated Physician Practice Information Survey (PPIS) PE/HR data. To

ease the impact of payment reductions for some specialties, this gradual transition was completed in 2013.
- **Relative Value Units (RVU) for Malpractice (M):** The RVUs for malpractice (or professional liability insurance) were revised for 2015 as part of the revised five year update cycle. At the time of printing, MP RVUs for chiropractic services remained generally unchanged. According to the 2015 MPFS Final Rule, only 98941 decreased by 0.01.

Updates to RVUs

The RVUs are updated on five year review cycles. The Relative Value Update Committee (RUC) makes recommendations to CMS for their review and endorsement/correction. CMS makes the final determinations for all RVUs.

No RVUs for Supplies and Lab (Non-Physician) Services

Not all codes are subject to RVUs and their calculations (e.g., laboratory and supplies). When there is resource data regarding fees other than the RVU, the fee is shown in the *ChiroCode DeskBook* as a dollar amount with the dollar ($) sign (e.g., $ 36.20).

DOLLAR CONVERSION FACTORS

Since January 1, 1992, Medicare has paid for physician services under section 1848 of the Social Security Act ("The Act"), "Payment for Physicians' Services." This section contains three major elements:

1. A fee schedule for the payment of physician services.
2. A method to control the rate of increase in Medicare expenditures for physicians' services.
3. Limits on the amounts that non-participating physicians can charge beneficiaries. The Act requires that payments under the fee schedule be based on national uniform Relative Value Units (RVUs) based on the resources used in furnishing a service. Section 1848(c) of the Act requires that national RVUs be established for physician work, practice expense, malpractice expense, and be reviewed every 5 years.

Unlike the RVU update process, the United States Congress, through CMS, makes its own determination for the annual dollar Conversion Factor (CF). This is the pivotal component in the fee calculation process. Without a proper dollar conversion factor, fees will be depressed. Because of the Balanced Budget laws in the past, Congress is determined to limit the total dollar amount that would be spent on the Medicare program. If the total dollars spent exceed the arbitrary spending limits that have been set, the "pie" will have to be cut into smaller pieces.

See Resource 171 for additional information and resources.

Dollar Conversion Factor Changes

2011: The House passed legislation in December 2010 to continue the current Medicare Physician Fee Schedule freeze through the end of 2011. The scheduled Dollar Conversion Factor for 2011 would have taken the conversion factor from $36.87 to $25.52, a 30.8% decrease.

2012: The 27% mandated fee decrease was temporarily frozen at $34.0376 until March 2012. Then it was frozen again through December 31, 2012.

2013: The 26.5% fee reduction was averted by the January 2, 2013 American Taxpayer Relief Act (ATRA) of 2012 which revised the conversion factor from $25.0008 to $34.0320.

2014: The mandated conversion factor of $26.82 was averted by the Protecting Access to Medicare Act (PAMA) of 2014 which set the conversion factor for 2014 as $35.8228.

2015: The PAMA has established a zero percent increase for the first quarter of 2015 (January 1-March 31). At the time of publication, there was no legislation to halt a mandated conversion factor *decrease* of 21.2 percent after the first quarter. However, it seems likely that Congress will once again halt this conversion factor decrease.

Note: Register for free ChiroCode Alerts, sent by email, to be notified when such changes occur. Go to ChiroCode.com/register

CHIROCODE FEE CALCULATIONS

The conventional approach to the fee calculation process is to adjust the three components (physician work, practice expense, and malpractice expense) for each procedure code by the Geographic Practice Cost Index (GPCI) for each area of the country. After each of the three components are adjusted and tallied, they are multiplied by a national conversion factor to convert the adjusted (local) relative value into a fee. The dollar conversion factor for 2015 is 35.8013 for the first quarter (January 1 – March 31, 2015). Watch for further announcements regarding the conversion factor for the remainder of the year. This methodology is used

FIGURE 2.3
ChiroCode Fee Calculator: Sample Screen

CHIROCODE FEE CALCULATOR WORKSHEET

My Account > ChiroCode Fee Calculator Worksheet

ChiroCode Fee Calculator Worksheet

To calculate fees for your area please enter your ZIP Code: 85021
You may also calculate two other fees based on a percentage of the Medicare fee.
The fee worksheet will show calcuations of 150 % and 200 %.

Create Worksheet (Please allow 30-60 seconds for worksheet generation.)

Common Chiropractic Codes and Fees
Medicare fees are based on the most recent information available to ChiroCode.
Exact Medicare fees may be obtained directly from your local Medicare office.
(NE - Not Established by Medicare/CMS)

Calculated for Arizona (85021) - Conversion Factor (CF): 34.0376

ChiroCode Short List (Most Common Chiropractic Codes)

Code	Medicare	Med (150%)	Better (200%)
Chiropractic Manipulation/Adjustment			
98940	$25.14	$37.70	$50.27
98941	$35.09	$52.64	$70.19
98942	$44.72	$67.07	$89.43
98943	$23.64	$35.46	$47.28

by Medicare/Medicaid, etc., and many other private payers. For the most up-to-date fees use the ChiroCode Fee Calculator (see Figure 2.3).

To eliminate this complicated process, the ChiroCode Institute developed the *ChiroCode Fee Calculator*, available online to current *ChiroCode DeskBook* subscribers. **This is an industry innovation**. It allows you to use a simple one-step process to calculate fees. While not an exact science, it is a quick and easy starting point. It will produce fees that based on a percentage of the Medicare Fee Schedule (MFS) for your geographic area.

The *ChiroCode Fee Calculator* calculates fees for all of the codes with RVUs in the book, based on your geographic location. It uses a three column format. Column 1 is for a Medicare fee schedule in your area. The other columns are for higher amounts, such as 150% and 200% of column 1. These amounts tend to be closer to the expected payments; see Figure 2.3.

See Resource 172 to use the *ChiroCode Fee Calculator*.

OTHER FEE SCHEDULES

Most chiropractors try to remain competitive in the market place and keep the cost of their care affordable to their patients. However, depending on their cost reduction methods, they may get into trouble. For example, some doctors may have developed a varying scale of fees, with numerous types of discounts: maybe a pastoral discount, a child discount, a friend discount, etc. Each of these discounts is different. Not every state has a rule regarding this practice, but some do. If your state does not have a specific rule as to how you can charge for your care then you need to make sure you are justified in your action. If your argument is purely financial then the legality is, at best, questionable.

Many allegations of fraud and abuse allegations come from having more than one fee schedule. Medicare policy mandates that payment is determined by the lowest of either the Medicare Fee Schedule (MFS) or the lowest fee schedule in the doctor's office. For example, if the Medicare schedule for a specific service is $30 and the doctor's lowest schedule is $15, Medicare could claim the $15 as their proper fee. Conversely, if a non-participating doctor in the Medicare program charges more than the **limiting charge,** it is considered aberrant and subject to fines and penalties for fraud and abuse.

See also the segment "Healthcare Discount Programs" on page B-27.

Warning: Usage of the term "cash discount" in a fee schedule is inappropriate and discouraged because it is about more than just cash. Most payments come in the form of checks or credit cards, so the safest method is to entirely eliminate the words "cash discount" from your vocabulary. Cash discounts could invite allegations that you are increasing the fees billed to insurance carriers.

Instead of offering a cash discount, offer patients and insurance companies your Time of Service (TOS) fee schedule. Payment at time of service reduces costs for all parties. Under this scenario, the patient chooses to submit their charges to their insurance carrier. The amount submitted must reflect the TOS fee schedule, and not your regular fee schedule.

If you are a participating provider, you may be precluded from collecting anything other than deductibles and co-payments directly from the patient, and you may be required to file claims on their behalf. Refer to your Provider Agreement for applicable rules.

Discounts

An unprecedented shift is occurring in health care. Deductibles are increasing and insurance is paying less. The number of underinsured and uninsured Americans continues to rise. The line between insurance and patient responsibility is clearly moving, with patients having to shoulder more of the costs for their care. Additionally, more patients are now in control of their healthcare dollars with health savings accounts (HSA), medical savings accounts (MSAs), and flexible spending accounts (FSAs), health reimbursement arrangements (HRAs) with their employers.

Because of this shift, patients are increasingly asking important financial questions, such as:

- How much is my insurance going to pay (insurance portion)?
- How much is this care going to cost me (patient portion)?
- What payment arrangements can you make for me?
- Can you discount your fees?

> **ACA Time of Service (TOS) Disclaimer:** The ACA does not officially recommend that doctors of chiropractic use TOS discounts. This is due to the possibility of violating state and/or federal law. Before implementing a TOS discount, doctors of chiropractic should consult with a health care law attorney.

Can You Discount Your Fees?

This question is applicable to any practice that provides covered health care to insured patients, especially those practices that might describe themselves as "out-of-network." The answer to this question is dependent upon properly following guidelines and documentation protocols. Fees may be appropriately discounted in two ways: 1. Financial need, or 2. Time of Service. Both have different requirements, but both must be properly documented in order to avoid allegations of fraud or abuse.

Hardship and Prompt Pay discounts are clearly recognized by the federal government. There may be other types of discounts which are permitted under federal and/or state laws.

> **Alert:** As noted earlier in this chapter, blanket waivers for coinsurance, co-pays and deductibles violates many federal statues, as well as third-party payer contracts.

Financial Hardship Policy

It is improper and illegal to waive co-payments and/or deductibles. For this reason, if you wish to offer some sort of assistance to a patient, the proper way to do so is through an official "Financial Hardship Policy".

Caution is advised when implementing hardship waivers. For example, waivers and reductions for co-pays, coinsurances, and deductibles should not be routine and should not be advertised in any way. Hardship waivers should be used only in cases where hardship is clearly indicated and documented. Clinics should have a written policy regarding determinations of financial hardship and a clear guideline on what qualifies as a hardship (e.g. by using federal poverty guidelines). The Financial Hardship Policy and Application provides both the official policy, and the application which is completed by the patient.

As a reminder, routine waivers or reductions of the patient's responsibility can violate the federal False Claims Act, Medicare Exclusion Statute, Anti-Kickback Statute, and the Civil Monetary Penalties Law. Additionally, many commercial insurers have provisions within their provider contracts that prohibit routine waiver or reductions of co-pays, deductibles or coinsurances.

FINANCIAL HARDSHIP DISCOUNT

For years, federal and state authorities have stated that providers can discount their fees based on patient financial need (hardship). These discounts (hardship policies) must be in writing and consistently applied. ChiroCode Institute has created the necessary template to create your own financial hardship policy and application. This form should be used sparingly and only in accordance with the policy.

> See Resource 146 for a full-size version of this form, with instructions.

> See Resource 173 for more information from the Health Resources and Services Administration (HRSA).

Sample: Financial Hardship Policy and Application

Prompt Pay Discounts (TOS)

Prompt pay discounts, also referred to as a Time-of-Service Fee Schedule, are different than hardship discounts. Whereas a hardship discount refers to a discount granted for financial need, the "prompt pay discount" refers to situations where the provider is seeking to avoid the costs of debt collection.

According to the Office of Inspector General (OIG), a prompt pay discount is "designed to reduce the Health System's accounts receivables and costs of debt collection, and to boost its cash flow." It's a discount that "bear(s) a reasonable relationship to the amount of collection costs that would be avoided."

The term, "Time of Service" can and should be defined by the individual office. In some cases it could mean that care is paid for within two working days, to others it means immediately. To make it legal, the Time of Service discount is available to all sources of payment, which includes third party payers, personal injury and Workers' Compensation. Some of these payers will not meet the deadline for this fee schedule, but nonetheless it should be available to them.

Once you have created your standard rate, you then choose your discount percentage for your Time of Service fee schedule. The rate you select is your choice; however, it must be considered "reasonable," such as 20-40% of your standard rates. Be aware of any applicable state laws and regulations regarding this practice. The key is you must take a flat percentage discount of your standard rate. You cannot have different rates for different procedures. If you give a 30% discount on your manipulation you must do so on your mechanical traction and so on.

This system will simplify your fee schedules and eliminate any accusation that you are discriminating to any specific payer.

> See Resource 174 for more information.

PLAN

1. Establish a standard fee schedule for 2015. This standard fee includes routine practice overhead expenses for the additional costs associated with claims processing, collecting and follow-up.
2. Establish a Time of Service (TOS) Fee Schedule. This schedule, which is your lowest schedule, is for those who pay in full at the time of service. It passes the savings on to

patients and insurance companies. Append the modifier -52 for a "reduced service" because your overhead costs for billing and claim management (included in the total RVU) are reduced.

3. Make your TOS fee schedule **available to all.** Treat patients and insurance companies alike. All have an equal opportunity to participate in reducing health care costs and to share in the savings. Payments can be made in any form: check, cash, credit card, debit card, etc. However, all must meet the same expectation and standard: Pre-payment or Payment At Time Of Service.

4. Determine if there are any local state laws that may apply. Consult with an experienced health care attorney specializing in contract law, your professional association, or legal counsel who belongs to the National Association of Chiropractic Attorneys (NACA).

5. Consider participating in a medical discount program. These programs can promote doctor-patient relationships without third party hassles and costs. However, be aware of specific state requirements (see page B-27).

> See Resource 110 for additional comments, resources, networks, and opinions, on discounts.

> **ACA Time of Service (TOS) Disclaimer:** The ACA does not officially recommend that doctors of chiropractic use TOS discounts. This is due to the possibility of violating state and/or federal law. Before implementing a TOS discount, doctors of chiropractic should consult with a health care law attorney.

Review: Establishing Fees

- What does "Usual, Customary, and Reasonable (UCR)" refer to? *B-40*
- Are RVUs a mathematical expression or a dollar amount? *B-41*
- What are the three components in the RBRVS methodology? *B-42*
- How is the Dollar Conversion Factor a pivotal component in the fee calculation process? *B-43*
- Where is a simple one-step process to calculate fees located? *B-44*
- What is the correct way to handle your fee schedule and reduce your legal risk? *B-45*
- What are the two ways to appropriately discount fees? *B-46*

1. Understanding Medicare
Page C-3

2. Medicare Coverage
Page C-15

3. Medicare Fees
Page C-30

4. Medicare Appeals
Page C-36

5. Physician Quality Reporting System (PQRS)
Page C-44

C MEDICARE GUIDELINES

MEDICARE GUIDELINES

OBJECTIVES

As the largest healthcare payer in the United States, Medicare policies, fees, and regulations are closely monitored and mimicked in the industry. This section helps you understand and apply these key concepts, whether or not you choose to treat Medicare beneficaries.

OUTLINE

1. Understanding Medicare *C-3*
    - What Is Medicare? *C-3*
    - How Medicare Payment Works *C-6*
    - Medicare Administrative Contractors *C-11*
    - Medicare Terms to Understand *C-13*
    - Review *C-14*

2. Medicare Coverage *C-15*
    - Medicare Coverage of Chiropractic Services *C-15*
    - Billing Help *C-20*
    - Medicare CMT Coding Flowchart *C-23*
    - Medicare Benefit Policy Manual, Chapter 15 *C-27*
    - Review *C-29*

3. Medicare Fees *C-30*
    - Medicare Fee Schedule *C-30*
    - Understanding Medicare Fees *C-32*
    - Review *C-35*

4. Medicare Appeals *C-36*
    - Medicare Appeals Process *C-36*
    - Review *C-43*

5. Physician Quality Reporting System (PQRS) *C-44*
    - PQRS *C-44*
    - Review *C-49*

1. Understanding Medicare

WHAT IS MEDICARE?

The Medicare program is administered by the Centers for Medicare and Medicaid Services (CMS), a division of the U.S. Department of Health and Human Services (HHS). It is the country's largest health insurance plan and provides coverage for an estimated 55 million beneficiaries. And as the baby boomer population continues to age, it will cover, and your practice will likely treat, an increasing number of Medicare patients.

There are four different "parts" to the Medicare program, each of which covers specific services.

- Medicare Part A covers expenses incurred at hospitals, some Skilled Nursing Facilities (SNF), home health, and hospice care.
- Medicare Part B covers physician and other healthcare provider services, outpatient care, durable medical equipment and home health care.
- Medicare Part C is also known as Medicare Advantage and offers Part A and Part B benefits, and may offer prescription drug coverage (Medicare Part D), through private health plans. Some plans offer additional benefits that Medicare does not generally cover.
- Medicare Part D covers prescription drugs. Beneficiaries may need to pay a separate monthly premium for Part D unless it is included as part of a Medicare Advantage plan.

Chiropractic services are covered under either Part B or Part C.

> **Caution**: There are situations where a Medicare benficiary will have Part A, but NOT Part B coverage. In these cases, the patient is responsible for Part B services, such as chiropractic care. For this reason, it is important to carefully review their insurance card to ensure coverage of services.

See ChiroCode.com/medicare (Resource 210) for the latest articles and webinars.

ACA Medicare Section Disclaimer: At the time of printing, the federal government had not yet released its changes for 2015. Every effort was made to update the information in the 2015 DeskBook with information available at the time of review. Ongoing updates on CMS-related topics will be posted on the ACA website at (www.acatoday.org/Medicare) and through its articles and publications.

The Need for Understanding

A major issue facing the chiropractic profession is not fully understanding Medicare regulations. According to the Medicare Improper Payment Report for 2013, 51.7% of chiropractic claims were paid improperly and 92.5% of those were due to insufficient documentation. In order to maintain credibility as a healthcare profession, our standards must improve!

> *Section D–Documentation* outlines best practice standards for medical record documentation.

In addition to professional credibility, there are two other very important reasons why every provider needs to understand how Medicare works. First, Medicare is frequently used as a standard in the insurance industry. Decisions from CMS are carefully observed, and often adopted, by other payers and state agencies. Second, you must carefully adhere to rules and regulations in order to avoid federal allegations of fraud and/or abuse.

If you treat a Medicare beneficiary, you are required to bill Medicare for all covered services—this is true whether you are a participating or a non-participating provider. In addition, you are also required to submit a claim for non-covered services, when requested by the patient.

Participation status is a major source of confusion regarding Medicare. The terms **participating** and **non-participating** apply mostly to payment methods, NOT whether or not you want to be a Medicare provider. See "Provider Enrollment" below for more information.

Provider Enrollment

To bill services for Medicare beneficiaries, you must enroll with CMS. In order to streamline the enrollment process, CMS has established an internet-based Provider Enrollment, Chain

---

E-Health Initiative

CMS has launched an initiative to improve the quality and efficiency of the Medicare program "by simplifying the use of electronic standards and the adoption of health information technology." The following programs are part of this initiative:

1. Medicaid and Medicare EHR Incentive Program
2. Quality Measurement
   - Hospital Inpatient Quality Reporting Program (IQR)
   - Physician Quality Reporting System (PQRS)
   - Maintenance of Certification Program Incentive
3. Administrative Simplification Operating Rules
   - Health Plan Identifier (HPID)
   - Electronic Funds Transfer (EFT) and Remittance Advice (ERA)
   - ICD-10
4. Patient Outcomes and Payment Reform
   - Comprehensive Primary Care (CPC) Initiative
   - Physician Feedback/Value-Based Payment Modifier Program
5. eRx Incentive Program

> See Resource 211 and 212 for additional information on this intitiative.

and Ownership System (PECOS) for physicians, non-physician practitioners, and provider and suppliers organizations. PECOS allows providers to electronically enroll, revalidate, and make changes to their Medicare enrollment.

If you do not know if you are enrolled in PECOS, check the national listing of PECOS providers or call your local A/B Medicare Administrative Contractor (MAC) provider enrollment line.

Although you may **treat** Medicare patients up to 30 days prior to your enrollment application being officially *received* by your MAC, you cannot **bill** Medicare until you have received all of your numbers. Before treating a Medicare beneficiary, contact your A/B MAC to 1) confirm that they are processing the enrollment application and 2) ascertain their official policy on when an applying provider may begin treating Medicare beneficiaries. You may also monitor the status of your application online from the MAC website enrollment status link.

TIP: One common enrollment mistake is when the provider's PTAN does not match the NPI expected by CMS. This generally happens when the provider has more than one NPI number (i.e. a group NPI and an individual NPI). This can significantly delay the enrollment process so pay close attention if you have more than one NPI.

Note: There is no cost to a healthcare provider for either enrollment or revalidation.

Note: Students preparing to graduate may want to create log-in accounts for the NPPES and PECOS systems. This may speed up the enrollment process once graduation is complete.

See Resource 213 for more information about provider enrollment.

Revalidation

Every five years, providers are required to revalidate their enrollment information or risk being removed from the system. As part of the revalidation process, providers are required to switch to Electronic Funds Transfer (EFT) for payment, if they are not already doing so.

See Resource 390 for more information about revalidation.

FIGURE 3.1
PAR/Non-PAR Comparison

Participating Providers	Non-Participating Providers
■ Signed agreement/contract with Medicare	■ No signed agreement with Medicare
■ Accept assignment on ALL claims	■ May choose to accept or not accept assignment
■ Payments are made directly to the provider	■ Non-assigned payments go to the patient
■ Medigap insurance automatically billed	■ Medigap insurance billed by provider or patient *(Item 27 on the 1500 form)*
■ Secondary insurance is automatically billed (if it is contracted with Medicare)	■ Secondary insurance is billed by provider or patient
■ Allowed Fees are 5% higher than Non-PAR assigned claim Allowed Fees	■ Charges cannot be more than the Limiting Charge

Screening Process

Effective March 25, 2011, Medicare began a new screening program. All new applicants, as well as those going through the revalidation process, will now go through this screening process program. Doctors of chiropractic will have a limited screening which includes license verification and database checks. However, "moderate risk" providers will also have unscheduled/unannounced site visits. As of March 25, 2012, all currently enrolled doctors are now screened. The screening happens during the revalidation process. This is why your compliance efforts are critical.

> *Section F–HIPAA Compliance* discusses more about EFT requirements and includes important cautions and tips.

> Are you properly registered with Medicare?

- See Resource 214 to determine if your office is on the PECOS listing. If not, get started right away. There are tutorials on this page to help with the process.

- If you have been seeing patients who qualify as a Medicare beneficiary, and you have not been billing Medicare, then you are in violation of the law. Get enrolled today.

- Many providers have found that their NPI taxonomy designation is incorrect. This leads to payment problems. First, see Resource 197 to review current taxonomy codes and their definitions. Then go to Resource 215 and do a provider search on your own practice to review your taxonomy code(s).

How Medicare Payment Works

Every doctor has an annual choice regarding their participation status in the Medicare program. You can change your status only once a year, usually between November 15 and December 31. See Figure 3.1 for a general comparison between Participation and Non-Participation in Medicare.

Participation

Participating (PAR) providers are those who have signed an agreement to participate. They are required to take assignment on every Medicare patient. Medicare sends 80% of the Allowed Amount directly to the provider, once the Part B deductible has been met. The patient portion

FIGURE 3.2
Medicare Fees Participation vs. Non-Participation Comparison Table
Example: Assignment impact if regular fee is $100 and the Medicare Allowed Amount is $50.

		PARTICIPATING Assigned Claims			NON-PARTICIPATING Assigned Claims			NON-PARTICIPATING Unassigned Claims			
Usual Fee	Amount Billed	Allowed Amount	Medicare Portion (80%)	Patient Portion* (20%)	Allowed Amount (95% of Par Allowed)	Medicare Portion (80%)	Patient Portion* (20%)	Limiting Charge (115% of Non-Par Allowed)	Medicare Portion (80%)	Patient Portion* (20%)	Provider Loss
$100	$100	$50.00	$40.00	$10.00							$50.00
$100	$54.63				$47.50	$38.00	$9.50				$52.50
$100	$54.63							$54.63 ‡	$38.00 §	$16.63	$45.37

*Supplemental insurance could apply if there is coverage for the 20% patient portion.
§ Paid directly to the patient.
‡ Patient pays provider $54.63 (both the Medicare Portion and the Patient Portion).

under Part B, which is the annual deductible and then 20% of the Allowed Amount, should be collected at the time of service or it will have to be collected later.

The Annual Part B deductible for 2015 is $147. It is the provider's responsibility to collect the deductible, as well as the coinsurance, from the patient. Failure to do so could be considered fraud and abuse. Exceptions can be made, but they are rare and must be documented as bonafide financial hardship cases.

> **Note:** Some supplemental policies pay the annual Part B deductible. Be sure to verify coverage before billing the patient erroneously.

Section A–Practice Management discusses the proper way to implement a Financial Hardship Policy (Resource 146) for your office. Without a policy and its proper use, it is improper and illegal to waive co-payments and/or deductibles.

The inducements for being a participating provider are many, such as: more patients coming to the physician because they have fewer hassles with Medicare, lower out-of-pocket costs for your patients, the physician receiving direct payment from Medicare for the 80% portion of the allowed amount, and having an automatic cross over (transmittal) of claim information for qualified Medigap policies (supplemental insurance).

Misinformation on Chiropractic Services

CMS has published a fact sheet (Resource 216) to correct misinformation about chiropractic services.

> Misinformation: If you are a non-participating **(non-par) provider, you do not have to worry about billing Medicare**
>
> ***Correction:*** Being non-par does not mean you don't have to bill Medicare. All Medicare Part B covered services must be billed to Medicare by the provider or the provider could face penalties. This is known as the "Mandatory Claim Submission Rule" (an exception to this is when the beneficiary has signed a valid Advance Beneficiary Notice of Noncoverage (ABN), Form CMS-R-131, with Option #2 selected (see page C-18 for further information).
>
> A non-par provider is actually someone who has enrolled to be a Medicare provider but chooses to receive payment in a different method and amount than Medicare providers classified as participating. Non-par providers may receive reimbursement for rendered services directly from their Medicare patients; however, they still must submit a bill to Medicare so the beneficiary may be reimbursed for the portion of the charges for which Medicare is responsible.
>
> It is important to note that non-par providers may also choose to accept assignment; therefore, the amount paid by the beneficiary must be reported in Item 29 of the CMS 1500 claim form or its electronic equivalent. This ensures that the beneficiary is reimbursed (if applicable) prior to Medicare sending payment to the provider. Whether or not non-par providers choose to accept assignment on all claims or on a claim-by-claim basis, Medicare reimbursement is five percent less than for a participating provider, as reflected in the annual Medicare Physician Fee Schedule.
>
> You can find a copy of the Medicare Participating Provider Agreement at www.cms.gov/Medicare/CMS-Forms/CMS-Forms/downloads/cms460.pdf on the CMS website. The form contains important information regarding the participation process and the annual opportunity you have to make or change your participation decision. Additional information is available in the Medicare Benefit Policy Manual (Chapter 15; Covered Medical and Other Health Services) at www.cms.gov/manuals/Downloads/bp102c15.pdf and the Medicare Claims Processing Manual (Chapter 12; Physician/ Nonphysician Practitioners) at www.cms.gov/manuals/downloads/clm104c12.pdf on the CMS website.

The Medicare Physician Fee Schedule (MPFS) has fluctuated wildly in the last few years. For this reason, one very important benefit of being a participating provider is that you can bill your usual fee to Medicare. When you bill your usual fee to Medicare, you are paid 80% of the allowed amount, you collect 20% from the patient and you write off the balance. However, should Medicare retroactively increase the MPFS, as they did in 2010, you are automatically paid the increase on all previously billed claims.

One down side to participation is that PAR physicians receive about 9% less reimbursement overall than NON-PAR providers who do not accept assignment.

Figure 3.2, *Medicare Fees Participation vs Non-Participation Comparison Table* clarifies this concept of payment for both types of providers.

Non-Participation

Non-Participating (NON-PAR) physicians are those who have not signed the Medicare Participation agreement. They are only a registered provider with a number. With Medicare NON-PAR status and an unassigned claim, the maximum a physician can charge the patient for covered services is an amount known as the "Limiting Charge". It is a little more than the

---

Misinformation on Chiropractic Services (continued)

Misinformation: If you are a non-par provider, you will never be audited nor have claims reviewed, etc.

Correction: Any Medicare claim submitted can be audited/reviewed; the participation status of the physician does not affect the possibility of this occurring. CMS audits/reviews are intended to protect Medicare trust funds and also to identify billing errors so providers and their billing staff can be alerted of errors and educated on how to avoid future errors. Correct coverage, reimbursement, and billing requirements are readily available to assist you in understanding Medicare requirements.

This information is in Medicare manuals that are at www.cms.gov/Manuals on the CMS website. In addition, an excellent way to stay informed about changes to Medicare billing and coverage requirements is to monitor MLN Matters® Articles, which are available at www.cms.gov/MLNMattersArticles on the same site.

Misinformation: Non-par providers do not have the same documentation requirements as par providers

Correction: Chiropractic care has documentation requirements to show medical necessity. The participating status of the provider is irrelevant to the documentation requirements.

Specific details regarding documentation requirements are in the Medicare Benefit Policy Manual (Chapter 15, Sections 30.5 and 240) at www.cms.gov/manuals/downloads/bp102c15.pdf on the CMS website. Also, see the Medicare Claims Processing Manual (Chapter 12, Section 220) at www.cms.gov/manuals/downloads/clm104c12.pdf on the CMS website.

Misinformation: You can opt out of Medicare

Correction: Doctors of Chiropractic (DC) may not opt out of Medicare. Note that opting out and being non-participating are not the same things. Chiropractors may decide to be participating or non-participating with regard to Medicare, but they may not opt out. (Opt out refers to physicians' ability to decide not to bill Medicare at all and then entering into private contracts with Medicare beneficiaries they treat. Services furnished under these private contracts that meet the opt out requirements are not covered services under Medicare and no payment is made for those services by Medicare.)

For further discussions of the Medicare "opt out" provision, see the Medicare Benefit Policy Manual (Chapter 15, Section 40; Definition of Physician/ Practitioner) at www.cms.gov/manuals/downloads/bp102c15.pdf on the CMS website.

Allowed Amount for participating providers. Exceeding the "Limiting Charge" could result in a $10,000 fine per occurrence.

With NON-PAR status, you can accept assignment (or not) on a claim-by-claim basis. NON-PAR offices typically do not take assignment, but might have reason to make exceptions. Either way, you must still file the claim with the Medicare Administrative Contractor (MAC). In addition, please note that being a NON-PAR provider will not keep you from being reviewed or audited or from refunding overpayments.

> **Note:** Non-participation is NOT the same thing as "opting out." See "Misinformation on Chiropractic Services" on page C-8 for a more detailed explanation.

Section F–Compliance discusses reviews, audits, and refund requests in greater detail.

Go to ACAtoday.org/content_css.cfm?CID=3138 (Resource 217) to read Medicare: To Participate or Not to Participate? by the ACA.

Insurance Secondary to Medicare

If a patient has insurance coverage under more than one plan (or "payer"), "coordination of benefits" rules decide which one pays first. The one that is responsible for paying first is called the "primary payer" and the one that pays second is called the "secondary payer." Bill the primary payer first, they pay what they owe on your bills and then you send the claims to the secondary payer. The secondary payer will then process the claims, taking into consideration what the primary payer has already paid, and the secondary payer will then pay the portion for which they are responsible. In some cases, there may also be a third payer (tertiary plan.)

> **TIP:** When billing the secondary or supplemental payer, the primary remittance needs to be included with the secondary claim. This allows the claim to be processed properly, thus minimizing the possibility of problems with overpayments/underpayments, etc.

Every office must stay alert to a patient's insurance status and conditions which could change the primary payer, especially with Medicare. There are different types of policies which are secondary to Medicare and they may need to be treated differently. Correctly identifying the type of secondary policy potentially reduces errors in billing as well as the amount collected from the patient.

Medigap (Supplemental)

A Medicare supplemental insurance policy is commonly referred to as a Medigap policy and is used to help pay some of the costs not paid by original Medicare, such as copays, coinsurance and deductibles. It fills in the payment "gaps" of original Medicare. In addition, for a PAR provider, if all the appropriate information is included on the claim form, once Medicare has finalized its payments, the claim may be automatically forwarded to the Medigap policy carrier along with any applicable explanation of benefits. The Medigap policy payer then reviews the claim and pays its portion of the charges. On assigned claims, this kind of insurance provides timely payment to the physician and can eliminate the patient's immediate out-of-pocket costs.

Other Secondary Insurance

Another type of secondary insurance policy is independent from Medicare and is often a group health plan supplied by a patient's employer. These types of policies may pay for services which are not normally covered by Medicare, such as exams and x-rays. A secondary insurance plan only pays if there are costs that the primary insurer did not cover. However, it is possible that the secondary payer might not pay all the unpaid costs because coverage is based on payer policy.

Medicare as the Secondary Payer (MSP)

Medicare Secondary Payer (MSP) is the term generally used when the Medicare program does not have primary payment responsibility - that is, when another entity has the responsibility for paying before Medicare. MSP concerns are complex and involve a thorough understanding of both patient and provider responsibilities, rules for PAR vs. Non-PAR, conditional payments and more. Resources 218 and 219 help to clarify these important concepts. It is important to note that the Medicare program is accelerating audits to recoup payments when Medicare was billed in error as the primary payer.

See Resource 218 and 219 for more information by CMS on MSP.

See Chapter 2–Medicare Coverage of this section for information about properly establishing the MSP using the "Medicare Status Questionnaire" (Resource 220).

Part C – Medicare Advantage

Medicare Advantage (MA) is also known as Medicare Part C. An MA plan is an alternative to original fee-for-service Medicare (Parts A and B). MA plans are sponsored by Medicare, who pays private insurance companies to provide coverage for health services to beneficiaries enrolled in these plans.

In order to join an MA plan, the patient must be enrolled in both Medicare Part A and Part B, and must continue to pay the Part B premium. Beneficiaries who elect an MA plan are still on Medicare and retain the full rights and protections entitled to all beneficiaries.

MA plans may give coverage and cost sharing options for beneficiaries beyond the traditional Part A and Part B fee-for-service program. Patients can have more benefits than Parts A and B but not less. Each plan is different, so it is important to verify the coverage and the patient cost-sharing for each patient. Please note that CMS does not process Part C claims. Those claims are processed directly through the Medicare Advantage insurance payer.

Part C patients will have a different card from traditional Medicare which usually has the word "Advantage" somewhere on it.

There are four main types of Medicare Advantage Plans:

- Health Maintenance Organization (HMO) Plans
- Preferred Provider Organization (PPO) Plans
- Private Fee-for-Service (PFFS) Plans
- Special Needs Plans (SNP)

Other less common types of Medicare Advantage Plans include:

- Medical Savings Account (MSA) Plans – A high deductible plan combined with a bank account. Medicare deposits funds to this account and the beneficiary uses the money from that bank account (a medical savings account) to pay for health care services.

    See Resource 222 to learn more about MSAs.

- HMO Point of Service (HMOPOS) Plans – A HMO plan in which you may be able to get some services out-of-network for a higher cost.

Most of the plans have doctor networks, and sometimes patients must stay in the network in order to have coverage – except for emergencies. Doctors of chiropractic do not need to be enrolled in Medicare to provide treatment to Part C beneficiaries. However, they may need to be an in-network provider with the Medicare Advantage payer (Resource 315). Call the payer listed on the card and verify the in-network/out-of-network (whichever applies to you) coverage as well as any applicable patient cost-sharing, prior to treating the patient.

> **Cost Sharing Limits**: For chiropractic services, Medicare Advantage plans may not require beneficiaries to pay more than $20 for plans requiring copayments or 50% for coinsurance plans. See ACAtoday.org/pdf/cms_ma_response.pdf (Resource 223) for more information about Medicare cost-sharing limits.

Accountable Care Organizations (ACOs)/Shared Savings Program

As part of healthcare reform, some new types of patient care models with unique forms of reimbursement are emerging in the marketplace. ACOs are groups of doctors, hospitals, and other health care providers who voluntarily come together to provide coordinated high quality patient care. These models are being used in Medicare as well as other settings. It is important for doctors of chiropractic to become involved in these groups to demonstrate the effectiveness of chiropractic care for musculoskeletal conditions. The number of Medicare ACOs is increasing and many include chiropractic care. According to CMS, there are three types of Medicare ACOs:

1. Medicare Shared Savings Program—a program that helps a Medicare fee-for-service program providers become an ACO.

2. Advance Payment ACO Model—a supplementary incentive program for selected participants in the Shared Savings Program.

3. Pioneer ACO Model—a program designed for early adopters of coordinated care.

See Resource 126 and ACAtoday.org/pdf/MSSP_ACO_Requirements.pdf (Resource 127) for more information.

Go to ChiroCode.com/hcr and ACAtoday.org/HCR for a more thorough review of the impact of healthcare reform on chiropractic care.

Medicare Overpayment/Provider Recoupment

There may be situations when a healthcare provider realizes they have received an improper Medicare payment. Voluntary refunds should be reported to CMS and made within 60 days of when the provider discovers the error on their own. Solicited refunds are refunds requested from providers by Medicare. In the case of voluntary refunds, it is best to follow the guidelines and use the forms found on your local MAC website. It may be called a "Voluntary Refund Form" or a "Overpayment Refund Form". For refunds requested by Medicare, follow the guidelines received from them.

MEDICARE ADMINISTRATIVE CONTRACTORS (MACs)

Medicare has divided the country into jurisdictions, each with its own A/B Medicare Administrative Contractor (MAC) – formerly known as "intermediaries" and "carriers" – to process Part A and Part B claims. Most MACs publish a Local Coverage Determination (LCD) for the jurisdiction(s) they serve. According to CMS:

> "The LCDs specify under what clinical circumstances a service is considered to be reasonable and necessary. They are administrative and educational tools to assist providers in submitting

correct claims for payment. Contractors publish LCDs to provide guidance to the public and medical community within their jurisdictions. Contractors develop LCDs by considering medical literature, the advice of local medical societies and medical consultants, public comments, and comments from the provider community.

"...Contractors shall consider a service to be reasonable and necessary if the contractor determines that the service is:

- Safe and effective.
- Not experimental or investigational.
- Appropriate, including the duration and frequency that is considered appropriate for the service, in terms of whether it is:
  - Furnished in accordance with the accepted standards of medical practice for the diagnosis or treatment of the patient's condition, or to improve the function of a malformed body member.
  - Furnished in a setting appropriate to the patient's medical needs and condition.
  - Ordered and furnished by qualified personnel.
  - One that meets, but does not exceed, the patient's medical need.
  - At least as beneficial as an existing and available medically appropriate alternative."

TIP: Many LCDs contain a list of primary and secondary diagnoses that the MAC considers the only diagnoses which justify medical necessity. LCDs may also indicate the specific order in which diagnoses should appear on the claim form.

Consolidated MAC Jurisdictions

As part of CMS' ongoing efforts to streamline operations to increase operational savings, the number of A/B MAC contracts is being reduced. What this means to providers is that they need to pay close attention to Medicare notices regarding who the Medicare Administrative Contractor (MAC) is for their location.

In March 2014, CMS announced their decision to postpone the final two remaining A/B MAC contract area consolidations for up to five years.

See Resource 396 for more information on MACs including an interactive tool to review state specific information.

MEDICARE TERMS TO UNDERSTAND:

Abuse Abuse describes practices that, either directly or indirectly, result in unnecessary costs to the Medicare Program. Abuse includes any practice that is not consistent with the goals of providing patients with services that are medically necessary, meet professionally recognized standards, and are fairly priced.

Examples of Medicare abuse may include:

- Misusing codes on a claim,
- Charging excessively for services, and
- Billing for services that were not medically necessary.

Accept Assignment Assignment means that the provider is paid the Medicare-allowed amount as payment in full for all Part B claims for all covered services for all Medicare beneficiaries.

Actual Charge The amount of money a doctor or supplier charges for a certain medical service or supply. This amount is often more than the amount Medicare approves. It is also referred to as the usual and customary charge or fee.

Allowed Amount The maximum amount on which payment is based for covered health care services. This may be called "eligible expense," "payment allowance," or "negotiated rate." It is usually less than the provider's actual charge.

Claims Submission Mandate By law, Medicare claims must be submitted by providers - this includes both PAR and NON-PAR providers.

Coinsurance The patient portion of the Medicare Allowed Amount after the deductible has been met.

Coordination of Benefits When a beneficiary is covered by more than one type of insurance that covers the same health care services, one pays its benefits in full as the primary payer and the others pay a reduced benefit as a secondary or tertiary (third) payer. When the primary payer doesn't cover a particular service but the secondary payer does, the secondary payer will pay up to its benefit limit as if it were the primary payer.

Copayment A fixed amount (for example, $15) the patient pays for a covered health care service, usually when they receive the service. The amount can vary by the type of covered health care service.

Deductible The amount that the beneficiary is responsible for during each calendar year before Medicare benefits begin to apply ($147 in 2015). This applies only to services and supplies covered by Medicare. The amount is based on the Medicare-approved amounts and not necessarily the charges billed by the provider.

Exacerbation An exacerbation is a temporary, marked deterioration of the patient's condition because of an acute flare-up of the condition being treated.

Fraud The intentional deception or misrepresentation that the individual knows to be false or does not believe to be true, and the individual does this knowing that the deception could result in some unauthorized benefit to themselves or someone else.

Limiting Charge A cap on how much Non-Participating physicians may bill Medicare patients on non-assigned claims. The limiting charge is 115% of the allowed amount for Non-Participating physicians (which is 95% of the Participating provider allowed amount).

Medigap A Medigap policy is offered by a private company to those entitled to Medicare benefits and provides payment for Medicare charges not payable because of the applicability of deductibles, coinsurance amounts, or other Medicare imposed limitations.

Non-Participating Provider A provider who chooses not to sign the Participation agreement. These providers can choose to accept assignment on a claim-by-claim basis; however, services that are unassigned are subject to the "Limiting Charge" restriction.

Offset The recovery by Medicare of a non-Medicare debt by reducing present or future Medicare payments and applying the amount withheld to the debt incurred.

Medicare Terms to Understand - continued

Opt Out An official designation for a provider who agrees to operate outside the Medicare system. When a provider opts out of Medicare, he or she opts out of all Medicare programs and plans for a two year period and treats patients under a private contract. **This option is currently not available to doctors of chiropractic**.

Overpayment Assessment A decision that an incorrect amount of money has been paid for Medicare services and a determination of what that amount is.

Part A Hospital Insurance Benefits (Fee for Service) Hospital insurance covers institutional services for inpatients that are then billed by the hospital to the Medicare contractor. Individual providers do not submit claims for Part A services.

Part B Medical Insurance Benefits (Fee for Service) Medical insurance coverage which helps to pay for all physician services that are medically necessary, outpatient hospital care and some other medical services that Part A does not cover.

Part C Medicare Advantage Health plans run by Medicare-approved private insurance companies. Medicare Advantage Plans include Part A and Part B benefits, and usually additional coverage like Medicare prescription drug coverage, sometimes for an extra cost. With this program, there could be overall lower costs and extra benefits for the beneficiary.

Participating Provider A provider who agrees to "accept assignment" for all covered services provided to all Medicare patients for the following year. The provider signs a Participation agreement and accepts the Participating provider fee schedule.

Patient Portion For participating providers, the beneficiary pays 20% of the allowed amount plus any deductible. For NON-PAR, the beneficiary pays up to the limiting charge, or 20% of the NON-PAR allowed amount plus any deductible.

Private Contract A contract between a Medicare beneficiary and a provider who has opted out of Medicare. The beneficiary agrees to give up all Medicare payments for services furnished by the provider and to pay the provider directly without regard to any limits that would otherwise apply to what the provider could charge. The contract must be in writing and must be signed before any service is provided. **This is currently not available to chiropractic physicians**.

Recoupment The recovery by Medicare of Medicare debt by reducing present or future Medicare payments and applying the amount withheld to the debt incurred.

Recurrence A return of symptoms from a previously treated condition that has been quiescent for a period of time.

Secondary Payer When coordinating benefits, the health plan that pays benefits only after the primary payer has paid its full benefits. It will pay the lesser of a) its benefits in full, or b) an amount that when added to the benefits payable by the primary payer equals 100% of covered charges.

Unassigned Claim NON-PAR providers can charge more than the Medicare-approved amount but no more than the limiting charge. If it is a covered service the physician is required to submit the claim to Medicare, but the program pays the patient.

Review: Understanding Medicare

- What are the four parts of the Medicare program? *C-3*
- How often are providers required to revalidate? *C-5*
- Are you properly registered with Medicare? *C-6*
- How does Medicare payment work? *C-6 to C-8*
- How is Participation different from Non-Participation? *C-6 to C-8*
- What are MACs, and how do they function? *C-11 to C-12*

2. Medicare Coverage

MEDICARE COVERAGE OF CHIROPRACTIC SERVICES

Coverage of Chiropractic services is not the same thing as payment, although it does determine if payment will be made. Actual coverage for Chiropractic services depends on the answers to the following questions:

1. Is the patient a Medicare Beneficiary? If so, to which Plan(s) do they belong?
2. What services were rendered?
3. Is the purpose of the visit for maintenance care or active care?
4. Is there sufficient supporting documentation to justify coverage of the services?

1. Establishing Eligibility

The first step in determining coverage is establishing eligibility. You need to find out if your patient has Medicare coverage as well as which type of coverage they have. Not all Medicare Beneficiaries have Part B, which is what pays for chiropractic care. Carefully review the patient's Medicare card. For them to have coverage, it should specifically state that they have Part B or a Medicare Advantage plan (also known as Part C). Also, since Medicare is not always the primary payer, it is your responsibility to ask about other coverage and determine which plan is the primary policy.

Alert: High on the OIG target list is recovering funds when Medicare was billed as the primary when they were actually the secondary payer.

MEDICARE STATUS QUESTIONNAIRE

Routinely use the *Medicare Status Questionnaire* form to help to identify Medicare as a Secondary Payer (MSP) situations and avoid billing errors.

See Resource 220 for a full-size version of this form, with instructions.

See also "Establish Patient Financial Responsibility" (page B-10) in *Section B–Insurance and Reimbursement* for more information.

Sample: *Medicare Status Questionnaire*

2. Maintenance Care vs. Active Care

All chiropractic providers need to fully understand the Medicare definition of active care. **Active care** provides a reasonable expectation of recovery or improvement of function.

The intake process should consider this definition and proper documentation in the patient record will establish medical necessity. According to Medicare, Chiropractic services are considered to be **Maintenance Care** when any of these conditions are met:

- "Further clinical improvement cannot reasonably be expected from continuous ongoing care, and the chiropractic treatment has become supportive rather than corrective in nature."
- "The treatment plan seeks to prevent disease, promote health, and prolong and enhance the quality of life."
- "Therapy is performed to maintain or prevent deterioration of a chronic condition."

Billing Maintenance Care

Once the provider ceases to anticipate any further improvement in function, explain to the patient that Medicare no longer considers their treatment to be payable and that they will have to pay for any further care out of their own pocket. Next, give the patient an Advance Beneficiary Notice of Noncoverage (ABN), fully explaining the form and their options. If the patient chooses Option 1, submit a claim to Medicare for the adjustment with the GA modifier appended (indicating a properly delivered Advance Beneficiary Notice). If the patient chooses Option 2, you cannot submit further claims to Medicare for maintenance care services. Modifiers are explained in greater detail on page C-21.

> **Note**: If the patient presents with a new condition or there is a recurrence of the old condition, it is considered a new episode of care and is no longer considered maintenance care. With proper documentation, it is appropriate to bill Medicare for this subsequent course of active care.

Misinformation on Chiropractic Services

Misinformation: Maintenance care is not a covered service under Medicare

Correction: Spinal manipulation is a covered service under Medicare. However, maintenance care is not considered by Medicare to be medically reasonable and necessary, and is not reimbursable by Medicare.

Only acute and chronic spinal manipulation services are considered active care and may, therefore, be reimbursable. Maintenance therapy is defined (per Chapter 15, Section 30.5.B. of the Medicare Benefit Policy Manual) as a treatment plan that seeks to prevent disease, promote health, and prolong and enhance the quality of life; or therapy that is performed to maintain or prevent deterioration of a chronic condition. When further clinical improvement cannot reasonably be expected from continuous ongoing care, the treatment is then considered maintenance therapy.

See MM3449 (Revised Requirements for Chiropractic Billing of Active/Corrective Treatment and Maintenance Therapy) at www.cms.gov/MLNMattersArticles/downloads/MM3449.pdf on the CMS website. This article contains important information on completing claims and how to identify acute and chronic adjustments as opposed to maintenance adjustments. When a maintenance spinal manipulation treatment is being provided, the ABN must be issued before the service is rendered. Additional details are available in the Medicare Benefit Policy Manual, Chapter 15, Section 30.5 (Chiropractor's Services) at www.cms.gov/manuals/Downloads/bp102c15.pdf on the CMS website.

- For official Medicare definitions, see the *"Medicare Benefit Policy Manual"* excerpt at the end of this segment (page C-27).

- For help understanding how clinical decision making and claims coding come together, refer to *Medicare CMT Coding Flowchart* (page C-23).

3. Supporting Documentation

Properly documenting the service can include more than just the typical visit documentation. It can also include other compliance-supporting forms such as Medicare's *Advance Beneficiary Notice of Noncoverage (ABN)*.

ADVANCE BENEFICIARY NOTICE OF NONCOVERAGE (ABN)

The *Advance Beneficiary Notice of Noncoverage (ABN)* is one of the most critical Medicare forms that you can utilize. It is mandated for use when any of the following criteria are met:

- You believe Medicare may not pay for an item or service.
- Medicare usually covers the item or service.
- Medicare may not consider it medically reasonable and necessary for this patient *in this particular instance*.

It can also be used voluntarily to notify patients of their financial responsibility for statutorily non-covered services and items.

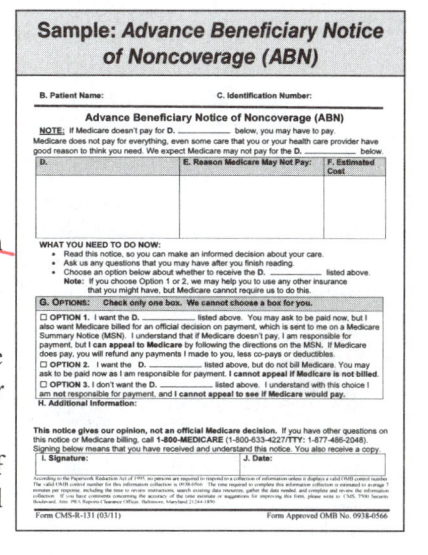

Tip: In the event a patient receives more than one CMT (spinal adjustment) on the same date of service, the ABN must be used for the second CMT visit as Medicare will not cover more than one chiropractic treatment per date-of-service.

The ABN is proof that you have told the patient that these services/supplies will most likely not be reimbursable by Medicare. As an informed consumer they can then decide whether or not to receive your services as an out-of-pocket expense, or through other insurance, if they have it.

Alert: It is a requirement to provide a completed copy of the ABN to the beneficiary or their representative. The original must be kept on file by the provider.

See Resource 224 to download the complete ABN instructions.

If you use it properly, you will be able to collect your full fee from the patient if Medicare determines that the care you provided is not reasonable or necessary. Without a properly executed ABN on file for that patient, you will have to refund any money that Medicare and/or the patient paid.

Note: A revised version of the ABN became mandatory for use in January 2012. According to the Medicare Claims Processing Manual, Chapter 30 Section 50.3, "The revised ABN is used to fulfill both mandatory and voluntary notice functions." Thus, this version of the ABN should eliminate any widespread need for the Notice of Exclusion from Medicare Benefits (NEMB) in voluntary notification situations.

See Resource 225 for a Spanish version ABN.

Are you using the correct ABN form? Look at the lower left hand corner of the form, it should say "03/11."

ADVANCE BENEFICIARY NOTICE OF NONCOVERAGE (ABN) FOR CHIROPRACTIC MAINTENANCE CARE

This is the ChiroCode Institute adaptation of the *ABN for Chiropractic Maintenance Care* only. The full-size version should be customized to include your practice information and your estimated cost per treatment. The prices listed should be your usual and customary charges.

It should be utilized when discussing and confirming maintenance care with the patient. They will typically check Option #2, but in rare cases they might still want you to submit a claim to Medicare for denial purposes (see Option #1).

In the rare occurrence that the patient selects Option #3, the provider should note the patient chart accordingly and not provide those items/services. Also, it should be noted that the patient retains the right to change their mind, in which case, a new ABN should be obtained and filed as applicable.

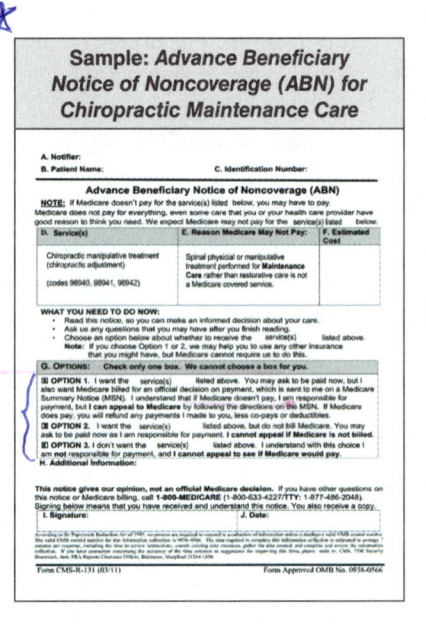

See Resource 226 for a full-size version of this form, with instructions.

Other Supporting Forms

The ChiroCode Institute has developed some other optional supporting forms. They are: *Notice of Medicare Coverage for Chiropractic Care* and the *Maintenance Care Notice*.

NOTICE OF MEDICARE COVERAGE FOR CHIROPRACTIC CARE

This form is designed to help patients understand their Medicare coverage. Coverage for services provided by a chiropractic physician is limited to spinal subluxations only. The bottom portion is for their signatures of **understanding** and **authorization**.

See Resource 227 for a full-size version of this form, with instructions.

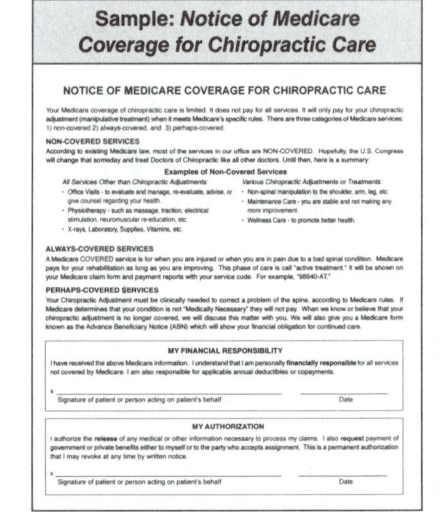

Misinformation on Chiropractic Services

Misinformation: You should get an Advance Beneficiary Notification (ABN) signed once for each patient, and it will apply to all services, all visits

Correction: The decision to deliver an ABN to a beneficiary must be based on the expectation that Medicare will not pay for a particular service because that service will not be considered medically reasonable and necessary in this instance. The ABN then allows the beneficiary to make an informed decision about receiving and paying for the service.

The ABN has 3 option boxes, and the beneficiary must choose one before signing the ABN for it to be considered a valid liability notification.

- **Option #1:** If the beneficiary selects option #1, s/he is agreeing to pay out of pocket for the service in question and requests that the chiropractor file a claim for that service with Medicare. With option #1 selected, the beneficiary retains appeals rights if s/he disagrees with Medicare's claim decision. The chiropractor is permitted to ask for payment from the beneficiary before the claim is filed if option #1 is chosen. (Beneficiaries who have secondary insurance may need a Medicare denial on a claim to enable reimbursement from their secondary insurance plan.)

- **Option #2:** A beneficiary selects option #2 when s/he agrees to pay out of pocket for the service in question and does not want a claim sent to Medicare. In accordance with the ABN, the provider would not file a claim, and the beneficiary would not have appeal rights since no claim is being submitted. (Please note that the patient can change his/her mind at a future time and request the claim be submitted.)

- **Option #3:** Option #3 is selected by the beneficiary who chooses not to receive and pay for the service. No service is rendered, and no claim is filed. Since no claim is filed, the patient cannot appeal to Medicare for a payment decision.

An ABN is issued each time a patient receives a Medicare covered service that the provider believes might be considered not medically reasonable and necessary and thus not payable by Medicare. Providers may issue a single ABN to a patient receiving the same service multiple times on a continuing basis (e.g., lumbar spinal manipulation monthly for a year). ABNs for repetitive services can be effective for up to one year. The ABN for ongoing services must describe the specific service(s) and frequency of delivery. If delivery of the repetitive service exceeds one year or the service provided changes, a new ABN must be issued. When a beneficiary with an ABN on file for repetitive services receives a different service that is not listed on the ABN, and for which Medicare payment is not expected, a separate ABN must be issued for the service which is not listed.

For further information, see the Medicare Claims Processing Manual (Chapter 30) at www.cms.gov/manuals/downloads/clm104c30.pdf and the Medicare Benefit Policy Manual (Chapter 15) at www.cms.gov/manuals/Downloads/bp102c15.pdf on the CMS website. Also see the booklet titled "Advance Beneficiary Notice of Non-Coverage (ABN) Part A and Part B" at www.cms.gov/MLNproducts/downloads/abn_booklet_icn006266.pdf on the CMS website.

MAINTENANCE CARE NOTICE (OPTIONAL)

This optional form can be used to help communicate with the patient about **maintenance care.** It could be used prior to completing the official Advanced Beneficiary Notice (ABN) form. This is only an example.

> See Resource 181 for a full-size version of this form, with instructions.

Learn More

> See *Section D–Documentation* for Medical record documentation requirements.

Sample: *Maintenance Care Notice*

BILLING HELP

This section identifies some problem areas and offers guidance on billing both covered and non-covered services. Carefully review the following sections and pay close attention to the proper use of modifiers to appropriately bill Medicare and avoid allegations of fraud and/or abuse.

Code by Subluxation First

All MACs (except First Coast Service Options) require that the primary diagnosis code billed is spinal subluxation.

The next diagnosis code entry on the claim is the presenting problem or chief complaint (e.g., headache) which is the associated or resultant problem from the causal subluxation. This diagnosis should be supportive of the primary diagnosis. See Figure 3.4.

This pattern continues with the third diagnosis which is often also a subluxation, in which case, the fourth diagnosis would be the neuromusculoskeletal complaint that is directly related to the third diagnosis and so on.

As a reminder, an LCD is an excellent resource for reviewing covered diagnoses and rules for the proper placement of diagnoses on claims.

Tip: First Coast Service Options (FCSO), does not require the 739 code series as subluxation codes in the first diagnostic position. You may bill the presenting problem or chief compliant as the primary diagnosis code on the claim.

FIGURE 3.4
Box 21, 1500 Claim Form Example

21. DIAGNOSIS or NATURE of ILLNESS or INJURY Relate A-L to Service Line Below			ICD Ind.	9
A. Subluxation	B. Chief Complaint (supports A)	C. Subluxation	D. Chief Complaint (supports C)	
E.	F.	G.	H.	
I.	J.	K.	L.	

Active Treatment

When submitting claims for spinal chiropractic manipulative therapy (CMT), doctors of chiropractic must append an AT modifier to identify services that are active/corrective treatment of an acute or chronic subluxation. Although the official description of the modifier seems to imply it is used only for acute care, the Medicare Manual states that the modifier should be used in all cases where active/corrective spinal manipulation is being performed.

By using the AT modifier, doctors of chiropractic indicate that the treatment provided is active/corrective in nature. Once the patient reaches "Maximum Therapeutic Benefit," the AT modifier should no longer be used. This indicates to Medicare that the care is now maintenance in nature. Medicare will deny claims without the AT modifier.

Medicare Modifiers

It is critical for every office to clearly understand the proper use of modifiers. Currently, the only **covered** codes by Medicare are the CMT codes (98940, 98941, and 98942) when they are "medically reasonable and necessary."

Here are the basics for coding and billing modifiers (see figure 3.5 for coding examples):

- *No modifier appended*

    No Medicare payment or patient responsibility.

- *AT modifier appended to spinal CMT*

    Active Treatment for the corrective phase of acute or chronic care.

- *GA modifier appended to spinal CMT*

    Your declaration that a Waiver of Liability Statement (ABN) has been properly delivered as required by payer policy.

- *GZ modifier appended to spinal CMT (optional)*

    You failed to deliver a mandated ABN, as is required by payer policy. In such cases, the patient does not have to pay. Please note that some providers have reported that the use of this modifier resulted in an audit.

- *GY modifier appended to 98943 and non CMT*

    Must be appended to all statutorily non-covered services.

- *GX modifier appended to non-covered services*

    Indicates that the ABN was used to voluntarily inform the patient that Medicare will not pay for a service because it is excluded from coverage by statute. Check your LCD to determine if your MAC accepts or requires this modifier.

Modifiers GX, GA, and GP

The GX modifier is used to signify that the ABN was voluntarily given to a patient to inform them that they will be financially liable for statutorily non-covered services. Since the GX modifier is used only with statutorily non-covered services, it should be used in combination with the GY modifier. Contact your Medicare Administrative Contractor (MAC) for usage instructions.

The GA modifier should be used when the "Waiver of Liability Statement Issued as Required by Payer Policy" has been provided to the patient. The GA modifier should only be used in conjuction with CPT codes 98940, 98941, and 98942 and only when appropriate.

The GP modifier is used to indicate that physical medicine services have been used as part of a treatment plan and is typically only used by physical therapists. However, some MACs require the use of this modifier by doctors of chiropractic as well. It would be used in combination with the GY modifier.

- **GP modifier appended to therapy services**
  Indicates that therapy services were delivered under an outpatient physical therapy plan of care. Some MACs, such as Palmetto GBA, require the GP modifier to be added to therapy services provided by a chiropractor. These services are not covered, but without the modifier, they will be rejected as unprocessable, which may not be acceptable to a secondary payer.

Recommendations

- Indicate the phase of care. AT modifier = Active Treatment. No AT modifier = Maintenance Care.
- Document the functional improvement of the patient in order to determine when the patient reaches Maximum Medical Improvement/Maximum Therapeutic Benefit (MMI/MTB).
- Counsel with the patient when they have reached Maximum Therapeutic Benefit and begin their maintenance phase of care.
- If you enter a statutorily non-covered code on the claim, append the GY modifier. This is a requirement.

Are you using modifiers properly? Review the recommendations and coding examples above and compare to your own submitted claims, office policies and procedures to ensure compliance.

See Chapter 4 (page C-36) for more information on Medicare appeals.

Other Tips

- Generally speaking, only bill a therapy, x-rays or exam code if the patient needs a rejection from Medicare in order to bill a secondary insurance.
- If Palmetto is your MAC: Use the GP modifier on therapy codes (if you bill them) to avoid potential denial problems with CMT services. However, when the GP modifier is used, the claim will be denied if items 17 and 17b are not completed.

FIGURE 3.5
Coding Examples for Medicare Modifiers

CMT Active Treatment (Modifier AT)
98940 | AT

CMT Maintenance Care with ABN (Modifier GA)
98940 | GA

Electrical Stimulation with Voluntary ABN (Modifiers GY and GX)
G0283 | GY | GX

CMT Maintenance Care without ABN (no modifier)
98940 |

E/M Service (Modifier GY)
99213 | 25 | GY

X-Rays (Modifier GY)
72010 | GY

Trigger Point Therapy when billed with CMT (Modifier GY)
97140 | 59 | GY

Medicare CMT Coding Flowchart

The flowchart in Figure 3.6 outlines a suggested sequence of care flowchart for Chiropractic Manipulative Treatment (CMT) codes (98940-98942). Medicare coverage for spinal CMT is according to their guidelines. If the AT modifier has not been used it means an automatic denial, and the patient has no financial responsibility to pay, unless the ABN has been properly delivered. If the AT modifier is missing due to a clerical error, use the "reopening" process to correct the claim. Other denials should be appealed in accordance with Medicare rules.

Flowchart Notes

1. PRESENTING PROBLEM

- Use box 14 on the 1500 Claim Form (or electronic equivalent) to indicate a new injury or condition. For doctors of chiropractic, box 14 (or electronic equivalent) is the date of initiation for this course of care.

  Note: The 1500 Claim Form includes a "Qualifier" field in this box. At the time of publication, Medicare policies have not been updated regarding the use of this field. Leave the "Qual" field blank unless otherwise instructed. One possible scenario, as shown in the example below, is National Uniform Claim Committee (NUCC) qualifier 431, which is "Onset of current symptoms or illness."

  Example:

14. DATE OF CURRENT ILLNESS, INJURY, or PREGNANCY (LMP)		
MM	DD	YY
01	12	2014 QUAL. 431

  Tip: Medicare requires this date to be the initial date the patient presented to be treated for the current symptoms/condition.

2. EXACERBATION OR RECURRENCE

The following are some general definitions of these terms. Some MACs may have their own definitions. Be aware of individual payer definitions.

- An **exacerbation** is a temporary, marked deterioration of the patient's condition because of an acute flare-up of the condition being treated. When an exacerbation occurs, note the occurrence and cause in the patient's chart and increase the visit frequency until the patient returns to their pre-exacerbation status.
- A **recurrence** is a return of symptoms from a previously treated condition that has been quiescent for 30 or more days (Novitas defines this as 90 days or more.) When the patient has a recurrence, do a history update, exam, new Outcomes Assessment, new treatment plan, and a new initial date of treatment.

3. EVALUATION AND MANAGEMENT

- Presence of subluxation is determined by either physical examination or x-ray. If documented by physical examination, the P.A.R.T. system must be used.

  See *Section D–Documentation,* Chapter 5, for more information about P.A.R.T.

- Orthopedic and neurological exams need to be performed to rule out pathological processes and because they are the standard of care within the profession.

FIGURE 3.6
Medicare CMT Coding Flowchart

MEDICARE CMT CODING
(See instructions on next page)

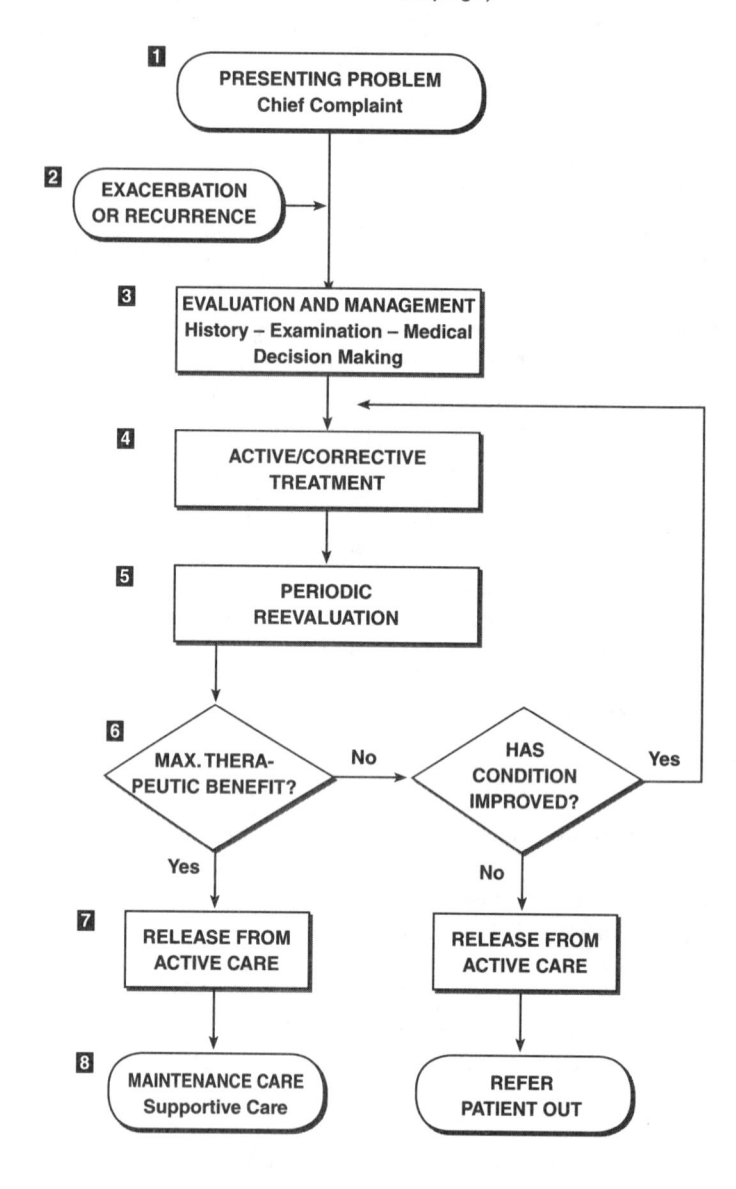

1. PRESENTING PROBLEM — Chief Complaint

2. EXACERBATION OR RECURRENCE

3. EVALUATION AND MANAGEMENT — History – Examination – Medical Decision Making

4. ACTIVE/CORRECTIVE TREATMENT

5. PERIODIC REEVALUATION

6. MAX. THERAPEUTIC BENEFIT?
- No → HAS CONDITION IMPROVED?
  - Yes → (return to Active/Corrective Treatment)
  - No → RELEASE FROM ACTIVE CARE → REFER PATIENT OUT
- Yes → RELEASE FROM ACTIVE CARE

7. RELEASE FROM ACTIVE CARE

8. MAINTENANCE CARE — Supportive Care

- Outcomes Assessment tools should be used to determine baseline impairment.
  - See *Section D–Documentation*, Chapter 5, for more information about outcomes assessment.
  - See Chapter 5 of this section to learn how to report the use of Outcome Assessments via the Physician Quality Reporting System.
- All services other than the three spinal CMT codes (98940-98942) are not covered. Therefore, a GY modifier should be appended, if the service is billed to Medicare.
- Append modifer -25 to the E/M code if CMT is performed on the same day and the E/M service is significantly and separately identifiable.
- The GX modifier indicates that you have a voluntary ABN on file and have notified the patient of their financial responsibility for statutorily non-covered services.

Examples of initial and reevaluations:

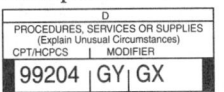

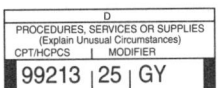

PROCEDURES, SERVICES OR SUPPLIES (Explain Unusual Circumstances) CPT/HCPCS	MODIFIER
99204	GY GX

PROCEDURES, SERVICES OR SUPPLIES (Explain Unusual Circumstances) CPT/HCPCS	MODIFIER
99213	25 GY

4. ACTIVE/CORRECTIVE TREATMENT

- Spinal CMT, in this phase of care, is billed with the AT modifier.
- The clinical necessity/rationale for this active/corrective phase of CMT service must be documented.
- The AT modifier indicates that your records demonstrate active corrective treatment. Outcomes Assessment tools are valuable to objectively measure progress and improvement.
- Active/corrective treatment continues until maximum therapeutic benefit is reached.

Example of 1-2 regions of active care CMT service:

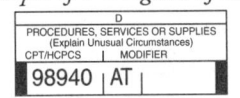

PROCEDURES, SERVICES OR SUPPLIES (Explain Unusual Circumstances) CPT/HCPCS	MODIFIER
98940	AT

5. PERIODIC REEVALUATION

- Reexamine the active care patient when clinically indicated.
- An Outcomes Assessment Tool (OAT) can be a valuable part of a reevaluation and care plan update. An OAT should be administered when clinically indicated at least every 30 days.
- Use an appropriate E/M code for reevaluation, when you perform a separately identifiable E/M service, however, keep in mind that the fee is the patient's responsibility.

6. DECISION MAKING

- Functional improvement is paramount in determining whether or not to continue with active treatment.
- The patient has reached Maximum Therapeutic Benefit when there is no significant improvement (30% or better is an industry standard) between two Outcomes Assessment Tools when they are administered 30 days apart.

7. RELEASE FROM ACTIVE CARE

- Corrective treatment for the presenting problem is complete.

8. MAINTENANCE CARE

- Clinical status has "stabilized"
- Further clinical improvement cannot reasonably be expected.
- This phase of care is billed with no AT modifier.
- The GA modifier is appended if a an ABN has been properly provided to the patient and is on file. GA only means an ABN has been provided to the patient. It does not mean "maintenance care." No AT on the CMT means "maintenance care."

Example:

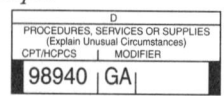

D PROCEDURES, SERVICES OR SUPPLIES (Explain Unusual Circumstances)	
CPT/HCPCS	MODIFIER
98940	GA

Tip: When the doctor believes the patient is still under active care, but knows the MAC may deny it because the patient has reached the MACs published review guideline threshold, it may be necessary to append both GA and AT on the claim. Be aware of individual MAC policies regarding this matter.

Go to ACAtoday.org/medicare (Resource 228) to review an FAQ by the ACA regarding the use of the GA and AT modifiers together.

Direct Submission to Secondary Insurance for Medicare Non-Covered Services

Direct Submission could be an effective way to avoid payment delays for secondary payers. This letter is for direct submission to these payers via paper claims. Use this letter for services that are not covered by Medicare but will be covered by a secondary payer. However, be aware that most payers require a denial letter from the primary before they will make a payment.

See Resource 397 for a full-size version of this form, with instructions.

Sample: *Direct Submission to Secondary Insurance for Medicare Non-Covered Services*

Common Misconceptions about Medicare Participation

Misinformation: There is a 12 visit cap or limit for chiropractic services

Correction: There are no caps/limits in Medicare for covered chiropractic care rendered by chiropractors who meet Medicare's licensure and other requirements as specified in the Medicare Benefit Policy Manual, Chapter 15, Section 30.5 (this manual is available at www.cms.gov/manuals/IOM/list.asp on the CMS website). Your claims contractor may have review screens (numbers of visits at which the Medicare Carrier or A/B MAC may require a review of documentation before allowing further care), but caps/limits are not allowed.

Misinformation: DME ordered by a DC will be reimbursed by CMS

Correction: A chiropractor may act as supplier of durable medical equipment (DME) if they have a valid supplier number assigned by the National Supplier Clearinghouse, but a chiropractor will not be reimbursed if they order DME.

Medicare Benefit Policy Manual, Chapter 15

The following are official regulations regarding Medicare coverage of chiropractic services. Sometimes, when you are trying to resolve a particular issue, it is helpful to quickly find and read the actual phrases and words directly from the policy. See Resource 331

30.5 – Chiropractor's Services
B3-2020.26

A chiropractor must be licensed or legally authorized to furnish chiropractic services by the State or jurisdiction in which the services are furnished. In addition, a licensed chiropractor must meet the following uniform minimum standards to be considered a physician for Medicare coverage. Coverage extends only to treatment by means of manual manipulation of the spine to correct a subluxation provided such treatment is legal in the State where performed. All other services furnished or ordered by chiropractors are not covered.

If a chiropractor orders, takes, or interprets an x-ray or other diagnostic procedure to demonstrate a subluxation of the spine, the x-ray can be used for documentation. However, there is no coverage or payment for these services or for any other diagnostic or therapeutic service ordered or furnished by the chiropractor. For detailed information on using x-rays to determine subluxation, see §240.1.2.

In addition, in performing manual manipulation of the spine, some chiropractors use manual devices that are hand-held with the thrust of the force of the device being controlled manually. While such manual manipulation may be covered, there is no separate payment permitted for use of this device.

A. Uniform Minimum Standards

Prior to July 1, 1974

Chiropractors licensed or authorized to practice prior to July 1, 1974, and those individuals who commenced their studies in a chiropractic college before that date must meet all of the following three minimum standards to render payable services under the program:

- Preliminary education equal to the requirements for graduation from an accredited high school or other secondary school;

- Graduation from a college of chiropractic approved by the State's chiropractic examiners that included the completion of a course of study covering a period of not less than 3 school years of 6 months each year in actual continuous attendance covering adequate course of study in the subjects of anatomy, physiology, symptomatology and diagnosis, hygiene and sanitation, chemistry, histology, pathology, and principles and practice of chiropractic, including clinical instruction in vertebral palpation, nerve tracing, and adjusting; and

- Passage of an examination prescribed by the State's chiropractic examiners covering the subjects listed above.

After June 30, 1974

Individuals commencing their studies in a chiropractic college after June 30, 1974, must meet all of the above three standards and all of the following additional requirements:

- Satisfactory completion of 2 years of pre-chiropractic study at the college level;

- Satisfactory completion of a 4-year course of 8 months each year (instead of a 3-year course of 6 months each year) at a college or school of chiropractic that includes not less than 4,000 hours in the scientific and chiropractic courses specified in the second bullet under "Prior to July 1, 1974" above, plus courses in the use and effect of x-ray and chiropractic analysis; and

- The practitioner must be over 21 years of age.

B. Maintenance Therapy

Under the Medicare program, chiropractic maintenance therapy is not considered to be medically reasonable or necessary, and is therefore not payable. Maintenance therapy is defined as a treatment plan that seeks to prevent disease, promote health, and prolong and enhance the quality of life; or therapy that is performed to maintain or prevent deterioration of a chronic condition. When further clinical improvement cannot reasonably be expected from continuous ongoing care, and the chiropractic treatment becomes supportive rather than corrective in nature, the treatment is then considered maintenance therapy. For information on how to indicate on a claim if a treatment is or is not maintenance, see §240.1.3.

240 – Chiropractic Services – General
B3-2250, B3-4118

The term "physician" under Part B includes a chiropractor who meets the specified qualifying requirements set forth in §30.5 but only for treatment by means of manual manipulation of the spine to correct a subluxation.

Effective for claims with dates of service on or after January 1, 2000, **an x-ray is not required to demonstrate the subluxation.**

Implementation of the chiropractic benefit requires an appreciation of the differences between chiropractic theory and experience and traditional medicine due to fundamental differences regarding etiology and theories of the pathogenesis of disease. Judgments about the reasonableness of chiropractic treatment must be based on the application of chiropractic principles. So that Medicare beneficiaries receive equitable adjudication of their claims based on such principles and are not deprived of the benefits intended by the law, carriers may use chiropractic consultation in carrier review of Medicare chiropractic claims.

Payment is based on the physician fee schedule and made to the beneficiary or, on assignment, to the chiropractor.

> **Note:** CPT code 98943 (CMT, extraspinal/non-spinal, one or more regions) is not a Medicare benefit.

240.1 - Coverage of Chiropractic Services

240.1.1 – Manual Manipulation
B3-2251.1

Coverage of chiropractic service is specifically limited to treatment by means of manual manipulation, i.e., by use of the hands. Additionally, manual devices (i.e., those that are hand-held with the thrust of the force of the device being controlled manually) may be used by chiropractors in performing manual manipulation of the spine. However, no additional payment is available for use of the device, nor does Medicare recognize an extra charge for the device itself.

No other diagnostic or therapeutic service furnished by a chiropractor or under the chiropractor's order is covered. This means that if a chiropractor orders, takes, or interprets an x-ray, or any other diagnostic test, the x-ray or other diagnostic test, can be used for claims processing purposes, but Medicare coverage and payment are not available for those services. This prohibition does not affect the coverage of x-rays or other diagnostic tests furnished by other practitioners under the program. For example, an x-ray or any diagnostic test taken for the purpose of determining or demonstrating the existence of a subluxation of the spine is a diagnostic x-ray test covered under §1861(s)(3) of the Act if ordered, taken, and interpreted by a physician who is a doctor of medicine or osteopathy.

Manual devices (i.e., those that are hand-held with the thrust of the force of the device being controlled manually) may be used by chiropractors in performing manual manipulation of the spine. However, no additional payment is available for use of the device, nor does Medicare recognize an extra charge for the device itself.

Medicare Benefit Policy Manual, Chapter 15 (cont'd)

Effective for claims with dates of service on or after January 1, 2000, an x-ray is not required to demonstrate the subluxation. However, an x-ray may be used for this purpose if the chiropractor so chooses.

The word "correction" may be used in lieu of "treatment." Also, a number of different terms composed of the following words may be used to describe manual manipulation as defined above:

- Spine or spinal adjustment by manual means;
- Spine or spinal manipulation;
- Manual adjustment; and
- Vertebral manipulation or adjustment.
- In any case in which term(s) used to describe the service performed suggests that it may not have been treatment by means of manual manipulation, the carrier analyst refers the claim for professional review and interpretation

Note: In July 2013, Medicare asked for public comment regarding possible changes in coverage for Evaluation and Management services. Several national organizations responded to this request. At the time of printing, no announcements have been made by CMS regarding this matter.

Review: Medicare Coverage

- What does actual coverage of chiropractic services depend on? *C-15*
- What is the first step in determining Medicare coverage? *C-15*
- What is is important to understand MSP? *C-15*
- When are Chiropractic services considered to be maintenance care? *C-16*
- Which form is used to notify Medicare patients that a normally covered service or supply might not be covered this time? *C-17*
- How is the CMT service for acute treatment coded? *C-21*
- Which modifier is your declaration that a Waiver of Liability Statement has been properly provided to the patient and is on file? *C-21*
- Must a doctor of chiropractic use an x-ray for Medicare documentation? *C-27*

3. Medicare Fees

MEDICARE FEE SCHEDULE

Annual Medicare Fees

Every chiropractic office should receive its annual Medicare Physician Fee Schedule (MPFS) from its Medicare Administrative Contractor (MAC) prior to the new year. The MPFS is also available on the internet. Every provider needs to know the local Medicare **allowed amounts** and **limiting charges** for the coming calendar year.

The MPFS lists the **allowed amounts** for participating providers and non-participating providers, as well as the **limiting charges** for non-participating providers not accepting assignment. Fees for all codes in your MPFS are already adjusted by the Geographic Adjustment Factor (GAF) for your area. These published fees become an excellent basis for evaluation and calculation of your other fees. Non-PAR are not allowed to exceed the limiting charge for Medicare covered services (98940-98942) by any amount for any reason.

Your Medicare fee schedule is probably a good minimum standard. Traditionally, a majority of payers across the nation use the MFS as a baseline and then add a percentage to it to set their own fee schedules. Most notably, Florida law mandates that auto claims are paid at 200% of Medicare. The rationale behind this practice is that Medicare fees are known to be far below a provider's usual and customary fees. Unfortunately, a few payers have low fee schedules that are less than the Medicare fee schedule.

Enter below your 2015 Medicare fees from your Medicare Administrative Contractor (MAC)–recording it here makes a handy and convenient reference for you throughout the year. These are your Medicare fees for the three spinal CMT codes for 2015. See Resource 229 to use the CMS Physician Fee Schedule look-up. You may also use the *ChiroCode Medicare Fee Calculator* (Resource 170).

2015 MEDICARE FEE SCHEDULE

Enter your local Medicare data here:

CMT Code	Participating Allowed Amount	Non-participating Limiting Charge
98940	_____	_____
98941	_____	_____
98942	_____	_____

Fee Calculations for Medicare

Medicare fees are calculated annually. They are a combination of:

- An adjusted Relative Value Unit (RVU) assigned by CMS to each procedure for each area/locality.
- The adjusted RVU is multiplied by Medicare Physician Fee Schedule (MPFS) Conversion Factor (CF) to calculate the MPFS into a dollar amount, which is the **allowed amount** for participating providers. Non-participating providers have a different payment rate which is called the **limiting charge.**

> **Alert:** At the time of publication, Congress was considering proposals to repeal the Sustainable Growth Rate (SGR) formula which is used to calculate the MPFS Conversion Factor. Watch for further announcements regarding the proposed SGR formula repeal and Medicare physician payment reform.

For your Medicare Fee Calculations use the *Medicare Fee Calculator for Chiropractic Codes* (Resource 170).

CMS (Medicare) Conversion Factor

The annual Medicare Conversion Factor (CF) is the pivotal component in the fee calculation process. Without a proper conversion factor, fees will be depressed. Although originally set to significantly decrease in 2014, the MPFS Conversion Factor for CY 2014 ended up as $35.8228. Historically speaking, the CF has only fluctuated mildly over the past several years due to Congressional action which averted the cuts mandated by the SGR (see above). At press time, the 2015 Medicare Conversion Factor (as published in the November 13, 2014 Federal Register) is set to decrease to $28.2239 after the first quarter of 2015, unless Congress intervenes once again.

Go to ChiroCode.com/onlinetools (Resource 330) for current fee updates, including RVUs.

Impact of Submitted Fee Amounts

Providers need to be very careful to collect only what Medicare regulations allow because the law states that to charge more than that is fraud. To avoid fraud allegations, many providers submit their claims with the allowed amount or even less, just to be safe. However, this creates an unintended consequence—a lower fee standard throughout the nation. Why? When a national or regional fee analysis is performed by using the submitted fees and they are not the provider's 'list price', the resulting average is lower than it should be. Historically, payers and data vendors used these national averages from submitted claims as part of their formula for calculating UCR fees.

If you are a **participating provider**, the fee amount submitted on a claim is not bound by law to be the Medicare allowed amount. PAR providers may bill whatever they wish on the claim.

CMT Fee Increase

A demonstration project to evaluate the feasibility and advisability of expanding coverage for chiropractic services had higher than expected costs and CMS had been deducting 2 percent from payments for chiropractic services. Effective July 1, 2014, this *2 percent reduction* for CMT (codes 98940, 98941, and 98942) was *eliminated.*

However, only the allowed amounts for covered services may actually be collected. Therefore, anything beyond the allowed amount must be written off and never billed to the patient!

If you are a NON-participating provider, not accepting assignment, the fee for covered services on the submitted claim cannot be more than the limiting charge.

See Figure 3.7 Medicare Fees Decision Chart for more information.

Participation Status

Participating (PAR): This means that a provider **has signed** an agreement with Medicare to bill them directly with assignment on all claims for direct payments, according to the **allowed amount** on the Medicare fee schedule. Names of participating providers are published by Medicare for patients to use.

> **Alert:** Failure by PAR providers to attempt collection of either the patient's 20% co-insurance portion, or the annual deductible, could be considered fraud.

Non-Participating (Non-PAR): This means that a provider has not signed the participation agreement to take assignment on all claims. Assignment is an option. Non-PAR providers can collect from a patient at the time of service, up to the **limiting charge** amount, when not accepting assignment.

If a doctor of chiropractic does not accept assignment on the claim, Medicare will reimburse the patient 80% of the Non-PAR fee allowance. If a non-participating provider accepts assignment, they must accept the Non-PAR fee allowance as payment in full.

> *Medicare for Chiropractors* (Resource 231) is a comprehensive resource for chiropractic offices to understand Medicare requirements.

UNDERSTANDING MEDICARE FEES

This Medicare Fees Decision Chart (Figure 3.7) includes examples and helps outline the decision process for billing the appropriate fees for Medicare patients. Be aware that the fees included here are only examples which are used for demonstration purposes **only**.

Flowchart Notes

1. **IS THIS ACTIVE CARE?**
   - Maintenance care does not go through the standard claims process. Since it is a non-covered Medicare service, you **cannot** bill the patient unless you have a properly delivered ABN on file. See step 2 for more information on the ABN.

2. **VERIFY ABN AND IF APPROPRIATE PROVIDE THE TREATMENT SERVICE**
   - Treatment may only be provided if the patient has a current, properly delivered ABN on file, and they have chosen either option #1 or #2. If they have chosen option #3, no treament may be provided.
   - If you have an ABN on file, it must be **less than a year old** to be valid (see alert below).
   - You **cannot** bill the patient if Medicare decides that the service/supply is medically unnecessary unless you have a properly delivered ABN on file.

FIGURE 3.7
Medicare Fees Decision Chart

MEDICARE FEES DECISION CHART

Note: Examples are based on Medicare PAR Allowable Amount of $50

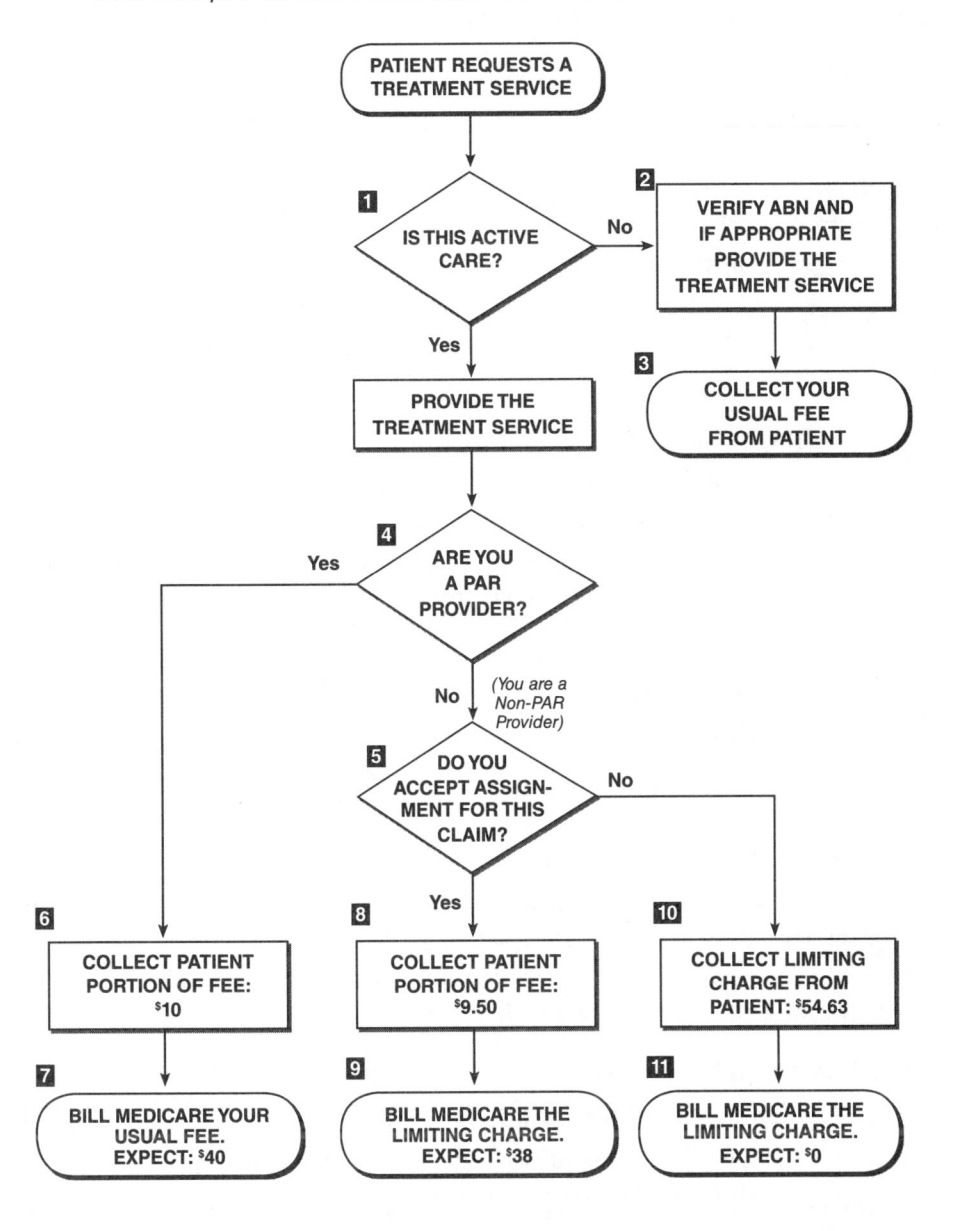

```
                    PATIENT REQUESTS A
                    TREATMENT SERVICE
                            │
                            ▼
            [1]                         [2]
        IS THIS ACTIVE    No    VERIFY ABN AND
            CARE?        ───►   IF APPROPRIATE
                                PROVIDE THE
                                TREATMENT SERVICE
            │ Yes                       │
            ▼                           ▼
        PROVIDE THE                 [3]
        TREATMENT SERVICE       COLLECT YOUR
            │                   USUAL FEE
            ▼                   FROM PATIENT
            [4]
    Yes  ARE YOU
    ◄──  A PAR
         PROVIDER?
            │ No  (You are a Non-PAR Provider)
            ▼
            [5]
         DO YOU
         ACCEPT ASSIGN-    No
         MENT FOR THIS   ───►
         CLAIM?
            │ Yes
```

[6] COLLECT PATIENT PORTION OF FEE: $10	[8] COLLECT PATIENT PORTION OF FEE: $9.50	[10] COLLECT LIMITING CHARGE FROM PATIENT: $54.63
[7] BILL MEDICARE YOUR USUAL FEE. EXPECT: $40	[9] BILL MEDICARE THE LIMITING CHARGE. EXPECT: $38	[11] BILL MEDICARE THE LIMITING CHARGE. EXPECT: $0

Participating providers should bill their usual fee and write-off the balance.
Non-PAR providers should bill the limiting charge.

- The ABN is only needed for services/supplies usually covered by Medicare that they deem not reasonable or necessary (e.g., maintenance care). It can also be used as a method to explain statutorily non-covered services/supplies for which the patient will be required to pay out of pocket.

> **Alert:** Once an ABN has been signed for the purpose of indicating maintenance therapy, that ABN is valid for that series of maintenance treatment, until there is any provision of active care, for up to one year. Once there is an exacerbation or new active treatment, any maintenance care following would require a newly delivered ABN.

Refer to the segment "3. Supporting Documentation" on page C-17 for more information about when an ABN is needed and when it should be used.

3. COLLECT YOUR USUAL FEE FROM PATIENT

- As long as you have a properly delivered and current ABN, you may collect your usual and customary fee from the patient. Medicare Allowed Amounts and Limiting Charges do not apply.

4. ARE YOU A PAR PROVIDER?

- A participating provider (PAR) takes assignment on all Medicare claims and accepts the Medicare allowed amount as payment in full.
- Payment for Non-Participating (Non-PAR) Providers is 95% of the allowed amount on assigned claims and up to the limiting charge (115% of the Non-PAR allowed amount) on unassigned claims.

5. DO YOU ACCEPT ASSIGNMENT?

- If you are Non-PAR and accept assignment you can expect 80% of the allowed amount from your MAC. If you are Non-PAR and do not accept assignment you can charge the patient up to the limiting charge which is 115% of the Non-PAR allowed amount.

6. COLLECT THE PATIENT PORTION OF THE FEE

- When collecting the patient portion, **if there is an unmet deductible**, this amount would be more than $10.
- The patient coinsurance, for a PAR-provider, is 20% of the allowed amount for assigned claims. Medicare pays the other 80% directly to the provider.

7. BILL MEDICARE YOUR USUAL FEE

- Expect $40, **unless the patient deductible has not** been met.
- Bill your usual fee and write off any difference over the PAR allowed amount. Expect 80% of the Medicare allowed amount from your local MAC.

> **Note**: If the patient has supplemental or secondary coverage which covers the deductible and/or patient co-insurance, do not charge the patient these amounts.

8. COLLECT THE PATIENT PORTION OF THE FEE

- When collecting the patient portion, **if there is an unmet deductible**, this amount would be more than $9.50.

- The patient coinsurance is 20% of the Non-PAR allowed amount. Your local MAC pays 80% directly to you.

9. BILL MEDICARE THE LIMITING CHARGE

- Bill Medicare no more than the Limiting Charge. Your local MAC will adjust and pay you 80% of the Non-PAR allowed amount.

> **Note:** If the patient has supplemental or secondary coverage which covers the deductible and/or patient co-insurance, do not charge the patient these amounts.

10. COLLECT THE LIMITING CHARGE

- Collect up to the limiting charge from the patient. You may collect less if you choose. The limiting charge is 115% of the Non-PAR allowed amount. Your local MAC pays 80% of the Non-PAR allowable to the patient.

11. BILL MEDICARE THE LIMITING CHARGE

- The limiting charge is 115% of the Non-PAR allowed amount. Your local MAC is billed in order to reimburse the patient.

Review: Medicare Fees

- Which amounts from the MPFS do doctors of chiropractic need to use in determining their fees? *C-30*
- How are Medicare fees calculated? *C-31*
- What does it mean to be a Participating Provider? *C-32*
- At what point do you need to have an ABN form signed? *C-34*
- What amount do you bill Medicare? *C-35*

4. Medicare Appeals

MEDICARE APPEALS PROCESS

Medicare Law provides an appeals process for providers and beneficiaries dissatisfied with the initial claim determination made by the Medicare Administrative Contractor (MAC). Because re-submitting a corrected claim that has been denied is not the same thing as the formal Medicare appeals process, it is important to understand the differences between a reopening and an appeal. Appeals can only be filed under the following scenarios:

- PAR: Participating physician (required to accept assignment on all claims)
- NON-PAR:
    - Non-Participating physicians who accepted assignment.
    - Non-Participating physicians who did not accept assignment, but may be responsible for refunding money to the beneficiary.
    - A physician who otherwise does not have appeal rights may appeal when the beneficiary dies and there is no one else to make the appeal.
    - Non-Participating physicians, who did not accept assignment may appeal on behalf of a patient, but only when they have valid transfer of appeal rights (see page C-39).

Caution: According to Medicare: "If you submit more than one claim for the same item or service, you can expect your duplicate claims to be denied. In addition, duplicate claims: 1) may delay payment; 2) could cause you to be identified as an abusive biller; or 3) if a pattern of duplicate billing is identified, may generate an investigation for fraud."

See Resource 285 for more information by CMS regarding duplicate claims.

Unprocessable Claims

Claims that are "unprocessable" should be corrected and re-submitted instead of using the appeals or reopening process. Carefully review the Medicare Summary Notice or the Remittance Advisory for two specific codes: CO16 and MA130. Code CO16 indicates that the claim is unprocessable, while code MA130 means there are no appeal rights. Typically, there is a third code which varies and will be the reason that the claim is unprocessable. If you see these codes simply correct the error and promptly re-submit the claim.

Before Submitting a Medicare Appeal

There are three situations which should be resolved through a reopening - NOT through the formal appeals process. In the following situations, contact your local MAC by either telephone or letter and request a reopening:

1. Correcting incomplete or invalid claims submission. For example, a missing provider NPI or an incorrect patient ID number.
2. A minor error or omission which caused the claim to be denied. For example, an improper modifier.
3. Failure to respond within 45 days to an Additional Documentation Request (ADR) has resulted in a denial. The reopening must be requested within 120 days from the initial determination to be considered.

The following time frames for a reopening are outlined in the Medicare Claims Processing Manual:

- Within one year from the date of the initial determination or redetermination for any reason; or
- Within four years from the date of the initial determination or redetermination for good cause as defined in §10.11; or
- At any time if the initial determination is unfavorable, in whole or in part, to the party thereto, but only for the purpose of correcting a clerical error on which that determination was based. Third party payer error does not constitute clerical error as defined in §10.4.

If the reopening results in an unfavorable determination, then the appeals process may be initiated.

Medicare Appeals – After the Initial Determination

The Medicare appeals process has five levels. Each level must be completed for each claim before proceeding to the next level. The entire process could take up to 780 days.

1. **Redetermination** – by the Medicare contractor
2. **Reconsideration** – by a Qualified Independent Contractor (QIC)
3. **Hearing** – by an Administrative Law Judge (ALJ)
4. **Review** – by the Medicare Appeals Council
5. **Review** – by the Federal District Court

On the following pages are instructions for proper Medicare appeals. They are sufficient for most offices. Providers and billers will want to master all components and steps, especially when large dollar amounts are involved.

Alert: In 2012, only 2.6% of Part B claim denials were appealed. Of these claims, 51% were overturned and ruled to be in provider's favor.

Figure 3.8 on the next page summarizes the appeals levels process. Pay close attention to timing deadlines and monetary amounts.

When do payments to providers become non-recoverable?

Medicare uses the same four-year regulation to reopen claims for recovery of overpayments. However, a provision in the American Taxpayer Relief Act of 2012 extends this time frame to five years, after which payments to providers are considered non-recoverable.

FIGURE 3.8
The Medicare Part B Appeals Process

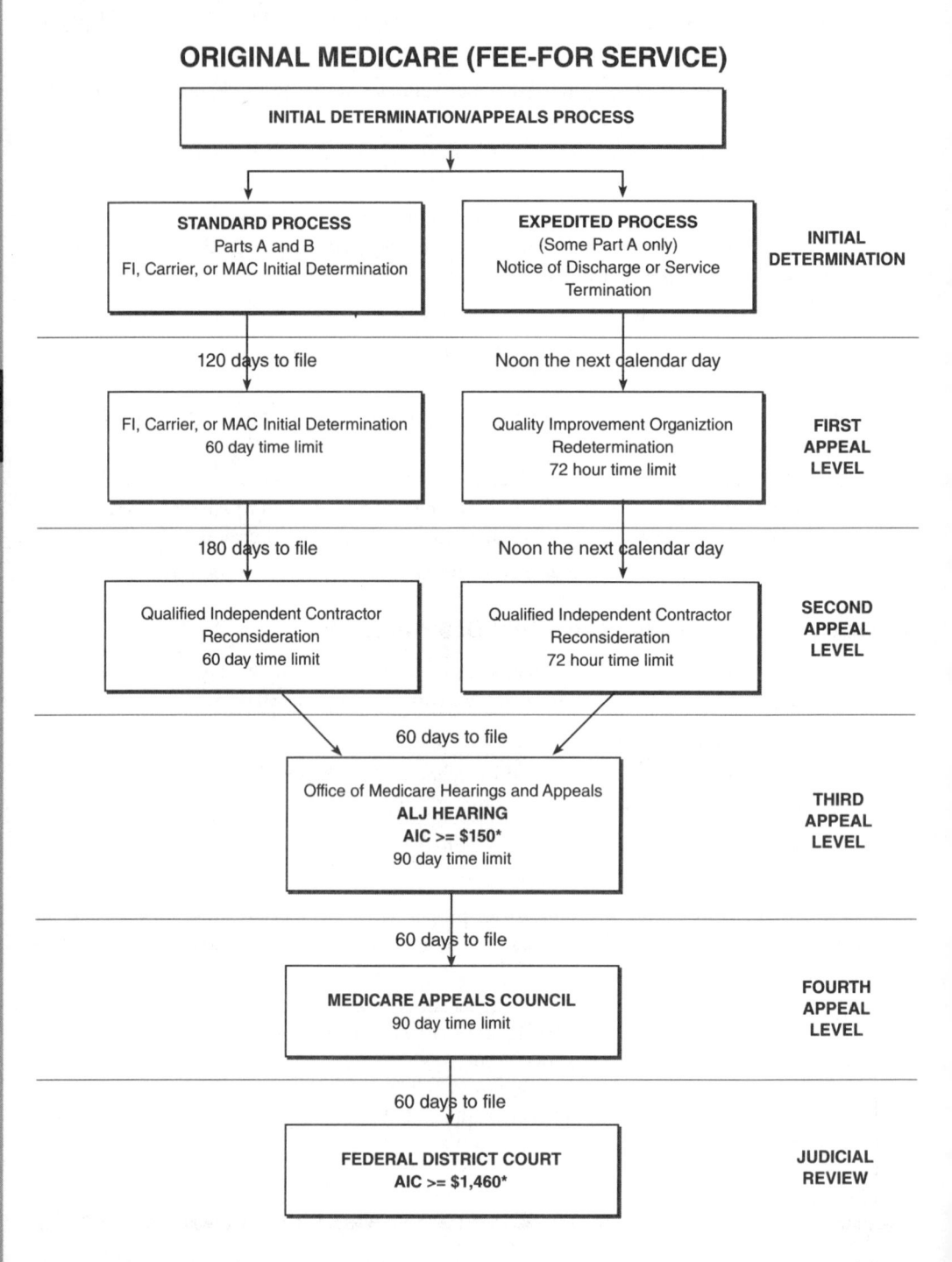

ORIGINAL MEDICARE (FEE-FOR SERVICE)

INITIAL DETERMINATION/APPEALS PROCESS

INITIAL DETERMINATION
- STANDARD PROCESS — Parts A and B — FI, Carrier, or MAC Initial Determination
- EXPEDITED PROCESS — (Some Part A only) — Notice of Discharge or Service Termination

FIRST APPEAL LEVEL
- 120 days to file → FI, Carrier, or MAC Initial Determination — 60 day time limit
- Noon the next calendar day → Quality Improvement Organiztion Redetermination — 72 hour time limit

SECOND APPEAL LEVEL
- 180 days to file → Qualified Independent Contractor Reconsideration — 60 day time limit
- Noon the next calendar day → Qualified Independent Contractor Reconsideration — 72 hour time limit

THIRD APPEAL LEVEL
- 60 days to file → Office of Medicare Hearings and Appeals — **ALJ HEARING** — AIC >= $150* — 90 day time limit

FOURTH APPEAL LEVEL
- 60 days to file → **MEDICARE APPEALS COUNCIL** — 90 day time limit

JUDICIAL REVIEW
- 60 days to file → **FEDERAL DISTRICT COURT** — AIC >= $1,460*

AIC = Amount In Controversy
ALJ = Adminstrative Law Judge
FI = Fiscal Intermediary
MAC = Medicare Administrative Contractor

*The AIC requirement for an ALJ hearing and Federal District Court is adjusted annually in accordance with the medical care component of the consumer price index. The chart reflects the amounts for calendar year (CY) 2015.

TRANSFER OF APPEAL RIGHTS (FOR NON-ASSIGNED CLAIMS)

The *Transfer of Appeal Rights* form (#CMS-20031) allows you to pursue payment through the appeals process. Keep each completed form on file. The form includes a second page with patient information.

Note: When the provider makes the appeal, they give up the right to bill the patient for that claim if their appeal fails. The patient is still responsible for any deductibles or coinsurance.

See Resource 240 for a full-size version of this form, with instructions.

Redetermination and Reconsideration

Step 1. Redetermination

After the initial determination and denial, the Redetermination review process is performed by your contractor. Your request must be submitted in written form. Your MAC generally makes a decision within 60 days from the time they receive your request. This decision will be in the form of a letter, Medicare Summary Notice (MSN), or Remittance Advice (RA).

File the *Medicare Redetermination Request Form* (#CMS-20027) with your Medicare Administrative Contractor (MAC) within 120 days of their **initial determination**. Be sure to attach all evidence if you check item #14 on the form.

See Resource 241 for a full-size version of this form, with instructions.

TROUBLE SHOOTING BY USING THE EOMB

One of the most valuable tools available to a practice for the reimbursement process is the Explanation of Medicare Benefits (EOMB) or payment report. The effectiveness of the entire billing process can be monitored by carefully reading these forms. If the claims in your practice are consistently being down-coded, bundled, or denied as medically unnecessary or unreasonable, you could be on the road to an audit. Corrective action in the practice can prevent many of these types of denials.

Additionally, contact the patient and ask what reasons were given to him/her for the denial. There are different standards about what information goes to the patient and what goes to the provider. You may find out information that can help you in the appeal process.

CHECKLIST FOR SUBMITTING A REDETERMINATION

Correspondence should include the items on the following checklist. Keep a checked copy with the *Redetermination Request Form* in the patient record for easy reference.

- A cover letter explaining why the Redetermination is being requested. However, according to Claims Processing Manual, Chapter 29, Section 310.1(B)(2), you do not need a letter if you use form CMS-20027.
- A copy of the claim and a copy of the remittance notice, or EOMB, as evidence of prior payment or denial.
- The patient's name and Medicare number.
- The Health Insurance Claim (HIC) or claim control number for the claim in question (circle this number on the remittance number or EOMB).
- The date of service for the claim in question.
- The physician provider number (NPI) and that of the organization (if applicable).

Tip: Frequently, the primary reason for denial is that Medicare does not consider the care to be "medically reasonable or necessary". In this situation, your appeal letter and supporting documents should clearly indicate **your** rationale for medical necessity.

SUPPORTING DOCUMENTATION

In addition to the above, include supporting documentation. Highlight information that you want to be considered. The goal is to support your position in reversing the original determination. You will want to enclose the patient's medical history, examination findings, documentation of severity or acute onset, radiology reports, test results, treatment plans, consultation reports, referral requests and reports, and/or copies of communication between provider and patient, as well as the daily notes. The submission of the Electronic Health Record (EHR) can assist in this process if your Medicare Administrative Contractor (MAC) is able to receive it. If you use handwritten notes or use your own style of shorthand or abbreviations, it is appropriate to transcribe and/or translate your notes before submitting them for review. You cannot add information but can interpret the information that is there into a more readable format. Be sure to include copies of the originals along with the transcribed information.

Tip: When making copies of records, if different colored ink is utilized by the provider for documentation and it is necessary for accurate interpretation, you should make color copies.

For more information on documentation and the EHR, see page D-8 in *Section D–Documentation*.

SIGNATURE REQUIREMENTS

The only acceptable signatures are:

- handwritten (this is defined as a mark or sign by an individual on a document to signify knowledge, approval, acceptance, or obligation),
- electronic,
- digital,
- facsimiles of original written signature,
- and/or digitized.

Do not use "Signature on File" or a stamp signature. If the signatures are not legible, or if you used initials, be sure to include a signature log which could also include an attestation statement. Additionally, if you have **not** signed your notes, be sure to include an attestation statement. See the CMS "Medicare Program Integrity Manual" (Pub. 100-08), Chapter 3, Section 3.3.2.4.C for guidance on attestation statements.

Step 2. Reconsideration

Reconsiderations are processed by Qualified Independent Contractors (QICs). File the *Medicare Reconsideration Request* form (#CMS-20033) with the QIC within 180 days of your local Medicare Administrative Contractor (MAC)'s Redetermination denial. Use the Medicare Reconsideration Form and be sure to review the Checklist for Submitting a Redetermination in Step 1. Evidence submitted should include a clear explanation of why you disagree with the redetermination, a copy of the MRN and any other useful documentation. This is the last level at which you can submit new evidence to reinforce your case.

Additional documentation submitted at this step could increase the time allotted for the QIC to make a decision.

See Resource 242 for a full-size version of this form, with instructions.

Sample: *Medicare Reconsideration Request Form*

Clinical Review Judgment

Clinical Review Judgment impacts all physicians, providers, and suppliers who provide services to Medicare beneficiaries and then bill Medicare contractors.

As a result of CR 6954, Section 3.14 (Clinical Review Judgment) has been added to the Medicare Program Integrity Manual. Medicare claim review contractors must now instruct their clinical review staffs to use clinical review judgment when making complex review determinations about a claim.

Clinical review judgment involves two steps:

1. The synthesis of all submitted medical record information (e.g. progress notes, diagnostic findings, medications, nursing notes, etc.) to create a longitudinal clinical picture of the patient; and
2. The application of this clinical picture to the review criteria to determine whether the clinical requirements in the relevant policy have been met.

This is very important to doctors of chiropractic, because previously, auditors could demand certain records that had very little to do with the patient's progress. Further, reviewers could choose to ignore submitted records that demonstrated positive outcome. Now, "all submitted medical record information" must be considered in determining if the treatment goals have been met.

You can find more information about clinical review judgment by going to CR 6954, located at www.cms.gov/Transmittals/downloads/R338PI.pdf on the Centers for Medicare & Medicaid Services (CMS) website.

Hearings and Reviews

If there is not satisfaction at levels one and two of your appeals, you can advance through these last three steps. Please note that these reviewers cannot review any new evidence, but only review the evidence which was submitted to the QIC (Level 2). At this level, it may be wise to retain the services of a qualified healthcare attorney to assist with this process.

> If you advance to these final levels of appeal, see Resource 243 for more information and forms.

Step 3. Hearing by an Administrative Law Judge (ALJ)

If after Step 2, the disputed amount is at least $150 (for 2015), you may request an ALJ hearing within 60 days of receipt of the reconsideration decision. Use the *Request for a Medicare Hearing by an Administrative Law Judge* form. The ALJ is employed by the Social Security Administration and not CMS/Medicare. Only the documentation from the second level (Reconsideration) and the law is considered. Detailed instructions regarding this step are included in the reconsideration decision letter.

> See Resource 244 for a full-size version of this form, with instructions.

> See Resource 245 for additional information about the ALJ level of appeal.

Sample: *Request for a Medicare Hearing by an Administrative Law Judge (ALJ)*

Step 4. Review by the Medicare Appeals Council (MAC)

The Departmental Appeal Board (DAB), also known as the Medicare Appeals Council, provides the final review by the Social Security Administration. The purpose of the DAB review is to correct any errors that might be made by the ALJ in Step 3. Use the *Request for Review of Administrative Law Judge (ALJ) Medicare Decision/Dismissal* form to submit your request.

> See Resource 246 for a full-size version of this form, with instructions.

Sample: *Request for Review of Administrative Law Judge (ALJ) Medicare Decision/Dismissal*

Step 5. Review by a Federal District Court

This Federal judicial review is the final step in the appeals process. Its mission is to correct any errors by the Social Security Administration's hearing and review. To request a review, follow the instructions in the MAC decision letter from Step 4.

> See Resource 247 to review the official CMS instructions regarding Medicare Appeals.

Medicare "Advantage" Part C Appeals

Medicare Advantage is the beneficiary option for a traditional fee-for-service (FFS) plan. Providers and patients who participate in these entities have the same rights as if they were in the traditional Part B plans. Accordingly, Medicare appeal rights are included in these programs too.

Late Filing Exceptions

As a general rule, providers have one year from the date of service to file a claim. However, it should be noted that there are exceptions to the rule. The Medicare Claims Processing Manual (Section 240, Chapter 29) outlines the general procedure for establishing any unusual **good cause** for late filing.

> See also "Timely Filing" on page E-5 of S*ection E–Claims and Appeals*.

Review: Medicare Appeals
■ What is a "reopening"? How much time is allowed for a reopening? *C-37*
■ What are the five steps for Medicare Appeals? *C-37*
■ In 2012, what percent of claims appealed were found to be in the providers favor? *C-37*
■ How must a redetermination be submitted? *C-39*
■ Which steps must be taken in a clinical review judgment? *C-42*
■ How many days do you have to request an ALJ hearing? *C-42*
■ What is the function of the DAB? *C-42*

5. Physician Quality Reporting System

PQRS

The American health care system offers millions of patients access to high-quality care, but at times the system is marked by serious and pervasive deficiencies in quality.

Quality problems affect patients of all ages, gender, financial status and race, and occur across all delivery systems and payment systems. Such deficiencies result in increased mortality and morbidity, lead to a lower quality of life and a less productive workforce while incurring billions of dollars in unnecessary costs. However, advances in the science of quality measurement, improvements in health information systems, and increases in our understanding of how to effect change in clinical practice, now present unprecedented opportunities for improvement. Health care consumers, purchasers, and providers all have an interest in building capacity for quality improvement and measurement.

The Physician Quality Reporting System (PQRS) of the Centers for Medicare and Medicaid Services (CMS) is one step in a continuing effort to improve health care. This system currently includes an incentive payment for eligible professionals (EPs) who satisfactorily report on quality measures for covered professional services furnished to Medicare beneficiaries. Licensed Doctors of Chiropractic who possess a National Provider Identifier (NPI) are recognized as eligible professionals.

Some professionals may be eligible, *but not able* to participate in PQRS due to their billing method. These would be professionals who do not bill Medicare at an individual National Provider Identifier (NPI) level, where the rendering provider's individual NPI is entered on specific line-item services (Item 24J) on either paper or electronic claims.

See Resource 316 for additional information about who is eligible to particpate.

Performance measurement in healthcare is the quantitative assessment of health care processes and outcomes. Eligible professionals (EPs), health care organizations, and/or heath care systems are scored using metrics called performance measures. Performance measures describe a process or outcome of care, in terms of whether, when, or how often it occurs.

Each year, CMS publishes the measures applicable for the upcoming year in the Federal Register. In 2014, there were 285 individual measures and 25 measures groups. Three of those individual measures were available for use by doctors of chiropractic: "Pain Assessment and Follow Up," "Functional Outcome Assessment" and "Preventive Care and Screening: Screening for High Blood Pressure and Follow-Up Documented". For 2015, there are 20 new individual measures, 2 new measures groups, and the deletion of 50 individual measures for a total of 255 individual measures.

Go to ChiroCode.com/PQRS or ACAtoday.org/PQRS for the most current information on performance measurements.

No advance registration is required to participate in the PQRS, but providers need a National Provider Identifier (NPI). To participate in the 2014 PQRS, individual EPs may choose to report information on individual PQRS quality measures or measures groups using the following methods:

1. Medicare Part B Claims
2. Registry
3. Direct Electronic Health Record (EHR): using certified EHR technology (CEHRT)
4. Qualified Clinical Data Registry (QCDR)
5. CEHRT via Data Submission Vendor

> **Alert**: It is important to note that at the time of printing, claims-based reporting is the ONLY method available to DCs to report PQRS measures.

Please note that not all reporting methods are available for all PQRS measures. For example, in 2014, **only the claims-based reporting option** was available for doctors of chiropractic reporting the three PQRS measures applicable to chiropractic services.

In 2014, doctors of chiropractic, considered to be Eligible Professionals (EPs), were required to report satisfactorily on all three individual measures applicable to chiropractic services during the 12-month reporting period (January 1 - December 31, 2014). Through satisfactory reporting, DCs will be able to avoid the 2016 PQRS payment reduction.

See page C-48 for information on determining the status of an EP's PQRS reporting.

> **Alert**: This is actually a situation of potentially great non-monetary benefit to chiropractic. The data gathered by reporting these codes will go far towards validating the long-argued advantages of chiropractic care.

See Resource 317 for additional information, articles and webinars.

Payment Adjustments

The Patient Protection and Affordable Care Act (PPACA) changed this previously voluntary program to a mandatory one for Medicare and Medicaid programs. At this time, Medicaid does not allow reporting all of the measures that Medicare allows. The bonus only continued through 2014. From here on, payment adjustments (penalties) will be assessed for providers who did not successfully and satisfactorily report data on quality measures for covered professional services two years prior. For example, if you did not successfully and satisfactorily report on PQRS quality measures in 2013, you will be assessed a penalty in 2015. Further, if you did not successfully and satisfactorily report on PQRS quality measures in 2014, you will be assessed the penalty in 2016, and so on.

The following penalty structure will be assessed through a reduction in the base payment amount for providers who do not successfully/satisfactorily report PQRS quality measure data:

- 2015 = 1.5% penalty based on participation in 2013. Providers will be paid at 98.5% of the fee schedule.
- 2016 and after = 2.0% penalty based on participation in 2014. Providers will be paid at 98% of the fee schedule.

See Resource 318 for additional information about payment adjustments.

Certification Bonus

Another provision of the PPACA is the introduction of the Maintenance of Certification Program (MOC or MOCP). As of 2014, the MOC did not apply to doctors of chiropractic because they are not included on the Qualified Maintenance of Certification Program Incentive Entities for 2014. It is included here for informational purposes because it is part of the PQRS program.

Providers eligible for PQRS are also eligible for an additional 0.5% bonus if all the following conditions are met:

- Be a board-certified physician and satisfactorily report PQRS measures for the specified reporting year.
- Participate in a Maintenance of Certification Program (MOC) more frequently than is required to qualify for or maintain board certification (at least once more).
- Successfully completed a qualified MOC practice assessment.

See Resource 323 for further information about the MOC.

Value Based Modifier (VBM)

Beginning in 2015, CMS is phasing in a new program to assess the quality of care furnished by providers as well as the cost of that care. This program represents a shift from the current payment methodology to a performance-based reimbursement model where **both** participating and non-participating providers will be required to demonstrate higher quality care at a lower cost with better patient satisfaction.

This program will begin with large groups (those with more than 100 eligible professionals (EPs). By 2017, all EPs will be affected by this modifier. For practices with fewer than 10 EPs, beginning in 2017, payments may be either increased or decreased by up to 2% depending on how well they meet the quality-tiering methodology, which is used for evaluating performance on quality and cost measures. At the time of publication, there was a proposed rule to change the maximum payment adjustment percentage from 2% to 4%.

Payment adjustments based on this modifier are in addition to the PQRS payment adjustments.

Alert: Because the VBM is largely based on PQRS reporting, this means that when the adjustments begin in 2017, it will be based on an EPs PQRS reporting during the 2015 calendar year. Therefore, if you have not done so already, we encourage you to begin implementing PQRS now in order to successfully demonstrate value before this program begins for smaller practices.

- See Resource 324 for information by CMS on value based modifiers.
- See Resource 325 to review additional information including the quality-tiering methodology.

Measure Applicability Validation (MAV)

Claims and registry based reporting are subject to a Measure Applicability Validation (MAV) if less than nine measures are reported. Providers using the other reporting options (Direct EHR, CEHRT via Data Submission Vendor) do not need to worry about this validation process. As part of this process, Clusters of Clinically Related Measures are used to determine relationships between measures. In 2014, a chiropractic cluster was added to the MAV process which means that claims are reviewed to see if additional measures should have been reported by the provider, but were not. For example, if measure #131 was reported, then measure #182 is also expected to be reported by doctors of chiropractic.

- See Resource 319 for a helpful 2014 MAV process flowchart created by CMS to help EPs determine if they were meeting the requirements for claims based reporting.
- See Resource 320 to take CMS's online MAV Training course.

About Performance Measurement (PM) Codes

As a result of PQRS, special codes have been created in the HCPCS code set to report Performance Measurement (PM) services and events. The intent of these codes is to facilitate the collection and reporting of evidence-based performance measures at the time of service, rather than from labor intensive retrospective chart reviews.

These codes are not intended as a replacement for CPT Category I codes, (all numeric), nor are these codes required for all billing situations. Proper use of these codes can **help to establish standards** and promote evidence-based best practices. Accordingly, no RVUs or fees are associated with these information codes which are updated each January 1st and July 1st.

Performance Measurement Codes for Chiropractic

Although there are hundreds of Performance Measurement (PM) services and events, three could be reported by doctors of chiropractic for the 2014 reporting year:

Measure #131 Pain Assessment and Follow Up

Measure #182 Functional Outcome Assessment

Measure #317 Preventive Care and Screening: Screening for High Blood Pressure and Follow-Up Documented

> **Alert**: At the time of publication, the 2015 PQRS measurements have not been released. Visit the ChiroCode Institute or the ACA website for the most current information.
>
> Go to ChiroCode.com/PQRS or ACAtoday.org/PQRS for any updates to performance measurement codes or information.

Claims Based Reporting Example

If you participate in the PQRS program, measures which are reported via submitted claims need to use the required CPT code and its applicable "G-code". As a reminder, in 2014, DCs were required to report on the three applicable measures for at least half of their Medicare patients treated with spinal CMT and CPT code 98940, 98941, or 98942 was reported on the claim form.

> **Reminder**: PQRS measures and their associated G-codes are updated every year. The codes listed in the example below were the appropriate PQRS G-codes for the 2014 reporting period, which ended on December 31, 2014.

To demonstrate how claims based reporting works, we will use 2014 information. Each measure has several G-codes, one for each possible finding that relates to the measure. For example, in 2014, for Measure #131—Pain Assessment and Follow Up, there were these six G-codes:

G8442 Pain assessment NOT documented as being performed, documentation the patient is not eligible for a pain assessment using a standardized tool

G8509 Pain assessment documented as positive using a standardized tool, follow-up plan not documented, reason not given

G8730 Pain assessment documented as positive using a standardized tool AND a follow-up plan is documented

G8731 Pain assessment using a standardized tool is documented as negative, no follow-up plan required

G8732 No documentation of pain assessment, reason not given

G8939 Pain assessment documented as positive, follow-up plan not documented, documentation the patient is not eligible

The appropriate G-code is to be included on line 24 in a paper 1500 claim form, and on service line 24 on an electronic 1500 claim. When reporting performance codes, use a charge of either $0.00 or $0.01, depending on payer and/or billing software requirements. CMS strongly encourages providers to use $0.01 instead of $0.00.

2014 Example:

D. PROCEDURES, SERVICES, OR SUPPLIES (Explain Unusual Circumstances) CPT/HCPCS	MODIFIER	E. DIAGNOSIS POINTER	F. $ CHARGES
98940			120 00
G8730			0 01

REMITTANCE ADVICE CODES

Reviewing your Remittance Advice (RA)/Explanation of Benefits (EOB) can show if submitted codes are valid for the current PQRS reporting year. Until July 1, 2014, denial code N365 was used to indicate the validity of 2014 PQRS codes submitted. However, in an effort to streamline reporting of quality data codes across multiple quality programs, CMS deactivated this remittance advice code.

Effective April 1, 2014, EPs who bill on a $0.00 Quality Data Code (QDC) line item will receive the N620 code. EPs who bill on a $0.01 QDC line item will receive the CO 246 N572 code.

Verification of PQRS Reporting Status

How does a provider know if they have reported all the expected quality measures necessary in order to successfully participate in PQRS? CMS makes this determination based on the codes listed in the individual quality measures. It is up to the provider to verify their status by reviewing the individual quality measurement data and by reviewing published reports.

Interim status reports are available through the PQRS Dashboard, which allows eligible professionals to log-in to a web-based tool and access interim PQRS data on a quarterly basis in order to monitor the status of claims-based individual measures. Please note the Dashboard does **not** provide final data analysis for full-year reporting or indicate PQRS incentive eligibility. The Dashboard will only provide claims-based data for interim feedback.

Quarterly interim feedback reports are available for every Taxpayer Identification Number (TIN) for which at least one eligible professional (identified by his/her NPI) reported at least one valid PQRS measure during the reporting period.

See Resource 326 to access the secure PQRS portal. Use the PQRS Verify Report tool to access reports. User guides are also available.

Unlike interim reports, PQRS Final Feedback Reports are issued by the A/B MAC for each provider upon request and are based on provider participation the previous year. Individuals must request a report based on their NPI number. If your practice is part of a group, you must request reports individually. PQRS feedback reports are made available to providers annually, usually in the fall of the following year (i.e. reports for 2014 should be available around October 2015.) The report will include statistics about how many quality codes you submitted and your reporting success rate.

- See Resource 327 to review detailed information on each individual quality performance measurement for chiropractic.
- See Resource 321 and 322 for answers to commonly asked questions about PQRS.
- The QualityNet help desk is available at 1-866-288-8912 (M-F 7:00 am-7:00 pm, and by email at Qnetsupport@hcqis.org.

Review: PQRS

- What is PQRS and how does it work? *C-44*
- What has been created to report Performance Measurement (PM) services and events? *C-47*
- What were the most appropriate PM codes for doctors of chiropractic in 2014? *C-47*
- On which line of the claim form is the appropriate "G" code inserted? *C-48*

NOTES

D DOCUMENTATION GUIDELINES

1. The Documentation Challenge
Page D-3

2. Record Keeping
Page D-7

3. Assessment Visits
Page D-18

4. Treatment Visits
Page D-28

5. Treatment Plans and Assessments
Page D-33

DOCUMENTATION GUIDELINES

OBJECTIVES

Documentation is the most highly scrutinized component of the Reimbursement Life Cycle, and as such, it should be fully understood and practiced. Documentation establishes the medical necessity of patient care. This section explains what payers and auditors are looking for when they examine records and what providers need to do to maintain compliance. Additionally, the importance of proper treatment plans and assessments in the patient medical record is discussed.

OUTLINE

1. The Documentation Challenge *D-3*
   - About Documentation and Charts *D-3*
   - Review *D-6*

2. Record Keeping *D-7*
   - Standards for Proper Record Keeping *D-7*
   - Abbreviations *D-16*
   - Review *D-17*

3. Assessment Visits *D-18*
   - Documentation Requirements for the Initial Visit *D-18*
   - Review *D-27*

4. Treatment Visits *D-28*
   - Medicare Documentation Requirements for Subsequent Visits *D-29*
   - Transitioning from Active Care *D-31*
   - Review *D-32*

5. Treatment Plans and Assessments *D-33*
   - The Treatment Plan *D-33*
   - Outcomes Assessment *D-43*
   - Review *D-46*

1. The Documentation Challenge

About Documentation and Charts

Years ago, documentation was not submitted to Medicare or other payers. The chances of a medical record becoming a legal document in a malpractice case were minimal. Since most patient records were only seen by the doctor and staff, documentation was done with the assumption that no one else needed to understand the examination notes. No standards existed for recording patient information.

Times have changed dramatically. Documentation is now a critical component in both the Reimbursement Life Cycle and as evidence of care for medical malpractice cases.

When it comes to the Reimbursement Cycle, documentation is the recording of pertinent facts and observations about a patient's health history and physical examination of the system(s) applicable to the current encounter. It includes testing, decision making, treatment planning, treatment, and outcomes assessment. If third-party reimbursement is needed, a claim is submitted for each patient encounter.

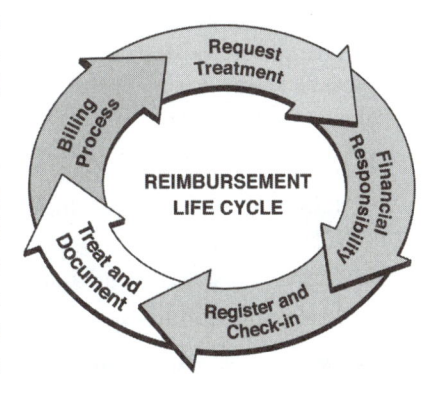

Additionally, the entire third party insurance payer industry, including government and private enterprises, uses the health care record to determine whether they consider the services on the submitted claims to be medically necessary.

To summarize, the medical record performs several functions. Not only does it support medical necessity, support insurance billing and reduce your exposure to audits, it also reduces medical errors and professional liability exposure, facilitates claims review, provides clinical data for both education and research, promotes continuity of care among providers, serves as a measure of patient safety, and demonstrates quality of care.

See Resource 365 for the latest information, webinars and articles on documentation.

See *Section B–Insurance and Reimbursement* for more about claims submission requirements.

ACA Documentation Section Disclaimer: The American Chiropractic Association has developed a comprehensive Clinical Documentation Manual (3rd edition) apart from the ChiroCode DeskBook. The ChiroCode Documentation section refers to the ACA Clinical Documentation Manual (3rd edition), where appropriate, for additional examples and clarification which illustrate ACA's current and official policies and opinions regarding Documentation.

The Role of Medical Necessity

Medicare defines **medical necessity** as services or items reasonable and necessary for the diagnosis or treatment of illness or injury, or to improve the functioning of a malformed body member. Consequently, the medical record became the vital determining factor when assessing what is medically reasonable and necessary.

Although this definition from Medicare sounds like a hard and fast rule, keep in mind that there are almost as many versions of "medical necessity" as there are payers, laws, and courts to interpret them. Generally speaking, most definitions incorporate the principle of providing services which are "reasonable and necessary" or "appropriate" in light of clinical standards of practice in one's medical community. The lack of objectivity inherent in these terms often leads to widely varying interpretations by physicians and payers, which in turn can result in the care provided not meeting the payer definition of necessity. Last, but not least, the decision as to whether the services were medically necessary was often made by a payer's reviewer, who had never seen the patient.

CMS/Medicare began determining medical necessity, and correct billing practices by providers, by requiring its Medicare Administrative Contractors (MACs) to perform current and postpayment reviews. These reviews checked claims against chart documentation to ensure that dollars spent were administered appropriately.

If a payer determines that services were medically unnecessary after payment has been made, it is treated as an overpayment, for which payments are demanded to be refunded immediately and with interest. Moreover, if a pattern of claims appears to demonstrate that the healthcare provider knows, or should have known, that the services were not medically necessary, they may also face allegations of fraud which can include large monetary penalties and/or exclusion from government programs such as Medicare. Additionally, criminal prosecution could be considered.

See Resource 365 for the latest information, webinars and articles on documentation.

See *Section F–Compliance and Audit Protection* for more information about other fraud concerns beyond documentation.

Did It Really Happen?

"If it is not documented it did not happen" has been used for years by payers for denial purposes. However, from a legal perspective it could have happened. In a recent court case this often used quote was used by the prosecution. The patient and doctor both testified that it did happen. The insurance prosecution lost.

Conclusion: This common myth can be negated/voided in court. However, it's better to document because it can save you future stress, time and legal fees.

The following terms are used interchangeably in this section of the *ChiroCode DeskBook*:
- Clinical and Medical
- Clinical Chart and Medical Record
- Medically Necessary and Clinical Necessity
- Electronic Health Record (EHR) and Electronic Medical Record (EMR)
- Treatment Plans and Care Plans

Chiropractic Services Targeted

The government has been taking a closer look at chiropractic, due to past errors in documentation and coding. This began when the 2004 Comprehensive Error Rate Testing (CERT) program revealed that chiropractic had the highest percentage of errors in claims submitted to Medicare. Despite education initiatives, claims for chiropractic services continues to rank at or near the top of the list for the number of errors among health care professionals. According to the 2013 CERT Annual Improper Payment Report, there was a 51.7% improper payment rate for chiropractic services; 92.5% of those improper payments were due to insufficient documentation.

To properly assess the situation, it is prudent to review the findings of the 2009 report by the Office of the Inspector General (OIG) which found that of the claims studied:

- Forty seven percent were for maintenance care, were not coded properly, or had insufficient documentation to justify the care provided.
- Only 76% of records contained *some* form of treatment plan. Of these 76%:
  - ◆ 43% lacked treatment goals,
  - ◆ 17% lacked objective measures, and
  - ◆ 15% lacked the recommended level of care.

Many of the infractions uncovered by the OIG were focused on the transition point between active care and maintenance care. It has been indicated that part of this problem is that doctors of chiropractic did not document the date services began along with any changes such as new injuries.

This illustrates the reason doctors of chiropractic should be serious about documenting the date of initial service. Keep in mind that payers often have estimates of how long a given illness should require treatment and reviewers are looking for claims which do not meet the payers established criteria or benchmarks. For this reason, it is very important to fully document dates of exacerbation, regression, re-injury, or the occurrence of new injuries which support a continuation of service as active care rather than maintenance care. See Figure 4.1.

See Resource 366 to review the OIG report on Medicare payments.

See Chapter 3–Assessment Visits of this *Documentation* section for more about properly documenting active vs. maintenance care.

FIGURE 4.1
Documentation Errors by Doctors of Chiropractic

Element	Percentage of Documentation Errors by Doctors of Chiropractic
Evaluation: Improper or missing	34%
Diagnosis: Improper or missing	33%
Treatment plan: Insufficient	83%
Medical necessity not shown or miscoded	67%
Contraindications not checked	66%

Figure 4.1 outlines the most prevalent problems as indicated in the comprehensive 2005 OIG report on chiropractic services in the Medicare program. Although the error rate has improved from 94% in 2005 to 52% in 2013, it appears that the same types of problems continue to afflict the documentation of chiropractic services. These national numbers may differ from local levels, so it is helpful to review available local data, where available, to understand the focus of reviewers in your area.

Proper documentation is not just for Medicare. It should be standardized within a practice, regardless of the payer or the type of patient case. Failure to find supporting documentation in the chart is frequently the rationale for medical necessity denials and state board complaints. Therefore, providers must respond with excellent documentation standards.

This section of the *ChiroCode DeskBook* includes information on general medical record standards as well as more specific information for documentation requirement for different types of patient encounters.

How Much Documentation?

Documenting every detail of a service is not necessary, reasonable or practical. The extent of documentation required depends on many factors. The higher the level of service billed, the more detailed the documentation should be. A claim may be denied or downcoded if the documentation is borderline. It is just as important to document routine medical services as it is to document unusual medical services. Even the specialty of the physician providing the services has an effect. A normal "head and neck exam" means different things to an orthopedic surgeon, an otolaryngologist (ear, nose, and throat specialist) and a doctor of chiropractic.

For each service provided, the documentation must support the patient's chief compliant, diagnosis and medical necessity. Additionally, there are two distinct types of chiropractic visits: assessment visits and treatment visits. The purpose of each type of visit is different, and therefore, the requirements for properly documenting each type of visit are also different.

- See Chapter 2–Record Keeping of this *Documentation* section for more about documentation standards.
- See Chapter 3–Assessment Visits of this *Documentation* section for more about documenting assessment and re-assessment visits.
- See Chapter 4–Treatment Visits of this *Documentation* section for more about documentating these types of visits.
- See Chapter 5–Treatment Plans and Assessments of this *Documentation* section for more information about treatment planning and outcomes assessments.

See Resource 367 for a review of the OIG report on Medicare payments.

See Resource 368 for documentation resources available in the ChiroCode Institute online store.

Review: The Documentation Challenge

- What is "Medical Necessity"? *D-4*
- According to the OIG and CERT, what are the main reasons for improper payments to chiropractors? *D-5*
- What are the two types of office visits for doctors of chiropractic? Are the recording requirements different for each? *D-6*

2. Record Keeping

STANDARDS FOR PROPER RECORD KEEPING

The medical record/patient chart should have already begun to be organized during "Step 3. Registration," as part of the *Reimbursement Lifecycle* (see page B-13). This chapter identifies general record keeping standards and guidelines relevant to either electronic or paper records. Specific requirements for the different types of visits (assessment vs. treatment) are covered in their own chapters.

Benefits of a Well-Organized Chart

In this era of value-based health care, doctors of chiropractic are held accountable by payers and the patient for clinical outcomes. As such, practitioners are stewards and co-authors of the patient's clinical record.

A well-organized chart enhances the ability of anyone reviewing the record to rapidly assess the present status of the patient's care with a high degree of accuracy in a matter of seconds. It demonstrates the practitioner's ability to give effective care in an appropriate and timely manner. It demonstrates to the healthcare community that we use (and speak the language of) quality records. It provides the rationale for prompt, fair payment, and the justification for extended care when needed. It is the precursor to being prepared for effective appeals if denied.

Organizing the Chart

The objective in chart organization is to create a picture of the chiropractic-appropriate care the patient has received from the presentation of their initial problem through every patient encounter and treatment session. Anyone reviewing the chart should be able to quickly understand your logic and the course of treatment(s). Reports should be filed in chronological order. When outside reports are received, acknowledge that you have reviewed them with your initials and the date. In addition to maintaining all pertinent clinical data, the patient's chart also has

---

Do it Once – But Do it Correctly

It is preferable to complete your daily chart for each patient while in the treatment room because that is the best time to accurately recall pertinent case information. Avoid doing only partial charting during the patient encounter and then waiting until the end of the day to finish. It is like waiting for a "root canal" at the end of each day. Psychologically you know that if you get five more patients, your "root canal" is just that much longer at the end of the day. Stalling the documentation diminishes your incentive to grow your practice and the accuracy of your records.

associated financial and other supporting data (e.g., forms for patient registration, assignment, authorizations, releases, consent to treat, HIPAA privacy, etc.).

Electronic Health Record (EHR)

What is an Electronic Health Record? Simply stated, an EHR refers to storing patient information in a way that keeps it private, and allows the information to be shared easily with others who may need it to perform their functions, such as third party payers or consulting practitioners.

These systems often help providers create more thorough documentation; however, with this benefit comes an increased caution about "canned" or "cloned" records. Clinical documentation should reflect each patient encounter independently, and no two encounters are exactly alike. Thus, the notes for two separate visits should not be exactly alike, unless they completely and accurately describe the encounter.

In spite of many doctors' desire to "keep things simple" by avoiding electronic patient record keeping, the option to do so may be expiring. Some states already require such records, and for a time, the federal government attempted to increase quality care standards by offering monetary incentives to providers who adopted certified electronic health record programs. Now, federal programs are beginning to penalize (reduce payments to) providers who do not successfully adopt EHRs. Continuing to use paper records might be compared to using a rotary phone. It might still work, but sooner or later it will become necessary to upgrade in order to continue to do business and maintain profitability.

> See Resource 382 for an article by Noridian regarding chiropractic computer generated documentation.

> See *Section F–Compliance and Audit Protection* for more information about record cloning and other auditor red flags.

FEDERAL EHR PROGRAM

Providers who submit claims to government programs need to be aware of how EHR impacts their practice. The Medicare EHR incentive program offered a limited number of American Recovery & Reinvestment Act of 2009 (AARA) stimulus payments for providers who successfully demonstrate EHR "meaningful use" within their practice. Eligible Professionals (EPs) – this includes all doctors of chiropractic – who adopt a certified EHR according to the EHR Incentive Program requirements and attest to its "meaningful use," were eligible for federal incentives for a limited time.

On August 29, 2014, CMS announced in a final rule that certain providers and eligible professionals are allowed an additional year to meet Stage 2 meaningful use requirements. This final

---

Meaningful Use

Meaningful Use (MU) is achieved when a provider has shown CMS that they are using their EHR in ways that can positively affect the care of their patients. Eligible Professionals must meet all the required objectives, such as recording specified patient data, and establishing patient privacy /security safeguards. There are three stages of meaningful use with varying requirements for each level. A qualified EHR program can help guide providers through the process to ensure that the appropriate steps are taken to attest to meaningful use.

> See Resource 387 for more information by CMS regarding meaningful use.

rule came in response to considerable feedback regarding software vendors having difficulty upgrading their EHR products, receiving certification and upgrading customer's systems in time to meet meaningful use attestation deadlines. Additional announcements in this final rule also allow for the following:

- Providers will be able to attest to meaningful use under the 2014 reporting year definition and use the clinical quality measures from 2013.
- Providers will not be penalized (see the "EHR Penalty" segment below) for failing to move to meaningful use Stage 2 during the 2014 reporting period.
- All eligible providers will be required to use the 2014 edition of certified EHR technology beginning in 2015.
- The Meaningful Use Stage 3 deadline has been delayed from January 1, 2016 to January 1, 2017, giving participants an additional year to meet Stage 2 requirements and take steps toward Stage 3 implementation.
- Meaningful Use Stage 2 reporting period for 2015 is a year-long reporting period. This differs from the 90 day reporting period during any quarter that has previously been allowed.

- See Resource 385 for more about the updated meaningful use timeline.
- See Resource 386 to read the Federal Register announcement.

EHR PENALTY

All Eligible Professionals (EPs) participating in Medicare must successfully demonstrate "meaningful use" of a certified EHR to avoid a reimbursement reduction penalty beginning in 2015. Even though the requirement for Stage 2 meaningful use requirements has been halted, this is not the same thing. If you wish to avoid a penalty in the future, you must begin using EHR and meet meaningful use requirements as indicated above.

Those who first demonstrated meaningful use in 2012 or 2013 must demonstrate meaningful use for a full year in 2014 to avoid payment adjustments in 2016. They must continue to demonstrate meaningful use every year to avoid payment adjustments in subsequent years.

This is an increasing penalty which will be assessed through a reduction in the base payment amount for providers who fail to attest to meaningful use. This must be done every year in order to avoid the following penalties:

- 2015 = 1% penalty. Providers will be paid at 99% of the fee schedule.
- 2016 = 2% penalty. Providers will be paid at 98% of the fee schedule.
- 2017 = 3% penalty. Providers will be paid at 97% of the fee schedule.

A hardship exception exists to avoid these "payment adjustments," but these exceptions are limited to very specific circumstances.

- See Resource 369 for details about the EHR program.
- See Resource 370 for more information about the EHR hardship exemption.
- See Resource 318 for additional information about EHR payment adjustments.

The Problem-Oriented Medical Record (POMR)

The Problem Oriented Medical Record (POMR) is one well-established medical record standard. It is currently the basis of standards used by accrediting organizations such as the National Committee for Quality Assurance (NCQA), the Utilization Review Accreditation Commission (URAC), and the Joint Commission of Accreditation Healthcare Organizations (JCAHO).

The purpose of POMR is to make it easy for anyone reviewing the record to quickly and thoroughly answer some basic questions:

1. Why did the patient begin care?
2. What did the provider find wrong?
3. What did he/she do about it?
4. How did care end?

With an understanding of the key elements and concepts upon which the POMR documentation method is based, the forms used in the charting system may be customized to meet each provider's individual needs. Here are the six elements of the POMR:

1. Complete the problem list with each item dated and numbered.
   - Use the patient's own words whenever possible. For example, when the patient says, "I have headaches and neck pain on the left side," that is the problem list. It is the number one problem because it is the most significant to the patient. Additional problems will be numbered thereafter: 2, 3, 4, etc.
2. Determine the diagnoses for each problem being treated.
3. Establish specific treatment goals for each condition/problem.
   - With three problems, there could be three goals and three clinical end points.
4. Prepare a written Treatment Plan for each active problem.
5. Use the SOAP format for the ongoing treatment(s). It is not necessary to restate all of the initial information in daily notes. The SOAP notes should refer back to each individual complaint, being sure to note progression through the treatment plan toward the previously determined goals.
6. Document the resolution and/or referral dates for each complaint. It should be noted that one problem may resolve while treatment continues for the other problems and thus, a new priority/primary problem may be addressable as patient progresses through care.

SOAP and the POMR

SOAP is an abbreviation for the **S**ubjective data, **O**bjective data, **A**ssessment, and **P**lan. Although SOAP is only 1/6th of POMR, it is an essential part. **It is the heart and body of the chart.** Its

---

A Perfect SOAP Note

There is no such thing as a perfect SOAP note that meets medical necessity requirements. This is because one purpose of a SOAP note (or any documentation) is to communicate what is going on with your patient to someone who is not there. While there are certain elements that should be part of every good SOAP note, it also should be flexible enough to change with the patient. For example, you have three patients who complain of neck pain. Even though their presenting problem is the same, they range from 5 to 85 years of age. Therefore, their documentation should look different. Simplification can be good, but there is a danger in too much simplification. As such, is it unwise to utilize a single 'perfect' SOAP note as a template for all your patients.

format encourages comprehensive records and organization of the notes, with rapid and easy retrieval of information.

The SOAP format was designed for medical doctors (MD) and their practice style. Both an MD and a doctor of chiropractic (DC) assess the patient at the initial visit and "prescribe" the necessary therapy. The difference is that the MD's treatment plan for many medical conditions, including back or neck pain, often consists of prescribing medication and/or home care instructions. Since the patient administers his or her own treatment, there is no treatment encounter to document until the patient returns for a re-assessment. Conversely, a chiropractic treatment plan usually includes a record of the encounters for each treatment delivered, followed by a more thorough record when the patient is reassessed. This difference could suggest a modified use of the SOAP format to better suit the chiropractic paradigm.

Quality Patient Records

Here are points to ponder for better records:

- Maintain one separate chart with a unique medical record number for each patient. Do not use the same record for other family members.
- The patient's name must be on each page or both sides of the page as applicable.
- Anything that relates to the patient encounter should be in the patient record. Remember that from the reviewer's perspective: "If it's not written, it didn't happen."
- Noncompliance with doctor recommendations, missed appointments, displeasure and negative events and reactions must be documented.
- Patient records should tell the complete story of the patient. Can the patient's past and current health concerns be understood by a person seeing the record for the very first time?
- Patient records may provide significant evidence in lawsuits, hearings, or inquests when the care provided is in question. Regardless of the type of assessment or investigation, a good or bad patient record may have a significant positive or negative impact on the outcome of the process.
- Recommendations for home care, exercises, and referrals (to and from other providers) must be documented.
- All recommended tests must have a report in the file.
- If records are handwritten, they must be in blue or black ink. Do not use different colored pens on the same day's notes.
- Only standard abbreviations should be used. If you have developed an individualized style of reporting and documenting using acronyms, you should ensure that a key with your full meaning is readily available (see "Abbreviations" on page D-16).
- All records must be legible. If you, your staff, or colleagues are having difficulty with the legibility of your records, you should consider alternate means of note-taking such as transcription and/or EHRs.
- Each patient encounter must be thoroughly documented.
- Blank spaces may not be used to imply that a test result was normal. Consider using acronyms such as "WNL" for "within normal limits" or "NAD" for "no abnormality detected".
- Entries must be written or dictated within 24 hours of the patient encounter.
- All entries must be dated and signed by the doctor.

Common Errors

Providers need to be aware of the most common documentation errors. Establish procedures to ensure that common errors are avoided. Although not a comprehensive list, here are some common errors to be aware of:

- Illegible records
- Missing dates
- Missing signature
- Missing informed consent
- Missing re-assessment
- Missing patient identifiers
- Missing metrics/objective
- Blanks used to indicate "Within Normal Limits" (WNL)
- Missing legend for abbreviations
- Missing care plan
- Diagnoses that do not support the service(s) rendered

Other Important Considerations

Detailed and thorough documentation should be kept for all patient case types. It is also essential to be aware of and adhere so specific payer guidelines or documentation requirements. Remember that even for non-insurance (cash) patients, your records might be requested for review or reference.

> **Alert**: HIPAA rules mandate that providers must comply with the rules regarding the proper uses and disclosures of Protected Health Information (PHI). For example, if a payer wishes to review records for a patient who is not their client, they must have the required releases in order to view them.
>
> See Chapter 2–HIPAA Compliance in *Section F–Compliance and Audit Protection* for more information about PHI.

Date and Time

Since the medical record is a legal document, a patient encounter is invalid without a date. Time could also be important when reconstructing services provided to a patient on the same date. When recording services in which a time element is in the code description, be sure to record the amount of time spent with the patient for those particular procedures.

Do not leave blank spaces in the chart because this encourages entering information out of order. Information should always be entered in the patient chart chronologically. Results of x-rays or other tests should be entered when received rather than on blank lines left by the date of service information. This practice could give the impression that the physician saw the information at the time of service which creates an inaccurate picture of the patient encounter. If data is pending, make a note in the chart stating that results are expected.

Signatures

The individual who ordered/provided services must be clearly identified in the medical records. Each chart entry must be legible and should include the practitioner's first and last name. For clarification purposes, Medicare recommends you include your applicable credentials (e.g., DC).

The purpose of a provider signature in the medical record is to demonstrate the services have been accurately and fully documented, reviewed and authenticated. Furthermore, it confirms the provider has certified the medical necessity and reasonableness for the service(s) submitted for payment consideration.

MEDICARE REQUIREMENTS FOR VALID SIGNATURES

Acceptable methods of signing records/test orders and findings include:

- Handwritten signature.
- Electronic signatures may be acceptable in several forms:
    - Digitized signature - an electronic image of an individual's handwritten signature reproduced in its identical form using a pen tablet.
    - Electronic signatures (contain date and timestamps and include printed statements, e.g., 'electronically signed by,' or 'verified/reviewed by,') followed by the practitioner's name and preferably a professional designation.
    - Digital signature - an electronic method of a written signature that is typically generated by special encrypted software that allows for sole usage.

UNACCEPTABLE SIGNATURES

The following have been declared unacceptable by Medicare and most third party payers:

- Signature 'stamps' alone in medical records are NO LONGER recognized by Medicare as valid authentication.
- Reports or any records that are dictated and/or transcribed, but do not include valid signatures 'finalizing and approving' the documents are not acceptable.
- Indications that a document has been 'Signed but not read' are not acceptable as part of the medical record.

Electronic Signatures

While EHR may simplify and automate the signature process, be aware that electronic and digital signatures are not the same as "auto-authentication" or "auto-signature" systems, some of which do not mandate or permit the provider to review an entry before signing or do not meet the requirements noted above.

CMS has cautioned that both computer systems and software products (the EHR program) must include protections against modification. Be sure to implement appropriate administrative safeguards which meet state and federal laws. Finally, check with your malpractice insurance regarding their requirements for electronic signatures.

See Resource 371, 372 and 373 for references and exceptions regarding electronic signatures.

Dictation

The growth of EHRs and voice recognition technology are permitting healthcare providers to have instant documentation. As such, dictation is becoming less commonly used in health care offices. For those practices still using this technology, be aware that it may take several days for dictation to be transcribed. The physician must review transcription for accuracy and sign it, and where corrections are necessary, they should be completed before the transcription is put in the patient's chart. Someone must make sure the transcription is placed in the patient's chart, and a summary should be written in the patient's chart in case the dictation or transcription is lost or misfiled.

Computer Generated Notes

There has been a great deal of abuse and misuse of software generated notes and their randomization function. When documentation is worded exactly like or similar to previous entries from visit to visit on a single patient or from patient to patient, it is referred to as cloned documentation. Even though it appears to be related to patient cases, in reality it does not have an accurate story to tell to allied professionals, or to those who may take over a case.

Computer generated notes must be specific to the particular patient on each day of service. Cloned records could lead to claim denials because the notes are not specific enough. They do not demonstrate why services were necessary on each day of service or why they were required by an individual patient. Regional contractors such as Palmetto GBA have warned that if cloned records are detected, it could result in denial of services for lack of medical necessity and recoupment of all overpayments made.

Alternatively, there is the problem of using "spinner" or "random text generator" software to produce "cloned records with a difference." With a spinner, the words flow, with the order switched and synonyms mixed in. In an industry such as chiropractic, where at the end of the day what you do to one patient closely resembles what you will do to the others, spinners save time but could create documentation problems.

Notes should be patient specific for each date of service, and as detailed as possible. Factors that should be taken into account should be:

- Age
- Severity of condition
- Past response to treatment
- Frequency of treatment
- Complicating factors

Again, it is important to demonstrate why the service was necessary on that particular day.

On September 24, 2012, the Department of Health and Human Services (HHS) issued a letter condemning "cloning" software and EHR software which inappropriately up-code documentation. They said, "False documentation of care is not just bad patient care; it is illegal." As a result, they are now more closely scrutinizing medical records.

See Resource 374 to read this letter in its entirety.

Guidelines for Corrections

Sometimes the patient record needs to be corrected. This is acceptable as long as the change is clearly indicated as such, and you date and initial it. A medical record should not be changed if it is subpoenaed for possible legal action. Any alterations at this time could damage the physician's credibility in court. Most attorneys state they would rather defend a physician with no medical record than defend a physician with an inappropriately altered record.

- It is important that corrections only be in the form of additions.
- There must be no erasures, white-out or overwriting on the record, such that the original entry is lost.
- To make additions or corrections to a paper record, draw a single line through inaccurate information to make sure a reviewer can still read it and then sign and date the correction.
- Add omitted information chronologically by the date the information is actually entered in the chart.

- When necessary, attach an addendum with additional information, such as accidentally left out documentation of a procedures step.
- Cross-reference the incorrect and correct entries.

Illustrations

Drawings, illustrations, and pictures may be used when appropriate. These are effective methods of medical shorthand which can quickly and clearly demonstrate the location of a symptom or verify a completed service. Illustrations may be hand-drawn or be commercially purchased illustrations. The chart should include the patient's name, date of birth, medical record number, and date. The physician's signature or initial is an appropriate confirmation.

Subjective Judgments and Statements

Patient medical information should be entered in an unemotional and objective manner. Personal opinion and subjective judgment about the patient or the patient's behavior have no place in the medical record. A patient who is slurring, staggering, and smells of alcohol should not be labeled as intoxicated unless a blood test establishes this fact. As an alternative, describe the patient with objective statements about the way the person speaks, walks, and smells. Some medical conditions are misleading. For example, ketoacidosis, which can occur in patients with diabetes, can cause symptoms similar to intoxication.

Avoid any written or verbal statements which could be interpreted as a guarantee. Use "75 percent of patients see improvement" rather than "the patient should see improvement."

Communications and Unusual Circumstances

All interactions between a patient and staff members (physician, receptionist, other staff) that could potentially affect the patient's care should be recorded in the patient chart. This includes not only patient/staff conversations, but also less obvious interactions such as a staff member overhearing a patient express unwillingness to follow the physician's treatment plan. What may seem like an offhand comment should be recorded because the patient's intent not to follow the physician's instructions has the potential to impact future care. In addition, any unusual circumstance, such as a patient who does not speak English, uses a wheelchair, or is uncooperative, may influence the patient's medical care and therefore should be documented.

Telephone calls between the patient and staff, cancellations, and no shows should also be documented. If there should be a legal action for a bad outcome, the physician will be in a much better position when it can be shown that the patient did not show up for appointments or follow the recommended course of treatment.

ABBREVIATIONS

Utilizing standardized abbreviations can help to lessen the time required to write daily visit notes. The notes need to be readable to any medical professional that should need to review them, so it is wise to limit your abbreviations to those that are common in the health care professions. If you do develop our own set of abbreviations, you need to provide a key.

Common acronyms and abbreviations are listed below:

symbol	meaning
A	assessment
@	at
a. c.	before eating
c̄	with
CC	chief complaint
cm	centimeter
D	day
Disp	disposition
DOB	date of birth
Dx	diagnosis
E/M	evaluation and management
Fx	fracture
HPI	history of present illness
ht	height
HTN	hypertension
Hx	history
ICS	intercostal space
Ⓛ	left
LE	lower extremity
MCL	midclavicular line

symbol	meaning
NKMA	no known medical allergies
p̄	after
P	plan
p. c.	after eating
PE	physical examination
PMHx	past medical history
PMI	point of maximum intensity
PRN	as needed for
Pt	patient
Ⓡ	right
R/O	rule out
ROS	review of systems
s̄	without
SOB	shortness of breath
Sx	sign/symptom
Tx	treatment
UE	upper extremity
WNL	within normal limits
Wt	weight
x̄	except

Descriptive Terms

The following are examples of acceptable descriptive terms, for describing the nature of an abnormality/subluxation.

off-centered	incomplete dislocation	motion:
misalignment	rotation	limited
malpositioning	lithesis:	lost
spacing:	antero	restricted
abnormal	postero	flexion
altered	retro	extension
decreased	lateral	hyper mobility
increased	spondylo	hypomotility
		aberrant

Other terms may be used if they clearly mean bone/joint space, position or motion changes of the vertebral elements. A statement of "pain" is insufficient. The location must be described, and noted if the particular vertebrae is capable of producing the pain in the stated area.

Symptoms should refer to the location:

Spine:	Nerve:	Muscle:
pondylo	neuro	myo
vertebral		
Bone:	Rib:	Joint:
osseo	costo	arthro
osteo	costal	

The symptoms should be reported as type. Such as:

Pain:	Inflammation:	Swelling
algia	itis	Spasticity

Symptoms should then be labeled as outcome/causing, for example:

headaches	hand problems	numbness
arm problems	leg pain	rib pain
shoulder problems	foot pain	

Rib and chest pain must relate to the spine

The precise level of subluxation is made in relation to the part of the spine in which the subluxation is identified. See the Medicare Benefit Policy Manual for the proper names and abbreviations for these spinal areas.

See *Section F–Compliance and Audit Protection* for additional documentation concerns as it relates to audits and reviews.

Review: Record Keeping

- What does EHR mean? *D-8*
- What are the six components of the POMR? *D-10*
- How is an electronic form signed? *D-13*
- What is considered "cloned documentation"? *D-14*
- How may a patient's record be corrected? *D-14*
- What communication with a patient needs to be recorded? *D-15*
- If standard abbreviations are not used, what must your documentation include? *D-16*

3. Assessment Visits

One of the keys to successsul payer communication is to implement protocols in your office that ensure compliance. Properly utilizing these protocols can result in documentation which justifies the medical necessity of care rendered in compliance with Medicare's regulations and those of other payers.

The first assessment, or initial intake visit is a key element to "getting it right." During an assessment visit, information is collected regarding the patient's history and condition through history forms and examinations. The training and professional judgment of a doctor of chiropractic is used to develop a diagnosis and a treatment plan.

The following documentation requirements for the assessment visit would be the same for a medical doctor or doctor of chiropractic: all subjective findings from the patient are noted, all objective test results and observations are recorded, the patient's condition is assessed and noted, a diagnosis is documented, and a plan of treatment is formulated with measurable goals. The findings are then communicated to the patient and treatment is initiated.

- See Chapter 5–Treatment Plans and Assessments in this *Documentation* section for more information about treatment plans.
- See Chapter 6– Physician's Quality Reporting System in this *Documentation* section for the required documentation components of an initial back pain visit.

DOCUMENTATION REQUIREMENTS FOR THE INITIAL ASSESSMENT VISIT

Documentation for the initial assessment visit should clearly identify all of the components for which payers and medical record reviewers are seeking. Make it easy for reviewers by clearly identifying each component. The initial exam documentation should address **all** of the following components:

1. History
   A. Chief Compliant (CC)
   B. History of Present Illness (HPI)
   C. Review of Systems (ROS)
   D. Past, Family, Social History (PFSH) (as applicable)
2. Physical Examination
3. Medical Decision Making (MDM)
4. Treatment Plan – See Chapter 5 of this *Documentation* section.

1. History

A. CHIEF COMPLAINT (CC)

The chief complaint is the patient's stated reason for the encounter. It should be concise and clearly indicate the symptom, problem or condition.

B. HISTORY OF PRESENT ILLNESS (HPI)

The History of Present Illness should be a chronological development of the current condition as it relates to the chief complaint. It is **not** the patient medical history (see D. Past, Family, Social History (PFSH) for medical history). This is the patient's point of view which includes their pain level, perception of function level, etc. The description needs to include all the following:

- Mechanism of trauma
- Quality and character of symptoms/problem
- Onset, duration, intensity, frequency, location and radiation of symptoms
- Aggravating or relieving factors
- Prior interventions, treatments, medication, secondary complaints
- Symptoms causing patient to seek treatment

The symptoms causing the patient to seek treatment should be specific and should be the primary problem of the patient at the time care was sought. If there are secondary problems or chronic problems, they should be listed separately with the same type of information as the primary problem.

For documentation purposes, labeling patient records with each of these subheadings makes it easier for an auditor to identify required elements from either a CMS or CPT guideline perspective.

> **Alert:** According to the Medicare Benefit Policy Manual, chapter 15, paragraph 240.1.2;
>
> "**These symptoms must bear a direct relationship to the level of subluxation**. The symptoms should refer to the spine (spondyle or vertebral), muscle (myo), bone (osseo or osteo), rib (costo or costal) and joint (arthro) and should be reported as pain (algia), inflammation (itis), or as signs such as swelling, spasticity, etc." See page D-23.

The symptoms must be linked to the spine or nervous system in a way that shows that the patient can benefit from chiropractic manipulative therapy.

- Review of medications (as appropriate)
- Review of laboratory and procedure results (if applicable)
- Review of outside consultation reports (if applicable)
- Presenting complaint, including the severity and duration of the symptoms
- Whether this is a new concern or an ongoing/recurring problem
- Changes in the patient's progress or health status since the last visit

> **Alert:** Medicare requires Item #14 of the 1500 claim form to indicate the date the treatment *began*, not the date of the initial occurrence.

Hint: Utilizing the prefixes and suffixes shown in the Medicare documentation could be helpful to reviewers who may be looking for them. See page D-16.

C. REVIEW OF SYSTEMS (ROS)

For E/M services, a review of systems is required. Review of Systems (ROS) should use the Health History Form as a beginning point.

See page H-24 in *Section H–Procedure Codes* for the elements of a ROS.

D. PAST, FAMILY, AND SOCIAL HISTORY (PFSH)

A proper PFSH includes: prior interventions, treatments, medications, secondary complaints.

Medicare Benefit Policy Manual, Chapter 15

240.1.3 – Necessity for Treatment

The patient must have a significant health problem in the form of a neuromusculoskeletal condition necessitating treatment, and the manipulative services rendered must have a direct therapeutic relationship to the patient's condition and provide reasonable expectation of recovery or improvement of function. The patient must have a subluxation of the spine as demonstrated by x-ray or physical exam, as described above.

Most spinal joint problems fall into the following categories:

- Acute subluxation-A patient's condition is considered acute when the patient is being treated for a new injury, identified by x-ray or physical exam as specified above. The result of chiropractic manipulation is expected to be an improvement in, or arrest of progression, of the patient's condition.

- Chronic subluxation-A patient's condition is considered chronic when it is not expected to significantly improve or be resolved with further treatment (as is the case with an acute condition), but where the continued therapy can be expected to result in some functional improvement. Once the clinical status has remained stable for a given condition, without expectation of additional objective clinical improvements, further manipulative treatment is considered maintenance therapy and is not covered.

For Medicare purposes, a chiropractor must place an AT modifier on a claim when providing active/corrective treatment to treat acute or chronic subluxation. However the presence of the AT modifier may not in all instances indicate that the service is reasonable and necessary. As always, contractors may deny if appropriate after medical review.

A. Maintenance Therapy

Maintenance therapy includes services that seek to prevent disease, promote health and prolong and enhance the quality of life, or maintain or prevent deterioration of a chronic condition. When further clinical improvement **cannot reasonably be expected** from continuous **ongoing care,** and the chiropractic treatment **becomes supportive** rather than corrective in nature, the **treatment** is then considered **maintenance therapy.** The AT modifier must not be placed on the claim when maintenance therapy has been provided. Claims without the AT modifier will be considered as maintenance therapy and denied. Chiropractors who give or receive from beneficiaries an ABN shall follow the instructions in Pub. 100-04, Medicare Claims Processing Manual, chapter 23, section 20.9.1.1 and include a GA (or in rare instances a GZ) modifier on the claim.

Past Health History

This includes general health, prior illness, injuries, hospitalizations, medications or surgeries. This is important to identify any possible contraindications. This information is best obtained when the patient first arrives.

According to AMA guidelines, a past history should include significant information regarding:

- Prior major illness and injuries
- Prior operations
- Prior hospitalizations
- Current medications
- Allergies (eg, drug, food)
- Age appropriate immunization status
- Age appropriate feeding/dietary status

When the patient first enters the office, you need to obtain basic information on a medical history form. According to the Medicare manual, you should obtain:

- Social history (not required but advisable)
- Ongoing/recurring health concerns (as appropriate)
- Patient risk factors (as appropriate)

Family History (As Applicable)

For the Family History, only include any relevant family history as it relates to the patient condition or chiropractic care. The following may be noted:

- health status or cause of death of parents, siblings, and children
- specific diseases related to problems identified in the Chief Complaint or History of the Present Illness, and/or Systems Review
- diseases of family members that may be hereditary or place the patient at risk

---

Alert: The initial history requirements for Medicare patients are organized differently than the history that is mandated by the CPT codebook and the 1997 CMS documentation guidelines. Failure to document any of these items may result in repayment of funds to Medicare for all services.

- Chief complaint/symptoms causing patient to seek treatment
- Family history if relevant
- Past health history (general health, prior illness, injuries, hospitalizations, medications and surgical history)
- Mechanism of trauma
- Quality and character of symptoms/problem
- Onset, duration, intensity, frequency, location and radiation of symptoms
- Aggravating or relieving factors
- Prior interventions, treatments, medications, secondary complaints

Social History

The social history requirements for E/M services are revised for 2015. A social history includes significant information regarding

- Marital status and/or living arrangements
- Current employment
- Occupational history
- Military history
- Use of drugs, alcohol, and tobacco
- Level of education
- Sexual history

Medical and Health History Form

The *Medical and Health History* form covers these areas and a brief social history.

See Resource 144 for a full-size version of this form, with instructions.

2. **Physical Examination**

The physical examination needs to closely mirror the chief complaint(s). Limit the exam to only those areas required to objectively assess the chief complaint. This is what the doctor can measure, as objectively as possible. Medicare, and most other payers, classify the spine into 5 areas: neck, back (thoracic), low back, pelvic, and sacral. The exam should include the following:

See Chapter 2–Evaluation and Management in *Section H–Procedure Code*s for all the elements required to code a physicial examination.

- Range of motion, level of muscle spasm, performance relative to neurological and orthopedic testing, and whatever else is an objective finding. Orthopedic tests, reflexes, and pin prick sensitivity tests are primarily for the purpose of ruling out pathological processes. The range of motion and muscle strength tests are primarily for functional assessment of the area of the spine being tested. Range of motion testing is where changes in sectional mobility are noted for P.A.R.T. (Pain, Asymmetry/misalignment, Range of motion abnormality, and Tissue/tone changes).

    See the segment "Evaluation of Musculoskeletal/Nervous System Through Physical Exam" on the following page for more about P.A.R.T.

- Relevant vital signs.

medicare

- Physical examination, focusing on the presenting complaint. Palpation is the manual inspection of the area of the spine indicated in the complaint. This is where the pain/tenderness, asymmetry/misalignment, changes in segmental mobility, tissue, and tone changes are noted for P.A.R.T.
- Positive physical findings.
- Significant negative physical findings as they relate to the problem.

> **Audit Alert:** Auditors check closely for how well the exam mirrors the chief complaint. It is a red flag to examine areas that are not considered medically relevant.

Evaluation of Musculoskeletal/Nervous System Through Physical Exam

The physical examination is a critical component to the initial documentation requirements. For Medicare purposes, a subluxation may be demonstrated by either an x-ray or by a physical examination using the P.A.R.T. criteria (Pain, Asymmetry/misalignment, Range of motion abnormality, and Tissue/tone changes). The P.A.R.T. is simply a list of those items that are to be identified during the palpation portion of the physical examination. Two of the four criteria are required, one of which must be Asymmetry/misalignment or Range of motion abnormality. It should be noted that this thinking could ignore two critical elements: the standard of care and necessity of diagnosis.

Use the outcomes assessment questionnaires to gauge the functional ability of the patient as a whole and to assess progress. This is a key element of the treatment plan and should be utilized with all patients, not just Medicare patients.

Standard of Care: Standard of Care is the benchmark used to evaluate and guide the practice of medicine encompassing the learning, skill and clinical judgment ordinarily possessed and used by providers of good standing in similar circumstances. Standard of Care is defined as "that course of action that a reasonably prudent [physician] in the defendant's specialty would have taken under the same or similar circumstances." -Washington v. Washington Hospital Center, 579 A2d 177 (DC App 1990).

Necessity of Diagnosis: The other consideration is the necessity of diagnosis. Essentially, these are the tests, signs and observations, both subjective and objective, that are needed to properly formulate a diagnosis. For example, if you do not have lumbar series x-rays and a written x-ray report that states disc thinning, you cannot justify a diagnosis of 722.52–Degeneration of

---

Medicare Benefit Policy Manual, Chapter 15

240.1.2 – Subluxation May Be Demonstrated by X-Ray or Physician's Exam
B3-2251.2

Subluxation is defined as a motion segment, in which alignment, movement integrity and/or physiological function of the spine are altered although contact between joint surface remains intact.

A subluxation may be demonstrated by an x-ray or by physical examination, as described below:

1. **Demonstrated by X-Ray**

    An x-ray may be used to document subluxation. The x-ray must have been taken at a time reasonably proximate to the initiation of a course of treatment. Unless more specific x-ray evidence is warranted, an x-ray is considered reasonably proximate if it was taken not more than 12 months prior to or 3 months following the initiation of a course of Chiropractic treatment. In certain cases of chronic subluxation (eg, scoliosis), an older x-ray may be accepted provided the beneficiary's health record indicates the condition is permanent. A previous CT scan and/or MRI is acceptable evidence if a subluxation of the spine is demonstrated.

lumbosacral intervertebral disc. Therefore, the physical examination that you conduct must be sufficiently thorough to provide the information necessary to justify the diagnosis that you utilize.

P.A.R.T. DOCUMENTATION FORM

This sample *P.A.R.T. Form* has the essential History and Examination (P.A.R.T.) and Decision Making (assessment and treatment plan) components as required by Medicare. It expresses a probable E/M level three code for a new patient (99203).

See Resource 400 for a full-size version of this form, with instructions.

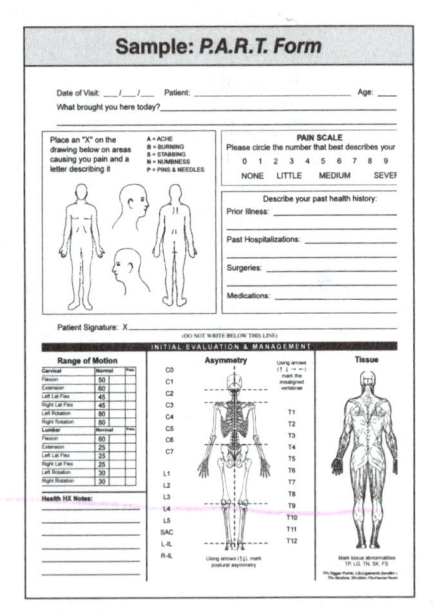

DIAGNOSTIC IMAGING

X-Rays: While x-rays are not required by Medicare to prove the existence of subluxation, they are necessary to justify some diagnoses. X-rays should be taken of the affected area of the spine, if the doctor suspects the presence of osseous changes such as disc narrowing or arthritic changes. If disc bulging is suspected, the patient should be referred to their MD for evaluation and CT or MRI.

Recurrence

If the patient returns with the same symptoms 31 or more days later, they have had a recurrence according to Medicare's definition. If the patient suffers a recurrence, take a new history, and perform a new exam (similar to the re-exam, with positives and significant negatives). Develop new diagnoses and a new treatment plan based on two weeks of care rather than four and a new initial date of treatment. Treat the patient in two-week blocks until they reach maximum therapeutic benefit. See the Council on Chiropractic Guidelines and Practice Parameters (CCGPP) algorithms (on page D-35) for more guidance. Repeat these procedures with each occurrence. When you have documentation demonstrating a recurrence or exacerbation, Item Number 14 on the 1500 claim form should be updated to reflect the start of a new or altered treatment plan.

See Chapter 5–Treatment Plans and Assessments in this *Documentation* section for more information about Treatment Plans.

3. **Medical Decision Making**

   Medical Decision Making (MDM) includes the following elements:

   A. diagnosis/management options (see below)

   B. complexity of data to review (see Chapter 3–Evaluation and Management in *Section H–Procedure Codes*)

   C. risks of treatment (see Chapter 3–Evaluation and Management in *Section H–Procedure Codes*)

A. DIAGNOSIS/MANAGEMENT OPTIONS

The diagnosis is the method whereby you communicate to payers what is wrong with the patient and where the problem is located using ICD-9-CM codes (ICD-10-CM codes on October 1, 2015). These codes are designed to be specific; every condition should be coded to the highest level of specificity possible.

- See *Section G–Diagnosis* for more information about diagnosis codes.
- See Chapter 3–Evaluation and Management in *Section H–Procedure Codes* to review the required elements for diagnosis/management options.

There are some general rules that apply when determining a diagnosis. Knowing these rules will generally help you to better determine the best diagnosis for your patient's condition. Each carrier handles the diagnosis a little differently. Some payers will provide you with a list of diagnoses that they will accept and some will allow you to use whatever diagnosis you feel is appropriate to document medical necessity.

> **Alert**: When you use a particular diagnosis make sure that you have performed the appropriate test(s) necessary to substantiate that diagnosis and that you have the report on file for the test(s) (e.g., a prolapsed disc can only be visualized with a CT or MRI).

The diagnosis is part of the "Assessment" section of the visit notes and reflects the doctor's professional opinion and judgment. The current diagnoses should be documented in the patient record as well as on the claim form and should be updated as necessary to reflect improvement (or lack thereof) at each re-assessment.

Each area of the spine that is to be adjusted generally requires a primary diagnosis of subluxation, a secondary diagnosis based on the presenting problem (the condition that brought the patient to your office), and, if appropriate, a diagnosis of any complicating factors. Some states vary from this protocol. Prior to January 2014, the old 1500 claim form only allowed four diagnostic codes. That is no longer the case. All appropriate diagnoses should be listed on the claim.

See Chapter 2–1500 Claim Form of *Section E–Claims and Appeals* for more information about the claim form.

A subluxation(s) diagnosis must be demonstrated by x-ray or physical examination (See the segment "Evaluation of Musculoskeletal/Nervous System Through Physical Exam" on page D-23 for more information.)

Diagnosing Notes:

- Claims for procedure code 98940, must have primary *and* secondary diagnoses listed for one to two spinal areas in the documentation and on the claim.
- Claims for procedure code 98941 must have primary *and* secondary diagnoses for three to four spinal areas listed in the documentation.
- Claims for procedure code 98942, must have primary *and* secondary diagnoses for all five spinal areas listed in the documentation. Also note that in most Medicare jurisdictions, claims at this level are generally audited; therefore, extensive documentation is necessary.

When documenting the secondary diagnoses, there is a hierarchy of codes that should be noted based on severity:

1. Neurological diagnoses
2. Structural diagnoses and acute injuries
3. Functional diagnoses
4. Soft tissue, extremity
5. Complicating factors/comorbidities

4. Treatment Plan

See Chapter 5–Treatment Plans and Assessments in this *Documentation* section for more information about Treatment Plans.

Complicating Factors

Medicare treatment parameters state:

"Acute subluxations (e.g., strains or sprains) problems may require as many as three months of treatment but some require very little treatment. In the first several days, treatment may be quite frequent but decreasing in frequency with time or as improvement is obtained."

This guideline is for an uncomplicated case. A complicated case would be expected to require more time.

The following complicating factors can increase the time required for recovery:

- Symptoms present for more than 8 days can increase recovery time by 1.5
- 4 to 7 previous episodes can increase recovery time by 2
- Presence of skeletal anomaly can increase recovery time by 2
- Presence of structural pathology can increase recovery time by 2
- Presence of severe pain can increase recovery time by 2
- Injury superimposed on the following conditions can increase recovery time by 2:
  - Pre-existing conditions
  - Underlying pathologies
  - Congenital anomalies

RE-ASSESSMENT VISITS

The re-assessment in a typical chiropractic care plan should generally occur after two weeks of care and then every four weeks thereafter. This communicates to the payer the patient's progress on the goals set during the initial assessment. It includes the same elements described above, but in the context of an update, rather than an initial assessment.

The patient's history should be updated. Typically, however, the history does not need to be duplicated, just updated to reflect relevant changes since the previous assessment.

The exam should be performed, but it typically will not need to be as extensive, unless something changed, or the patient did not progress as expected. Emphasis can be placed on positive findings from the initial assessment.

The care plan should then be evaluated and the following questioned answered:

- Were goals met?
- Are there new goals?
- Are the treatments going to change in any manner?

Tip: Because re-assessment visits do not require as much work as initial assessments, the RVUs for established patients (99211-99215) reflect a lower reimbursement value than for the same level for new patients (99201-99205).

- See Chapter 2–Evaluation and Management in *Section H–Procedure Codes* for more information about documenting E/M visits.
- See Chapter 3–Establishing Fees in *Section B–Insurance and Reimbursement* for more information about RVUs.

Review: Assessment Visits

- Which components should the initial exam address? *D-17*
- What is "Necessity for Treatment"? *D-20*
- Does Medicare require the date that treatment began, or the date of the initial occurrence? *D-21*
- Into which five areas does Medicare and most payers classify the spine? *D-22*
- What is P.A.R.T.? *D-24*
- What is the hierarchy of codes that should be noted on diagnoses? *D-26*

4. Treatment Visits

Once you have assessed the patient, documented the condition of the patient, and commenced treatment, you are required to document what happens at each treatment visit. Treatment visits differ from assessment visits in that they briefly assess progress, but do not include a significant and separately identifiable Evaluation and Managment visit.

When a patient encounter is documented properly, another doctor can read the notes and know exactly what happened during that encounter and why. The notes should be readable and the most recent patient record should not read like the first patient record. Good documentation will concisely record the patient's condition, both subjectively from the patient's point of view and objectively from the doctor's point of view, what treatment was performed, why the treatment was performed, and how well the patient is progressing toward the treatment goals.

It should be noted that all patient encounters should be recorded in the patient's file. This includes telephone calls and encounters with staff members as they relate to patient care.

> See page H-32 of *Section H–Procedure Coding* for details about when it is appropriate to bill an E/M visit at the same encounter as a CMT.

Treatment Visits

The treatment visits are where the plan developed during the assessment visit is put into action. A schedule of visits is established for the patient leading up to the next assessment visit, and the patient's condition is treated utilizing the adjustment techniques and therapies that would be most effective.

The recording requirements for the treatment visits would be different than those for the assessment visits. The subjective statements from the patient are still noted regarding changes in their condition and objective findings from palpation. The assessment would be limited to determining if the patient is "on course" or not. Since the plan was already established during the assessment visit, few, if any, comments regarding the plan would be required during the treatment visit sequence.

During the treatment visit, the treatments and therapies administered to the patient and the patient's response to them should be noted.

Utilizing the SOAP format in this manner allows for more accurate record keeping by eliminating the need for redundant entries in the patient records. It also means that to develop an accurate picture of patient care another doctor or a reviewer would need a "block" of records, including the records of the assessment visits before and after the date in question, as well as all of the treatment visit records for the visits that occurred between those assessment visits.

Medicare Documentation System (Resource 375) by Dr. Ron Short contains training and forms based on the assessment and treatment visit concept. The information presented in the book is valuable for all patient encounters, not just Medicare.

MEDICARE DOCUMENTATION REQUIREMENTS FOR SUBSEQUENT VISITS

For subsequent treatment visits, Medicare requires specific documentation. These are good standards for other payers as well. These elements blend quite well within the standard SOAP note format. The following documentation requirements apply whether the subluxation is demonstrated by x-ray or by physical examination.

> **B. Documentation Requirements: Subsequent Visits**
>
> The following documentation requirements apply whether the subluxation is demonstrated by x-ray or by physical examination:
>
> 1. History
>   - Review of chief complaint;
>   - Changes since last visit;
>   - System review if relevant.
> 2. Physical exam
>   - Exam of area of spine involved in diagnosis;
>   - Assessment of change in patient condition since last visit;
>   - Evaluation of treatment effectiveness.
> 3. Documentation of treatment given on day of visit.

It is important to note here that there is no provision in the published regulations that state that each of these elements must be performed and documented on each subsequent visit. Most of the elements will, by their nature, be performed and recorded on each visit and others will not. For risk management, it is recommended that the physician list the segments adjusted and the technique used in the treatment. An example would be: CMT C7, T3, T7, L3 and L5 – Diversified.

1. History

Review of Chief Complaint

The chief complaint is what caused the patient to seek care. A review of the chief complaint gives a good indication of how the patient perceives their progress. The review is as simple as asking the patient, "How does your low back pain (neck pain, etc.) feel today?"

Changes since Last Visit

Monitoring changes in the patient's condition on a visit-by-visit basis is a sound medical procedure. This allows you to quickly determine if any adverse reactions are occurring and to take the appropriate corrective action. A simple question, "Is anything different today than it was last visit?" will accomplish this goal.

2. Physical Exam

Exam of area of spine involved in diagnosis

It is important to physically examine the specific area(s) of the spine involved in the diagnosis. There has been much confusion as to the nature of this examination. Careful examination of the section of the Medicare manual pertaining to P.A.R.T. reveals that all elements can be determined by palpation. The examination of the area involved in the diagnosis can be accomplished by palpating the area.

Assessment of Changes in Patient Condition since Last Visit

If changes are revealed during the examination, the doctor should note these. Both positive and negative changes should be noted.

Evaluation of Treatment Effectiveness

It is important to evaluate the effectiveness of the treatment that the patient is receiving, but doing this at every treatment visit would be the equivalent of a medical doctor evaluating a patient after they take each pill in a course of antibiotic therapy. The treatment needs time to work before its effectiveness can be evaluated. The treatment's effectiveness should be evaluated at the initial visit, two weeks into the treatment plan, at each subsequent re-exam, or every 30 days after that, whichever is sooner.

3. Documentation of Treatment Given on Day of Visit

The type(s) of treatment(s) performed on the patient should be documented as well as which segmental levels were treated. Treatment visit notes should be divided into three parts to coincide with Medicare's three areas of information that they require: history, physical examination, and documentation of treatment given on the day of the visit. This can still be reported in a traditional SOAP note format where the S=history, O=physical examination, and P= treatment given.

The notes should also have an area for doctor's comments and a notation of the day and time of the next visit. Additionally, specific items should be included **every** time with **no** exceptions:

1. The patient's name
2. The date
3. The doctor's signature

Maintenance Therapy Is Not Medically Necessary

"...Chiropractic maintenance therapy is not considered to be medically reasonable or necessary, and is therefore not payable. Maintenance therapy is defined as a treatment plan that seeks to prevent disease, promote health, and prolong and enhance the quality of life; or therapy that is performed to maintain or prevent deterioration of a chronic condition. When further clinical improvement **cannot reasonably be expected** from continuous **ongoing care**, and the chiropractic treatment **becomes supportive** rather than corrective in nature, the **treatment** is then considered **maintenance therapy**."

-Medicare Benefit Policy Manual, Chapter 15, 30.5

Transitioning from Active Care

At some point during the subsequent treatment visits, the patient will no longer be in the active care stage. They may have reached their optimum level of improvement or they may need to be referred to another provider. Pay particular attention to HIPAA requirements for release of medical records and carefully follow payer specific provider referral requirements.

> See the CCGPP algorithms in Chapter 5–Assessment and Treatment Planning for more guidance on when to transition from active care and/or refer patient elsewhere.

Patient Progress

Most third party payers do not cover situations where the patient is not progressing. At each visit, progress should be noted. If there is no improvement, or no further improvement could be reasonably anticipated, then the patient either moves into a maintenance care situation or else they need to be referred to another provider.

> See Chapter 5–Assessment and Treatment Planning for more information about assessing patient progress.

Maintenance Care/Wellness Visits

When the patient's chief complaint has been addressed, he/she may want to continue treatment to maintain their current state. These maintenance visits are considered "wellness visits." Wellness visits, while beneficial for the patient, are not covered by most payers, including Medicare.

The documentation for these visits needs to clearly identify that this is not active care. For Medicare patients, it is important to include a signed ABN in the patient chart.

> - See *Section C–Medicare* for more about the ABN.
> - See code S8990 in Chapter 2–Commonly Used Codes of *Section H–Procedure Codes* for tips on using this code for *non-Medicare* wellness visits.

Release From Care

There may be two unique situations when it becomes necessary to release the patient from your care. 1) the patient may need to be referred to another provider or specialist or 2) when the patient has reached their therapeutic goals.

When the patient is not progressing or their condition warrants review by another professional, the documentation clearly needs to indicate why they are being referred. If the patient no longer benefits from active treatment, an official "discharge" needs to be clearly indicated in the medical record. Lack of an end date could suggest that the patient is no longer under active treatment and care is not medically necessary. Further visits are considered wellness or maintenance visits and must be documented as such.

Review: Treatment Visits

- What are the Medicare specific requirements for documentation? *D-29*
- What requirements do you need to pay particular attention to when releasing medical records to referred providers? *D-31*
- Are "wellness visits" covered by most payers? *D-31*

5. Treatment Plans and Assessments

After the physician has conducted a thorough history, performed a physical examination, and ordered the relevant studies (x-rays), the next step is to create a treatment plan. It is very difficult to defend treatment denials from third party payers when there are no plans or goals for the outcome of care. If you needed to build a house you would have to select a blueprint, order materials, hire a contractor, etc. The house would never come together if you just started pounding nails into random 2x4s. Likewise, third parties want to see that there is a plan to get the patient better, and perhaps equally important, a way to measure improvement.

Because these needs for treatment plans and outcome assessment measurements are integral components of both the "Initial Examination" and the "Subsequent Examination", they are addressed in this chapter.

See Resource 365 for the latest information, webinars and articles on treatment plans.

Evidence Based Treatment Planning

Once an initial diagnostic assessment has been established, a care plan must be formulated for every condition. It should include the estimated duration and frequency of care, technique selection, indicated modalities and procedures, use of any structural supports, exercise/rehabilitation recommendations, instructions regarding activities of daily living, and the establishment of any total or partial disability period.

Functional and symptomatic responses of the patient to the care provided should be documented before proceeding from one phase of care to another (therapeutic to continuing). This process allows the practitioner to move towards evidence-based care which is a systematic approach designed to establish more objective criteria upon which to base clinical decisions. This is the basis for the CCGPP algorithms included later in this section.

Assessment of the patient will become more refined and streamlined to reflect clinical changes in response to care which can be measured (e.g. range of motion metrics, muscle function and strength metrics, patient questionnaires, etc). This is the language that payers expect when assessing medical necessity. Providers who understand and communicate clearly in this language will minimize claims delays and denials.

The benefits of this approach transcends mere cost savings, as the ultimate benefactor to the public and patient through the delivery of high quality value-based care that is provided in a clinically efficient and effective manner.

THE TREATMENT PLAN

The written treatment plan is one of the key elements to proving medical necessity. It includes a recommended level of care, specific treatment goals, and objective measures to evaluate treatment effectiveness. A treatment plan should never be set in stone. It is a dynamic plan that can frequently change based on the patient's progress. Medical reviewers look negatively on static, non-customized treatment plans.

The proper use of the treatment plan cannot be over-emphasized. Insurance reviewers are looking for this document in the records that they request. The Problem Oriented Medical Record (POMR), as discussed in Chapter 1 of this section, clearly communicates the plan to any third party reviewer. Without a viable treatment plan, the care that you rendered will be considered medically unnecessary and you will be required to refund the money that you have been paid.

The real key to a treatment plan based on objective outcome assessments is that it gives third parties very little ammunition with which to deny your claims. Essentially you are playing by their rules, and it will work to your advantage if you do it right. The idea is simple: take something subjective and make it objective, or measurable. There are numerous tools available and they nearly all provide you with a score. For example, a perfectly healthy person might score a "0" on an outcome assessment, but someone who just suffered some significant injuries in a car accident might have a score of "75." This makes it easy to communicate with the payer. "75" is easier for them to understand than "the patient says it hurts a lot." They can now objectively see why a certain level of care was recommended.

The Council for Chiropractic Guidelines and Practice Parameters (CCGPP) developed three consensus documents regarding treatment plans in December 2012. The publication titled, "Algorithms for the Chiropractic Management of Acute and Chronic Spine-Related Pain" includes definitions of terms related to acute and chronic care, and evaluation components in addition to the algorithms for acute and chronic care. It is an excellent resource for reviewing treament plans.

The next segment of this book are the flowcharts from these CCGPP Algorithms which may also function as a resource for providers seeking to establish effective protocols in their practice.

Medicare Documentation System (Resource 375), by Dr. Ron Short includes detailed information about properly documenting treatment plans and assessments.

INFORMED CONSENT FOR CHIROPRACTIC TREATMENT

For appropriate risk management, every office needs to have a signed Informed Consent Agreement prior to treatment. Consult with your legal counsel and your malpractice insurance carrier for specific forms that they might recommend for your office (e.g., decompression therapy, pediatrics, etc.). Here is a basic and general consent form for those who have none. Generally, there is no legally required expiration date on this consent, however, one year would be a good standard since a patient could forget details.

The patient needs to sign this form BEFORE treatment begins.

- See Resource 376 for a full-size version of this form, with instructions.
- See Resource 377 for a sample treatment plan.

Algorithms for the Chiropractic Management of Acute and Chronic Spine-Related Pain

The Council on Chiropractic Guidelines and Practice Parameters (CCGPP) Algorithms (Figures 4.2-4.4) were developed through a consensus process and are being reviewed by many professional organizations for adoption as clinical policy. The ACA has adopted the "CCGPP Acute and Chronic Care Guidelines." Using evidence-based clinical algorithms such as these, supports effective standardized care. It has been reprinted here by permission.

The introduction to these algorithms by CCGPP states the following:

> "These algorithms are only a guide, and are not appropriate for all patients and conditions. In particular, it should be noted that they relate specifically to spine-related pain, so are not applicable to other chiropractic treatment objectives. Furthermore, these algorithms are designed to guide the DC in planning the stages of care. They do not dictate the type of treatment procedures provided.
>
> The algorithms are not designed for the management of other clinical objectives, such as non-painful functional or structural spinal care. They are also not appropriate for wellness care or

FIGURE 4.2
Treatment of Spine Related Pain

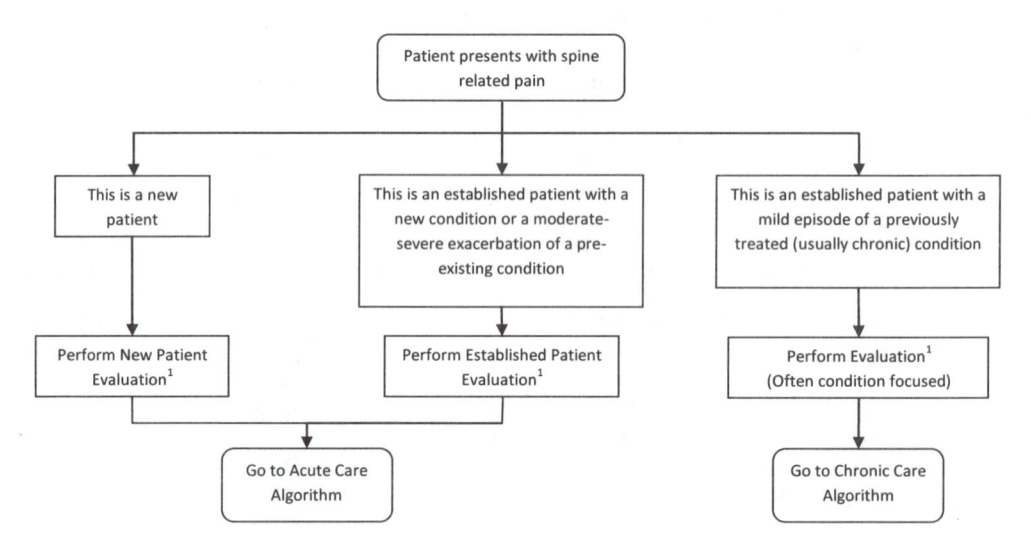

```
                    Patient presents with spine
                         related pain
                              |
        ┌─────────────────────┼─────────────────────┐
        │                     │                     │
  This is a new    This is an established    This is an established
     patient       patient with a new        patient with a mild
                   condition or a moderate-  episode of a previously
                   severe exacerbation of    treated (usually chronic)
                   a pre-existing condition  condition
        │                     │                     │
  Perform New       Perform Established      Perform Evaluation¹
  Patient           Patient Evaluation¹      (Often condition focused)
  Evaluation¹
        │                     │                     │
        └──────────┬──────────┘                     │
                   │                                │
          Go to Acute Care                 Go to Chronic Care
             Algorithm                         Algorithm
```

¹**Evaluation components**

- History
- Examination
- Outcomes Assessment Tools
    - Pain intensity scales
    - Pain diagrams
    - Pain and disability questionnaires
    - Functional outcomes questionnaires
    - General health questionnaires
    - Psychological profiles
- Imaging if warranted

other types of prevention and/or health promotion. If the algorithm suggests the release or referral of a patient, then the patient has either recovered or the clinical objective is outside the scope of this algorithm."

Algorithm Notes

Begin with figure 4.2 and proceed through each succesive flowchart.

1. **Evaluation Components**

    The components listed below Figure 4.2 need to happen on the initial visit.

    - **Outcomes Assessment Tools** (OAT) allow you to establish the baseline functional ability of the patient. This results of the OAT(s) should be part of the patient medical record.

        > **Tip:** Administer the same tool twice during their visit. Ask the patient to respond once for their current status and the second time for their status BEFORE the incident or episode of care started. This helps to distinguish if any of the functional loss was pre-existing.

2. **Definitions**

    > **TOPICS IN INTEGRATIVE HEALTH CARE [ISSN 2158-4222] – VOL 3(4) - Page 2**
    >
    > The terms "supportive care" and "maintenance care," which are frequently used within the chiropractic health care arena, are not consistent with general healthcare industry lexicon. Instead of "supportive care," we use the more descriptive term, "ongoing/recurrent" care. Chronic pain management can be divided into three categories:
    > (1) those who can home manage;
    > (2) those who can be managed with episodic care; and
    > (3) those who need "scheduled" ongoing care, which is a very small proportion of chronic pain sufferers. Those patients require proper documentation of responses to care and procedures, including therapeutic withdrawal response, multi-modal, multi-disciplinary consideration, patient education, etc.
    >
    > **Other related consensus-based terms:**
    > *Medically necessary care of acute conditions:* "care that is reasonable and necessary for the diagnosis and treatment of a patient with a health concern and for which there is a therapeutic care plan and a goal of functional improvement and/or pain relief."
    >
    > *Medically necessary care for recurrent/chronic conditions*: "care that is provided when the injury/illness is not expected to completely resolve after a treatment regimen but where continued care can reasonably be expected to result in documentable improvement for the patient."
    >
    > *Chiropractic management of chronic/recurrent conditions*: "Chiropractic care provided for the purpose of preventing relapse and/or exacerbations of the original complaint(s) as well as associated comorbidities."
    >
    > *Chiropractic wellness care or preventive care*: "Chiropractic care provided for the purpose of preventing disease, optimizing function, and supporting the patient's wellness-related activities."

FIGURE 4.3
Acute Care Algorithm

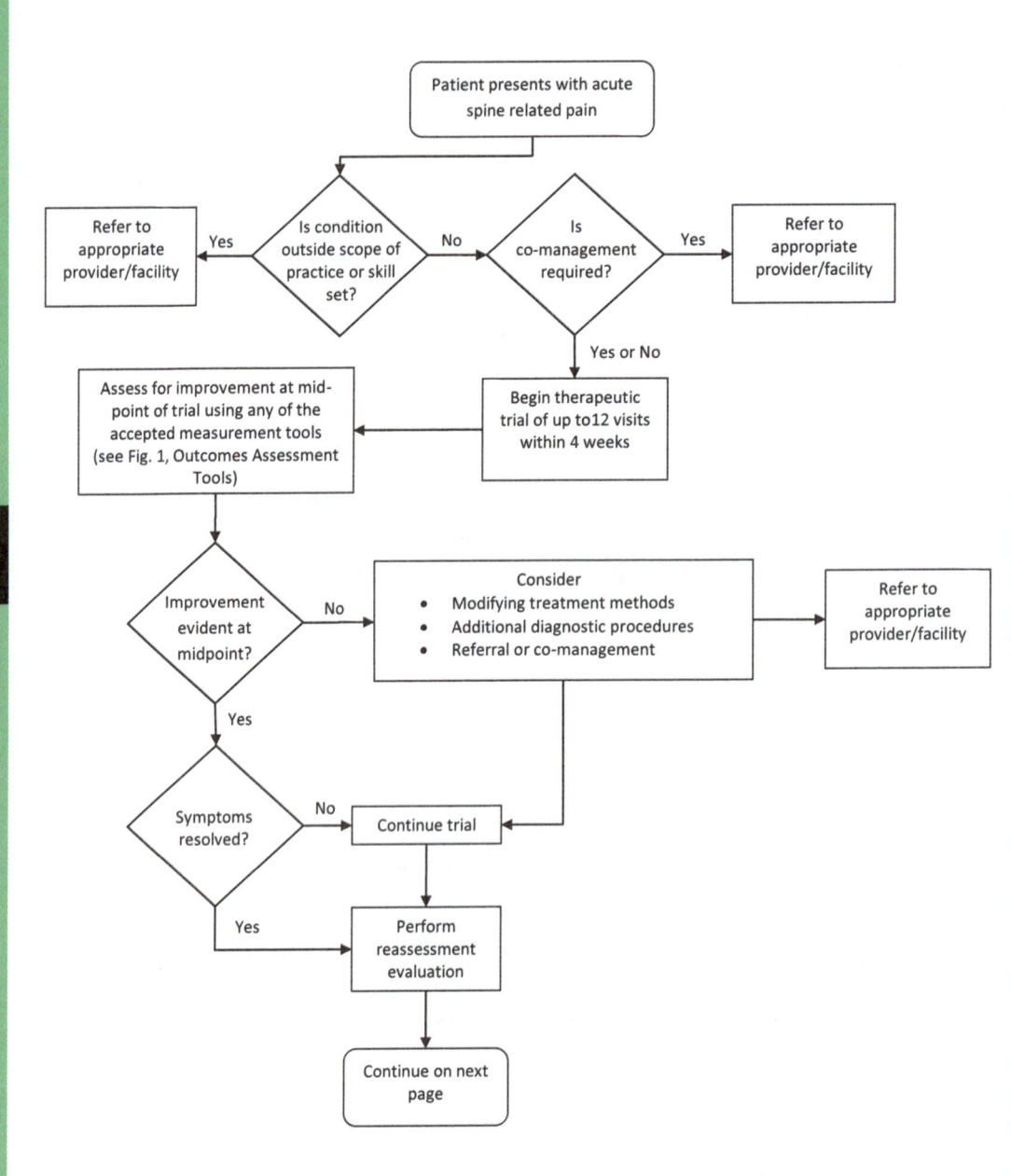

```
                    Patient presents with acute
                         spine related pain
                                 |
                                 v
  Refer to        Yes    Is condition      No        Is            Yes      Refer to
  appropriate  <------  outside scope of  ------> co-management  ------>  appropriate
  provider/facility     practice or skill          required?              provider/facility
                        set?
                                                     |
                                                  Yes or No
                                                     v
  Assess for improvement at mid-          Begin therapeutic
  point of trial using any of the  <----  trial of up to 12 visits
  accepted measurement tools              within 4 weeks
  (see Fig. 1, Outcomes Assessment
  Tools)
        |
        v
  Improvement   No       Consider                              Refer to
  evident at  ------>  • Modifying treatment methods   ----> appropriate
  midpoint?            • Additional diagnostic procedures     provider/facility
        |              • Referral or co-management
       Yes                       |
        v                        |
  Symptoms      No                |
  resolved?  ------> Continue trial <---
        |                        |
       Yes                       |
        v                        v
              Perform reassessment
              evaluation
                        |
                        v
              Continue on next
              page
```

Reprinted with permission. Baker GA, Farabaugh RJ, Augat TJ, Hawk C. Algorithms for the chiropractic management of acute and chronic spine-related pain. Top Integrative Health Care 2013;3(4).

http://tihcij.com/PubView.aspx?vol=3&is=4

C Cheryl Hawk, DC, PhD
Editor, TIHC

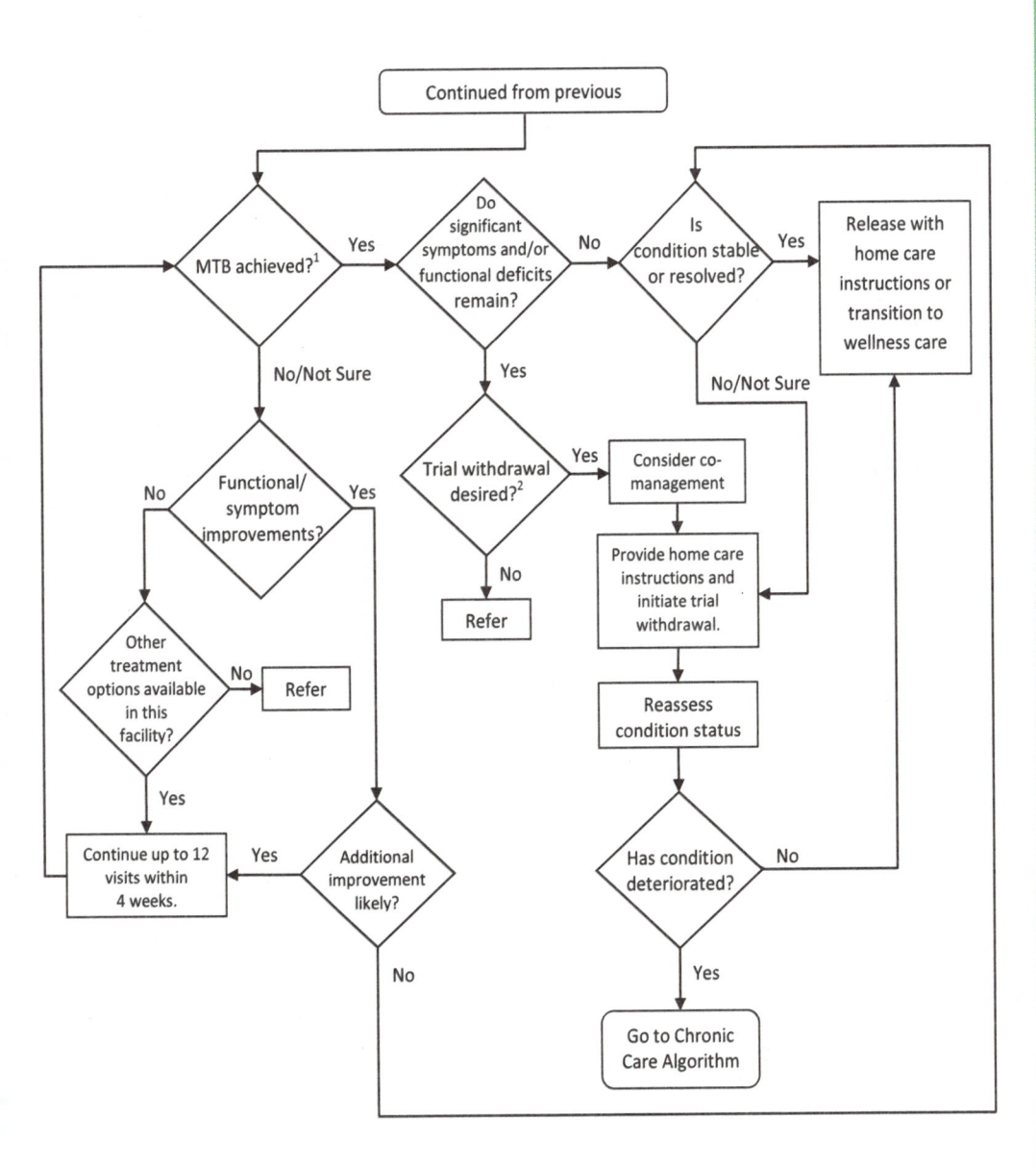

```
                        Continued from previous
                                │
        ┌───────────────────────┴─────┐
        ▼                             ▼
   ┌─────────┐   Yes   ┌──────────────┐   No   ┌──────────────┐   Yes   ┌─────────────┐
   │   MTB   │────────▶│      Do      │───────▶│      Is      │────────▶│ Release with│
   │achieved?¹│         │  significant │        │condition stable│      │  home care  │
   └─────────┘         │ symptoms and/or│       │ or resolved? │         │instructions or│
        │              │functional deficits│    └──────────────┘         │ transition to│
        │ No/Not Sure  │   remain?    │              │                   │ wellness care│
        ▼              └──────────────┘              │ No/Not Sure       └─────────────┘
                              │ Yes                  │
   ┌─────────┐                ▼                      │
   │Functional/│        ┌──────────────┐   Yes   ┌──────────────┐
   │ symptom  │         │    Trial     │────────▶│  Consider co-│
   │improvements?│      │  withdrawal  │         │  management  │
   └─────────┘         │   desired?²  │         └──────────────┘
   No │    │ Yes        └──────────────┘                │
      ▼    │                   │ No                     ▼
 ┌────────┐│                   ▼                 ┌──────────────┐
 │ Other  ││              ┌────────┐             │ Provide home │
 │treatment││             │  Refer │             │    care      │
 │options ││  No ┌──────┐ └────────┘             │instructions and│
 │available│────▶│Refer │                        │initiate trial │
 │in this  ││    └──────┘                        │  withdrawal. │
 │facility?││                                    └──────────────┘
 └────────┘│                                            │
   │ Yes   │                                            ▼
   ▼       │                                    ┌──────────────┐
┌──────────┐│  Yes  ┌──────────┐                │   Reassess   │
│Continue up│◀──────│Additional│                │condition status│
│to 12 visits│      │improvement│               └──────────────┘
│within 4    │      │  likely? │                       │
│weeks.     │      └──────────┘                        ▼
└──────────┘            │                      ┌──────────────┐  No
                        │ No                   │Has condition │──────▶
                        ▼                      │deteriorated? │
                                               └──────────────┘
                                                       │ Yes
                                                       ▼
                                               ┌──────────────┐
                                               │ Go to Chronic│
                                               │Care Algorithm│
                                               └──────────────┘
```

¹MTB=maximum therapeutic benefit

²Trial withdrawl:

A trial withdrawal may be necessary once a patient reaches maximum therapeutic improvement. This helps to determine if the condition recovery is stable. If the condition has deteriorated after the trial, then chronic or ongoing care may be necessary to maintain function and minimize symptoms. The therapeutic withdrawal can be gradual, where the patient's care is tapered off. It can also be abrupt, with the patient instructed to return if the symptoms recur; or the patient can be scheduled for an evaluation at a later date to determine if there is any regression.

FIGURE 4.4
Chronic Care Algorithm

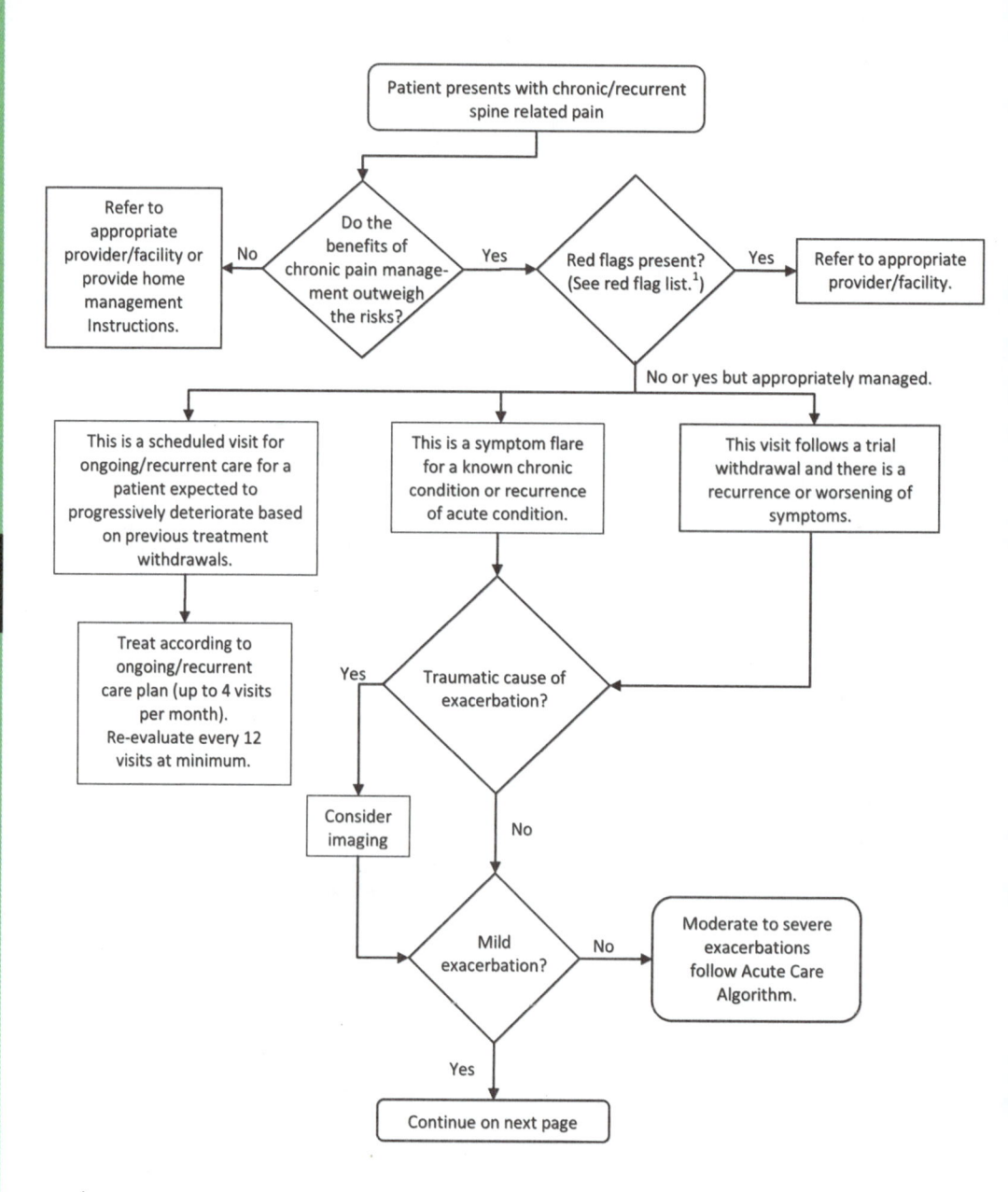

```
Patient presents with chronic/recurrent spine related pain
                    ↓
        Do the benefits of chronic pain management outweigh the risks?
   No ←                                    → Yes
   ↓                                           ↓
Refer to appropriate                    Red flags present?
provider/facility or                    (See red flag list.¹)
provide home                            No or yes but appropriately managed ← → Yes → Refer to appropriate provider/facility.
management Instructions.
```

- **This is a scheduled visit for ongoing/recurrent care for a patient expected to progressively deteriorate based on previous treatment withdrawals.**
  → Treat according to ongoing/recurrent care plan (up to 4 visits per month). Re-evaluate every 12 visits at minimum.

- **This is a symptom flare for a known chronic condition or recurrence of acute condition.**

- **This visit follows a trial withdrawal and there is a recurrence or worsening of symptoms.**

Traumatic cause of exacerbation?
- Yes → Consider imaging
- No → Mild exacerbation?
  - No → Moderate to severe exacerbations follow Acute Care Algorithm.
  - Yes → Continue on next page

¹Red flags
- Progressive neurological disorders
- Cauda equina syndrome
- Bone weakening disorders; i.e.; acute spinal fracture, spinal infection, spinal or extra-vertebral bony malignancies
- Tumor
- Articular derangements indicating instability; i.e., active avascular necrosis in weight-bearing joints

Treatment Plans and Assessments

Flowchart (continued from previous page):

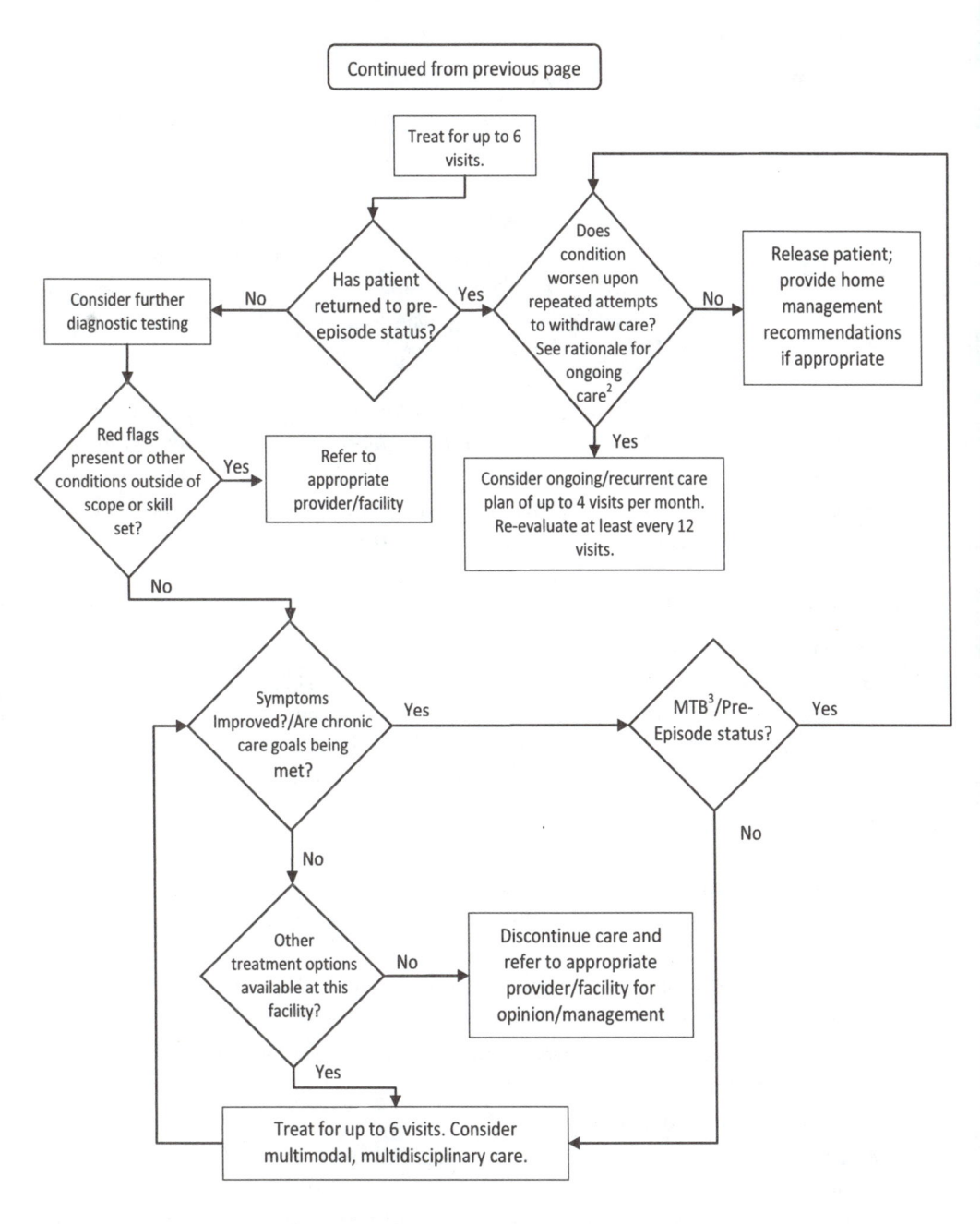

- Continued from previous page → Treat for up to 6 visits.
- **Has patient returned to pre-episode status?**
  - No → Consider further diagnostic testing
    - **Red flags present or other conditions outside of scope or skill set?**
      - Yes → Refer to appropriate provider/facility
      - No → (go to Symptoms Improved?)
  - Yes → **Does condition worsen upon repeated attempts to withdraw care? See rationale for ongoing care[2]**
    - No → Release patient; provide home management recommendations if appropriate
    - Yes → Consider ongoing/recurrent care plan of up to 4 visits per month. Re-evaluate at least every 12 visits.

- **Symptoms Improved?/Are chronic care goals being met?**
  - Yes → **MTB[3]/Pre-Episode status?**
    - Yes → (Release patient path)
    - No → Treat for up to 6 visits. Consider multimodal, multidisciplinary care.
  - No → **Other treatment options available at this facility?**
    - No → Discontinue care and refer to appropriate provider/facility for opinion/management
    - Yes → Treat for up to 6 visits. Consider multimodal, multidisciplinary care.

[2]Documentation of necessity of ongoing care (in addition to standard documentation):*
- Clinically meaningful response to initial treatment
- Maximum therapeutic benefit (MTB)
- Significant residual activity limitations
- Attempts to transition to self-care
- Consideration of alternative treatment approaches
- Factors affecting likelihood that self-care alone will sustain MTI (see Complicating Factors, next page

COMPLICATING FACTORS

This list of complicating factors* by CCGPP for Figure 4.4 is not all-inclusive:

Patient Characteristics	Injury Characteristics	History
■ Older age	■ Severe initial injury	■ Pre-existing pathology/surgery
■ Psychosocial factors	■ > 3 previous episodes	
■ Delay treatment >7 days	■ Severe signs and symptoms	■ History of lost time
■ Non-compliance		■ History of prior treatment
■ Lifestyle habits	■ Number/severity previous exacerbations	■ Congenital anomalies
■ Obesity**		■ Symptoms persist despite previous treatment
■ Type of work activities	■ Treatment withdrawal fails to sustain MTI	

* *Source: Farabaugh RJ, Dehen MD, Hawk C. Management of chronic spine-related conditions: Consensus recommendations of a multidisciplinary panel. J Manipulative Physiol Ther 2010;33(7):484-492.*

** *Source: Harvard Health Letter. Drop pounds to relieve back pain. Strengthening your core muscles can also help. Harv Health Lett 2012;37(10):4.*

Algorithm Notes - Cont from page D-35

3. Maximum Therapeutic Benefit (MTB)
- When the patient has reached their treatment goals, they no longer require active care. Most payers only cover care that is active and shows progress which means that the third-party payers should no longer be responsible for reimbursing the provider.
- At this stage, it is important to discuss options with the patient.

4. Referring Patients
- If the patient is not making progress, then it may be necessary to have them obtain additional care. They may need to be referred to another provider of a different specialty or with different equipment or training. Maybe they need to have an MRI or even benefit from physical therapy.
- When referring a patient, remember that HIPAA requires that medical records require an official Release of Information Authorization from the patient.
- Create the necessary referral paperwork and give to the patient. Include a copy in the medical record. Note: A pre-authorization may be required.

5. Releasing Patients from Active Care
- Once the patient has reached the maximum expected improvement, they need to be released from active care.
- Consider whether Maintenance Care or other wellness care services would benefit the patient. Discuss the options with the patient and note these recommendations in their record. Be sure they understand their financial obligations for these types of care.

Effective Treatment Plan Components

An effective treatment plan, which is consistent with POMR, should include the following:

1. A list of each complaint, with their relevant diagnoses (for example, neck pain 723.1)
2. Treatments and modalities selected (for example, neck stretches-with diagrams in the notes)
3. Duration and frequency of care (for example, supervised stretching exercises 12 minutes three times per week for one week, two times per week for three weeks, etc., then continued at home)
4. Treatment goals (for example, improve flexibility of the bilateral trapezius and suboccipitals. expect 50% improvement within three to four weeks)
5. Objective measures to show progress (for example, ROM exam findings and neck pain disability index scores)

Plan

When creating individual patient treatment plans, there are various treatment options which may be appropriate to include. Different payers may have different requirements or policies, however, here is a generally accepted list of what to do about their condition. It is based upon specific clinical endpoint(s), i.e., resolution, referral, re-evaluation of clinical trial, etc.

Example

The treatment plan includes a line that says "A re-exam will be performed in four weeks. Outcomes assessment score is anticipated to improve by 30%." During the re-exam, there are only three possible scenarios: 1) The score improves, 2) The score worsens or falls short of the goal 3) The score improves more than anticipated or reaches "0" depending on the measurement tool(s) used.

In the first scenario, you have proven that the patient's treatment plan worked. You were able to reach the goals as outlined, therefore you should be able to continue until the patient reaches maximum therapeutic benefit. The third party payer would have no logical reason to disagree.

In the second scenario, you would need to alter the original plan. Either get more aggressive, take a different approach, or refer out to another provider for different care. This demonstrates that you are not going to provide care that does not help the patient, and the third party again thinks of you as a very skilled health care provider. The payer would have no reason to disagree.

In the third scenario, you have shown that the plan was even better than anticipated. The care plan should be altered accordingly. Perhaps you decrease the frequency of care. Perhaps you continue with the same plan, but you bump up the goal. Perhaps, shoot for 50% improvement by the next re-exam rather than 30%. The payer would still have no reason to disagree and should be impressed with your clinical skills. If the new score is "0", release the patient from care for that complaint. If maintenance/wellness care is recommended, make it clear that it is no longer part of the plan. Update your diagnosis. Don't charge the third party for maintenance/wellness visits.

Medicare Requirements

The above examples are general guidelines for all treatment plans. While these guidelines should suffice for Medicare, it should be noted that CMS requires care plans to include three elements. Also, the date of the initial treatment **must** also be included for the initial visit.

> **240.1.2 – Subluxation May Be Demonstrated by X-Ray or Physician's Exam**
> **B3-2251.2**
> A. **Documentation Requirements: Initial Visit**
>   5. Treatment plan: The treatment plan should include the following:
>   - Recommended level of care (duration and frequency of visits);
>   - Specific treatment goals; and
>   - Objective measures to evaluate treatment effectiveness.

1. Recommended level of care (duration and frequency of visits) – how long and how often are you going to see the patient?
   - Acute treatment may be up to three months at a relatively high frequency (i.e 3x/week for 4 weeks, 2x/week for 4 weeks, etc.)
   - Chronic treatment may take longer, but should be at a lower frequency.
2. Specific treatment goals—What are you trying to accomplish?
3. Objective measures to evaluate treatment effectiveness—How do you know when you have accomplished the goal?

The Medicare manual also includes the following guidelines regarding recommended levels of care.

> **240.1.5 – Treatment Parameters**
> **B3-2251.5**
> The chiropractor should be afforded the opportunity to effect improvement or arrest or retard deterioration in such condition within a reasonable and generally predictable period of time. **Acute subluxation** (e.g., strains or sprains) problems may require as many as three months of treatment but some require very little treatment. In the first several days, treatment may be quite frequent but decreasing in frequency with time or as improvement is obtained.
>
> **Chronic** spinal joint condition implies, of course, the condition has existed for a longer period of time and that, in all probability, the involved joints have already "set" and fibrotic tissue has developed. This condition may require a longer treatment time, but not with higher frequency.
>
> Some chiropractors have been identified as using an "intensive care" concept of treatment. Under this approach multiple daily visits (as many as four or five in a single day) are given in the office or clinic and so-called room or ward fees are charged since the patient is confined to bed usually for the day. The room or ward fees are not covered and reimbursement under Medicare will be limited to not more than one treatment per day.

OUTCOMES ASSESSMENT TOOLS (OAT)

An important key element to an effective treatment plan is the the proper use of outcomes assessment tools (or questionnaires). This is because they help to establish reliable, objective measures which make them effective communication methods for the patient record.

The OAT provides the ideal objective measure for documenting improvement of function. Reviewers can easily determine the patient's improvement, or lack thereof. The number of visits is objectively limited by the medical necessity of the patient's condition rather than subjective opinions and policy limits. As long as the outcomes assessment tools utilized continue to demonstrate improvement of function, Medicare considers the care medically necessary. While not a

Medicare requirement, it is advisable to re-administer the outcomes assessment questionnaires after two weeks of care to confirm that the patient is progressing, and then every 30 days thereafter.

Outcomes Assessment scores most frequently measure the degree of "functional impairment." This is the objective measure of impairment in the patient's activities of daily living (ADL). When comparing the original score to the subsequent score, usually measured as part of the re-assessment, although there is no official standard, a clinically significant improvement might be a 30% reduction in the OAT score in a 30 day period. When used properly, OATs can establish the necessity of care that has been received while simultaneously establishing the need for further treatment, which is communicated in a language clearly understood by most payers and reviewers.

Common Assessment Tools

There are many outcomes assessment tools on the market today. Keep in mind that personal preferences do play a significant role in the choice of assessment tools used. Some of the most commonly used questionnaires are the following:

- Revised Oswestry Low Back Disability Questionnaire
- Neck Disability Index (NDI)
- Roland-Morris Low Back Pain and Disability Questionnaire
- Subjective and Objective Numerical Outcome Measure Assessment (SONOMA)
- Bournemouth questionnaires
- Functional Rating Index (FRI)
- McGill Pain Questionnaire (MPQ)

There are other questionnaires that are for specific complaints such as the Headache Disability Inventory (HDI), or Disabilities of Arm, Shoulder, and Hand (DASH).

Example: Revised Oswestry Low Back Pain Questionnaire

In Figure 4.5, note that the patient indicated in Section 1, "The pain is moderate and does not vary much," and in Section 6, "I cannot stand for longer than ½ hour without increasing pain." In this example, the treatment goals should be "To decrease the patients pain in the affected area from moderate to mild," and "To allow the patient to stand for longer than ½ hour without increasing pain." Figure 4.6 shows how the questionnaire could look during the re-exam.

You have accomplished the goals that you set forth in your initial treatment plan. This does not mean that you are done. The patient still has deficiencies, as is noted in Section 6 where the patient indicated, "I cannot stand for longer than one hour without increasing pain." The new treatment goal would be "To have the patient able to stand for more than one hour without increasing pain."

FIGURE 4.5

The Revised Oswestry Low Back Pain Questionnaire: Initial visit

SECTION 1 - Pain Intensity	SECTION 6 - Standing
A The pain comes and goes and is very mild.	A I can stand as long as I want without pain.
B The pain is mild and does not vary much.	B I have some pain on standing but it does not increase with time.
C The pain comes and goes and is moderate.	C I cannot stand for longer than one hour without increasing pain.
D **The pain is moderate and does not vary much.**	D **I cannot stand for longer than 1/2 hour without increasing pain.**
E The pain comes and goes and is severe.	E I cannot stand for longer than 10 minutes without increasing pain.
F The pain is severe and does not vary much.	F I avoid standing because it increases the pain immediately.

ROWLAND-MORRIS LOW BACK PAIN AND DISABILITY QUESTIONNAIRE

See Resource 378 for a full-size version of this form, with instructions.

Sample: Rowland-Morris Low Back Pain and Disability Questionnaire

PATIENTS' GLOBAL IMPRESSION OF CHANGE (PGIC) SCALE

The "Patients' Global Impression of Change" (PGIC) scale is completed by the patient and can be critically important evidence in the patient's record. The PGIC shows the patient's perspective as to what degree of change (improvement vs. no change or worse) they have experienced compared to the initial date of service. As such, it is a useful tool for patients, doctors and payers.

See Resource 379 for a full-size version of this form, with instructions.

Sample: Patients' Global Impression of Change (PGIC) Scale

FIGURE 4.6

The Revised Oswestry Low Back Pain Questionnaire: Re-Exam

SECTION 1 - Pain Intensity	
A	<u>The pain comes and goes and is very mild.</u>
B	The pain is mild and does not vary much.
C	The pain comes and goes and is moderate.
D	The pain is moderate and does not vary much.
E	The pain comes and goes and is severe.
F	The pain is severe and does not vary much.

SECTION 6 - Standing	
A	I can stand as long as I want without pain.
B	I have some pain on standing but it does not increase with time.
C	<u>I cannot stand for longer than one hour without increasing pain.</u>
D	I cannot stand for longer than 1/2 hour without increasing pain.
E	I cannot stand for longer than 10 minutes without increasing pain.
F	I avoid standing because it increases the pain immediately.

SONOMA

The Subjective and Objective Numerical Outcome Measure Assessment (SONOMA) is an outcome measurement tool that evaluates pain perception, activities of daily living or function, and physical parameters separately and combines values for a reliable and diversified clinical picture. It is simple and practical for both the patient and the provider. Developed by chiropractors to specifically assess spinal function, it is a highly effective tool for the chiropractic setting.

SONOMA forms in both English (Resource 388) and Spanish (Resource 389) are available in the ChiroCode store.

Outcomes and Chiro-Appropriate Value-Based Care

The past lack of understanding by conventional health care payers of chiropractic philosophy, methodology, and value has hindered their coverage policies and reimbursements. As insurance payers and managed care organizations respond to the increasing market pressure from their clients (employers, unions and trusts), they are examining and eliminating costs of clinically unnecessary services. Quality standards for "necessity" are generally determined by evidence in the literature and the patient's clinical outcomes. Consequently, accurate and thorough documentation with outcomes assessment will continue to become more important to patients, payers and physicians.

Incorporating outcomes data into patient documentation provides the following benefits. It:

- Demonstrates the value of care provided according to patient-specific condition classification and severity ratings
- Establishes the ability to self-manage without managed care oversight
- Supports special studies, e.g., supportive care
- Opens a "seat at the table" to decision makers
- Protects the integrity and future of chiropractic

Review: Treatment Plans and Assessments

- What elements are required to meet Medicare's requirements for a treatment plan? *D-42 to D-43*
- What is the expiration date on the Informed Consent Agreement? *D-43*
- What is the suggested minimal percent of improvement for an objective measure to be considered clinically significant? *D-42*
- Where can questionnaires be found to conduct Outcomes Assessment? *D-43 to D-44*

Notes

E CLAIMS AND APPEALS

1. Claims Processing
Page E-3

2. 1500 Claim Form
Page E-11

3. Guidelines for Unpaid Claims
Page E-37

4. ERISA Appeals
Page E-47

CLAIMS AND APPEALS

OBJECTIVES

Claims and Appeals are the central components of the Billing Process which is the final step of the "Reimbursement Life Cycle" as introduced in *Section B—Insurance and Reimbursement*. Once a patient encounter has been properly documented, this process begins with the submission of a claim that meets all the necessary requirements for reimbursement by a third-party payer. This section teaches how to properly submit a claim including guidelines and tips. It also includes valuable chapters on Guidelines for Unpaid Claims and ERISA Appeals.

OUTLINE

1. Claims Processing *E-3*
   - Overview of Claims Processing *E-3*
   - How to File Claims *E-6*
   - Filing Tips *E-8*
   - Review *E-10*

2. 1500 Claim Form *E-11*
   - Changes to the 1500 Claim Form *E-11*
   - 1500 Health Insurance Claim Form Instructions *E-14*
   - Review *E-36*

3. Guidelines for Unpaid Claims *E-37*
   - Claim Followup Procedures *E-37*
   - Claim Denial Management *E-39*
   - General Guidelines for Unpaid Claims *E-39*
   - Appeals Guidelines *E-41*
   - Reducing Denials *E-44*
   - Review *E-46*

4. ERISA Appeals *E-47*
   - ERISA Appeals (for Health Plans by Employers in the Private Sector) *E-47*
   - First Steps with ERISA *E-49*
   - Erisa Law Excerpts *E-52*
   - Review *E-55*

1. Claims Processing

Proper claim processing is the keystone of the Reimbursement Life Cycle—without claims payment or reimbursement, the practice will not survive. Although payment from an insurance company used to be the end of this process, that is no longer the case. Post-payment reviews and audits are placing an ever-increasing burden on all medical providers.

This section of the *ChiroCode Deskbook* explains how to file claims correctly, using the 1500 claim form, how to properly appeal denied claims, and how to manage unpaid claims.

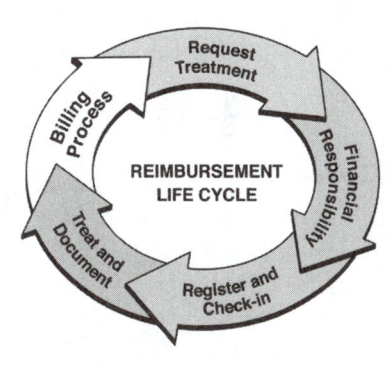

- See *Section C–Medicare* for information on appealing Medicare claims.
- See *Section F–Compliance and Audit Protection* for more about post-payment audits and reviews.

See Resource 199 for additional resources including links, articles and webinars.

Overview of Claims Processing

Submitting a clean claim is vital to the process of claims processing. Additionally, your treatment and documentation must meet medical necessity standards (establishing clinical need), and include all required elements for proper claims processing. It may seem strange to include documentation as a part of claims processing, but claims auditors closely examine the medical record and thus it becomes an important, and often neglected, component of ensuring that claims are paid correctly without fear of recoupment.

See *Section D–Documentation* for more information about this important part of claims processing and appeals.

When it comes to reimbursement issues, a clean claim is of paramount importance. A "clean claim" is defined as one that meets all the necessary requirements for the insurance carrier to process the claim. The "cleaner" the claim, the faster you will receive payment. It is the responsibility of the provider (you) to understand what is needed by the carrier. Your claim needs to meet insurance carrier guidelines, and provide all other information required in order to process the claim (e.g. proper claimant identification numbers). Attend third party payer workshops or obtain and review their instructions for claims processing which are often accessible online. The specific written guidelines are typically found within the carrier or provider manual. Remember that not all insurance contracts and policies are alike. You need to understand the differences between companies and contracts.

Accurate Information Is Key

Pay particular attention to these items to ensure a clean claim.

- Place the beneficiary's name and ID number on each piece of documentation submitted. Always use the beneficiary's name **exactly** as it appears on the beneficiary's insurance card.
- Include all applicable National Provider Identifiers (NPI) on the claim, including the NPI for the referring provider.
- Indicate the correct address, including the valid ZIP code where the service was rendered to the beneficiary. Any missing, incomplete or invalid information in the Service Facility Location Information field will cause the claim to be rejected. **Never** use a post office box address in the field for the location where the service was rendered.
- Ensure that the number of units/days and the date of service range are not contradictory.

See Resource 175 for additional information about billing units.

Clinical Need

Clinical need is demonstrating to third party payers that treatment was appropriate and necessary. Even though payers often have limits on the number of allowed visits, there could be situations where the number of visits is changed based on what is considered medically necessary. This need is demonstrated with appropriate documentation, including, but not limited to, patient history, clinical findings and objective outcome assessments.

- See *Section C–Medicare* for more about Medicare's clinical need requirements.
- See *Section D–Documentation* for more about appropriate documentation.

Diagnosis Code Pointing

Diagnosis code pointing is required by insurance companies in order to delineate which services were provided with which diagnosis. This is where the diagnosis listed in box #21 on the 1500 claim form is paired with a specific procedure code listed in box # 24D. Such pointing or pairing is standard within the insurance reimbursement industry. Since most claims are now processed by computer software programs which examine claim forms and transfer the information for processing in the carrier's system, there must be a valid diagnosis match (link) to each procedure or supply. The diagnosis is an essential part of the patient's medical record, and it is the driving force that justifies your treatment plan and payment.

Warning: When listing more than one diagnosis in the "diagnosis pointer box," Box 24E, always have the procedure "point" to only the diagnosis that is most clinically significant for that particular service line.

In addition, when a modifier such as "59" is appended to the CPT code 97140 to indicate that a separately identifiable procedure was rendered, the pointer must point to the diagnosis which is related only to the area in which the procedure was rendered.

- Many Medicare carriers require that subluxation be coded first. For Medicare, or any other payers that require subluxation as the principle diagnosis code, see *Section C–Medicare* for more information on how to do those claims.
- See *Section G–Diagnosis Codes* for more about diagnosis coding standards.

Multiple Diagnoses on a Claim Form

The new paper 1500 claim form was revised to match the electronic 5010 format and accommodate twelve diagnoses codes on a claim. Even though there is room for twelve codes, different insurance carriers have different requirements. Not all allow the maximum of twelve diagnosis codes on a claim so it is important to be aware of individual payer preferences. Even though there are now more places on the paper claim to report additional diagnoses, only include those which are **relevant** to the patient's treatment plan. Keep in mind that even though there may be twelve diagnosis codes on a claim, both the paper and electronic claim only allow four diagnosis codes to "point" to a single claim procedure line (see Item Number 24E, Diagnosis Pointer on page E-33).

In the past, many payers wanted only one ICD-9 diagnostic code: the primary code, which directly relates to the service/treatment. Although this protocol for some payers might fill their immediate processing needs, it comes with big risks, because it fails to tell the complete story, which could lead to allegations of false claims. Always identify all applicable diagnosis codes on the 1500 form, even if a payer will only look at one code. When you document services correctly, you protect your practice.

See Chapter 2–1500 Claim Form in this *Claims and Appeals* section for more about using the claim form.

Multiple Page Claims

The following general guidelines from the NUCC explain how to handle claims that span more than one page. However, be aware of individual payer requirements. Some may have different standards.

> "When reporting line item services on multiple page claims, only the diagnosis code(s) reported on the first page may be used and must be repeated on subsequent pages. If more than twelve diagnoses are required to report the line services, the claim must be split and the services related to the additional diagnoses must be billed as a separate claim."

Tip: Instead of using "Page XX of YY" for multiple pages, one way to avoid confusion is to simply split the claim. Bill related charges only on one claim form and put additional days of service on a separate claim form.

Timely Filing

Most insurance payers have a specific time period, commencing after the date of service, during which a health insurance claim must be submitted. If the claim arrives after this date, the claim is denied. Providers must obtain this information from each payer and make sure that claims are submitted within the time frame allowed.

To be eligible for Medicare reimbursement, claims must be filed with Medicare no later than one calendar year (basically 12 months) from the initial date of service or the claim will be denied.

Some payers follow the Medicare standard on the one calendar year filing deadline. However, it is always best to verify their standards by contacting their Provider Relations Department to find out about individual policies.

Late Filing Exceptions

Most providers are unaware that there are some late filing exceptions. Most payers allow claims to be filed late, but only under certain circumstances. Contact the payer to find out their particular policy regarding late filing. The following may be some accepted reasons for fighting a late filing denial:

- Errors on the original claim.
- Claim filed with the incorrect carrier.
- Missing authorizations or referrals.
- Claims that were filed by the provider in the correct time frame, but lost by the carrier.

Refiling/Resubmitting Claims

There are several reasons to refile or resubmit a claim. The carrier could lose them, they could be lost by the postal service or there could be a problem during the electronic transmission. Whatever the reason, follow-up is important. Keeping a detailed log or printing reports of sent claims is essential. Some payers may have specific protocols which must be followed such as using a special form or printing "refiled claim" on paper claims. To avoid duplication errors, determine the insurer's policy before resubmitting a claim. Include this information in the "Daily Policies and Procedures Manual" for easy reference.

Claims Adjudication

Claims processing describes the action of submitting claims to the payer and the resulting determination. The process by which the payer makes a determination about a claim based on benefits and coverage information is known as adjudication. When a payer receives a claim, adjudication follows a predetermined route.

Upon arrival at the payer, each claim is dated. Usually, paper claims are also scanned or photocopied for long-term storage. Data is then entered into the payer's computer system. While proceeding along the "claims processing" route, claims go through a series of edits to verify the patient's coverage and eligibility and to check for medical necessity and non-covered services. If the claim is "clean", it is paid. If the claim fails the edits it could be denied; or, the payer marks the claim as unprocessable and contacts the provider's office or the patient.

See Resource 178 for official 1500 claim form instructions.

How to File Claims

Providers have only two options for filing claims: paper or electronic. There are pros and cons to either option. For example, electronic claims are paid faster, but you must meet all HIPAA requirements, which requires additional software and training costs. Evaluate both options to determine which one is an appropriate "fit" for your practice.

Data Mining

Computer information technology has made claims processing (adjudication) a science instead of a guessing game. Computerized data analysis, also called data mining, allows payers to profile physicians and review services and their billing patterns.

As Medicare analyzed these patterns to discover implications of fraudulent behavior, their fraud and abuse activities dramatically increased. It didn't take long for private payers to recognize the financial impact of Medicare's fraud and abuse initiatives. They also began to monitor and audit claims to verify the performance and necessity of billed services.

See the Fraud and Abuse segment in *Section F—Compliance and Audit Protection* for more information.

Other important factors to consider are state law and individual carrier contracts. Even though HIPAA does **not** require all claims to be submitted electronically (there are exceptions available), there are some states which do **not** have exceptions. Also, some payers are now requiring electronic claims submission. Pay special attention to your contract renewals to ensure compliance.

Paper Claims

Paper claims are submitted using the 1500 claim form. The form should be submitted using the red ink version that can be scanned by payers. A typical copy machine or printer cannot duplicate the red ink used to print the 1500 form. Therefore, if you attempt to print the red ink version of the 1500 form from your printer many carriers will not be able to process your claims.

For those wishing to maintain exemption from HIPAA mandates (which is rare) and continue to bill paper claims, you must not send or receive any electronic transactions (eligibility, coordination of benefits, payments, payment reports, etc.). However, be aware of any contract with any payer that might require that you submit electronic claims. Medicare, for example, mandates electronic claims submission; however, if you are a small provider with less than 10 full-time equivalent employees, you can be exempt from their electronic claims mandate. Make sure they have your exemption status on file.

> **Caution:** Read the segment "HIPAA Exempt Offices (Paper)" in Chapter 2–HIPAA Compliance in *Section F–Compliance and Audit Protection* for detailed information on what is required for exemption from HIPAA.

See *Section F–Compliance and Audit Protection* for help with HIPAA.

Official 1500 claim forms (Resource 179) may be purchased from the ChiroCode Store.

See Resource 194 for information about the Medicare electronic claims exemption.

Eletronic Claims

Electronic claims are 1500 claims in an electronic (837) format and are subject to all HIPAA standards for transactions, privacy and security. When submitting an electronic claim you automatically become a HIPAA entity. Make sure that your office, your software billing company, vendors, subcontractors and the receiving payer are all HIPAA compliant.

As of January 1, 2012, the official HIPAA transaction standard is HIPAA 5010. Version 5010 is the X12 standard (837p and 837i) for all HIPAA electronic claims submission. HIPAA 5010 allows for the longer ICD-10-CM codes that will be implemented in October 2015 along with other changes. Everyone should be using version 5010 at this time.

HIPAA 6020

The change from version 4010 to 5010 was problematic to say the least. As an attempt to avoid having the same thing happen again, in March 2013, CMS partnered with a company called Emdeon to begin the process of mapping version 5010 to version 6020 and testing the resulting conversion process.

This testing project was scheduled for completion in September 2013. It appears that CMS is preparing for version 6020, but no official announcements have been made.

Paperwork Segment

The paperwork segment (PWK) is a new tool for providers to help claims be paid properly the first time instead of going through an appeals process. In order to facilitate the need for "linkage" between electronic claims and additional documentation which is needed for claims adjudication, the 837 format has a special segment refered to as the paperwork segment (PWK). As of October 1, 2012, many payers were accepting PWK. PWK is different than electronic submission of medical documentation (esMD) in that an electronic claim indicates that paper documentation is being sent. Most payers require the completion of a specific cover sheet to be included with documentation which is submitted via fax or mail. Generally, you only have 7-10 days to successfully submit the necessary documentation once the electronic claim has been filed.

Be aware of individual payer differences and requirements. For example, WPS Medicare is requiring PWK when electronic claims are submitted with modifiers 22 or 52. Talk to your claims software vendor to see if they are ready to implement the PWK.

> **Tip:** Your business associates and subcontractors must be HIPAA compliant, this includes your clearinghouse and billing software. The Omnibus Final Rule changed the definition of a business associate and new "Business Associate Agreements" will need to be executed in accordance with that rule.
>
> For Business Associate Agreements see *Complete & Easy HIPAA Compliance* (Resource 116).
>
> See *Section F–Compliance and Audit Protection* for detailed information regarding HIPAA.
>
> Go to ACAtoday.org/HIPAA for information by the ACA regarding HIPAA.

FILING TIPS

General Filing Tips

The following tips apply to both paper and electronic claims.

Coding Tips

- Use current, valid diagnosis codes and code to the highest level of specificity (maximum number of digits) available. Also make sure that the diagnosis codes used are appropriate for the gender of the beneficiary.
- Use current valid procedure codes as described in the Current Procedural Terminology (CPT) or Healthcare Common Procedure Coding System (HCPCS) manuals.
- Use current and valid modifiers when necessary.

Lost Claims

Lost claims are a dreaded but inevitable part of health care claims processing. The best way to avoid them is to file claims electronically. This removes a lot of pitfalls that can go wrong with paper. If a claim is lost after being filed electronically then re-submit on paper. If you have talked to someone at the insurance company, ask to send it directly to their attention. To assure delivery, send the claim either by certified mail, with proof of service, or with delivery confirmation.

- Follow the written guidelines of individual payers. If there is an issue with their policies, work with your professional association, such as the ACA, to resolve the problem. Professional associations are often successful in overturning incorrect coding policies.

> See *Section G–Diagnosis Codes* for current ICD-9-CM and ICD-10-CM codes.
> See *Section H–Procedure Codes* for current CPT codes.
> See *Section I–Supply Codes* for current HCPCS codes for supplies.

Common Errors to Avoid

- Different patient names or addresses than the insurers' records.
- Incorrect patient ID number.
- Incomplete patient information.
- Incorrect or missing provider ID number or Social Security number.
- Incorrect dates of service.
- Incorrect dates, or dates entered with an incorrect number of digits.
- Insufficient information regarding primary or secondary coverage.
- Invalid procedure, supply or diagnostic codes.
- Invalid or missing modifiers.
- Unit of service errors.
- Invalid or missing Place of Service (POS) codes.
- Invalid diagnostic codes that do not point to the correct procedure or service.
- Failure to enter the fee (left blank); fees not itemized and totaled.
- Missing patient and/or provider signatures.
- Ineligible claims (expired or canceled insurance contract).
- Late filing errors.

Tips for Error-Free Paper Claims

Troubleshooting Basics

- Use only an original 1500 claim form that has red print on white paper.
- Use dark ink for entering claim information.
- Do not print, hand-write, or stamp any extraneous data on the form.
- Do not staple, clip, or tape anything to the 1500 claim form.
- Remove pin-fed edges at side perforations.
- Use only lift-off correction tape to make corrections.
- Place all necessary documentation in the envelope with the claim form.

Format Hints

- Do not use italics or script.
- Do not use dollar signs, decimals or punctuation.
- Use only upper case (CAPITAL) letters.
- Use 10- or 12-pitch (pica) characters and standard dot matrix fonts.
- Do not include titles (e.g. Dr., Mr., Mrs., Rev., M.D.) as part of the beneficiary's name.
- Enter all information on the same horizontal plane within the designated field.

- Follow the correct Health Insurance Claim Number (HICN) format. No hyphens or dashes should be used. The alpha prefix or suffix is part of the HICN and should not be omitted. Be especially careful with spouses who have a similar HICN with a different alpha prefix or suffix.
- Ensure data is in the appropriate field and does not overlap into other fields.
- Use an individual's name in the provider signature field, not a facility or practice name.

Review: Claims Processing

- What makes a "clean claim"? *E-3*
- How many diagnosis codes may be entered on either a paper claim or an electronic claim? *E-5*
- Does an error on an original claim qualify it for a late filing exception? *E-6*
- How many employees do you need to be exempt from the electronic claims mandate? *E-7*

2. 1500 Claim Form

This section covers the 1500 claim form (See Figure 5.2), which was implemented on April 1, 2014. Only those claim form items which are new, revised or need special attention are included here. Detailed instructions for all claim form items can be found in the Claim Form Appendix which is available online.

See Resource 178 for official 1500 claim form instructions.

See Chapter 1– Claims Processing of *Section E–Claims and Appeals* for general claim completion tips and information regarding electronic claims.

CHANGES TO THE 1500 CLAIM FORM

In order to have the paper claim form more closely match the electronic claim form standards, the NUCC proposed changes to the 1500 claim form which were approved by CMS for paper claims beginning on January 1, 2014 (see Figure 5.2.) As of April 1, 2014, version 08/05 of the 1500 Claim Form is discontinued; only version 02/12 of the 1500 Claim Form is to be used. All rebilling of claims will be on the (02/12) 1500 Claim Form from this date forward, even though earlier submissions may have been on the version (08/05) 1500 Claim Form.

The changes to this form were considered "minor" in that all proposed changes are within the current lines of the claim form. The exception is Item 21, "Diagnosis or Nature of Illness or Injury." That change is major enough to require most providers to update any billing software (see the "Listing of Changes" that follows). By now, you should have updated your software to utilize the revised form.

Figure 5.2 outlines all the changes to the 1500 claim form. Revised items are outlined in gray.

About the NUCC

The NUCC is a voluntary organization whose members represent major providers, payers, health researchers, or other organizations representing billing professionals and electronic standard developers. The NUCC maintains the National Uniform Claim Committee Data Set designed for non-institutional claims (Hospitals and other institutions use a different form.) The NUCC is one of four national organizations named in the 1996 HIPAA Administrative Simplification legislation for a consultative role in establishing administrative standards for health care.

FIGURE 5.2

Changes to the1500 Health Insurance Claim Form

HEALTH INSURANCE CLAIM FORM

APPROVED BY NATIONAL UNIFORM CLAIM COMMITTEE (NUCC) 02/12

PICA — PICA — CARRIER

1. MEDICARE (Medicare#) | MEDICAID (Medicaid#) | TRICARE (ID#/DoD#) | CHAMPVA (Member ID#) | GROUP HEALTH PLAN (ID#) | FECA BLK LUNG (ID#) | OTHER (ID#)

1a. INSURED'S I.D. NUMBER (For Program in Item 1)

2. PATIENT'S NAME (Last Name, First Name, Middle Initial)

3. PATIENT'S BIRTH DATE MM DD YY — SEX M F

4. INSURED'S NAME (Last Name, First Name, Middle Initial)

5. PATIENT'S ADDRESS (No., Street)

6. PATIENT RELATIONSHIP TO INSURED — Self Spouse Child Other

7. INSURED'S ADDRESS (No., Street)

CITY — STATE

8. RESERVED FOR NUCC USE

CITY — STATE

ZIP CODE — TELEPHONE (Include Area Code) ( )

ZIP CODE — TELEPHONE (Include Area Code) ( )

9. OTHER INSURED'S NAME (Last Name, First Name, Middle Initial)

10. IS PATIENT'S CONDITION RELATED TO:

11. INSURED'S POLICY GROUP OR FECA NUMBER

a. OTHER INSURED'S POLICY OR GROUP NUMBER

a. EMPLOYMENT? (Current or Previous) YES NO

a. INSURED'S DATE OF BIRTH MM DD YY — SEX M F

b. RESERVED FOR NUCC USE

b. AUTO ACCIDENT? YES NO — PLACE (State)

b. OTHER CLAIM ID (Designated by NUCC)

c. RESERVED FOR NUCC USE

c. OTHER ACCIDENT? YES NO

c. INSURANCE PLAN NAME OR PROGRAM NAME

d. INSURANCE PLAN NAME OR PROGRAM NAME

10d. CLAIM CODES (Designated by NUCC)

d. IS THERE ANOTHER HEALTH BENEFIT PLAN? YES NO *If yes*, complete items 9, 9a, and 9d.

READ BACK OF FORM BEFORE COMPLETING & SIGNING THIS FORM.

12. PATIENT'S OR AUTHORIZED PERSON'S SIGNATURE I authorize the release of any medical or other information necessary to process this claim. I also request payment of government benefits either to myself or to the party who accepts assignment below.

SIGNED ____ DATE ____

13. INSURED'S OR AUTHORIZED PERSON'S SIGNATURE I authorize payment of medical benefits to the undersigned physician or supplier for services described below.

SIGNED ____

PATIENT AND INSURED INFORMATION

14. DATE OF CURRENT ILLNESS, INJURY, or PREGNANCY (LMP) MM DD YY — QUAL.

15. OTHER DATE QUAL. MM DD YY

16. DATES PATIENT UNABLE TO WORK IN CURRENT OCCUPATION FROM MM DD YY TO MM DD YY

17. NAME OF REFERRING PROVIDER OR OTHER SOURCE — 17a. — 17b. NPI

18. HOSPITALIZATION DATES RELATED TO CURRENT SERVICES FROM MM DD YY TO MM DD YY

19. ADDITIONAL CLAIM INFORMATION (Designated by NUCC)

20. OUTSIDE LAB? YES NO — $ CHARGES

21. DIAGNOSIS OR NATURE OF ILLNESS OR INJURY Relate A-L to service line below (24E) — ICD Ind.

A. B. C. D.
E. F. G. H.
I. J. K. L.

22. RESUBMISSION CODE — ORIGINAL REF. NO.

23. PRIOR AUTHORIZATION NUMBER

24. A. DATE(S) OF SERVICE From MM DD YY To MM DD YY	B. PLACE OF SERVICE	C. EMG	D. PROCEDURES, SERVICES, OR SUPPLIES (Explain Unusual Circumstances) CPT/HCPCS MODIFIER	E. DIAGNOSIS POINTER	F. $ CHARGES	G. DAYS OR UNITS	H. EPSDT Family Plan	I. ID. QUAL.	J. RENDERING PROVIDER ID. #
1								NPI	
2								NPI	
3								NPI	
4								NPI	
5								NPI	
6								NPI	

25. FEDERAL TAX I.D. NUMBER SSN EIN

26. PATIENT'S ACCOUNT NO.

27. ACCEPT ASSIGNMENT? (For govt. claims, see back) YES NO

28. TOTAL CHARGE $

29. AMOUNT PAID $

30. Rsvd for NUCC Use

31. SIGNATURE OF PHYSICIAN OR SUPPLIER INCLUDING DEGREES OR CREDENTIALS (I certify that the statements on the reverse apply to this bill and are made a part thereof.)

SIGNED DATE

32. SERVICE FACILITY LOCATION INFORMATION — a. NPI b.

33. BILLING PROVIDER INFO & PH # ( ) — a. NPI b.

PHYSICIAN OR SUPPLIER INFORMATION

NUCC Instruction Manual available at: www.nucc.org — *PLEASE PRINT OR TYPE* — APPROVED OMB-0938-1197 FORM 1500 (02-12)

1500 Health Insurance Claim Form: Listing of Changes

- **Header**
  Replaced 1500 rectangular symbol with black and white two-dimensional Quick Response Code (QR Code).
  Added "(NUCC)" after "APPROVED BY NATIONAL UNIFORM CLAIM COMMITTEE."
  Replaced "08/05" with "02/12."

- **Item Number 1**
  Deleted "CHAMPUS" and changed "(Sponsor's SSN)" to "(ID#/DoD#)."
  Under "GROUP HEALTH PLAN," changed "(SSN or ID)" to "(ID#)."
  Under "FECA BLK LUNG," changed "(SSN)" to "(ID#)."
  Under "OTHER," changed "(ID)" to "(ID#)."

- **Item Number 8**
  Deleted "PATIENT STATUS" and content of field.
  Changed title to "RESERVED FOR NUCC USE."

- **Item Number 9b**
  Deleted "OTHER INSURED'S DATE OF BIRTH, SEX."
  Changed title to "RESERVED FOR NUCC USE."

- **Item Number 9c**
  Deleted "EMPLOYER'S NAME OR SCHOOL." Changed title to "RESERVED FOR NUCC USE."

- **Item Number 10d**
  Changed title from "RESERVED FOR LOCAL USE" to "CLAIM CODES (Designated by NUCC)."

- **Item Number 11b**
  Deleted "EMPLOYER'S NAME OR SCHOOL."
  Changed title to "OTHER CLAIM ID (Designated by NUCC)."
  Added vertical, dotted line in the left-hand side of the field to accommodate a 2-byte qualifier.

- **Item Number 11d**
  Changed "If yes, return to and complete Item 9 a-d" to "If yes, complete items 9, 9a, and 9d."

- **Item Number 14**
  Changed title to "DATE OF CURRENT ILLNESS, INJURY, or PREGNANCY (LMP)."
  Removed the arrow and text in the right-hand side of the field.
  Added "QUAL." and a vertical, dotted line to accommodate a 3-byte qualifier.

- **Item Number 15**
  Changed title from "IF PATIENT HAS HAD SAME OR SIMILAR ILLNESS. GIVE FIRST DATE" to "OTHER DATE."
  Added "QUAL." with two dotted lines to accommodate a 3-byte qualifier.

- **Item Number 17**
  Added a vertical, dotted line in the left-hand side of the field to accommodate a 2-byte qualifier.

- **Item Number 19**
  Changed title from "RESERVED FOR LOCAL USE" to "ADDITIONAL CLAIM INFORMATION (Designated by NUCC)."

- **Item Number 21**
  Added "ICD Ind." and two vertical, dotted lines in the upper right-hand corner of the field to accommodate a 1-byte indicator.
  Added 8 additional lines for diagnosis codes.
  Evenly spaced the diagnosis code lines within the field.
  Changed labels of the diagnosis code lines to alpha characters (A – L).
  Removed the period within the diagnosis code lines.

- **Item Number 22**
  Changed title from "MEDICAID RESUBMISSION" to "RESUBMISSION."

- **Item Number 30**
  Deleted "BALANCE DUE."
  Changed title to "Rsvd for NUCC Use."

- **Footer**
  Changed OMB approval numbers to OMB-0938-1197

1500 Health Insurance Claim Form Instructions

The following rules for the 1500 are excerpts from NUCC and Medicare instructions, but they are generally universal. Consult with your specific insurance payer for their adaptations. However, these instructions apply to claims submitted on paper or electronically and must be used when filing claims with Medicare. Please note that payment rules can change frequently for any payer.

The instructions included in this section are excerpts from the following documents along with commentary by ChiroCode Institute:

- *1500 Health Insurance Claim Form Reference Instruction Manual for Form Version 02/12 (version 2.0 07/14)*, by the National Uniform Claim Committee (NUCC).
- Medicare instructions by CMS (Rev. 3083, 10-02-14) are added to the NUCC instructions in shaded areas.

Please note that this section only contains instructions or information that have either changed, are new, or should be paid close attention to when submitting claims. Complete instructions are available online.

> See Resource 178 for the complete list of line items and their associated guidelines and revisions, including exclusive ChiroCode Institute tips.

Instruction Conventions

Item Number and Titles are in bold text.

NUCC descriptions are in italic text.

NUCC instructions are in regular text.

Additional instructions by Medicare are shaded.

| Alerts and commentaries by ChiroCode Institute are enclosed in this type of box. |

▶ ◀   Identifies new or revised text for this year.

Field specifications are omitted. (See the full instructions by the NUCC.)

Overall Instructions

Each item number includes the title, instructions, description, and example. The examples provided in the instructions are demonstrating how to enter the data in the field. They are not providing instruction on how to bill for certain services. **Please note:** Form images throughout this manual may not be to scale.

▶Multiple Page Claims

When reporting line item services on multiple page claims, only the diagnosis code(s) reported on the first page may be used and must be repeated on subsequent pages. If more than four diagnoses are required to report the line services, the claim must be split and the services related to the additional diagnoses must be billed as a separate claim. ◀

General Formatting Guidelines

- Do not use ▶punctuation (i.e. commas, periods) or other symbols ◀ in the address (e.g., 123 N Main Street 101 instead of 123 N. Main Street, #101). When entering a 9-digit ZIP code, include the hyphen.
- Enter all dates (i.e. birth date) as an 8-digit number (MM | DD | YYYY)

Medicare Instructions

▶ The Administrative Simplification Compliance Act (ASCA) requires that Medicare claims be sent electronically unless certain exceptions are met. Providers meeting an ASCA exception may send their claims to Medicare on a paper claim form. (For more information regarding ASCA exceptions, refer to Chapter 24.)

Providers sending professional and supplier claims to Medicare on paper must use Form CMS-1500 in a valid version. This form is maintained by the National Uniform Claim Committee (NUCC), an industry organization in which CMS participates. Any new version of the form must be approved by the White House Office of Management and Budget (OMB) before it can be used for submitting Medicare claims. When the NUCC changes the form, CMS coordinates its review, any changes, and approval with the OMB.

The NUCC has recently changed the Form CMS-1500, and the revised form received OMB approval on June 10, 2013. The revised form is version 02/12, OMB control number 0938-1197.

The revised form will replace the previous version of the form 08/05, OMB control number 0938-0999.

Throughout this chapter, the terms, "Form CMS-1500," "Form 1500," and "CMS-1500 claim form" may be used to describe this form depending upon the context and version. The term, "CMS-1500 claim form" refers to the form generically, independent of a given version.

Medicare will conduct a dual-use period during which providers can send Medicare claims on either the old or the revised forms. When the dual-use period is over, Medicare will accept paper claims on only the revised Form 1500, version 02/12.

For the implementation and dual-use dates, contractors shall consult the appropriate implementation change requests for the revised Form 1500. Providers and other interested parties may obtain the implementation dates on the CMS web site @ www.cms.gov.

Reminder: Regardless of the paper claim form version in effect: **Providers cannot submit ICD-10-CM codes for claims with dates of service prior to implementation of ICD-10.** ◀

The following instructions are required for a Medicare claim. ▶ They apply to both the 08/05 and 02/12 versions of the form except where noted. A/B MACs (B) and DME MACs should provide information on completing the CMS-1500 claim form ◀ to all physicians and suppliers in their area at least once a year.

▶ These instructions represent the minimum requirements for using this form to submit a Medicare claim. However, depending on a given Medicare policy, there may be other data that should also be included on the CMS-1500 claim form; if so, these additional requirements are addressed in the instructions you received for such policies (e.g., other chapters of this manual). ◀

Providers may use these instructions to complete this form. The CMS-1500 ▶claim form◀ has space for physicians and suppliers to provide information on other health insurance. This information can be used by A/B MACs ▶(B)◀ to determine whether the Medicare patient has other coverage that must be billed prior to Medicare payment, or whether there is another insurer to which Medicare can forward billing and payment data following adjudication if the provider is a physician or supplier that participates in Medicare. (See Pub 100-05, Medicare Secondary Payer Manual, Chapter 3, and Chapter 28 of this manual).

Providers and suppliers must report 8-digit dates in all date of birth fields (items 3, 9b, and 11a), and either 6-digit or 8-digit dates in all other date fields (items 11b, 12, 14, 16, 18, 19, 24a, and 31)

Providers and suppliers have the option of entering either a 6 or 8-digit date in items 11b, 14, 16, 18, 19, or 24a. However, if a provider of service or supplier chooses to enter 8-digit dates for items

11b, 14, 16, 18, 19, or 24a, he or she must enter 8-digit dates for all these fields. For instance, a provider of service or supplier will not be permitted to enter 8-digit dates for items 11b, 14, 16, 18, 19 and a 6-digit date for item 24a. The same applies to providers of service and suppliers who choose to submit 6-digit dates too. Items 12 and 31 are exempt from this requirement.

Legend	Description
MM	Month (e.g., December = 12)
DD	Day (e.g., Dec15 = 15)
YY	2 position Year (e.g., 1998 = 98)
CCYY	4 position Year (e.g., 1998 = 1998)
(MM | DD | YY) or (MM | DD | CCYY)	A space must be reported between month, day, and year (e.g., 12 | 15 | 98 or 12 | 15 | 1998). This space is delineated by a dotted vertical line on the Form CMS-1500.
(MMDDYY) or (MMDDCCYY)	No space must be reported between month, day, and year (e.g., 121598 or 12151998). The date must be recorded as one continuous number.

Field Specific Instructions

Items 1-13 Patient and Insured Information

Note: If the patient can be identified by a unique Member Identification Number, the patient is considered to be the "insured." The patient is reported as the insured in the insured data fields and not in the patient fields.

Item Number 1, Medicare; Medicaid; ▶TRICARE; CHAMPUS,◀ CHAMPVA; Group Health Plan; FECA Blk Lung; Other

Description: "Medicare, Medicaid, TRICARE, CHAMPVA, Group Health Plan, FECA, Black Lung, Other" means the insurance type to which the claim is being submitted. "Other" indicates health insurance including HMOs, commercial insurance, automobile accident, liability, or workers' compensation. This information directs the claim to the correct program and may establish primary liability.

Indicate the type of health insurance coverage applicable to this claim by placing an X in the appropriate box. Only one box can be marked.

> ▶**Medicare:** Shows the type of health insurance coverage applicable to this claim by the appropriately checked box; check the Medicare box. ◀

Item Number 1a, Insured's ID Number

Description: The "Insured's ID Number" is the identification number of the insured. This information identifies the insured to the payer.

Enter the insured's ID number as shown on insured's ID card for the payer to which the claim is being submitted. If the patient has a unique Member Identification Number assigned by the payer, then enter that number in this field.

▶**For TRICARE:** Enter the DoD Benefits Number (DBN 11-digit number) from the back of the ID card.

For Workers Compensation Claims: Enter Employee ID.

For Other Property & Casualty Claims: Enter the Federal Tax ID or SSN of the insured person or entity. ◀

▶**Medicare:** Enter the patient's Medicare Health Insurance Claim Number (HICN) whether Medicare is the primary or secondary payer. This is a required field. ◀

Item Number 5, Patient's Address (multiple fields)

5. PATIENT'S ADDRESS (No., Street)		
123 Main Street		
CITY		STATE
Anytown		IL
ZIP CODE	TELEPHONE (Include Area Code)	
60610	(312) 5551212	

Description: The ▶*Patient's Address is* ◀ *the patient's permanent residence. A temporary address or school address should not be used.*

Enter the patient's address. The first line is for the street address; the second line, the city and state; the third line, the ZIP code.

Do not use punctuation (i.e., commas, periods) or other symbols in the address (e.g., 123 N Main Street 101 instead of 123 N. Main Street, #101). When entering a 9-digit ZIP code, include the hyphen.

▶If reporting a foreign address, contact payer for specific reporting instructions. ◀

If the patient's address is the same as the insured's address, then it is not necessary to report the patient's address.

"Patient's Telephone" does not exist in 5010A1. The NUCC recommends that the phone number not be reported. Phone extentions are not supported.

For Workers Compensation and Other Property and Casualty Claims If required by a payer to report a telephone number, do not use a hyphen or space as a separator within the telephone number.

Medicare: Enter the patient's mailing address and telephone number. On the first line enter the street address; the second line, the city and state; the third line, the ZIP code and phone number.

ChiroCode Institute Tip: Verify this demographic information. The patient's address is not always the same as the insured's address. Using the incorrect address is a common cause of delayed payment.

Item Number 6, Patient Relationship to Insured

6. PATIENT RELATIONSHIP TO INSURED			
Self ☐	Spouse ☐	Child ☒	Other ☐

Description: The ▶ *"Patient Relationship to Insured" indicates* ◀ *how the patient is related to the insured.* "Self" would indicate that the insured is the patient. "Spouse" would indicate that the patient is the husband or wife or qualified partner as defined by the insured's plan. "Child" would indicate that the patient is the minor dependent as defined by the insured's plan. Other would indicate that the patient is other than the self, spouse, or child, which may include employee, ward, or dependent as defined by the insured's plan.

Enter an X in the correct box to indicate the patient's relationship to insured when Item Number 4 is completed. Only one box can be marked.

▶If the patient is a dependent, but has a unique Member Identification Number and the payer requires the identification number be reported on the claim, then report "Self", since the patient is reported as the insured. ◀

Medicare: Check the appropriate box for patient's relationship to insured when item 4 is completed

Item Number 8, Reserved for NUCC Use

```
8. RESERVED FOR NUCC USE
```

Description: This box is reserved for NUCC Use

This field was previously used to report "Patient Status." "Patient Status" does not exist in 5010A1, so this field has been eliminated.

This field is reserved for NUCC use. The NUCC will provide instructions for any use of this field.

▶**Medicare:** Form version 08/05: Check the appropriate box for the patient's marital status and whether employed or a student.

Form version 02/12: Leave blank. ◀

Item Number 9, Other Insured's Name

```
9. OTHER INSURED'S NAME (Last Name, First Name, Middle Initial)
   Doe, Mary, A
```

Description: The Other Insured's Name indicates that there is a holder of another policy that may cover the patient.

If Item Number 11d is marked, complete fields 9, 9a and 9d, otherwise leave blank. When additional group health coverage exists, enter other insured's full last name, first name, and middle initial of the enrollee in another health plan if it is different from that shown in Item Number 2. If the insured uses a last name suffix (e.g., Jr, Sr) enter it after the last name and before the first name. Titles (e.g., Sister, Capt, Dr) and professional suffixes (e.g., PhD, MD, Esq) should not be included with the name.

Use commas to separate the last name, first name, and middle initial. A hyphen can be used for hyphenated names. Do not use periods within the name.

Medicare: Enter the last name, first name, and middle initial of the enrollee in a Medigap policy if it is different from that shown in item 2. Otherwise, enter the word SAME. If no Medigap benefits are assigned, leave blank. **This field may be used in the future for supplemental insurance plans.**

NOTE: Only participating physicians and suppliers are to complete item 9 and its subdivisions and only when the beneficiary wishes to assign his/her benefits under a MEDIGAP policy to the participating physician or supplier.

Participating physicians and suppliers must enter information required in item 9 and its subdivisions if requested by the beneficiary. Participating physicians/suppliers sign an agreement with Medicare to accept assignment of Medicare benefits for **all** Medicare patients. A claim for which a beneficiary elects to assign his/her benefits under a Medigap policy to a participating physician/supplier is called a mandated Medigap transfer. (See chapter 28.)

Medigap - Medigap policy meets the statutory definition of a "Medicare supplemental policy" contained in §1882(g)(1) of title XVIII of the Social Security Act (the Act) and the definition contained in the NAIC Model Regulation that is incorporated by reference to the statute. It is a health insurance policy or other health benefit plan offered by a private entity to those persons entitled to Medicare benefits and is specifically designed to supplement Medicare benefits. It fills in some of the "gaps" in Medicare coverage by providing payment for some of the charges for which Medicare does not have responsibility due to the applicability of deductibles, coinsurance amounts, or other limitations imposed by Medicare. It does not include limited benefit coverage available to Medicare beneficiaries such as "specified disease" or "hospital indemnity" coverage. Also, it explicitly excludes a policy or plan offered by an employer to employees or former employees, as well as that offered by a labor organization to members or former members.

Do not list other supplemental coverage in item 9 and its subdivisions at the time a Medicare claim is filed. Other supplemental claims are forwarded automatically to the private insurer if the private insurer contracts with the ▶A/B MAC (B) or DME MAC◀ carrier to send Medicare claim information electronically. If there is no such contract, the beneficiary must file his/her own supplemental claim.

> **ChiroCode Institute Tip:** Some payers may want the name entered without commas. Be aware of individual payer differences.

> **ChiroCode Institute Tip:** For Medicare, item 9 should only be completed when the provider is a participating physician or supplier, and when the patient wishes to assign his/her benefits under a Medigap policy to the participating physician or supplier. Participating providers sign an agreement with Medicare to accept assignment of Medicare benefits for all Medicare patients. A claim for which a beneficiary elects to assign his/her benefits under a Medigap policy to a participating provider is called a mandated Medigap transfer.
>
> Other supplemental coverage should not be listed in item 9 or its subdivisions at the time a Medicare claim is filed. Other supplemental claims are forwarded automatically to the private insurer if the private insurer contracts with the carrier to send Medicare claim information electronically. If there is no such contract, the beneficiary must file his/her own supplemental claim.

> **ChiroCode Institute Tip:** Item 9: This is an important item to properly complete because incorrectly billing Medicare as primary when it should have been secondary is high on the list of red flags for OIG.
>
> See Chapter 4–OIG Compliance in *Section F–Compliance and Audit Protection*.

Item Number 9b, Reserved for NUCC Use

| 9b. RESERVED FOR NUCC USE |

Description: This box is reserved for NUCC Use

This field was previously used to report "Other Insured's Date of Birth, Sex." "Other Insured's Date of Birth, Sex" does not exist in 5010A1, so this field has been eliminated.

This field is reserved for NUCC use. The NUCC will provide instructions for any use of this field.

> **Medicare:** ▶Form version 08/05: Enter the Medigap insured's 8-digit birth date (MM | DD | CCYY) and sex.
>
> Form version 02/12: Leave blank. ◀

Item Number 9c, ▶Reserved for NUCC Use ◀

```
9c RESERVED FOR NUCC USE
```

Description: This box is reserved for NUCC Use

This field was previously used to report "Employer's Name or School Name." "Employer's Name or School Name" does not exist in 5010A1, so this field has been eliminated.

This field is reserved for NUCC use. The NUCC will provide instructions for any use of this field.

▶**Medicare:** Leave blank if item 9d is completed. Otherwise, enter the claims processing address of the Medigap insurer. Use an abbreviated street address, two-letter postal code, and ZIP code copied from the Medigap insured's Medigap identification card. For example:

1257 Anywhere Street
Baltimore, MD 21204

is shown as "1257 Anywhere St. MD 21204." ◀

Items Number 10a–10c, Is Patient's Condition Related To:

```
10. IS PATIENT'S CONDITION RELATED TO:

a. EMPLOYMENT? (Current or Previous)
       [ ] YES   [X] NO
b. AUTO ACCIDENT?
                      PLACE (State)
       [ ] YES   [X] NO  [____]
c. OTHER ACCIDENT?
       [ ] YES   [X] NO
```

Description: This information indicates whether the patient's illness or injury is related to employment, auto accident, or other accident. "Employment (current or previous)" would indicate that the condition is related to the patient's job or workplace. "Auto accident" would indicate that the condition is the result of an automobile accident. "Other accident" would indicate that the condition is the result of any other type of accident.

When appropriate, enter an X in the correct box to indicate whether one or more of the services described in Item Number 24 are for a condition or injury that occurred on the job or as a result of an automobile or other accident. Only one box on each line can be marked.

The state postal code where the accident occurred must be reported, if "YES" is marked in 10b for "Auto Accident." Any item marked "YES" indicates there may be other applicable insurance coverage that would be primary, such as automobile liability insurance. Primary insurance information must then be shown in Item Number 11.

Medicare: Check "YES" or "NO" to indicate whether employment, auto liability, or other accident involvement applies to one or more of the services described in item 24. Enter the State postal code. Any item checked "YES" indicates there may be other insurance primary to Medicare. Identify primary insurance information in item 11.

ChiroCode Institute Tip: Any item marked "yes" indicates there may be other insurance.

ChiroCode Institute Tip: Item 10: The OIG is taking severe measures to acquire information on claims they paid which may have been the liability of another party - secondary vs primary.

Item Number 10d, Claim Codes (Designated by NUCC)

```
10d. CLAIM CODES (Designated by NUCC)

```

Description: The "Claim Codes" identify additional information about the patient's condition or the claim.

When applicable, use to report appropriate claim codes. Applicable claim codes are designated by the NUCC. Please refer to the most current instructions from the public or private payer regarding the need to report claim codes.

When required by payers to provide the sub-set of Condition Codes approved by the NUCC, enter the Condition Code in this field. The Condition Codes approved for use on the 1500 Claim Form are available at 🌐 www.nucc.org under Code Sets.

When reporting more than one code, enter three blank spaces and then the next code.

For Workers Compensation: Condition Codes are required when submitting a bill that is a duplicate or an appeal. (Original Reference Number must be entered in Box 22 for these conditions). **Note:** Do not use Condition Codes when submitting a revised or corrected bill.

Medicare: Use this item exclusively for Medicaid (MCD) information. If the patient is entitled to Medicaid, enter the patient's Medicaid number preceded by MCD.

Item Number 11, Insured's Policy, Group, or FECA Number

```
11. INSURED'S POLICY GROUP OR FECA NUMBER
    A1234
```

Description: The "Insured's Policy, Group, or FECA Number" refers to the alphanumeric identifier for the health, auto, or other insurance plan coverage. For workers' compensation claims the workers' compensation carrier's alphanumeric identifier would be used. The FECA number is the 9-digit alphanumeric identifier assigned to a patient claiming work-related condition(s) under the Federal Employees Compensation Act 5 USC 8101.

Enter the insured's policy or group number as it appears on the insured's health care identification card. If Item Number 4 is completed, then this field should be completed.

Do not use a hyphen or space as a separator within the policy or group number.

Medicare: THIS ITEM MUST BE COMPLETED, IT IS A REQUIRED FIELD. BY COMPLETING THIS ITEM, THE PHYSICIAN/SUPPLIER ACKNOWLEDGES HAVING MADE A GOOD FAITH EFFORT TO DETERMINE WHETHER MEDICARE IS THE PRIMARY OR SECONDARY PAYER.

If there is insurance primary to Medicare, enter the insured's policy or group number and proceed to items 11a - 11c. Items 4, 6, and 7 must also be completed.

NOTE: Enter the appropriate information in item 11c if insurance primary to Medicare is indicated in item 11.

If there is no insurance primary to Medicare, enter the word "NONE" and proceed to item 12.

If the insured reports a terminating event with regard to insurance which had been primary to Medicare (e.g., insured retired), enter the word "NONE" and proceed to item 11b.

If a lab has collected previously and retained ▶Medicare Secondary Payer (MSP)◀ information for a beneficiary, the lab may use that information for billing purposes of the non-face-to-face lab service. If the lab has no MSP information for the beneficiary, the lab will enter the word "None" in Block 11 of Form CMS-1500, when submitting a claim for payment of a reference lab service. Where there has been no face-to-face encounter with the beneficiary, the claim will then follow the normal claims process. When a lab has a face-to-face encounter with a beneficiary, the lab is expected to collect the MSP information and bill accordingly.

Insurance Primary to Medicare - Circumstances under which Medicare payment may be secondary to other insurance include:

> **ChiroCode Institute Tip:** Call the Medicare Coordination of Benefits Contractor at 1-800-999-1118 and ask them who is the primary payer.

- Group Health Plan Coverage
    - ☐ Working Aged;
    - ☐ Disability (Large Group Health Plan); and
    - ☐ End Stage Renal Disease;
- No Fault and/or Other Liability; and
- Work-Related Illness/Injury:
    - ☐ Workers' Compensation;
    - ☐ Black Lung; and
    - ☐ Veterans Benefits

Note: For a paper claim to be considered for ▶MSP◀ benefits, a copy of the primary payer's explanation of benefits (EOB) notice must be forwarded along with the claim form. (See Pub. 100-05, Medicare Secondary Payer Manual, chapter 3.)

Item Number 11b, Other Claim ID (Designated by NUCC)

```
b. OTHER CLAIM ID (Designated by NUCC)
Y4 |112233445566
```

Description: The "Other Claim ID" is another identifier applicable to the claim.

Enter the "Other Claim ID." Applicable claim identifiers are designated by the NUCC.

▶When submitting to Property and Casualty payers, e.g. Automobile, Homeowner's or Workers' Compensation insurers and related entities, the following qualifier and accompanying identifier has been designated for use.

    Y4 Agency Claim Number (Property Casualty Claim Number) ◀

Enter the qualifier to the left of the vertical, dotted line. Enter the identifier number to the right of the vertical, dotted line.

For Workers Compensation and Other Property & Casualty Claims: Required if known. Enter the claim number assigned by the payer.

> ▶**Medicare:**
>
> Form version 08/05: Enter employer's name, if applicable. If there is a change in the insured's insurance status, e.g., retired, enter either a 6-digit (MM | DD | YY) or 8-digit (MM | DD | CCYY) retirement date preceded by the word "RETIRED."
>
> Form version 02/12: provide this information to the right of the vertical dotted line. ◀

Item Number 11d, Is there another Health Benefit Plan?

d. IS THERE ANOTHER HEALTH BENEFIT PLAN?
[X] YES   [ ] NO   *If yes*, return to and complete item 9 a-d.

Description: "Is there another health benefit plan" indicates that the patient has insurance coverage other than the plan indicated in Item Number 1.

When appropriate, enter an X in the correct box. If marked "YES", complete 9, 9a, and 9d. Only one box can be marked.

> Medicare: Leave blank. Not required by Medicare.

Item Number 12, Patient's or Authorized Person's Signature

> READ BACK OF FORM BEFORE COMPLETING & SIGNING THIS FORM.
> 12. PATIENT'S OR AUTHORIZED PERSON'S SIGNATURE I authorize the release of any medical or other information necessary to process this claim. I also request payment of government benefits either to myself or to the party who accepts assignment below.
>
> SIGNED __SOF_____ DATE _____

Description: The "Patient's or Authorized Person's Signature" indicates there is an authorization on file for the release of any medical or other information necessary to process and/or adjudicate the claim.

Enter "Signature on File," "SOF," or legal signature. When legal signature, enter date signed in 6-digit ▶ (MM|DD|YY) or 8-digit format (MM|DD|YYYY) ◀ If there is no signature on file, leave blank or enter "No Signature on File."

> **Medicare:** The patient or authorized representative must sign and enter either a 6-digit date (MM | DD | YY), 8-digit date (MM | DD | CCYY), or an alpha-numeric date (e.g., January 1, 1998) unless the signature is on file. In lieu of signing the claim, the patient may sign a statement to be retained in the provider, physician, or supplier file in accordance with Chapter 1, "General Billing Requirements." If the patient is physically or mentally unable to sign, a representative specified in Chapter 1, "General Billing Requirements" may sign on the patient's behalf. In this event, the statement's signature line must indicate the patient's name followed by "by" the representative's name, address, relationship to the patient, and the reason the patient cannot sign. The authorization is effective indefinitely unless patient or the patient's representative revokes this arrangement.
>
> **NOTE:** This can be "Signature on File" and/or a computer generated signature.
>
> The patient's signature authorizes release of medical information necessary to process the claim. It also authorizes payment of benefits to the provider of service or supplier when the provider of service or supplier accepts assignment on the claim.
>
> **Signature by Mark (X)** - When an illiterate or physically handicapped enrollee signs by mark, a witness must enter his/her name and address next to the mark.

> **ChiroCode Institute Tip:** The signed agreement(s) should be kept with the patient's records in the provider's files. The authorization may be on a lifetime agreement. It need not specify a period of time and the patient can cancel it at any time. This agreement is effective from the date of signing, and is effective indefinitely unless the patient or the patient's representative revokes this arrangement.
>
> During an audit, the payer may request that you provide them with a Signature on File or patient signature.

Item Number 13, Insured's or Authorized Person's Signature

```
13. INSURED'S OR AUTHORIZED PERSON'S SIGNATURE I authorize
    payment of medical benefits to the undersigned physician or supplier for
    services described below.

    SIGNED    SOF
```

Description: The "Insured's or Authorized Person's Signature" indicates that there is a signature on file authorizing payment of medical benefits.

Enter "Signature on File," "SOF," or legal signature. If there is no signature on file, leave blank or enter "No Signature on File."

Medicare: The patient's signature or the statement "signature on file" in this item authorizes payment of medical benefits to the physician or supplier. The patient or his/her authorized representative signs this item or the signature must be on file separately with the provider as an authorization. However, note that when payment under the Act can only be made on an assignment-related basis or when paymen is for services furnished by a participating physician or supplier, a patient's signature or a "signature on file" is not required in order for Medicare payment to be made directly to the physician or supplier.

The presence of or lack of a signature or "signature on file" in this field will be indicated as such to any downstream ▶coordination of benefits◀ trading partners (supplemental insurers) with whom CMS has a payer-to-payer coordination of benefits relationship. Medicare has no control over how supplemental claims are processed, so it is important that providers accurately address this field as it may affect supplemental payments to providers and/or their patients.

In addition, the signature in this item authorizes payment of mandated Medigap benefits to the participating physician or supplier if required Medigap information is included in item 9 and its sub-divisions. The patient or his/her authorized representative signs this item or the signature must be on file as a separate Medigap authorization. The Medigap assignment on file in the participating provider of service/supplier's office must be insurer specific. It may state that the authorization applies to all occasions of service until it is revoked.

NOTE: This can be "Signature on File" signature and/or a computer generated signature.

Items 14–33: Physician or Supplier Information

Medicare: Reminder: For date fields other than date of birth, all fields shall be one or the other format, 6-digit: (MM | DD | YY) or 8-digit: (MM | DD | CCYY). Intermixing the two formats on the claim is not allowed.

Item Number 14, Date of Current Illness, Injury, or Pregnancy (LMP)

```
14. DATE OF CURRENT ILLNESS, INJURY, or PREGNANCY (LMP)
    MM   DD   YY
    01   14   2014      QUAL.  431
```

Description: The "Date of Current Illness, Injury, ▶or Pregnancy" identifies the ◀ first date of onset of illness, the actual date of injury, or the LMP for pregnancy.

Enter the 6-digit (MM | DD | YY) or 8-digit (MM | DD | YYYY) date of the first date of the present illness, injury, or pregnancy. For pregnancy, use the date of the last menstrual period (LMP) as the first date.

Enter the applicable qualifier to identify which date is being reported.

    431 Onset of Current Symptoms or Illness
    484 Last Menstrual Period

Enter the qualifier to the right of the vertical, dotted line.

Medicare: Enter either an 8-digit (MM | DD | CCYY) or 6-digit (MM | DD | YY) date of current illness, injury, or pregnancy. For chiropractic services, enter an 8-digit (MM | DD | CCYY) or 6-digit (MM | DD | YY) date of the initiation of the course of treatment and enter an 8-digit (MM | DD | CCYY) or 6-digit (MM | DD | YY) date in item 19.

▶Additional information for form version 02/12: Although this version of the form includes space for a qualifier, Medicare does not use this information; do not enter a qualifier in item 14. ◀

ChiroCode Institute Tip: When there is a new course of treatment (e.g. exacerbations), this field may be used to indicate the new start date of the updated treatment plan.

Item Number 15, Other Date

15. OTHER DATE		MM	DD	YY
QUAL.	454	01	25	2014

Description: The "Other Date" identifies additional date information about the patient's condition or treatment.

Enter another date related to the patient's condition or treatment. Enter the date in the 6-digit (MM|DD|YY) or 8-digit (MM|DD|YYYY) format.

Enter the applicable qualifier to identify which date is being reported.

- 454 Initial Treatment
- 304 Latest Visit or Consultation
- 453 Acute Manifestation of a Chronic Condition
- 439 Accident
- 455 Last X-ray
- 471 Prescription
- 090 Report Start (Assumed Care Date)
- 091 Report End (Relinquished Care Date)
- 444 First Visit or Consultation

Enter the qualifier between the left-hand set of vertical, dotted lines.

Medicare: Leave blank. Not required by Medicare.

Item Number 17, Name of Referring Provider or Other Source

17. NAME OF REFERRING PROVIDER OR OTHER SOURCE
DN | Jane A Smith MD

Description: The name entered is the referring provider, ordering provider, or supervising provider who referred, ordered or supervised the service(s) or ▶supply(ies)◀ on the claim. The qualifier indicates the role of the provider being reported.

Enter the name (First Name, Middle Initial, Last Name) followed by the credentials of the professional who ▶referred, ordered, or supervised◀ the service(s) or supply(ies) on the claim.

If multiple providers are involved, enter one provider using the following priority order:

1. Referring Provider
2. Ordering Provider
3. Supervising Provider

Do not use periods or commas. A hyphen can be used for hyphenated names.

Enter the applicable qualifier to identify which provider is being reported.

1. DN   Referring Provider
2. DK   Ordering Provider
3. DQ   Supervising Provider

Enter the qualifier to the left of the vertical, dotted line.

> **ChiroCode Institute Tip:** If the name is very long, use the complete last name and as much of the first name as will fit in the remaining space.

Medicare: Enter the name of the referring or ordering physician if the service or item was ordered or referred by a physician. All physicians who order services or refer Medicare beneficiaries must report this data. ▶Similarly, if Medicare policy requires you to report a supervising physician, enter this information in item 17.◀ When a claim involves multiple referring ▶ordering, or supervising physicians, use ◀ a separate CMS-1500 ▶claim form ◀ for each referring or ▶supervising ◀ physician.

▶Additional instructions for form version 02/12: Enter one of the following qualifiers as appropriate to identify the role that this physician (or non-physician practitioner) is performing:

Qualifier	Provider Role
DN	Referring Provider
DK	Ordering Provider
DQ	Supervising Provider

Enter the qualifier to the left of the dotted vertical line on item 17.

NOTE: Under certain circumstances, Medicare permits a non-physician practitioner to perform these roles. Refer to Pub 100-02, Medicare Benefit Policy Manual, chapter 15 for non-physician practitioner rules. Enter non-physician practitioner information according to the rules above for physicians. ◀

The term "physician" when used within the meaning of §1861(r) of the Act and used in connection with performing any function or action refers to:

1. A doctor of medicine or osteopathy legally authorized to practice medicine and surgery by the State in which he/she performs such function or action;
2. A doctor of dental surgery or dental medicine who is legally authorized to practice dentistry by the State in which he/she performs such functions and who is acting within the scope of his/her license when performing such functions;
3. A doctor of podiatric medicine for purposes of §§(k), (m), (p)(1), and (s) and §§1814(a), 1832(a)(2)(F)(ii), and 1835 of the Act, but only with respect to functions which he/she is legally authorized to perform as such by the State in which he/she performs them;
4. A doctor of optometry, but only with respect to the provision of items or services described in §1861(s) of the Act which he/she is legally authorized to perform as a doctor of optometry by the State in which he/she performs them; or
5. A chiropractor who is licensed as such by a State (or in a State which does not license chiropractors as such), and is legally authorized to perform the services of a chiropractor in the jurisdiction in which he/she performs such services, and who meets uniform minimum standards specified by the Secretary, but only for purposes of §§1861(s)(1) and 1861(s)(2)(A) of the Act, and only with respect to treatment by means of manual manipulation of the spine (to correct a subluxation). For the purposes of §1862(a)(4) of the Act and subject to the limitations and conditions provided above, chiropractor includes a doctor of one of the arts specified in the statute and legally authorized to practice such art in the country in which the inpatient hospital services (referred to in §1862(a)(4) of the Act) are furnished.

Referring physician - is a physician who requests an item or service for the beneficiary for which payment may be made under the Medicare program.

Ordering physician - is a physician or, when appropriate, a non-physician practitioner who orders non-physician services for the patient. See Pub 100-02, Medicare Benefit Policy Manual, chapter 15 for non-physician practitioner rules. Examples of services that might be ordered include diagnostic laboratory tests, clinical laboratory tests, pharmaceutical services, durable medical equipment, and services incident to that physician's or non-physician practitioner's service.

The ordering/referring requirement became effective January 1, 1992, and is required by §1833(q) of the Act. All claims for Medicare covered services and items that are the result of a physician's order or referral shall include the ordering/referring physician's name. See Items 17a and 17b below for further guidance on reporting the referring/ordering provider's UPIN and/or NPI. The following services/situations require the submission of the referring/ordering provider information:

- Medicare covered services and items that are the result of a physician's order or referral;
- Parenteral and enteral nutrition;
- Immunosuppressive drug claims;
- Hepatitis B claims;
- Diagnostic laboratory services;
- Diagnostic radiology services;
- Portable x-ray services;
- Consultative services;
- Durable medical equipment;
- When the ordering physician is also the performing physician (as often is the case with in-office clinical laboratory tests);
- When a service is incident to the service of a physician or non-physician practitioner, the name of the physician or non-physician practitioner who performs the initial service and orders the non-physician service must appear in item 17;
- When a physician extender or other limited licensed practitioner refers a patient for consultative service, submit the name of the physician who is supervising the limited licensed practitioner.
- Effective for claims with dates of service on or after October 1, 2012, all claims for physical therapy, occupational therapy, or speech-language pathology services, including those furnished incident to a physician or nonphysician practitioner, require that the name and NPI of the certifying physician or nonphysician practitioner of the therapy plan of care be entered as the referring physician in Items 17 and 17b.

Items Number 17a and 17b (split field)

```
17a. 0B  ABC1234567890
17b. NPI 0123456789
```

Item 17a, Other ID#

Description: The non-NPI ID number of the referring, ordering, or supervising provider is the unique identifier of the professional or provider designated taxonomy code.

The Other ID number of the referring, ordering, or supervising provider is reported in 17a in the shaded area. The qualifier indicating what the number represents is reported in the qualifier field to the immediate right of 17a.

The NUCC defines the following qualifiers used in 5010A1:

0B	State License Number	G2	Provider Commercial Number
1G	Provider UPIN Number	LU	Location Number (This qualifier is used for Supervising Provider only.)

Medicare: Leave blank

> **ChiroCode Institute Tip:**
>
> - ▶Other◀ ID: Often providers ask which other ID number they should be using for a specific payer (e.g. State Farm, Cigna). Different payers have different requirements. Obtain this information directly from the payer.
>
> - Taxonomy codes are specific classifications for providers and are a component of NPI applications. The National Uniform Claim Committee (NUCC) is presently maintaining the Health Care Provider Taxonomy list. See Resource 197 for the taxonomy codes.

Item Number 19, Additional Claim Information (Designated by NUCC)

```
19. ADDITIONAL CLAIM INFORMATION (Designated by NUCC)
```

Description: "Additional Claim Information" identifies additional information about the patient's condition or the claim.

Please refer to the most current instructions from the applicable public or private payer regarding the use of this field. Some payers ask for certain identifiers in this field. If identifiers are reported in this field, enter the appropriate qualifiers describing the identifier. Do not enter a space, hyphen, or other separator between the qualifier code and the number.

The NUCC defines the following qualifiers used in 5010A1:

- 0B State License Number
- 1G Provider UPIN Number
- G2 Provider Commercial Number
- LU Location Number (This qualifier is used for Supervising provider only
- N5 Provider Plan Network Identification Number
- SY Social Security Number (The social security number may not be used for Medicare.)
- X5 State Industrial Accident Provider Number
- ZZ Provider Taxonomomy (The qualifier in the 5010A1 for Provider Taxonomy is PXC, but ZZ will remain the qualifier for the 1500 Claim form.

The above list contains both provider identifiers, as well as the provider taxonomy code. The provider identifiers are assigned to the provider either by a specific payer or by a third party in order to uniquely identify the provider. The taxonomy code is designated by the provider in order to identify his/her provider type, classification, and/or area of specialization. Both, provider identifiers and provider taxonomy may be used in this field.

▶Taxonomy codes reported in this field must not be reportable in other fields, i.e., Item Numbers 17, 24J, 32, and/or 33. ◀

When reporting a second item of data, enter three blank spaces and then the next qualifier and number/code/information.

For Workers' Compensation: Required based on Jurisdictional Workers' Compensation Guidelines.

When reporting Supplemental Claim Information, use the qualifier PWK for data, followed by the appropriate Report Type Code, the appropriate Transmission Type Code, then the Attachment Control Number. Do not enter spaces between qualifiers and data. The NUCC defines the following qualifiers, since they are the same as those used in 5010A1:

REPORT TYPE CODE

Code	Description
03	Report Justifying Treatment Beyond Utilization
04	Drugs Administered
05	Treatment Diagnosis
06	Initial Assessment
07	Functional Goals
08	Plan of Treatment
09	Progress Report
10	Continued Treatment
11	Chemical Analysis
13	Certified Test Report
15	Justification for Admission
21	Recovery Plan
A3	Allergies/Sensitivities Document
A4	Autopsy Report
AM	Ambulance Certification
AS	Admission Summary
B2	Prescription
B3	Physician Order
B4	Referral Form
BR	Benchmark Testing Results
BS	Baseline
BT	Blanket Test Results
CB	Chiropractic Justification
CK	Consent Form(s)
CT	Certification
D2	Drug Profile Document
DA	Dental Models
DB	Durable Medical Equipment Prescription
DG	Diagnostic Report
DJ	Discharge Monitoring Report
DS	Discharge Summary
EB	Explanation of Benefits (Coordination of Benefits or Medicare Secondary Payor)
HC	Health Certificate
HR	Health Clinic Reports
I5	Immunization Record
IR	State School Immunization Records
LA	Laboratory Results
M1	Medical Record Attachment
MT	Models
NN	Nursing Notes
OB	Operative Note
OC	Oxygen Content Averaging Report
OD	Orders and Treatments Document
OE	Objective Physical Examination (including vital signs) Document
OX	Oxygen Therapy Certification
OZ	Support Data for Claim
P4	Pathology Report
P5	Patient Medical History Document
PE	Parenteral or Enteral Certification
PN	Physical Therapy Notes
PO	Prosthetics or Orthotic Certification
PQ	Paramedical Results
PY	Physician's Report
PPZ	Physical Therapy Certification
RB	Radiology Films
RR	Radiology Reports
RT	Report of Tests and Analysis Report
RX	Renewable Oxygen Content Averaging Report
SG	Symptoms Document
V5	Death Notification
XP	Photographs

TRANSMISSION TYPE CODE

Code	Description
AA	Available on Request at Provider Site
BM	By Mail

Example: PWK03AA12363545465

Medicare: Enter either a 6-digit (MM | DD | YY) or an 8-digit (MM | DD | CCYY) date patient was last seen and the NPI of his/her attending physician when a physician providing routine foot care submits claims.

Enter either a 6-digit (MM | DD | YY) or an 8-digit (MM | DD | CCYY) x-ray date for chiropractor services (if an x-ray, rather than a physical examination was the method used to demonstrate the subluxation). By entering an x-ray date and the initiation date for course of chiropractic treatment in item 14, the chiropractor is certifying that all the relevant information requirements (including level of subluxation) of Pub. 100-02, Medicare Benefit Policy Manual, chapter 15, are on file, along with the appropriate x-ray and all are available for ▶A/B MAC (B)◀ review.

Enter the drug's name and dosage when submitting a claim for Not Otherwise Classified (NOC) drugs.

Enter a concise description of an "unlisted procedure code" or ▶a◀ NOC code if one can be given within the confines of this box. Otherwise an attachment shall be submitted with the claim.

Enter all applicable modifiers when modifier -99 (multiple modifiers) is entered in item 24d. If modifier -99 is entered on multiple line items of a single claim form, all applicable modifiers for each line item containing a -99 modifier should be listed as follows: 1=(mod), where the number 1 represents the line item and "mod" represents all modifiers applicable to the referenced line item.

Enter the statement, "Patient refuses to assign benefits" when the beneficiary absolutely refuses to assign benefits to a non-participating physician/supplier who accepts assignment on a claim. In this case, payment can only be made directly to the beneficiary

NOTE: Effective May 23, 2008, all provider identifiers submitted on the ▶CMS-1500 claim form◀ MUST be in the form of an NPI.

ChiroCode Institute Tip: This "Additional Claim Information" box is valuable but is often overlooked. It is one of the places on the form where explanatory information can be given. Supplemental information relating to a specific procedure code should use the shaded area of Item 24.

If there is not enough space, attach a report. Providers typically use this box to provide clarifying information (such as rationale for modifiers to procedure codes in item 21).

Item Number 21, Diagnosis or Nature of Illness or Injury

21. DIAGNOSIS OR NATURE OF ILLNESS OR INJURY Relate A-L to Service Line Below (24E)			ICD Ind.	9
A. 83902	B. 7840	C. 8470	D. E8130	
E.	F.	G.	H.	
I.	J.	K.	L.	

Description: The "ICD Indicator" identifies the version of the ICD code set being reported. The "Diagnosis or Nature of Illness or Injury" is the sign, symptom, complaint, or condition of the patient relating to the service(s) on the claim.

Enter the applicable ICD indicator to identify which version of ICD codes is being reported.

- 9   ICD-9-CM
- 0   ICD-10-CM

Enter the indicator between the vertical, dotted lines in the upper right-hand portion of the field.

Enter the codes ▶left justified on each line ◀ to identify the patient's diagnosis and/or condition. ▶Do not include the decimal point in the diagnosis code, because it is implied.◀ List no more than 12 ICD-9-CM or ICD-10-CM diagnosis codes. Relate lines A - L to the lines of service in 24E by the letter of the line. Use the ▶greatest◀ level of specificity. Do not provide narrative description in this field.

Medicare: Enter the patient's diagnosis/condition. With the exception of claims submitted by ambulance suppliers (specialty type 59), all physician and nonphysician specialties (i.e., PA, NP, CNS, CRNA) use ▶diagnosis codes ◀ to the highest level of specificity for the date of service. Enter ▶the ◀ diagnoses in priority order. All narrative diagnoses for nonphysician specialties shall be submitted on an attachment.

▶Reminder: Do not report ICD-10-CM codes for claims with dates of service prior to implementation of ICD-10-CM, on either the old or revised version of the CMS-1500 claim form.

For form version 08/05, report a valid ICD-9-CM code. Enter up to four diagnosis codes.

For form version 02/12, it may be appropriate to report either ICD-9-CM or ICD-10-CM codes depending upon the dates of service (i.e., according to the effective dates of the given code set).

- The "ICD Indicator" identifies the ICD code set being reported. Enter the applicable ICD indicator according to the following:

Indicator	Code Set
9	ICD-9-CM diagnosis
0	ICD-10-CM diagnosis

    Enter the indicator as a single digit between the vertical, dotted lines.

- Do not report both ICD-9-CM and ICD-10-CM codes on the same claim form. If there are services you wish to report that occurred on dates when ICD-9-CM codes were in effect, and others that occurred on dates when ICD-10-CM codes were in effect, then send separate claims such that you report only ICD-9-CM or only ICD-10-CM codes on the claim. (See special considerations for spans of dates below.)

- If you are submitting a claim with a span of dates for a service, use the "from" date to determine which ICD code set to use.

- Enter up to 12 diagnosis codes. Note that this information appears opposite lines with letters A-L. Relate lines A- L to the lines of service in 24E by the letter of the line. Use the highest level of specificity. Do not provide narrative description in this field.

- Do not insert a period in the ICD-9-CM or ICD-10-CM code. ◄

ChiroCode Institute Tip: Up to 12 diagnosis codes can be accepted by Medicare and most payers.

ChiroCode Institute Tip: There is a hierarchy of codes that should be used in box 21.

- **Neurological diagnosis** (such as radiculitis and sciatica). Some payers require that the subluxation be in the first position.
- **Structural diagnosis** (such as degenerative disc disorders and spondylolisthesis).
- **Functional diagnosis** (such as restricted range of motion and deconditioning syndrome).
- **Soft tissue** (such as fibromyalgia and myofascitis), **extremity** (such as carpal tunnel syndrome and adhesive capsulitis), and **complicating factor** diagnoses.

List additional diagnostic codes/descriptors in the patient's chart. Note also that the diagnoses should always represent the regions being treated (with supporting documentation).

ChiroCode Institute Tip: The following are common diagnosis coding problems that could possibly cause delay or denial of payments:

- Not coding to the highest level of specificity
- The code does not establish medical necessity
- Using a chronic diagnosis as the primary diagnosis when it is not the reason for the encounter
- Using an italicized ICD-9-CM (ICD-10-CM in October 2015) code alone or as the primary diagnosis
- Using an E code alone or as the primary diagnosis

Item Number 22, Resubmission and/or Original Reference Number

22. RESUBMISSION CODE	ORIGINAL REF. NO.
7	ABC1234567890

Description: "Resubmission" means the code and original reference number assigned by the destination payer or receiver to indicate a previously submitted claim or encounter.

List the original reference number for resubmitted claims. Please refer to the most current instructions from the public or private payer regarding the use of this field (e.g., code).

When resubmitting a claim, enter the appropriate bill frequency code left justified in the left-hand side of the field.

    7 Replacement of prior claim
    8 Void/cancel of prior claim

This Item Number is not intended for use for original claim submissions.

Medicare: Leave blank

Item Number 23, Prior Authorization Number

23. PRIOR AUTHORIZATION NUMBER
1234567890A

Description: The "Prior Authorization Number" is the payer assigned number authorizing the service(s).

Enter any of the following: prior authorization number, referral number, mammography pre-certification number, or Clinical Laboratory Improvement Amendments (CLIA) number, as assigned by the payer for the current service.

Do not enter hyphens or spaces within the number.

For Workers Compensation and Other Property & Casualty Claims: Required when a prior authorization, referral, concurrent review, or voluntary certification was received.

> ▶**ChiroCode Institute Tip:** This item can only contain one authorization code for one condition. Any additional conditions and authorization should be reported on a separate 1500 form. ◀

Medicare: Enter the Quality Improvement Organization (QIO) prior authorization number for those procedures requiring QIO prior approval.

Enter the Investigational Device Exemption (IDE) number when an investigational device is used in an FDA-approved clinical trial. Post Market Approval number should also be placed here when applicable.

For physicians performing care plan oversight services, enter the ▶NPI ◀ of the home health agency (HHA) or hospice when CPT code G0181 (HH) or G0182 (Hospice) is billed.

Enter the 10-digit Clinical Laboratory Improvement Act (CLIA) certification number for laboratory services billed by an entity performing CLIA covered procedures

▶For ambulance claims, enter the ZIP code of the loaded ambulance trip's point-of-pickup. ◀

NOTE: Item 23 can contain only one condition. Any additional conditions should be reported on a separate ▶CMS-1500 claim form. ◀

Section 24

24. A. DATE(S) OF SERVICE From MM DD YY To MM DD YY	B. PLACE OF SERVICE	C. EMG	D. PROCEDURES, SERVICES, OR SUPPLIES (Explain Unusual Circumstances) CPT/HCPCS MODIFIER	E. DIAGNOSIS POINTER	F. $ CHARGES	G. DAYS OR UNITS	H. EPSDT Family Plan	I. ID. QUAL	J. RENDERING PROVIDER ID. #
1									NPI
2									NPI
3									NPI
4									NPI
5									NPI
6									NPI

Supplemental information can only be entered with a corresponding, completed service line. The six service lines in section 24 have been divided horizontally to accommodate submission of both the NPI and another/proprietary identifier and to accommodate the submission of supplemental information to support the billed service. The top area of the six service lines is shaded and is the location for reporting supplemental information. It is not intended to allow the billing of 12 lines of service.

The supplemental information is to be placed in the shaded section of 24A through 24G as defined in each Item Number. Providers must verify requirements for this supplemental information with the payer.

Medicare: The six service lines in section 24 have been divided horizontally to accommodate submission of supplemental information to support the billed service. The top portion in each of the six service lines is shaded and is the location for reporting supplemental information. It is not intended to allow the billing of 12 service lines.

▶When required to submit NDC drug and quantity information for Medicaid rebates, submit the NDC code in the red shaded portion of the detail line item in positions 01 through position 13. The NDC is to be preceded with the qualifier N4 and followed immediately by the 11 digit NDC code (e.g. N499999999999). Report the NDC quantity in positions 17 through 24 of the same red shaded portion. The quantity is to be preceded by the appropriate qualifier: UN (units), F2 (international units), GR (gram) or ML (milliliter). There are six bytes available for quantity. If the quantity is less than six bytes, left justify and space-fill the remaining positions (e.g. UN2 or F2999999).◀

Item Number 24E, Diagnosis Pointer [lines 1–6]

E. DIAGNOSIS POINTER

ABCD

Description: The Diagnosis Pointer ▶is the◀ line letter from Item Number 21 that relates to the reason the service(s) was performed.

In 24E, enter the diagnosis code reference letter (pointer) as shown in Item Number 21 to relate the date of service and the procedures performed to the primary diagnosis. When multiple services are performed, the primary reference letter for each service should be listed first, other applicable services should follow. The reference letter(s) should be A – L or multiple letters as applicable. ICD-9-CM (or ICD-10-CM, once mandated) diagnosis codes must be entered in Item Number 21 only. Do not enter them in 24E.

Enter letters left justified in the field. Do not use commas between the letters.

Medicare: ▶This is a required field.◀ Enter the diagnosis code reference numbers ▶or letter (as appropriate, per form version)◀ as shown in item 21 to relate the date of service and the procedures performed to the primary diagnosis. Enter only one reference ▶number/letter◀ per line item. When multiple services are performed, enter the primary reference ▶number/letter◀ for each service, either a 1, or a 2, or a 3, or a 4.

▶When using form version 08/05, this reference will be either a 1, or a 2, or a 3, or a 4.

When using form version 02/12, the reference to supply in 24E will be a letter from A-L. Otherwise, the instructions above apply.◀

If a situation arises where two or more diagnoses are required for a procedure code (e.g., pap smears), the provider shall reference only one of the diagnoses in item 21.

> **ChiroCode Institute Tip:**
> - ▶Even though you can enter 12 diagnosis codes in item 21, you can still only enter 4 diagnosis pointers in item 24E.◀
> - It should be noted that in addition to avoiding the use of commas between letters, the use of spaces or dashes should also be avoided.

Item Number 27, Accept Assignment?

Description: The accept assignment indicates that the provider agrees to accept assignment under the terms of the payer's program.

Enter an X in the correct box. Only one box may be marked.

Report "Accept Assignment?" for all payers.

Medicare: Check the appropriate block to indicate whether the provider of service or supplier accepts assignment of Medicare benefits. If Medigap is indicated in item 9 and Medigap payment authorization is given in item 13, the provider of service or supplier shall also be a Medicare participating provider of service or supplier and accept assignment of Medicare benefits for all covered charges for all patients.

The following providers of service/suppliers and claims can only be paid on an assignment basis:

- Clinical diagnostic laboratory services;
- Physician services to individuals dually entitled to Medicare and Medicaid;
- Participating physician/supplier services;
- Services of physician assistants, nurse practitioners, clinical nurse specialists, nurse midwives, certified registered nurse anesthetists, clinical psychologists, and clinical social workers;
- Drugs and biologicals.

> **ChiroCode Institute Tip:** These are mandatory Medicare assignment situations. When billing any of the above services/supplies, the "Yes" box should be checked.

ChiroCode Institute Tip: Medicare *Participating* providers have signed an agreement with the Medicare program to accept assignment of Medicare Part B payment for all covered services provided to Medicare patients. *Non-participating* providers may accept or decline assignment of Medicare benefits on a claim-by-claim basis. However, they cannot accept assignment in item #27 if it is not authorized in item #13.

Note: It is very important to complete this field in accordance with Medicare requirements. Participating providers should always check 'yes.'. Non-participating providers have the option to check 'yes' or 'no' unless the supply/service is a mandatory assignment situation. If the provider makes no entry in Item 27, the carrier will automatically assume the following:

- Participating providers will be a "yes."
- Non-participating providers will be a "no."
- Mandatory assignment situations will be a "yes" (eg, labs, physician assistants, etc.)

See *Section C–Medicare* for detailed information regarding accepting assignment on Medicare claims.

ChiroCode Institute Tip: Only when assignment is **authorized** by the patient in item 13 can it be **accepted** (or rejected) by the provider in item 27.

Item Number 30, Reserved for NUCC Use

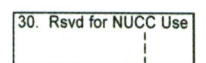

Description: ▶ This field is ◀ reserved for NUCC Use.

This field was previously used to report "Balance Due." "Balance Due" does not exist in 5010A1, so this field has been eliminated.

This field is reserved for NUCC use. The NUCC will provide instructions for any use of this field.

▶**Medicare:** Leave blank. Not required by Medicare.◀

Item Number 32b: Other ID#

Description: The non-NPI ID number of the service facility is the payer assigned unique identifier of the facility.

Enter the 2-digit qualifier identifying the non-NPI number followed by the ID number. Do not enter a space, hyphen, or other separator between the qualifier and number.

The NUCC defines the following qualifiers used in 5010A1:

- 0B   State License Number
- G2   Provider Commercial Number
- LU   Location Number

Medicare: Effective May 23, 2008, Item 32b is not to be reported.

Items Number 33, 33a, and 33b

```
33. BILLING PROVIDER INFO & PH #   ( 312 ) 5552222
    Physician Practice Inc
    1234 Healthcare Street
    Anytown IL 60610-1234
a. 9876543210    b. 1BZ5678901234
```

Item Number 33b, Other ID#

Description: The non-NPI ID number of the billing provider refers to the payer assigned unique identifier of the professional.

Enter the 2-digit qualifier identifying the non-NPI number followed by the ID number. Do not enter a space, hyphen, or other separator between the qualifier and number.

The NUCC defines the following qualifiers used in 5010A1:

- 0B State License Number
- G2 Provider Commercial Number
- ZZ Provider Taxonomy (The qualifier in the 5010A1 for Provider Taxonomy is PXC, but ZZ will remain the qualifier for the 1500 Claim Form.)

The above list contains both provider identifiers, as well as the provider taxonomy code. The provider identifiers are assigned to the provider either by a specific payer or by a third party in order to uniquely identify the provider. The taxonomy code is designated by the provider in order to identify his/her provider type, classification, and/or area of specialization. Both, provider identifiers and provider taxonomy may be used in this field.

Medicare: ▶Item 33b is not generally reported. However, for some Medicare policies you may be instructed to use this item; direction as to how to use this item will be in the instructions you received regarding the specific policy, if applicable. ◀

Review: 1500 Claim Form

- What are the changes to the 1500 claim form? *E-13*
- What should you avoid doing when entering an address on the claim form? *E-17*
- When should item 9 be completed? *E-18*
- When might Medicare be secondary to other insurances? *E-21*
- For item number 14, what date is used? *E-24*
- Where do you use provider identifiers? *E-25 to E-26*
- On item 21, how do you know which order to put the codes in? *E-31*
- What do you enter for item number 32b? *E-35*

3. Guidelines for Unpaid Claims

Resolving issues with unpaid claims falls under two categories. Either the claim is simply not paid, or it is denied. This section includes guidelines for resolving these types of problems and is an important component of the Billing Process of the "Reimbursement Life Cycle."

One of the most important factors for reducing the volume of unpaid claims is establishing effective office standards and followup policies.

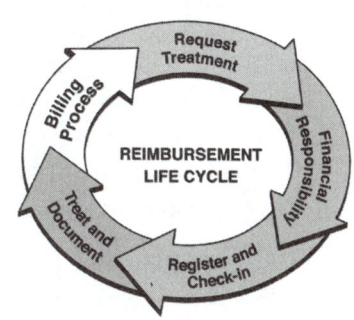

See the "Billing Process Flowchart" (figure 2.1) in Chapter 1–Understanding Insurance of *Section B–Insurance and Reimbursement*.

See Resource 199 for additional information on guidelines for unpaid claims.

Claim Followup Procedures

Every office should have a policy to review and keep track of claims that are unpaid as well as reviewing claim payments that are received. Designate a time each week for making appeals. At a minimum, all outstanding claims more than 30 days old should be reviewed to find out why they remain unpaid.

Some software programs automatically address this accounts receivables issue. However, specialized software is not a requirement for good claims followup procedure. Some offices simply use a paper filing system with the days of the month.

Regardless of the system used, if payment comes in, carefully review the claim and the EOB and make sure that all items are accounted for. If any of the claim is denied, then the appeals process should begin.

Review Payment Reports

Failure to review payment reports is a common oversight, however, this task must be done routinely. Some consultants suggest having at least one hour each week set aside for reviewing claims and filing appeals. This will help identify potential problems and increase cash flow. When claims are denied in whole or in part it is important to evaluate the reason. If it is a valid denial, learn from it and improve your billing. If it is an invalid denial, an appeal should be made.

Another reason to carefully review all denials is because repeating the same errors over and over establishes a pattern of bad billing. These patterns are precisely what the insurance carrier "data mining" programs are looking for. If there is a problem on your end, recognize and remedy it quickly in order to avoid negative profiling.

Handling Overpayments

If a provider discovers an overpayment or an error that could result in incorrect reimbursement, a corrected claim with a letter describing the error should be sent to the payer. Mark the claim "CORRECTED BILLING – NOT A DUPLICATE CLAIM." Include any additional documentation needed along with any refund for overpayments.

Some payers have their own Voluntary Refund (Overpayment) form which should be used for overpayments. Check their website to see if they require their own special form to accompany all submitted refunds. This sample Voluntary Refund Form could be used for payers not requiring the use of a specific form.

> See Resource 195 for a full-size version of this form, with instructions.

Medicare and others can prosecute practices which retain claim overpayments. Not returning an overpayment is considered fraud (see *Section F-Compliance and Audit Protection* for additional information). It may be possible to quickly resolve an overpayment issue with a telephone call, but this may vary by payer.

Prompt Pay Laws

Every state has their own prompt pay laws which state that insurance companies must meet specific deadlines in processing claims. As long as your claim is "clean" and there are not errors which prevent it from being processed by the carrier, then they are required to respond before these state deadlines or face penalties. Use the "Prompt Pay Letter" to follow up with claims which have been filed for more than 30 days, or what your state allows. Be prepared to include documented proof that the claim was filed promptly and cleanly.

Prompt Pay Letter

This sample letter should be used to fight late or slow paying carriers. It is important that you modify the letter for your specific state law. This sample letter includes text from the state of Utah.

Go to your state department of insurance website or consult with an attorney for additional assistance in finding your applicable state law.

> See Resource 196 for a full-size version of this form, with instructions.

Unprocessable Claims

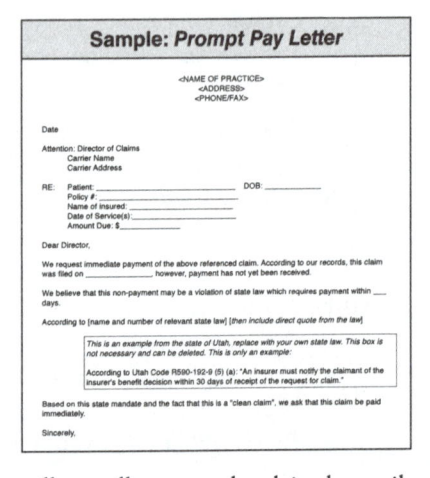

An unprocessable claim does not mean that the payer will actually return the claim by mail. The remittance advice will have a brief message identifying the problem so that the provider can correct the mistake and submit a corrected claim, either electronically, by fax, or by mail. Be sure to respond and correct unprocessable claims promptly. **Do not** appeal a claim when it has been denied because of incomplete or invalid information. Simply make the correction and submit a "corrected claim" for reconsideration.

CLAIM DENIAL MANAGEMENT

The most effective action providers can take for obtaining payment on a denied claim, and one that is often overlooked, is filing an appeal. The ability to successfully appeal a denied claim is an important skill set for providers in today's health care reimbursement landscape. No single strategy will prove successful every time. Success will often lie in a combination of approaches, depending on the case at hand.

All insurance payers have a process for adjudicating (reviewing) claims. Effective practices also have established protocols for dealing with unpaid and denied claims. According to Government Accountability Office (GAO) data on the outcomes of appeals filed with insurers in four states, 39% to 59% of appeals resulted in the insurer reversing its original coverage denial in favor of the health care provider.

> See *Section F–Compliance and Audit Protection* for OIG numbers on Medicare collections.

Here are three basic rules to help with your claim denials:

1. Understand the payer's rationale for the denial.
2. Determine the jurisdiction (who has the authority to decide your appeal).
3. Understand the appeal process for each type of claim.

Denials and appeals are subject to state or federal laws, and all payers have an appeals process if all or part of your claim is denied. Be aware that appeal protocols can vary by payer types.

Why Appeal?

Reimbursement revenue is what keeps the electricity on and the staff members paid. Yet, the typical practice loses thousands of dollars in reimbursements that are denied or paid incorrectly. Unpaid claims can be a challenge and an opportunity for every practitioner.

According to GAO statistics, only a small percentage of offices appeal their insurance denials for a variety of reasons. Unfortunately, many write-off the loss as a cost of doing business rather than make the effort to collect fees that are rightfully and legally due. The American Medical Association recommends that providers utilize the appeals process for all inappropriate denials.

It is important to realize that time spent on appeals is well worth the effort. You should appeal all denials and adverse benefit determinations. Realize that it's not just an issue of one case, but it's about the value of all the similar procedures you will perform during the next several years.

It will quickly become evident that the cost of additional hours by a staff member could be offset by successful appeals.

GENERAL GUIDELINES FOR UNPAID CLAIMS

These general guidelines are for dealing with unpaid claims with commercial payers. Note that specific payers may have specific appeals processes that must be followed.

1. **Review your contract.** Your contract may outline when the provider should expect to receive payment. Specifically review the part about payment obligations. Be able to answer the following questions:

- Do you have the right to appeal?
- Do you have the right to represent the patient?
- Do you have the right to litigate if the appeals process is unsuccessful?
- Does accepting assignment limit your right to pursue an appeal?
- Are there specific guidelines about their appeals processes or how to contact people about problems with claims?

> **Evergreen Contracts:** If your payer contracts are automatically renewed each year, when was the last time you reviewed your contract? There could be changes, new clauses or additional conditions in it which could limit your appeal rights.

2. **Ask questions and remain professional.** There could be many reasons why your claim has not been paid - do not assume that the delay is deliberate. Ask about the status of the claim first. If the delay is simply an administrative error, the person answering the phone may be able to correct the situation quickly.

    Please keep in mind that the first person you talk to on the phone may not know the solution, however, they may be able to steer you in the right direction. If the person you are speaking to cannot correct the situation or tell you who can, you will need to follow the chain of command to find someone who can help, therefore you may need to ask to speak with one or more of the following.

    - Supervisor or Benefits Supervisor
    - Provider Relations
    - Director of Provider Relations and/or the Medical Director

    Remember, it is important to fully document your calls. In the patient record, write down the contact individual's first and last name, date and time of the call, a reference number (if applicable) and the information given to you.

3. **Register complaints.** Send a written complaint to the director of provider relations. Read through it to ensure that the tone of the letter is professional and factual, not personal.

4. **Contact agencies and associations who advocate for providers and patients.** The following are some suggested groups that may be willing to help with unresolved issues. Understand who the key players are in your state, as they may be able to point you in the right direction. If your appeal efforts are unsuccessful, you may want to try one or all of the following:

    - **Local Associations.** Your local professional association can be an important resource for information. They may collect and aggregate data on local reimbursement problems. Legislative representatives will be able to tell you the status of recent legislation. Insurance representatives may be able to assist you with local payer issues. They may even be able to contact the payers on your behalf. Your documentation will be most helpful for your association to act as your advocate.
    - **National Associations.** National associations, such as the American Chiropractic Association (ACA), are also collecting written reports of problems their members are encountering, and one of their targeted issues is reimbursement. Send them a summary of your problem with supporting documentation. Remember to follow HIPAA rules to protect patient privacy.
    - **State Insurance Commissioner.** Depending on your state, the state insurance commissioner may take complaints from both providers and patients (consumers),

or only from the patient. If they are unable to help, ask them if there is some other department (i.e., the department of health or the department of labor) that can help.

See Resource 204 to find state-specific insurance commissioner information.

- **State Attorney General.** Like the insurance commissioner, some attorneys general are proactive when it comes to health care. It doesn't hurt to call or write them to find out. In fact, it might be helpful.
- **Consumer Advocacy Groups.** Patients can register complaints with the local chapters of these groups. A simple internet search for "patient advocacy" can help direct a patient to the appropriate resource.
- **Media.** Many state and national television broadcasters have consumer advocacy departments, and the media can be particularly sensitive to health care issues.
- **Congressional Representatives.** A sympathetic congressperson can be very effective on your behalf. Contact their local office by letter or phone to describe the problem and ask if they would be able to intervene on your or your patient's behalf.

5. **Stay informed.** Information is power. Your professional association may have newsletters or other forums designed to help their members stay current. The *ChiroCode Alerts* and the ACA *In Touch* newsletters are good resources. If you have other information that would be helpful to others, please send a letter or email message to ChiroCode Institute.

6. **Keep your patient** (or a responsible family member) **informed**. For employer sponsored health benefit plans, your patient should also inform their employer's Human Resources Department. In this situation, insurance carriers are under contract to employers to deliver medical services, and employers review these contracts periodically. If enough employees are dissatisfied, the employers may select another plan or advise the carrier to correct problem areas.

APPEALS GUIDELINES

Use Appeals to Your Advantage

Most practices think they are the ones who made the mistake when they get a denial from a carrier, so they don't appeal, fearing further denials. That is just not the case. Providers who follow proper appeals processes actually demonstrate to the payer that they understand proper billing procedures.

Know your appeal rights and the various steps involved with the process. Also, it is important to know the state and federal insurance laws and regulations, so that your appeal can be based on the regulatory environment in addition to billing guidelines. Individual plan documents regarding utilization review (UR) criteria are often available on their websites.

It is also critical to meet all appeal deadlines. If you do not, the merits of your case may not matter. Denials due to 'administrative noncompliance' are rarely overturned. If the case is denied on an administrative basis (i.e., a request for continued certification was not made within the specified time, pre-certification procedures were not followed, or there were benefit coverage exclusions), you will need to explain any extenuating circumstances in your appeal.

Under certain circumstances, a phone call to the payer requesting that the claim be reprocessed may be all that is needed to correct a denial or improperly processed claim. Carefully document the details of the call so that you can cite a reference if it is a written appeal or additional phone calls are necessary. If the phone call is not effective, then proceed with a formal, written appeal.

Here are a few additional appeals tips:

- Regularly follow-up on written appeals with a phone call.
- Record all communication with the payer: dates, names, titles, telephone numbers, reference numbers, and what was stated.
- If your appeal is denied, appeal again to the next highest level. Most payers offer at least two levels of appeal. Some states also require that payers have an external appeal process. Exhaust all levels of appeal before initiating litigation.
- Remember, it is required to get permission from your patients to release their information if authorization is not already on file. See "Designation of Authorized Representative" segment in Chapter 4–ERISA Appeals on page E-47 for more information.
- Ask the patient to contact his or her employer's Personnel/Human Resources Department with their concerns. Payers are often more responsive to employer complaints than to complaints from physicians or patients.

See Chapter 4–Medicare Appeals in *Section C–Medicare* for information on appeals for Medicare Claims.

Expedited Appeals

In an emergency or urgent care situation, it may possible to request an "expedited appeal" over the telephone with a qualified specialist. The majority of payers have such services. If possible, have them fax their approval later for inclusion in the medical record.

Because these types of appeals only apply in emergency situations, they are rarely used for chiropractic care. According to the requirements of the Patient Protection and Affordable Care Act (PPACA), these would only be situations in which delays could seriously jeopardize the life or health of the claimant, or jeopardize the claimant's ability to regain maximum function.

See Resource 205 for more infomation regarding appeals under PPACA.

Appeal Letters

Write letters routinely and create templates or keep copies of various types of appeals to reuse the language (See "Response Letter to 97110-97124 Denials" sample letter).

When submitting an appeal, there is no substitute for an effective cover letter. Keep this letter to a single page as much as possible and direct it to the appropriate address. Specific appeals templates or forms required by the payer often include the proper mailing address.

Be sure your letter includes the following:

- Request for a reviewer that is trained in your specialty.
- Be specific, with a clear and compelling case for medical necessity.
- Clarify any information from the chart as needed.
- Correct any diagnostic or procedural coding or other information on the claim form.

Response Letter to 97110-97124 Denials

This sample letter is designed to appeal your denial, when payment is denied for codes 97110 thru 97124 due to obsolete bundling edits by your payer. Use this to help correct and update the insurance company edits. This is a general template. Customize it to your specific claim denial.

See Resource 206 for a full-size version of this form, with instructions.

Sample: *Response Letter to 97110-97124 Denials*

```
<DATE>
<INSURANCE REPRESENTATIVE NAME – IF KNOWN>
<INSURANCE COMPANY NAME>
<INSURANCE STREET>
<INSURANCE CITY/ST/ZIP>

RE: Appeal of Denied Services for 97110-97124

Thank you for your payment report on claim <INSERT CLAIM#_____> for <PATIENT NAME>.
However, the claim was denied for our therapy procedure <INSERT CODE(S)#_____>. This
claim needs to be paid correctly.

Please be advised that our office strives to follow the CPT guidelines for 97110 (Therapeutic Exercise),
97124 (Massage), and 97112 (Neuromuscular Reeducation). We assume that your office also follows
those guidelines. As a courtesy, to expedite billing, we appended the modifier 59, which was an alert
to you that the service was a "distinct procedure" from the chiropractic manipulative treatment (CMT)
service code.

Whereas your denial of this service indicates that you might not have current and correct information on
this important coding and billing matter, you should know that the American Medical Association (AMA)
has clarified previous confusion and/or private interpretations about the bundling of this code with the
CMT. Here is their guideline in this matter:

"The physical medicine codes 97110-97124 represent distinctly separate and unrelated proce-
dures not considered inclusive of the CMT described by codes 98940-98943. Therefore when
clinically relevant, it would be appropriate to report codes 97110-97124 in addition to the CMT
when performed in the same anatomic site, (i.e. separate body regions are not required)."
-CPT Assistant, March 2006. Volume 15, Issue 3, page 15

Additionally, this guideline from the AMA is consistent with the Relative Value Units (RVUs) for CMT
codes (98940-98943) which do not include any RVUs for these 15 minute procedures.

Therefore, please reprocess this claim correctly using CPT guidelines. If, for any reason, this specific
therapy code is not a benefit in the patient's policy, please advise in writing. We will then bill them for
your denied payment.

Please forward this letter to your administrative department chairman who is responsible for the correct
coding software edits. Surely they will want to update your obsolete software edits as soon as possible.

Sincerely,

Dr. <PROVIDER NAME>

enc
cc: <CLAIMANT/PATIENT>
```

Additional Appeal Letter Tips

- Documentation is extremely important. Send supporting information such as test results and other clinical evidence. Refer to objective measurements, not opinions.

- Keep communications professional, not personal. Remember that the employees at the payer's office are just trying to do their jobs.

- If you are appealing on the basis of medical necessity, be sure to include a report(s), including outcome assessments, which indicate why treatment was necessary and have the doctor sign the letter.

See Chapter 5–Treatment Plans and Assessments in *Section D–Documentation* for information on outcome assessments.

Letters for Continued Care

If your claim is denied due to arbitrary visit limits, time screens or other reasons, an appeal for continued care as medically necessary is required. Here are some concepts to help in that process.

- Be candid about the patient's condition. Describe any changes in diagnosis, comorbidities, progression, or regression of the patient's condition. Objective Measurement Tools are very helpful in establishing necessity of care.

- Describe the next phase of treatment, providing goals and an approximate time frame for the completion of treatment. This will demonstrate that you have an action-oriented approach.

- Present evidence of similar cases where the care was approved.

- Include any literature that supports your case, including references to practice guidelines. This may help convince the reviewer that the requested or updated treatment plan will result in the desired outcome.

See *Section D–Documentation* for more about objective measures and treatment plans.

New Consumer Health Plan Appeals

As part of the Patient Protection and Affordable Care Act (PPACA) of 2010, patients now have expanded appeal rights in all states. These new regulations, which are effective for all plan years beginning on or after September 23, 2010, grant the right to both an internal appeal through the insurance plan, as well as an independent external appeal.

Some states already have some consumer protection laws; however, the PPACA sets the minimum standard. Other provisions of this law also further extend patient protection the following ways:

- Requiring insurance plans to give consumers detailed information about the denial along with information on how to appeal.
- Expedited appeals for urgent cases such as emergency room visits.
- Restricted appeal costs for the consumer. The health plan is responsible for the remainder of the appeal costs.

Plans that are currently in existence, that have not undergone substantial changes, are "grandfathered," and will not be covered under the new rules. Nevertheless, you should still follow every appeal possibility.

> See Chapter 4–ERISA Appeals of this *Claims and Denials* section for more about these types of appeals.

> See "Grandfathered Plans" in Resource 156.

External Appeals

External appeals may be available with the health plan or insurance company payer with whom you or the patient is contracted.

All states have various review boards to protect the public interest. External appeals or reviews refer to a formal dispute-resolution process that has the authority to evaluate and resolve disputes involving health care. Outside review panels are mandated to have no connection to the health plan. Each side in the dispute agrees to abide by the board's decision, although in some states, patients may still sue a company if they're not satisfied with the decision. You can check with your association to find out how review boards operate in your state.

External review **is not a substitute for first following the "internal" appeals** process established by individual third-party payers. Never consider using external appeals until after exhausting all internal appeal levels.

Patients and providers might be hesitant to use the external review process; however, patients and their physicians should take advantage of this process for resolving disputes that arise in obtaining appropriate care. Although this is still a relatively new concept, external review programs are popular with consumer and advocacy groups. Some state laws encourage such a mediation process.

REDUCING DENIALS

Basic Steps to Reduce Denials

Here are some basic proactive measures for health care providers to consider in order to reduce denials when billing third party payers:

1. Use the most current versions of the CPT, ICD-9-CM (ICD-10-CM when implemented in October 2015) and HCPCS. Many health care providers still bill codes that haven't

been in use for years. This is easily remedied: update your *ChiroCode DeskBook* annually and use it!

2. Ensure the proper usage of modifiers on your claims where appropriate. Many coding situations require that modifiers be used.
3. Utilize the National Correct Coding Initiative (NCCI) edits in your defense. If you are up to standard as far as the NCCI goes, use it when appealing denials and defending your billing.
4. Stay current on payer policies and coverage by signing up for their newsletters or email notifications. Changes in policies are often announced in these publications. Many payer websites allow you to search for billing and coding policies.
5. Review the OIG reports and change your billing policies as appropriate to avoid known coding problems.
6. Review documentation requirements and update as necessary to ensure that your records meet high standards.

- See *Section F–Compliance and Audit Protection* to review OIG reports.
- See *Section H–Procedure Codes* for more about NCCI edits.
- See *Section D–Documentation* for more about meeting necessary requirements.

Clinical Documentation Manual (Resource 151) by the ACA includes detailed documentation information.

Downcoded Denials

Downcoding is the practice of using a lower level code when a higher level should have been either 1) billed on a claim or 2) paid by a third-party payer. On the part of the payers, a lower level code is paid rather than the one that was billed. On the part of the providers, a lower level of service is billed than what was actually provided. Regardless of the reasons why the provider may decide to bill a lower level code, it is important to always select the code which most accurately describes the services rendered. Downcoding is not an effective strategy for avoiding audits.

One issue with the practice of downcoding is that it results in an inaccurate record of the patient encounter. When a payer downcodes, it can also result in lesser payments.

Many providers are unaware that insurance companies use specialized software that analyzes submitted claims. This software can determine frequency of codes billed by a provider, by professional classification, or even within a geographic area. Those providers who consistently down-code their own claims, create a false picture of the actual care that was needed and over time, this can distort statistical averages. It is essential for providers to always bill appropriate codes, and support billed charges with detailed documentation.

See *Section D–Documentation* for required information to support the codes billed.

Review: Guidelines for Unpaid Claims

- How do you mark a claim that has a corrected error? *E-38*
- What three basic rules help to avoid claim denials? *E-39*
- When making an appeal, is it better to make a phone call or write a letter? *E-41*
- What supporting information should and should not be sent with the appeal? *E-42 to E-43*
- How can the Affordable Care Act help with your appeal? *E-44*
- What are six things that can be done to reduce denials when billing insurance carriers? *E-44 to E-45*

4. ERISA Appeals

ERISA Appeals (for Health Plans by Employers in the Private Sector)

Most health insurance plans are governed by the Employee Retirement Income Security Act (ERISA) of 1974 and the Patient Protection and Affordable Care Act (PPACA) of 2010. ERISA is federal law that regulates private sector employee benefit plans in order to protect the individuals participating in these plans. Generally, ERISA applies to health plans that are sponsored by employers in the private sector (non-government or civic).

Most employer sponsored health insurance plans are ERISA-based plans. The employer is considered the plan sponsor and the employee is the participant. For the most part, unless a patient is covered by a government plan (Medicare, Medicaid, etc.), a church, auto or individual health plan, it is highly probable that your patient's health plan is an ERISA plan.

There are two types of ERISA health insurance plans – those that are self-funded and those that are fully funded. ERISA rules apply both to plans that are "fully-funded" (that is, a health insurer bears the risk for claims) and plans that are "self-funded" (that is, the employer bears the risk for employee's claims), though some self-funded plans may be exempt. For plans that are fully-funded, state laws may apply in addition to ERISA and may give consumers additional rights to appeal to an independent entity outside of their health plan such as to a department of insurance (external appeals).

This distinction is important because different federal or state regulations can apply depending on the type of ERISA plan, the first step of an ERISA appeal is to determine if the plan is in fact subject to ERISA, and to understand the type of plan that is in question.

Use the "Verification of Insurance Coverage Form" as discussed in *Section B–Insurance and Reimbursement* (page B-12) to assist in making this determination.

- Go to ChiroCode.com/erisa or ACAtoday.org/ERISA for additional information on ERISA and ERISA appeals.
- Go to ACAtoday.org/pdf/erisaflowchart.pdf (Resource 361) for a "ERISA Appeals Process Flowchart.

PPACA Grandfathered Exception

Group or individual plans that were purchased or implemented on or before March 23, 2010 are exempted from many of the required PPACA changes. These "grandfathered" health plans lose their exemption status if there are significant changes to benefits or premiums (as defined by PPACA). As such, according to the Kaiser Family Foundation's most recent Employer Health Benefits Survey, the number of grandfathered plans dropped an estimated 20% from 2011 to 2013, and will likely continue to decline.

See Resource 384 for more information and state listings.

Self-Funded Plan Exceptions

Under ERISA, employers offering self-funded plans are not insurers which means that they are not governed by most state insurance laws. Even though self-funded plans are considered an ERISA plan (unless they are government or church related employers), they fall under the regulatory authority of the U.S. Department of Labor's Employee Benefits Security Administration (EBSA). The EBSA does require self-funded plans to include a Summary Plan Description (SPD) for participants, however, benefits can and do vary. This is why the Insurance Verification process discussed in *Section B-Insurance* is so important.

Providers need to understand that although there are remedies for beneficiaries under ERISA such as appeals to a federal court, PPACA exempts self insured plans from some of its provisions. For example, essential health benefits do NOT apply to these types of plans. Also, self-funded plans do not have to comply with the Medical Loss Ratio requirements. Only these PPACA consumer protections apply to self-funded plans:

- Annual and lifetime plan limits are not allowed.
- Rescissions by insurers are not allowed.
- Discriminating against patients with pre-existing conditions is not allowed.
- Coverage of dependent children up to age 26 is required.
- Coverage of preventive screenings is required.
- External appeals are required.

Benefits for Your Patients

Health care providers and patients should understand that ERISA can provide an enormous benefit to them. Historically, patients and providers were denied an opportunity for full and fair review of claims denials. ERISA has specific procedures for appealing adverse benefit determinations and requires that participants and beneficiaries are provided notice and an opportunity for a full and fair review of the claims determinations. The PPACA also requires both internal and external appeals processes be implemented by health benefit plans. This is extremely important in the context of prepayment and post-payment claim reviews. For example, if a determination is made that a claim should be denied for lack of medical necessity, the ERISA claims procedures may apply and the patient, or provider (if the provider has a valid assignment), can seek to enforce the rights to a full and fair review under ERISA.

> See the segment "Step 4. Understand Claim Procedures and Appeal Rights" on page E-51 for more information.

ERISA also provides remedies under the civil enforcement provisions that may include equitable relief and civil penalties for violation of the claims procedures. Plan sponsors and plan fiduciaries can be held accountable. Specifically, some of the available rights and remedies include:

State vs Federal

The Patient Protection and Affordable Care Act (PPACA) is a federal statute which includes federal standards for external reviews and appeals. Individual states may have their own external review process as long as they meet or exceed the the federal standards. As of January 1, 2014, all states must be in compliance or have standards that exceed that of federal regulations.

> See Resource 183 for more information and state listings.

- The right to accurate coverage information as stated in the Summary Plan Description (SPD) by their employer.
- The right to a $110 per day penalty if the SPD is not provided.
- The right for a patient to designate the health care provider as their authorized representative.
- The right to appeal a denied or reduced claim when the plan says any of the following: (1) the care is not medically necessary or appropriate, (2) you are not eligible for the health plan or benefit, (3) you have a pre-existing condition, or (4) the care is experimental or investigational.
- The right to know the criteria and other information used for the claim denial, such as "lack of medical necessity."
- The right to know the name of the in-state reviewer.
- Injunctive relief and other equitable remedies.

Providers who do not wish to follow these steps in appealing an adverse determination, should inform the patient of their rights under ERISA. There are state run Consumer Assistance Programs (CAP) which could be of assistance to them during their appeal.

Accountability and Fiduciary Responsibility

As mentioned earlier, ERISA holds the third party administrators (TPA) and plan fiduciaries accountable, along with the plan sponsors, for abusive practices for failure to adhere to ERISA guidelines.

Understanding the rights and remedies under ERISA is important in the context of claims denials and it is prudent for patients and providers to seek the assistance of experienced counsel when faced with these types of claim denials.

See *Appeals Made Simple for ERISA Type Claims* (Resource 184) by attorney Rob Sherman, Esq. for help with reimbursement denials and refund demands.

First Steps with ERISA

The following steps will help you get paid according to your patient's summary plan description (SPD). There is no substitute for thoroughness in these basic steps. They are essential for proper protocols in making ERISA appeals. They also lay the foundation for any health care lawyer if you decide to take the matter to a federal court.

Go to ACAtoday.org/pdf/erisaflowchart.pdf (Resource 361) for an "ERISA Appeals Process Flowchart."

Step 1. Get the Summary Plan Description

This first step is essential. Only with the Summary Plan Description (SPD) can you determine if your service is a covered benefit. If it is not listed, there are no appeal rights and paying for the service is the patient's financial obligation. Only when your service is a covered benefit and the plan administrator makes an adverse benefit determination can the appeals process commence. The SPD is provided by the plan administrator. It is not an insurance policy, which is a phantom SPD. If the patient does not have an SPD, you have to obtain it with proper authorization from the patient.

Step 2. Become the Authorized Representative

The "Designation of Authorized Representative" form is a crucial document. You must obtain it in order to serve as the authorized representative of your patient and to pursue their rights under ERISA law.

The typical "assignment of benefits" that is generally given to a doctor is not sufficient for them to qualify as an Authorized Representative under ERISA. According to the Department of Labor, the official watchdog for ERISA and the courts, the usual "assignment of benefits" is limited to receiving a benefit payment under the terms of the health plan. It does not grant any authority to act in pursuing or appealing an adverse benefit determination. The validity of the designation of an authorized representative will depend on whether the designation has been made in accordance with the procedures established by the health plan, if any.

The "Designation of Authorized Representative" form (see next page) is primarily designed to designate you as the authorized representative of the patient. For that reason you could use this form in conjunction with whatever assignment of benefits/lien form you already use (as developed by legal counsel in your state). This form and your assignment/lien form should provide sufficient documentation for the ERISA plan administrator to allow you to pursue your patient's ERISA rights. Although it states that the plan administrator is required to deal with the doctor as the patient's designated representative, it does not incorporate the legal jargon that is found in many assignment/lien documents that are carefully drafted by legal experts in each state.

The plan should direct all information and notifications to which the claimant is entitled. You can then act on the claimant's behalf with respect to the initial determination of the claim, requests for documents, and appeals. Please note that a plan may establish reasonable procedures for determining whether an individual has been authorized to act on behalf of the claimant.

Designation of Authorized Representative

This sample form must be obtained in order to appeal ERISA claims.

See Resource 186 for a full-size version of this form, with instructions.

See ACAtoday.org/ERISA (Resource 187) for an additional sample letter by the ACA. It is also shown in the *ACA Template Letters Appendix* of this *ChiroCode DeskBook*.

Sample: *Designation of Authorized Representative*

DESIGNATION OF AUTHORIZED REPRESENTATIVE

I [PATIENT'S NAME], do hereby designate [Doctor's name and clinic name] to the full extent permissible under the Employee Retirement Income Security Act of 1974 ("ERISA") and as provided in 29 CFR 2560-503-1(b)4 to otherwise act on my behalf to pursue claims and exercise all rights connected with my employee health care benefit plan, with respect to any medical or other health care expense(s) incurred as a result of the services I receive from the above named doctor. These rights include all rights to act on my behalf with respect to initial determinations of claims, to pursue appeals of benefit determinations under the plan, to obtain records, and to claim on my behalf such medical or other health care service benefits, insurance or health care benefit plan reimbursement and to pursue any other applicable remedies.

Patient's Signature

Patient's Printed Name

Date

Use an Accompanying Cover Letter

Use an explanatory cover letter for your "Designation of Authorized Representative" form. It is essential for proper processing of your request. Explain that you are requesting the summary plan description (SPD) and not a third party insurance policy, and that you are providing two documents: (1) Your Designation of Authorized Representative form that designates you as the authorized representative of the patient to pursue all rights granted under ERISA, and (2) An assignment of benefits or other document (approved by legal counsel in your state) that secures payment for services you provide.

Note: Letters should be sent in a manner that provides proof of delivery. This is required to begin the clock count-down. This could be an overnight courier, or U.S. Mail, Return Receipt Requested.

This sample letter could be used to accompany your request for ERISA information.

See Resource 188 for a full-size version of this form, with instructions.

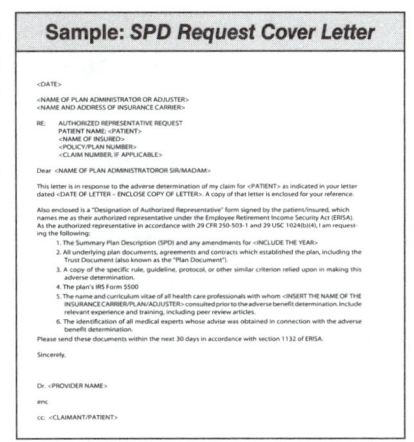

Sample: SPD Request Cover Letter

Step 3. Discover Who the Plan Administrator Is

Typically the Plan Administrator is the employer, or someone within its organization who oversees healthcare benefits. The employer could delegate this role with its fiduciary responsibilities to a third party administrator (TPA) or an insurance company. If so, the delegation and acceptance should be in a contract. Do not waste time in communicating or making appeals with anyone who is not the official Plan Administrator with fiduciary responsibilities.

Step 4. Understand Claim Procedures and Appeal Rights

The ERISA statute and regulations require ERISA plans to establish and maintain claims procedures under which entitlement benefits and/or disputes can be requested by the plan participants. Basic steps in any claims procedure include:

1. A claim for benefits by a claimant or an authorized representative;
2. A benefit determination by the plan, with required notification to the claimant;
3. An appeal by the claimant or authorized representative of any adverse determination; and
4. The determination on review by the plan, with required notification to the claimant.

Generally, the Plan Administrator shall notify the claimant of the plan's adverse benefit determination within a reasonable period of time, but usually not later than thirty (30) days after receipt of the claim. The notification must set forth, among other things, the specific reason or reasons for the adverse determination; a description of the plan's review procedures and the time limits applicable to such procedures; and the criterion upon which the adverse determination was based.

APPEALS

Once an adverse benefit determination is made, every employee benefit plan is required to establish and maintain a procedure by which a claimant shall have a reasonable opportunity to appeal such a determination. This includes both internal reviews and external appeals processes. The claims procedure must provide claimants at least sixty (60) days following receipt of a notification of an adverse benefit determination within which to appeal the determination. For group health plans, the claims procedures must allow claimants at least one hundred eighty (180) days to appeal the determination. The notification must provide claimants with an opportunity to submit information relating to the claim for benefits. The notification must also provide that a claimant is entitled to all documents, records, and other information relevant to the claimant's claim for benefits.

After the appeal, the plan administrator is required to notify the claimant of the plan's final benefit determination on review within a reasonable period of time. For group health plans, the notification must be provided not later than sixty (60) days after receipt by the plan of the claimant's request for review of an adverse benefit determination. The plan administrator is again required to notify the claimant of the specific reasons for the final adverse determination and must indicate that the claimant is entitled to all documents, records and other information relevant to the claimant's claim for benefits.

Since the claims procedures can vary depending on the type of claim and the type of plan, a wise claimant should proceed in this Step 4 with the assistance of an experienced ERISA subject matter expert (SME) and/or health care attorney.

In Conclusion

The Power of ERISA

It could be tempting to believe that ERISA has no teeth and never imposes penalties on plan fiduciaries and their duties—but the following cases confirm Congress' wisdom in enforcing those duties.

On January 4, 2013, in the case of Lifecare management Services v. Insurance Management Administrators, Inc., the Texas Court of Appeals ruled against the plan adminstrator in that they abused their discretion. The district court awarded LifeCare benefits payments in excess of $512,000 **and** attorneys' fees totaling more than $453,000.

In another case in 2007, (Cromer-Tyler v. Edward R. Teitel, M.D., P.C), a pension plan maintained by a health care clinic was assessed statutory penalties against the owner of the clinc for failure to respond to requests for relevant documentation. This resulted in a fine of $179,960 ($110 per day for 1,636 days). The original amount in dispute was less than $10,000.

Penalty awards can greatly exceed the amount of the basic benefits at stake in an ERISA lawsuit. These cases illustrate that courts, confronted with an egregious set of facts, have ruled in favor of the plantiff and have also chosen to use the statutory disclosure penalty as a way of punishing a "breach of fiduciary duty."

ERISA LAW EXCERPTS

The following excerpts from the ERISA law can be a valuable reference resource and could be cited in your communication with the plan administrator.

See Resource 193 for the ERISA law text.

"Adverse Benefit Determination" Definition:

According to ERISA and PPACA regulations, an "adverse benefit determination" means a denial, reduction, or termination of, or a failure to provide or make payment (in whole or in part) for a benefit in any of the following situations:
- based on a determination of a participant's or beneficiary's eligibility to participate in a plan
- for group health plans, resulting from the application of any utilization review
- for group health plans, failure to cover an item or service for which benefits are otherwise provided, because it is determined to be experimental or investigational or not medically necessary or appropriate (See 29 CFR 2560.503-1(m)(4).)
- any rescission of coverage as defined in 29 C.F.R. §2590.715-2712(a)(2)

§ 1022. Summary Plan Description

(a) A summary plan description of any employee benefit plan shall be furnished to participants and beneficiaries as provided in section 1024 (b) of this title. The summary plan description shall include the information described in subsection (b) of this section, shall be written in a manner calculated to be understood by the average plan participant, and shall be sufficiently accurate and comprehensive to reasonably apprise such participants and beneficiaries of their rights and obligations under the plan. A summary of any material modification in the terms of the plan and any change in the information required under subsection (b) of this section shall be written in a manner calculated to be understood by the average plan participant and shall be furnished in accordance with section 1024 (b)(1) of this title.

(b) The summary plan description shall contain the following information: The name and type of administration of the plan; in the case of a group health plan (as defined in section 1191b (a)(1) of this title), whether a health insurance issuer (as defined in section 1191b (b)(2) of this title) is responsible for the financing or administration (including payment of claims) of the plan and (if so) the name and address of such issuer; the name and address of the person designated as agent for the service of legal process, if such person is not the administrator; the name and address of the administrator; names, titles, and addresses of any trustee or trustees (if they are persons different from the administrator); a description of the relevant provisions of any applicable collective bargaining agreement; the plan's requirements respecting eligibility for participation and benefits; a description of the provisions providing for nonforfeitable pension benefits; circumstances which may result in disqualification, ineligibility, or denial or loss of benefits; the source of financing of the plan and the identity of any organization through which benefits are provided; the date of the end of the plan year and whether the records of the plan are kept on a calendar, policy, or fiscal year basis; the procedures to be followed in presenting claims for benefits under the plan including the office at the Department of Labor through which participants and beneficiaries may seek assistance or information regarding their rights under this chapter and the Health Insurance Portability and Accountability Act of 1996 with respect to health benefits that are offered through a group health plan (as defined in section 1191b (a)(1) of this title) and the remedies available under the plan for the redress of claims which are denied in whole or in part (including procedures required under section 1133 of this title).

§ 1104. Fiduciary Duties

(a) Prudent man standard of care

(1) Subject to sections 1103(c) and (d), 1342, and 1344 of this title, a fiduciary shall discharge his duties with respect to a plan solely in the interest of the participants and beneficiaries and—

(A) for the exclusive purpose of:

(i) providing benefits to participants and their beneficiaries; and

(ii) defraying reasonable expenses of administering the plan;

(B) with the care, skill, prudence, and diligence under the circumstances then prevailing that a prudent man acting in a like capacity and familiar with such matters would use in the conduct of an enterprise of a like character and with like aims;

(C) by diversifying the investments of the plan so as to minimize the risk of large losses, unless under the circumstances it is clearly prudent not to do so; and

(D) in accordance with the documents and instruments governing the plan insofar as such documents and instruments are consistent with the provisions of this subchapter and subchapter III of this chapter.

ERISA Law Excerpts (cont'd)

(2) In the case of an eligible individual account plan (as defined in section 1107(d)(3) of this title), the diversification requirement of paragraph (1)(C) and the prudence requirement (only to the extent that it requires diversification) of paragraph (1)(B) is not violated by acquisition or holding of qualifying employer real property or qualifying employer securities (as defined in section 1107(d)(4) and (5) of this title).

§ 1191b. Definitions

(a) Group health plan

For purposes of this part—

(1) In general

The term "group health plan" means an employee welfare benefit plan to the extent that the plan provides medical care (as defined in paragraph (2) and including items and services paid for as medical care) to employees or their dependents (as defined under the terms of the plan) directly or through insurance, reimbursement, or otherwise

(2) Medical care

The term "medical care" means amounts paid for—

(A) the diagnosis, cure, mitigation, treatment, or prevention of disease, or amounts paid for the purpose of affecting any structure or function of the body,

(B) amounts paid for transportation primarily for and essential to medical care referred to in subparagraph (A), and

(C) amounts paid for insurance covering medical care referred to in subparagraphs (A) and (B).

(b) Definitions relating to health insurance

For purposes of this part—

(1) Health insurance coverage

The term "health insurance coverage" means benefits consisting of medical care (provided directly, through insurance or reimbursement, or otherwise and including items and services paid for as medical care) under any hospital or medical service policy or certificate, hospital or medical service plan contract, or health maintenance organization contract offered by a health insurance issuer

(2) Health insurance issuer

The term "health insurance issuer" means an insurance company, insurance service, or insurance organization (including a health maintenance organization, as defined in paragraph (3)) which is licensed to engage in the business of insurance in a State and which is subject to State law which regulates insurance (within the meaning of section 1144(b)(2) of this title). Such term does not include a group health plan.

(3) Health maintenance organization

The term "health maintenance organization" means—

(A) a federally qualified health maintenance organization (as defined in section 1301(a) of the Public Health Service Act (42 U.S.C. 300e (a))),

(B) an organization recognized under State law as a health maintenance organization, or

(C) a similar organization regulated under State law for solvency in the same manner and to the same extent as such a health maintenance organization.

(4) Group health insurance coverage

The term "group health insurance coverage" means, in connection with a group health plan, health insurance coverage offered in connection with such plan.

ERISA Law Excerpts (cont'd)

§ 1371. Penalty for failure to timely provide required information

The corporation may assess a penalty, payable to the corporation, against any person who fails to provide any notice or other material information required under this subtitle, subtitle A, B, or C of this subchapter, or section 1083(k)(4) of this title [1], or any regulations prescribed under any such subtitle or such section, within the applicable time limit specified therein. Such penalty shall not exceed $1,000 for each day for which such failure continues.

Review: ERISA Appeals

- Which area of insurance does ERISA cover? *E-47*
- What are some specific rights under ERISA? *E-51*
- Name the four steps to take for ERISA appeals? *E-49 to E-51*
- What is the SPD, and where is it obtained from? *E-49*
- Who is the Authorized Representative? *E-50*
- Who is the official Plan Administrator? *E-51*
- What are the basic steps to take in any claims procedure? *E-51*
- What is an "Adverse Benefit Determination"? *E-52*
- According to ERISA law, what is "medical care"? *E-54*
- What are the ERISA penalties for failure to provide any required notice or other material information? *E-55*

1. The Need for Compliance
Page F-3

2. HIPAA Compliance
Page F-14

3. Medicare Compliance
Page F-30

4. OIG Compliance Program Guidance
Page F-35

5. Audit Protection
Page F-45

F COMPLIANCE AND AUDIT PROTECTION

COMPLIANCE AND AUDIT PROTECTION

OBJECTIVES

This section introduces important compliance issues and how they directly impact your practice. You will learn about:

- Why compliance plays an integral role in daily activities and how taking steps now mitigates your risks.
- Health Insurance Portability and Accountability Act (HIPAA), HITECH and Omnibus Final Rule compliance regulations regarding security, privacy and more.
- Changes to the Office of the Inspector General (OIG) compliance program.
- Other agencies, such as OSHA who are entering this compliance realm.
- Specific ways to avoid allegations of fraud and abuse.
- How to appropriately and effectively respond to refund demands and audits.

Compliance is about risk management – protecting your practice. Taking preventive actions now and being proactive by implementing these programs can demonstrate to enforcement officers that your practice is committed to excellence in both business practices and the healthcare services that you provide.

Compliance programs directed at reducing, preventing and deterring fraudulent and improper conduct are at the forefront of the healthcare industry's goals.

OUTLINE

1. The Need for Compliance *F-3*
    - ◆ About Compliance *F-3*
    - ◆ The Importance of Having a Compliance Plan *F-6*
    - ◆ Fraud and Abuse *F-7*
    - ◆ OSHA Requirements *F-10*
    - ◆ Review *F-13*
2. HIPAA Compliance *F-14*
    - ◆ Who Is Affected by HIPAA? *F-15*
    - ◆ Electronic Transactions and Code Set Requirements *F-18*
    - ◆ Privacy Requirements *F-20*
    - ◆ Security Requirements *F-23*
    - ◆ HITECH Enforcement Requirements *F-25*
    - ◆ National Identifier Requirements *F-28*
    - ◆ Review *F-29*
3. Medicare Compliance *F-30*
    - ◆ Automated Reviews *F-31*
    - ◆ OIG Reviews *F-31*
    - ◆ CMS Reviews *F-32*
    - ◆ MAC Reviews *F-33*
    - ◆ Review *F-34*
4. OIG Compliance Program Guidance *F-35*
    - ◆ OIG Compliance Program Guidance *F-35*
    - ◆ OIG Work Plan *F-42*
    - ◆ Review *F-44*
5. Audit Protection *F-45*
    - ◆ Audits Are Here to5 Stay *F-45*
    - ◆ General Audit Protection *F-47*
    - ◆ Avoiding an Audit *F-49*
    - ◆ Refund Requests and Demands *F-53*
    - ◆ Review *F-55*

1. The Need for Compliance

About Compliance

Compliance is a three step process.

1. Research and seek to understand which rules and regulations apply to your situation.
2. Create a plan of action regarding these rules. This is the policy and procedure portion of compliance.
3. Report your findings. If errors are found, corrections need to be made. Policies and procedures should be re-evaluated on a regular basis in order to stay current.

A compliance program is a powerful tool for staying abreast of regulations and avoiding trouble. It can also help protect your practice from implications of insurance abuse or fraud. Designing a compliance program can help every part of your business adhere to best practices, and present opportunities for process improvement which could lead to increased profitability. Most importantly, an essential part of your practice's compliance strategy is starting and maintaining a compliance program which includes regular refresher training sessions for staff. An active, effective compliance program can also demonstrate to regulating agencies or reviewers that there was intent to comply which may, in some cases, mitigate penalties. Compliance programs should be a source of continuous incremental improvement for your practice.

The odds of being audited have been increasing exponentially over the last several years. In February of 2014, HHS announced that in 2013 alone, a record $4.3 billion was recovered through their fraud prevention and enforcement efforts.

In July 2012, the Obama adminstration announced a ground-breaking fraud prevention partnership in which both private and government programs join forces. Now the federal government, state officials, several leading private health insurance organizations and other health care anti-fraud groups are working together and sharing data in order to prevent fraud. The need for provider compliance has never been greater.

See Resource 263 for additional information on compliance, including articles and webinars.

Some providers are unaware of the reality that a request for records from a payer is an audit. When you send your documentation to a payer, it is carefully reviewed (audited), and the results of this review will determine whether or not additional scrutiny and audits will take place.

Additionally, compliance is about more than just claims and payments. Standards in record keeping, business practices, patient privacy, and security also play an important role. The challenge for providers is to not only stay current with correct billing and documentation, but to understand all the additional legal requirements of practicing medicine.

In all fairness, newspaper headlines keep the problem of fraud and abuse within the health care system in the public eye. It is costing the system billions of dollars annually and payers in need of maintaining programs and services must find these offenders and hold them accountable. This puts a greater burden on providers to ensure that their practices hold up to increased scrutiny.

Steeper fines and ever-increasing audits have caused a financial strain on many providers. Some have gone out of business or even declared bankruptcy as a direct result of refund demands and audits. It has been said that the best defense is a good offense and this adage holds true for refunds and audits. Be proactive to resolve internal problems before an audit takes place.

Who is Being Targeted?

No type of provider is exempt. From sole proprietors to large corporations, a myriad of tools are being implemented by payers in order to find questionable billing practices. Statistically speaking, computer modeling trends tend to target smaller practices which do not fit into corporate medicine patterns.

A new tool being used by payers is "data mining," which is the process by which submitted claims are aggregated and statistically analyzed in order to summarize it into useful information. For payers, that means computer software can now find ways to increase revenues, cut costs, or discover fraudulent activities. If your billing patterns fall outside their established statistical pattern for chiropractic providers in your area, you may be flagged for an audit. Proper documentation should support the medical necessity for cases that do not conform to typical patterns.

Chiropractic practices tend to be targeted for a few reasons:

1. Solo practitioners tend to be specialty oriented and thus limit the number of codes used. Commonly, the vast majority of their claims only utilize a handful of diagnosis and procedure codes.

2. Practices are small, sometimes just a doctor and a receptionist or CA, who may well be a spouse or family member. Every activity that is not related to patient care is time spent away from earning, and patient care is a priority over paperwork. But if the records or the books are not done right or kept up to date, they do not stand up to inspection—which makes recoupment easy for auditors. Do not underestimate the importance of documentation and record-keeping.

> **Warning:**
> - Doctors of chiropractic should be aware that some business tactics taught by practice management companies could be considered fraudulent. Consider consulting a qualified health care attorney or a certified compliance specialist (see Resource 264) when implementing these business practices.
> - Doctors of chiropractic should be sure that their documentation justifies the services rendered.

Piggy-back Audits:

If you have been audited by a government entity and the outcome is not favorable, it becomes public record. The special investigation units of private payers review those public records and often will follow with their own audit. In some states they actually work with the government audit agencies.

Compliance Is Inevitable

This new climate for compliance inspection, in which agencies pay more attention to your documented procedures than to your claims, changes the game. This process can be highly invasive, but it will bring you certain advantages.

The weakest defense against mushrooming regulations and inspections is to resist and deny and wish they'd go away. The strongest defense is to create a proactive, comprehensive compliance system, as described in the following pages.

There is no "one size fits all" compliance program. Learn the components of compliance and implement a program that best suits your practice. Having a compliance program that is ill defined, not applicable to the practice or not followed by the practice poses significant risk and liability.

Who Demands Compliance?

Government and Private Insurance Companies

Insurance companies generally copy the actions of CMS and the OIG, although they often do not provide as many safeguards for providers. As the federal government shifts to inspecting offices for compliance, expect insurance companies to do the same.

ERISA and Non-ERISA

While speaking of insurance companies, it may be good to consider compliance as it relates to both ERISA and non-ERISA actions. ERISA cases are federal in nature. Non-ERISA cases are adjudicated on the state level. Be prepared for any differences this may inflict when you set up your compliance program.

State Departments of Labor and Industries

Doctors of chiropractic may also have to defend their practice against the Department of Labor and Industries if they provide services in workers' compensation cases. Workers' compensation laws vary from state to state.

U.S. Department of Justice

The U.S. Department of Justice, headed by the Attorney General, is responsible for federal law enforcement. As such, federal crimes, such as false claims, are often prosecuted by this department. Many of these cases are forwarded by investigators (and whistleblowers) to the HHS Office of the Inspector General (OIG). From there, the cases may be forwarded to the Justice Department.

See Resource 265 for more about this federal department.

Compliance Diminishes Fines

ChiroCode Institute industry consultants have confirmed with top officials that even an appearance of active, ongoing efforts of maintaining a compliance program can demonstrate intent and can be successful in reducing penalties. In the words of one of them, "Virtually every federal agency and the federal sentencing guidelines consider the existence of an effective compliance program as a mitigating factor in the imposition of fines and civil monetary penalties."

The Importance of Having a Compliance Plan

A compliance plan allows a practice to maintain consistency in the delivery of health care services and provides a written plan or outline of the appropriate actions for a practice. It also assures continuity of actions by employees even during staff turnover. In the circumstance of an audit with subsequent fines, a viable compliance plan may be used as a mitigating factor to avert or decrease fines and jail time. To realize the importance of having a viable compliance plan, consider the following averages of recoupment from an audit. The repayment amounts are based on the average patients seen per week in the office and the amounts typically recouped in an audit.

Over the last three years, the government recovered $8.10 for every dollar spent on fraud and abuse investigations, which is the highest three-year average return on investment in the 17-year history of the Health Care Fraud and Abuse (HCFAC) Program. They are serious about these programs and providers should be too.

Although compliance plans overseen by certified compliance officers have been implemented in hospitals, medical doctors' offices, nursing homes, and other health facilities, it has been largely ignored by the chiropractic profession. Certified compliance officers can effectively implement a compliance plan that will meet the OIG guidelines.

When considering hiring a compliance officer or consultant, keep in mind that many know compliance and others may know chiropractic. It is imperative that you hire a certified compliance specialist who knows the operation, documentation and coding for chiropractic. The compliance officer will aid in rectifying problems prior to an audit. By bringing each office into compliance, each physician will ultimately help to improve the quality of health care for all of our patients and simultaneously ensure the future of chiropractic.

See Resource 264 for assistance in selecting a certified compliance specialist.

Benefits of a Compliance Program

An effective compliance program is essential for physician practices of all sizes and does not have to be costly or resource-intensive. With the development of a formal program, a physician practice may find it easier to comply with its affirmative duty to ensure the accuracy of claims submitted for reimbursement. Numerous benefits can be gained by implementing an effective compliance program. These benefits may include:

- Development of effective internal procedures to ensure compliance with regulations, payment policies, and coding rules
- Improved medical record documentation
- Improved education for practice employees
- A reduction in the number of claim denials
- More streamlined practice operations through better communication and more comprehensive policies
- Avoidance of potential liability arising from noncompliance
- Reduced exposure to penalties
- Improved patient care resulting from an increased focus on safety, security, and quality

The OIG will consider the existence of an effective compliance program that predated any governmental investigation when addressing the appropriateness of administrative sanctions; however, the burden is on the physician's practice to demonstrate the operational effectiveness of the compliance program. In addition, an effective compliance program that was in place at the time of the criminal offense may mitigate criminal sanctions. It is widely held that if you hope for leniency during an audit or investigation, then you must follow these guidelines as closely as possible.

> **Alert:** A formal compliance program that is **not** enforced may create greater liability. Do not purchase a compliance product and then allow it to collect dust on the book shelf.

Summary

Compliance not only consists of HIPAA but also OSHA and other risk management and operational safety measures that must be evaluated regularly by practices in order to properly plan, train and maintain a successful compliance program. Every practice, including small offices, should be concerned about compliance.

Implementing a compliance program is preventive. An effective compliance program also sends an important message to a practice's employees that while the practice recognizes that mistakes can occur, employees have an affirmative, ethical duty to come forward and report fraudulent or erroneous conduct so it may be corrected.

See Resource 266 for more compliance information from the OIG.

Fraud and Abuse

Fraud and abuse is considered to be a huge and costly problem for Medicare, Medicaid, and other government and private health care programs. It is estimated that up to 10% of the projected $606 billion the federal government will pay in 2015 in health care reimbursements will be for fraudulent bills or non-compliant billing practices. The improper payment rate increased from 8.5% in 2012 to 10.1% in 2013. According to the 2013 CERT Annual Improper Payment Reports, chiropractic claims had one of the highest error rates of all Part B claim types. The error rate was 47.4% in 2012 and 51.7% in 2013.

See Resource 267 for more information about the Health Care Fraud and Abuse Control Program results.

According to CMS, the primary difference between fraud and abuse is intention. They are defined as follows:

> "Fraud: When someone intentionally executes or attempts to execute a scheme to obtain money or property of any health care benefit program."

> "Abuse: When health care providers or suppliers perform actions that directly or indirectly result in unnecessary costs to any health care benefit program."

What used to be referred to as abuse is now categorized as fraud because even if a provider did not know a certain practice was improper, they "should have known." The responsibility is now placed on providers to understand and follow all laws that affect their practice.

Monitoring

The government has an ongoing program to monitor settlement agreements with integrity provisions and corporate integrity agreements, Other pertinent facts include:

- Under the False Claims Act, a whistleblower ("relater") can be rewarded up to 25%-30% of the recovered fraudulent amount.

- Under the False Claims Act, the government does not need to prove that the provider intended to commit fraud. They only need to have reasonable suspicion.
- Under the False Claims Act, the definition of "knowingly" means: 1) actual knowledge; 2) reckless disregard for the truth; or 3) deliberate ignorance.
- More than 60% of the whistleblower cases brought under the False Claims Act involve health care fraud.
- The OIG encourages beneficiaries to be involved in the identification of fraudulent activities, which results in their hotline receiving a very high volume of calls.
- FBI funding for health care investigations in 2013 was $128.1 million.
- Federal funding for the Health Care Fraud and Abuse Program in 2013 was over $295 million with an additional $309 million in discretionary funding. Consequently, special units are well funded for aggressive investigations.

Six Important Fraud and Abuse Laws

According to the OIG, the following six federal fraud and abuse laws are very important to physicians: the False Claims Act (FCA), the Anti-Kickback Statute (AKS), the Physician Self-Referral Law (Stark law), the Exclusion Authorities, the Civil Monetary Penalties Law (CMPL), and the newly created Health Care Fraud statute.

Understanding these laws helps your office avoid potential problems.

1. ***False Claims Act [31 U.S.C. §§ 3729–3733]*** It is illegal to submit claims for payment to Medicare or Medicaid that you know or should know are false or fraudulent. No INTENT to defraud is required, reckless disregard or "deliberate ignorance" are also considered fraudulent.

   Penalty: Fines up to three times the programs' loss plus $11,000 per claim filed. Additionally, criminal charges and prison time are also a possibility.

   > **Overpayments:** If the provider does not repay an overpayment within 60 days, they may be liable under the False Claims Act.

2. ***Anti-Kickback Statute [42 U.S.C. § 1320a-7b(b)]*** Federal health care programs specifically prohibit any type of "remuneration" for patient referrals. You cannot receive any type of gift or anything of value for referring a patient to another provider. It is illegal.

   The Affordable Care Act changed the burden of proof standard. Now, providers can be held liable **without** specific knowledge of or specific intent to violate the law.

   Under this law, routinely waiving the patient co-payment is illegal.

   > See Chapter 3–Establishing Fees in *Section B–Insurance and Reimbursement* for more about properly discounting fee schedules.

   Penalty: Criminal and administrative penalties apply to both parties. Fines up to $50,000 per kickback plus three times the amount of the actual kickback value. Additionally, jail time and exclusion from participation in federal health care programs can be applied.

   Kickbacks are also pursued under the False Claims Act which carries a heftier penalty.

3. ***Physician Self-Referral Law [42 U.S.C. § 1395nn]*** Known as the Stark law, this law prohibits providers from referring patients for "designated health services" payable by Medicare or Medicaid to a business where the provider or an immediate family member has a financial relationship. Specific intent to violate the law is not required.

Penalty: Fines and exclusion from participation in federal health care programs.

The simplest way to avoid the Stark Law, or a state's version called a mini-Stark Law, is to always pay attention when referring patients to other practitioners or service providers.

Specifically pay attention to:

- Clinical laboratory,
- Physical therapy services,
- Mobile diagnostic units,
- Occupational therapy services,
- Radiology services, including magnetic resonance imaging (MRI),
- Computerized axial tomography scans and ultrasound services,
- Radiation therapy services,
- Durable medical equipment,
- Parenteral and enteral nutrients, equipment, and supplies,
- Prosthetics, orthotics, and prosthetic devices,
- Home health services,
- Outpatient prescription drugs,
- Inpatient and outpatient hospital services.

Most of these do not involve doctors of chiropractic, but some do. There are some ways to stay in a safe harbor (some organizations advise their doctors never to refer to just one entity, but to the three closest entities.) Working within a bona fide "physician group" can help you avoid possible violations of this law. Know the laws in your state before making referrals, and consult your attorney before entering into any practice agreements.

It is important to document your financial relationships with referring physicians in your Compliance Manual. Be careful about productivity bonuses and gifts as they could fall under Stark laws too.

4. ***Exclusion Statute [42 U.S.C. § 1320a-7]*** Providers who are specifically excluded from participation in federal health care programs because of several types of felony convictions as well as patient abuse or neglect, cannot bill Medicare or Medicaid for any items or services provided - either directly or indirectly (through an employer or group practice).

   Penalty: Employers who hire someone who is listed in the Exclusions Database, are assessed Civil Monetary Penalties of $10,000 for each item or service furnished by the excluded provider.

   > See Resource 268 and immediately check your employees against the Exclusions Database. Document your searches and self-disclose if you discover that you have unknowingly employed an excluded individual.

5. ***Civil Monetary Penalties Law [42 U.S.C. § 1320a-7a]*** This law, enforced by the OIG, applies to a broad range of activities such as violating Medicare assignment provisions or the Medicare physician agreement.

   Penalty: Penalties range from $10,000 to $50,000 **per violation** plus damages up to three times the amount of the improper claim. Depending on the type and number of violations, penalties have been reported that are well over a million dollars.

   > See Resource 269 to read more about this law.

6. ***Health Care Fraud Statute [18 U.S.C. § 1347]*** This federal law is part of HIPAA. The following is the official definition:

> TITLE 18 - CRIMES AND CRIMINAL PROCEDURE
> PART I - CRIMES
> CHAPTER 63 - MAIL FRAUD
> § 1347. Health care fraud
>
> Whoever knowingly and willfully executes, or attempts to execute, a scheme or artifice—
>
> (1) to defraud any health care benefit program; or
>
> (2) to obtain, by means of false or fraudulent pretenses, representations, or promises, any of the money or property owned by, or under the custody or control of, any health care benefit program, in connection with the delivery of or payment for health care benefits, items, or services, shall be fined under this title or imprisoned not more than 10 years, or both. If the violation results in serious bodily injury (as defined in section 1365 of this title), such person shall be fined under this title or imprisoned not more than 20 years, or both; and if the violation results in death, such person shall be fined under this title, or imprisoned for any term of years or for life, or both.

Penalty: Up to 10 years in prison for just one count of fraud, 20 years if a patient is injured and life in prison if the patient dies as a result of the fraud committed.

Erroneous or Fraudulent

According to the OIG, there is a distinction between mistakes and intentional deception or fraud. Their Program Integrity Reviews have identified various causes of improper payments ranging from innocent errors to intentional deception. The following list shows these different levels of improper payments as they increase in severity. Level 1 problems can often be resolved through the payers "corrected claim" process. However, higher levels can have penalties associated with them.

1. Mistakes/errors
2. Inefficiency/waste
3. Bending the rules/abuse
4. Intentional deception/fraud

OSHA Requirements

The Occupational Safety and Health Administration (OSHA) was created to assure safe and healthful working conditions for working men and women by setting and enforcing standards and by providing training, outreach, education, and assistance.

While generally associated with industrial facilities or construction sites, OSHA rules apply in chiropractic practices as well. If you have one employee, then you must have an OSHA plan in place. Some have tried to skirt the law by saying that independent contractors are not employees. As far as OSHA is concerned, if they work in your office, they are considered an employee, no matter what title they are given.

Like HIPAA rules, OSHA federal requirements are the minimum standard. At the time of publication, there were 25 states (and 2 territories) which have their own OSHA plans which may be different than federal rules. Be aware of your individual state requirements.

See Resource 270 for the list of states with their own OSHA requirements.

Quite often, an OSHA inspection begins with a complaint from either an employee or a patient. Your office will then be given an on-site visit. To help you avoid being blind-sided by these on-site visits, it is important to understand these requirements.

Fines and penalties for OSHA violations range from $3,000-$70,000 per violation, depending on several factors, including the severity of the incident, the type and size of the business entity and the provider's willingness to comply with the law. Penalties for small offices with up to 25 employees are reduced by 60%. Providers who have not had any previous violations and who can **demonstrate a good faith effort** may be able to **significantly** reduce those fines. For this reason, it is wise to implement an OSHA Compliance Program in your office in order to demonstrate a "good faith" effort.

See Resource 271 for OSHA penalty calculation information.

How to Begin

Be aware that there are entire books on the subject of OSHA and how to fully and properly meet OSHA requirements. The information presented here is only a beginning point. OSHA recommends taking the following steps in your compliance program:

1. Learn which requirements apply to health care.
2. Identify hazards at your facility and learn how to minimize the risks for those hazards.
3. Develop a comprehensive safety and health program.
4. Train your employees on safety.
5. Establish procedures for record keeping, reporting, and posting.

> **Alert:** If an illness or injury happens to a temporary employee - including those from a staffing agency, in most cases, the reporting entity is NOT the staffing agency - it is the office where the event occurred. See Resource 272 for more information.

Start by creating your own "OSHA Compliance Manual" in order to document your compliance steps. Include sections on:

- General Safety which can include areas such as fire safety, ergonomic hazards, radiation safety (if you have an x-ray machine) and an emergency action plan.
- Pathogen Standards which include procedures for disinfection and sterilization.
- Hazard Standards which include Material Safety Data Sheets (MSDS) for hazardous materials and how to properly handle those hazards.

> **Alert:** MSDS forms will be standardized and updated to Safety Data Sheets (SDS) as of June 1, 2015. Employers need to update their hazardous chemical labeling and hazard communication programs as necessary, and provide additional employee training for newly identified physical or health hazards by June 1, 2016. See Resource 273 and 274 for additional information.

- Record-keeping which includes reports of training as well as incidents with their associated incident response. At the time of printing, there was a proposed rule to make it easier to do this reporting online.

OSHA offers many free resources on their website including a "Compliance Assistant Quick Start" for the healthcare industry. These resources can assist providers who are setting up a compliance program on their own. On-site consultations to identify hazards and provide advice for small businesses may also be available in your area.

For those who desire professional assistance, there are compliance specialists who can come to your office and set up your program. There are also commercial products available to assist in the creation of a personalized OSHA Compliance Manual.

See Resource 328 for additional information including tips, a quick start guide, forms and other resources.

Quick Tips

Here are some quick steps you can take to get started with an OSHA compliance plan. Be sure to document these steps in your OSHA Compliance Manual.

- Obtain a poster that lists employee protections and applicable laws and hang it in a prominent staff area such as a lunchroom. These "Job Safety and Health Posters" can be found in many office supply stores.

    See Resource 277 to download a free "It's the Law" poster.

- Hang fire extinguisher(s) of the appropriate type in an accessible location. Assign a staff member to record the status of the gauge on a monthly basis in your OSHA Compliance Manual where it can be seen by an inspector.

- Provide an eyewash station (a gallon of clean water and an eye cup may do for starters) in areas where chemicals are stored (x-ray developer or cleaning supplies). Have a staff member record the condition and readiness of these facilities on a monthly basis. Keep this record in your Compliance Manual where it can be seen by an inspector.

- Obtain an OSHA spill kit. Cleaning up spills of OSHA covered items requires an official policy and procedure which should be included in your OSHA Compliance Manual. Train staff on how to safely clean spills and record that training in your manual.

    > **Tip:** Kits may be purchased from supply companies, but they can also be easily created on your own. To create your own spill kit, simply include the following items in a dated plastic baggie: kitty litter, scoop, gloves, goggles, brush and if mercury is used in your office, your kit also needs a thermometer. Place the kit close enough to places that might have spills so that it can be easily accessed by all staff.

- Provide emergency exit charts at each work area that illustrate the appropriate path out of the office.

- Post emergency numbers by telephones. Have policies regarding who should be called for what event. Keep a book labeled "Emergency Phone Numbers" in plain site in the office.

- Obtain Material Safety Data Sheets (MSDS) (Safety Data Sheets (SDS) beginning in June 2015) for any toxins in your office and keep them in a clearly labeled binder (your Compliance Manual is a good place). This includes printer ink, toner and cleaning supplies. Warning posters can typically be obtained for your darkroom chemicals from your supplier free of charge.

- Provide a secure lockbox in a public area for the submission of suggestions, and log the submissions in your OSHA Compliance Manual on a regular basis.

- Provide scrubs on site for employees for emergencies. They must change out of contaminated clothing BEFORE they leave the office! This is for all bio spills, including someone vomiting in your office.
- Understand and evaluate rules for proper ergonomics in each department and for each employee.
- Be sure that employees are properly trained in all areas of OSHA compliance as well as the reporting procedures for injuries and other safety related occurrences.

Review: The Need for Compliance

- What is the three step process for compliance? *F-3*
- Why are doctors of chiropractic easily targeted? *F-4*
- Which government departments demand compliance? *F-5*
- Why do doctors of chiropractic need compliance programs? *F-6*
- Other than a reduction in the number of claim denials, what are other benefits of having a compliance program? *F-6*
- What percent of claims for chiropractic services did Medicare determine were "improper"? *F-7*
- What are six important fraud and abuse laws? *F-8 to F-10*
- What is "deliberate ignorance"? *F-8*
- What is the penalty for violating the Medicare Physician Agreement? *F-9*
- What is the difference between a mistake and intentional deception or fraud? *F-10*
- What should be in a OSHA Compliance Manual? *F-11*

2. HIPAA Compliance

The legislation known as "HIPAA" stands for the Health Insurance Portability and Accountability Act of 1996. The intent of the Administrative Simplification, or Accountability portion, of this law was to establish standards and requirements to improve the efficiency and effectiveness of the health care industry and safeguard health information. Legislation enacted over the last few years has expanded and, in some case, changed the responsibilities of providers.

Alert: The HIPAA 2013 Omnibus Final Rule is now in effect. Providers need to ensure that they are meeting all new provisions.

- For more detailed information about the effect of the Omnibus Final Rule, see page F-21.
- For more information about the Breach Notification Rule, see page F-25.

See Resource 278 for additional resources including links, articles and webinars.

Go to ACAtoday.org/HIPAA to review information by the ACA regarding HIPAA.

This chapter only contains a cursory overview of HIPAA. For a complete do-it-yourself guide, including customizable policies, compliance plans and required forms, see the publication *Complete & Easy HIPAA Compliance* (Resource 116).

The five main components of HIPAA are:

1. Electronic Transaction and Code Sets
2. Privacy
3. Security
4. Enforcement
5. National Identifiers

HIPAA directly impacts almost all health care providers as well as their business partners. Providers who **must** comply with HIPAA requirements are those who transmit health care information electronically, or who have it sent electronically on their behalf.

ACA HIPAA Disclaimer: ACA recognizes that, as a federal regulation, HIPAA is complex. Providers should take care not only to be in compliance, but to assure they observe state laws and regulations which may provide similar protections/requirements. The information offered by ACA is provided as helpful tips and providers are encouraged to seek the counsel of a qualified healthcare law attorney licensed in their state for further guidance.

Who is Affected by HIPAA?

The HIPAA requirements apply directly to four specific groups commonly referred to as "Covered Entities." These groups include:

1. *Providers:* Those who transmit (or have a third party transmit) any health information electronically.
2. *Health Plans:* These include any government (Medicare, etc) or non-government organization (NGO) or private plan that provides or pays for medical care. An exception to the law was granted to state Workers' Compensation plans.
3. *Health Care Clearinghouses:* These are organizations that translate nonstandard information into a standard transaction or vice versa. Clearinghouses may include billing services and repricing companies.
4. *Business Partners:* All third party vendors and business partners that perform services on behalf of or exchange data with those organizations that create, receive, maintain or transmit protected health information. Examples are accountants, lawyers, medical answering services, consultants, billing agencies, etc.

Practitioners, including doctors of chiropractic, fall into the first category. A provider within this category is either a HIPAA Covered Entity, or is exempt from HIPAA. How you conduct Protected Health Information (PHI) transactions determines your status. Keep in mind, however, that the HIPAA standards have become the "gold standard" for storing and sending health information. Also, more states and payers are requiring electronic transactions and thus more providers need to abide by HIPAA regulations. The requirements for HIPAA compliance are covered on the following pages.

HIPAA Exempt Offices (Paper)

It is a common misconception that every doctor's office is (or must become) a HIPAA Covered Entity; however, those who still qualify for exemption from HIPAA is rapidly shrinking. There are exceptions to the HIPAA requirements; if a practice sends or receives no transactions electronically, it is not a covered entity. Offices must be careful to ensure they truly are not performing electronic transactions. While a provider may not submit claims electronically, the provider's staff could be using the internet to query patient information from a plan or payer source or a third party may submit payments electronically. Consequently, accessing this information electronically makes the practice a Covered Entity.

If you employ more than ten full-time employees (or full-time equivalents), you are required to submit Medicare claims electronically; therefore, you become a HIPAA Covered Entity. It is almost easier to become a Covered Entity than not to.

To be a HIPAA non-covered entity (exempt from HIPAA), you must, **at a minimum**, meet **all** of the following conditions:

HIPAA is Only the Federal Minimum Standard

If you are a HIPAA exempt office, you must still abide by any **state regulations** applicable to health care providers and all healthcare matters, including confidentiality of patient information. It is good business practice to always maintain policies and procedures aimed at protecting patient information.

- Keep records in your office on paper. Information in computers must only be output to paper and then mailed. No Protected Health Information (PHI) may be transmitted electronically to or from your office.
- Do not use a billing service, clearinghouse or other third party to conduct electronic transactions such as submitting electronic claims for you.
- Do not use any internet applications, direct data entry, or point of service application containing PHI from your computer.
- Do not become a HIPAA Covered Entity by function, contract, agreement, or certification.
- Do not have any contracts or business agreements that require HIPAA compliance. Many health plans are now including a requirement for electronic claim submission in their agreements. Read your contract renewals carefully.
- Do not fax PHI transactions from your computer (conventional, free-standing fax machines may be used).
- Your practice is **not** located in a state that requires all claims to be be electronically submitted.

Alert: All providers, even HIPAA non-covered entities, need to be concerned about protecting patient information. There are about 45 states which have laws regarding privacy of medical records. It is important to be aware of individual state requirements.

See Resource 279 for helpful information on who is a covered entity.

Covered Entity Offices

There are five HIPAA components for covered entities: Electronic Transactions, Privacy, Security, Identifiers, and Enforcement. Each has its own rules and dates of implementation. If you are a "Covered Entity," you are held accountable if you do **not** follow the minimum standards established by HIPAA. You need to comply with all laws, standards, rules, and regulations related to HIPAA. If you have state laws which exceed these HIPAA standards, they prevail (override). The following is an overview of the requirements for each of the **five** basic HIPAA areas:

1. **Electronic Transaction and Code Set Standards Requirements**

    The Transaction and Code Set rules provide national standards for the electronic exchange of health care information including formats and data content. HIPAA requires every provider who does business electronically to use the same health care transactions and code sets. Many of the electronic changes required under HIPAA are highly technical. It is important for you to know about these requirements and how they impact your office. Transaction and code set requirements were created to give the health care industry a

Mobile Devices & Breaches

Mobile devices such as cell phones, tablets and laptops have been linked to a significant number of HIPAA breaches. The problem is so widespread that the OIG has included this on their Work Plan and the Department of Health and Human Services (HHS) has created a special resource page for all healthcare professionals which includes web training. Be sure to document all training in your Compliance Manual.

- See Resource 280 for additional information and training by HHS.
- Go to ACAtoday.org/HIPAA for additional information.

common language to make it easier to transmit information electronically (e.g., a physician's office inquires about a patient's insurance eligibility, or submits a bill to a health plan for payment).

Transactions include: 1) claims or equivalent encounter information; 2) payment and remittance advice; 3) claim status inquiry and response; 4) eligibility inquiry and response; 5) referral certification and authorization inquiry and response; 6) enrollment or disenrollment in a health plan; 7) health plan premium payments; and 8) coordination of benefits.

The code sets required under the regulations are those that have been commonly used in the industry for many years. They include International Classification of Diseases, 9th Revision (ICD-9), Current Procedure Terminology, 4th Version (CPT-4), and Healthcare Common Procedure Coding System (HCPCS) codes.

> **Note:** ICD-10-CM and ICD-10-PCS will be replacing ICD-9-CM on October 1, 2015.

2. **Privacy Requirements**

The privacy requirements limit how patient Protected Health Information (PHI) may be used and/or disclosed. Patients are provided with basic rights related to the use and disclosure of information related to their past, present and future health. Confidential data must be securely guarded and carefully handled when conducting the business of health care.

It is critical for practices to have a solid understanding of HIPAA privacy requirements and patient rights in order to avoid costly mistakes. Proper staff training is essential to maintain compliance.

3. **Security Requirements**

The security requirements outline the minimum administrative, technical, and physical systems required to protect the availability, integrity, and confidentiality of Electronic Protected Health Information (ePHI). Security procedures must be put in place to prevent unauthorized access to ePHI. The requirements include both required and addressable activities that must take place.

> **Note:** The Breach Notification Rule expands and tightens the requirements of both the privacy and security requirements.

4. **HITECH Enforcement Rule**

The enforcement rule contains the regulations governing the investigation of probable violations and their associated penalties. The HITECH Act of 2009 expanded this rule by making penalties for violations more strict, creating tiered violation levels, and splitting the responsibility of HIPAA enforcement between the Department of Health and Human Services (HHS) and the Federal Trade Commission (FTC).

5. **National Identifier Requirements**

HIPAA requires all health care providers, health plans, and employers to have a national number that will identify them on standard transactions. Providers are required to use the NPI which is a unique 10-digit number which is required on electronic transactions.

In September 2012, new identifiers were announced for a unique health plan identifier (HPID and an "other entity" identifier (OEID)). Covered entities must use HPIDs in electronic transactions by November 7, 2016. Watch for health plans to begin requiring claims to include this new HPID in the future.

Omnibus 2013 Final Rule

On January 25, 2013, the Department of Health And Human Services (HHS) issued the long awaited final rule regarding multiple provisions of HIPAA Rules. The following areas are revised or added within this 563 page document. This is only a high level listing and therefore should not be considered an all inclusive list of the areas that providers should review:

- HITECH Privacy & Security
    - Business associates
    - Subcontractors
    - Marketing & Fundraising
    - Sale of PHI
    - Right to request restrictions
    - Electronic access
- HITECH Breach Notification
- HITECH Enforcement
- Genetic Information Nondiscrimination Act (GINA) Privacy
- Other (non-statutory) modifications
    - Research authorizations
    - Notice of Privacy Practices (NPP)
    - Decedents
    - Student immunizations

ELECTRONIC TRANSACTION AND CODE SET REQUIREMENTS

Code Sets

This HIPAA component required little or no adjustment by providers, as most doctors have already been using these code sets for many years—HIPAA has simply mandated their use. The greatest impact was on payers who have used non-standard codes; they were required to stop using them.

All providers are required to use updated codes on the effective date of the annual updates. New ICD-9 (ICD-10 beginning this fall) usage commences on October 1st of each year; new CPT and HCPCS codes become effective January 1st of each year.

An exception to the mandated use of the standard code sets is the state Workers' Compensation carriers. Most state agencies follow the national code sets, but they can and do have some unique code exceptions. Be aware of any differences.

Fax and Photocopier Caution

Recent OCR breach settlement announcements has brought attention to faxes and photocopiers. Todays machines typically scan the image and store it in memory before either copying or sending. Thus, these machines fall under HIPAA regulations because PHI is being stored. As such, they become an "electronic transaction".

You cannot dispose of these types of machines unless they have been destroyed or purged in accordance with HIPAA guidelines.

Electronic Transactions

HIPAA does not require that a health care provider conduct all transactions electronically; however, it can be a requirement by CMS or other payers. Even CMS has an exception for small businesses which use paper claims and have less than ten (full-time equivalent) employees. If they are going to conduct any business transactions electronically, they will need to follow the standard formats outlined under HIPAA. If you contract with a third party biller or clearinghouse to conduct any electronic transactions for you, it is up to the health care provider, to see that such transactions are conducted in compliance with HIPAA. Make sure you address the status of your compliance with your payers, billing service, clearinghouse, and/or software vendor. For HIPAA Covered Entities, there are financial implications for not submitting compliant transactions, including delayed payment, claim rejections, and contractual breach.

Electronic Funds Transfer (EFT) and Electronic Remittance Advice (ERA)

Electronic Funds Transfers (EFT) is one method by which payment for health care operations may take place. An Electronic Remittance Advice (ERA) is basically the electronic version of a paper explanation of benefits (EOB).

Section 1104(b)(2)(A) of the Patient Protection and Affordable Care Act (PPACA) included the requirement to implement operating standards for both EFT and ERA by January 1, 2014. These new standards were intended to streamline payment processing and resolve previous issues with "matching" an EFT to its ERA for reconciliation by health care providers.

There are advantages and disadvantages to implementing EFT. The interim final rule reported the following benefits were cited by respondents of an Association of Finance Professionals survey:

- **Cost savings:** Savings resulted from not printing checks, purchasing and stuffing envelopes, and manually depositing checks;
- **Fraud control:** Ninety percent of respondents that experienced payment fraud in 2008 were victims of paper check fraud, compared to 7 percent of organizations that experienced payment fraud who were victims of EFT fraud; and
- **Improved cash flow and cash forecasting:** Forty percent of respondents reported improved cash forecasting as a result of EFT payments.

Adoption of EFT may be disadvantageous as providers try to integrate existing systems into these new requirements. Accounts receivable or practice management software may need to be upgraded or installed in order to take full advantage of these enhancements. To avoid potential problems or disruptions to your practice, some health care consultants suggest maintaining a separate bank account dedicated specifically for EFT transactions.

Pay close attention to contractual arrangements with individual payers, especially as contracts are renewed. Remember, if you receive EFT payments or ERAs, you are receiving PHI electronically and your practice automatically become a HIPAA covered entity. If you wish to remain exempt from HIPAA, you **cannot** participate in EFT or ERA.

Virtual Cards

Under EFT rules, entities may choose either Automated Clearing House (ACH) or another payment network through which to receive reimbursement. However, health plans MUST transmit payments through ACH if requested by the provider. Although many payers utilize ACH, virtual card payments have recently emerged as an alternative to ACH. Virtual cards are basically a credit card that is run through the provider's credit card processing terminal.

One of the problems with virtual cards is that the cost of payment processing shifts from the payer to the provider. The provider is responsible for all credit card processing fees including interchange fees and per transaction charges. Check options thoroughly to choose what is best for your clinic.

See Resource 300 for more information about virtual cards.

Note: The compliance date for adopting standards for the Health Care Electronic Funds Transfers (EFT) and Electronic Remittance Advice transactions (ERA) was January 1, 2014.

Privacy Requirements

Compliance with the Privacy component of HIPAA is probably the most challenging issue for most offices, even though most have always had good common sense procedures in place.

Privacy is the right of an individual to control the use and disclosure of his/her Protected Health Information (PHI). Confidentiality is the obligation of providers; part of that obligation is putting measures into place to protect information and disclose the minimum necessary to conduct business and care for the patient.

Treatment, Payment, and Health Care Operations

It should be noted that no permission is required to use PHI for Treatment, Payment, and Health Care Operations (TPO). According to HHS, "To avoid interfering with an individual's access to quality health care or the efficient payment for such health care, the Privacy Rule permits a covered entity to use and disclose protected health information, with certain limits and protections, for treatment, payment, and health care operations activities."

A covered entity must develop policies and procedures that reasonably limit its disclosures of, and requests for, protected health information for payment and health care operations to the minimum necessary.

The Omnibus Final Rule included a significant modification to this exception. Now a patient has a right to prohibit disclosure of items and services to their health care plan when they have paid out of pocket and in full for those items or services. All members of your "workforce" need to excercise caution and be trained on how to properly identify these types of records to avoid an inadvertent disclosure when making other approved disclosures to health plans. Your policies and procedures will need to be updated to adequately address this change.

See Resource 281 for more information about HHS limits in this situation.

See *Complete & Easy HIPAA Compliance* (Resource 116) for editable disclosure forms, including one for patients requesting to restrict disclosures.

Privacy To-Do List

Every office needs a checklist to make sure there are no omissions. Here is a brief summary of some items that Covered Entities should address for compliance with HIPAA Privacy standards. It is also an excellent tool to use in identifying areas that may need auditing to determine the effectiveness of your office's compliance measures.

Has your office:

- Appointed or designated a Privacy Officer responsible for the development and implementation of office policies and procedures with regard to the Privacy Rule?

- Determined a Compliance Officer to serve as the HIPAA decision maker?
- Appointed or designated a contact person responsible for receiving complaints?
- Established a provider and office/practice workforce training program?
- Identified persons or classes of persons on the staff who need access to PHI?
- Developed and implemented appropriate administrative, technical and physical safeguards?
- Developed a process allowing patients or staff to file a complaint?
- Developed office/practice policies and procedures with respect to PHI that comply with HIPAA mandates? Have these policies been updated to meet the new Omnibus rule requirements?
- Instituted a procedure to verify the identity of anyone requesting PHI?
- Developed a procedure that ensures existing and new contracts with vendors includes appropriate HIPAA language? Have your business asssociate contracts been updated to meet Omnibus Rule standards?
- Developed a procedure or process that limits the use or disclosure of PHI to only those who need to know? Has this process been updated to meet Omnibus Rule provisions?
- Developed and updated your "Notice of Privacy Practices" that conforms to the requirements of the Rule 164.520 and the Omnibus Rule?
- Developed and implemented appropriate policies/procedures regarding patient authorizations?
- Developed a policy/procedure advising patients of their rights to request restrictions on PHI, including the new out-of-pocket restrictions?
- Developed a policy/procedure that recognizes a patient's right to access, inspect and copy PHI? Has this policy been updated to allow them to receive an electronic copy as required by the Omnibus Rule?
- Developed a policy/procedure that recognizes a patient's right to amend their PHI?
- Instituted policies/procedures recognizing the patient's right to an accounting of their PHI disclosures?

   - See Resource 260 for further guidance on Privacy Rules. The Office for Civil Rights (OCR) has released specific guidance, summaries, and frequently asked questions related to key HIPAA points.
   - See Resource 261 for HIPAA training materials by the Department of Health and Human Services.

Go to ACAtoday.org/HIPAA for additional information.

HIPAA Notice of Privacy Practices (Resource 262) is a patient brochure which explains the use and disclosure of their Protected Health Information.

Alert: If your practice has a website, you are required to post your Notice of Privacy Practices on the website. Additionally, because of Omnibus Rule mandated changes to this notice, you must also post notification on your website that your Notice of Privacy Practices has changed.

Omnibus Final Rule Modifications

The long awaited Final Rule was issued by the Department of Health and Human Services on January 25, 2013, and became effective on September 23, 2013.

Some of the biggest changes are:

- Requiring business associates to be held to the same standards as Covered Entities. A business associate is now a covered entity by definition when it comes to protecting PHI. As such, they are directly liable for breaches of PHI.

- Expanding the definition of "business associate" to include subcontractors along with provisions requiring business associates to have appropriate "business associate agreements" in place with their subcontractors.

- Redefining marketing, fundraising, and sale of PHI activities. Any activities for which the covered entity receives direct or indirect "financial remuneration" now require the patient to approve these types of disclosures before they happen.

- Expanding the rights of individuals to have access to their PHI and permitting Covered Entities to charge a "reasonable cost-based fee" for this service. A patient can even request to have their information emailed to them.

> See the publication *Complete & Easy HIPAA Compliance* (Resource 116) for full explanations of these Final Rule changes along with helpful guidance and implementation tips.

Privacy Protections and Rights

Here are some excerpts from an HHS fact sheet titled *Protecting the Privacy of Patients' Health*.

The Privacy rule ensures a national floor of privacy protections for patients by limiting the ways that health plans, pharmacies, hospitals, and other covered entities can use patients' personal medical information. The regulations protect medical records and other individually identifiable health information, whether it is on paper, in computers, or communicated orally. Some key provisions of these federal standards include:

- **Access to Medical Records.** Patients should generally be able to see and obtain copies of their medical records and request corrections if they identify errors. Health plans, doctors, hospitals, clinics, nursing homes, and other covered entities should generally provide access these records within 30 days and may charge patients a reasonable cost-based fee to cover their costs for copying and sending the records.

- **Notice of Privacy Practices.** Covered health plans, doctors, and other health care providers must provide a notice to their patients relating how they may use personal medical information and their rights under the new privacy regulations. Doctors, hospitals, and other direct-care providers will generally provide the notice on the patient's first visit and anytime thereafter upon request. Patients will generally be asked to sign, initial, or otherwise acknowledge that they received this notice. Health plans must generally mail the notice to their enrollees upon initial enrollment and again if the notice changes significantly. Patients may also ask covered entities to restrict the use or disclosure of their information beyond the practices included in the notice, but in most cases, the covered entities would not have to agree to the changes.

  > **Alert:** Patients need to be notified that there have been changes to your Notice of Privacy Practices due to the Omnibus Final Rule. They need to be made aware of changes to their rights since their last visit.

- **Limits on the Use of Personal Medical Information.** The Privacy rule sets limits on how health plans and covered providers may use individually identifiable health information. In order to promote the best quality care for patients, the rule does not restrict the ability of doctors, nurses, and other providers in sharing information needed to treat their patients. In other situations, though, personal health information may generally not be used for purposes unrelated to health care, and covered entities may use or share only the minimum amount of protected information needed for a particular purpose. In addition, patients would have to sign a specific authorization before a Covered Entity could release their medical information to a life insurer, bank, marketing firm, or another outside entity for purposes not related to their health care.

- **Prohibition of Marketing.** The Privacy rule sets restrictions and limits on the use of patient information for marketing purposes. Pharmacies, health plans, and other Covered Entities must first obtain an individual's specific authorization before disclosing their patient information for marketing. At the same time, the rule permits doctors and other Covered Entities to communicate freely with patients about treatment options and other health-related information, including disease management programs.

- **Stronger State Laws.** The federal privacy standards do not affect state laws that provide additional privacy protections for patients. The confidentiality protections are cumulative; the Privacy rule sets a national "floor" of privacy standards that protect all Americans; any state law providing additional protection continues to apply. When a state law requires a certain disclosure, such as reporting an infectious disease outbreak to the public health authorities, the federal privacy regulations do not preempt the state law.

- **Confidential Communications.** Under the Privacy rule, patients can request that their doctors, health plans, and other Covered Entities take reasonable steps to ensure that their communications with the patient are confidential. For example, a patient could ask a doctor to call his or her office rather than home, and the doctor's office should comply with that request if it can reasonably be accommodated.

- **Complaints.** Consumers may file a formal complaint regarding the privacy practices of a health plan or covered provider. Such complaints can be made directly to the covered provider or health plan or to HHS Office for Civil Rights (OCR), which is charged with investigating complaints and enforcing the privacy regulation. Information about filing complaints should be included in each Covered Entity's Notice of Privacy Practices.

> **Alert:** The Omnibus Final Rule gives individuals the right to request a report of all non-routine disclosures of PHI, including electronic PHI. Maintaining such a report was already required for all HIPAA compliant offices, but this rule gives the patient the right to see that report.

SECURITY REQUIREMENTS

The HIPAA standards for security refer to the means used to protect confidential electronic information. Effective security measures are essential for protecting health information. The Security rule outlines eighteen standards that your compliance efforts must address. The standards include specifications that are either "Required" or "Addressable." The Required elements are mandatory and must be implemented. The Addressable elements must be reviewed and

---

Overseas Billing Caution

Many companies have outsourced their billing overseas in order to cut costs. Keep in mind that there could be some costly side effects. As an example, a provider had PHI stolen by someone employed by an overseas billing company. The provider, who had a properly executed business associate agreement, is suing the billing company, but there is a significant problem—the backlog of lawsuits in that country can take up to 24 years. Fines imposed by the U.S. Government are payable **immediately**. Most businesses would find it difficult to wait 24 years to recoup their money.

evaluated for applicability to the covered entity. If it is not feasible to put into practice any Addressable element, the reason why and the alternative implementation strategy for it must be documented in your HIPAA Compliance Manual. Covered Entities and now business associates must evaluate and document their evaluation of these specifications.

> **Windows XP Alert:** As of April 8, 2014, Windows XP is no longer HIPAA compliant. It is recommended that providers update their computer operating systems as soon as possible.
>
> See Resource 312 or go to ACAtoday.org/HIPAA for detailed information about this important change.

Safeguards

Security is all about assessing the risks, then managing those risks. As a Covered Entity, there are two significant events in your security protocols. First, you must assess your current protocols, implement written policies and procedures, and then re-evaluate them regularly. Your implemented procedures are important for your defense if you are ever accused of breaching security standards. Second, you must educate your employees about the security standards. Education and enforcement are critically important. For any security technology to be effective, individuals must abide by the safeguards put in place.

How much security is enough? The Federal Register states that standards should "be scalable and flexible enough to allow different entities to implement the standards in a manner that is appropriate for their circumstances." All Covered Entities must implement the required specifications and explore the addressable ones, but the technology implemented and the exact "how to" are up to the individual provider.

Security To-Do List

In addition to a privacy checklist, it's also important to make sure that your office addresses specific security questions. Although not an exhaustive list, here are some of the tasks that must be done:

- Appoint a Security Officer
- Conduct a risk analysis/assessment

    See Resource 301 for additional information about security risk assessments.

Cloud Computing Caution

With the expansion of cloud computing comes additional risks that must be addressed. Make sure that your contract specifies that the servers remain in the USA! Data is being stolen from overseas servers and people are having a difficult time obtaining legal recourse. Also be sure that all of your contractors, including cloud services, are HIPAA compliant. Both the provider and contractor can be fined for HIPAA violations if it was found the proper security measures were not put into place.

At a bare minimum, before putting data in the cloud, you need to ask the cloud service provider if they are SSAE 16 (formerly SAS 70) compliant and HIPAA compliant. Most are not. SSAE 16 is an audit done of internal controls and measures to ensure proper security is in place and will weed most of the pretenders out.

Also, be sure to have all your contractors/vendors sign a business associate agreement (BAA) which discloses the patient security record requirements. If you don't have a signed BAA and a breach occurs at the fault of a contractor, you are in trouble.

- Develop policies and procedures to protect, detect, contain, and correct any security violations
- Develop data access controls
- Develop a user ID and password management process
- Develop a process to audit and evaluate security measures periodically
- Develop a process to control facility access
- Implement technical safeguards including authentication, automatic logoff, firewalls, virus protection, and encryption
- Develop a sanction policy
- Create a contingency plan
- Develop policies and procedures for workstation use
- Develop security incident procedures
- Develop policies for media disposal and re-use

Recent Modifications

It is important to realize that HIPAA rules and regulations are being reviewed and revised on a regular basis. Your policies and procedures must meet the new Omnibus Rule requirements and any other revisions made in the future. For example, here are some recent modifications that should have been implemented by your practice:

- Application of the Security Rule to include "business associates."
- Modifications to administrative safeguards, and organizational requirements.
- Changes to laboratories and patient access to lab results.

HITECH ENFORCEMENT REQUIREMENTS

Enforcement is the fifth component of HIPAA. There are numerous federal agencies involved in the enforcement of HIPAA, and penalties depend on the type of violation. The HHS Office for Civil Rights (OCR) is responsible for administering and enforcing HIPAA's privacy, security, and breach notification rules.

The Health Information Technology for Economic and Clinical Health Act (HITECH) made HIPAA rules even more strict and includes breach notification provisions. These regulations require health care providers, health care clearinghouses, health plans, and all business associates to keep PHI secure. The Omnibus Rule extends these requirements to business associates. Breaches require reporting to the government, notifying patients, and in cases involving more than 500 people, informing the media.

Breach Notification Rules

All HIPAA Covered Entities, including business associates, must be aware of and abide by the Health Information Technology for Economics and Clinical Health Act (HITECH) breach notification rules.

These regulations require health care providers, health care clearinghouses, health plans, and all business associates to keep PHI secure. Breaches must satisfy all reporting and notification regulations. See the "Who Must Be Notified?" segment later in this chapter for more information.

Breach Notification rules apply to ALL types of UNSECURED PHI including electronic records, papers, or even verbal communication. By definition, "Unsecured PHI" is any information that has **not** been rendered unusable or undecipherable by an approved security measure (for example, see exceptions 1 and 2 on the next page). Please note that this rule does NOT apply to PHI that has been de-identified in accordance with the Privacy Rule.

See Resource 200 for more information about de-identifiers.

Penalties

For breaches, the penalties depend on several factors including the severity of the breach. For both privacy and security violations, they range from civil penalties of $100.00 per violation to criminal penalties of up to $1,500,000.00 per identical violation and/or 10 years imprisonment for knowing or willful disclosure or misuse of information. This penalty cap applies to even those who "did not know" the breach was taking place, UNLESS they correct the violation within the 30 days from the "first date the person liable for the penalty knew, or by exercising reasonable diligence would have known". Now, the Omnibus Rule states that this 30 day correction time frame also extends to "a period determined appropriate by the Secretary based up on the nature and extent of the entity's failure to comply."

The sizable number of HIPAA settlements being announced by the OIG on a regular basis indicates that they are very serious about enforcing HIPAA breaches, even those made by smaller providers.

The Ominbus Rule also added that in cases of 'willful neglect', the HHS Secretary may immediately impose civil monetary penalties without going through the formal discovery process.

What Constitutes a Breach?

The Omnibus Rule modified the breach standard. Now, every "acquisition, access, use, or disclosure of protected health information in a manner not permitted is **presumed** to be a breach **unless** the covered entity or business associate, as applicable, demonstrates that there is a low probability that the protected health information has been compromised based on a *risk assessment*." The risk assessment should include, *at the very least*:

1. The nature and extent of the PHI involved, including the types of identifiers and the likelihood of re-identification;
2. The unauthorized person who used the PHI, or to whom the disclosure was made;
3. Whether the PHI was actually acquired or viewed; and
4. The extent to which the risk to the PHI has been mitigated.

Because a breach is now presumed unless proven otherwise, the risk assessment becomes very important tool for covered entities. It must be performed whenever a covered entity discovers that there is a possiblity of a breach of PHI.

State Breach Standards

This portion of the *ChiroCode DeskBook* only includes information on the Federal minimum standards for security breach notification. Most states also have their own security breach notification requirements. Be aware of any differences and consider consulting a healthcare attorney in your state to ensure that your compliance plan meets all your state requirements.

For instance, a cleaning person may straighten a stack of papers in the course of their duties. Even if there was PHI in the stack, if they did not record or use the information there, no breach has taken place. However, if they copy a patient's name, a breach has occurred. Theft or loss of computers or portable data devices like thumb drives or portable hard drives that DO NOT utilize approved encryption methods would be a reportable breach.

Exceptions

There are five breach notification exceptions: The Omnibus Rule modified the unintentional and inadvertent definitions.

1. **Encryption**: PHI is encrypted in accordance with 45 CFR 164.304's definition of encryption. PHI is secured using encryption methods approved by the National Institute of Standards and Technology (NIST). There are different guidelines for data at rest (databases, folder, etc.) versus data in motion (data moving through any network including internet).

    See Resource 208 for more information about encryption.

2. **Destruction**: PHI that has been destroyed according the following specifications:
    - Paper, film, or other hard copy media have been shredded or destroyed such that the PHI cannot be read or otherwise cannot be reconstructed.
    - Electronic media have been cleared, purged, or destroyed consistent with NIST Special Publication 800-88, Guidelines for Media Sanitization such that the PHI cannot be retrieved.

    See Resource 286 for more information about media sanitation. New guidelines have been proposed and may be announced sometime in 2015.

3. "**Unintentional** acquisition, access, or use of protected health information by a workforce member acting under the authority of a covered entity or business associate as long as it is within their scope of authority and is not further used or disclosed."

4. **Inadvertent** disclosure of protected health information "by a person who is authorized to access protected health information at a covered entity or business associate to another person authorized to access protected health information at the same covered entity or business associate, or organized health care arrangement in which the covered entity participates, and the information received as a result of such disclosure is not further used or disclosed in a manner not permitted."

5. **Good Faith Belief**: "The covered entity or business associate has a good faith belief that the unauthorized individual, to whom the impermissible disclosure was made, would not have been able to retain the information." For example, an office computer is stolen and when recovered, forensic analysis shows that the computer was never accessed.

Who Needs To Be Notified?

Security breaches need to be reported as soon as possible, but no later than 60 days after discovery that a breach occurred. If the breach involved more than 500 people, the affected individuals need to be notified immediately as well as the HHS Secretary and possibly even the media. Breaches involving fewer than 500 people can simply be logged as part of your HIPAA Security logs and then reported annually to the HHS secretary.

To notify the victims, generally a first-class letter is sufficient. However, if their addresses are outdated there are other alternatives, such as posting a legal notice in the paper of the last known location(s). In some cases, the media may also need to be notified.

> To make the proper notifications to the HHS, see Resource 288.

Alert: In cases where there is insufficient or out-of-date contact information for 10 or more individuals, then notification must be in **one** of the following ways: 1) a conspicuous posting for a period of 90 days on the home page of the Web site of the covered entity involved, or 2) conspicuous notice in major print or broadcast media in geographic areas where the individuals affected by the breach likely reside

Compliance Reviews

The Omnibus Rule created the option for the HHS Secretary to conduct compliance reviews in cases where a preliminary review indicates there is willful neglect (ignoring the HIPAA rules). There only needs to be a "possible" violation in order to initiate the review.

The investigation reviews all pertinent policies, procedures, or practices of the entity. Penalties can be assessed for every violation discovered.

Privacy and Security Audit Program Review

From November 2011-December 2012, an audit pilot program was conducted by the Office of Civil Rights (OCR) to assess privacy and security compliance efforts by covered entities and business associates. Of the 115 entities audited, **only 11%** were in full compliance. Small providers had the worst record with some showing a complete disregard of HIPAA regulations. Based on these results, it is highly likely that this program will be expanded during the coming years.

NATIONAL IDENTIFIER REQUIREMENTS

National Provider Identifier (NPI)

HIPAA requires all providers to obtain their own NPI number which is a unique 10 digit number used only by them for health care transactions. No longer will different payers have their own unique identifier for you. Like a Social Security number, this number never expires, and it goes with you as you move from one location to another. When there is a parent organization, such as a clinic, it might also need to have its own NPI.

> See Resource 289 to apply for an NPI.

Employer Identifier Number (EIN)

Historically, there could have been as many different identifiers for an employee as there were payers. However, with HIPAA there can now be only one identifier. HHS has mandated the national Employer Identifier Number (EIN), as issued by the Internal Revenue Service, to be used as the official employer identifier in health care transaction.

Taxonomy Codes

Another required component of your NPI application is your taxonomy code. Taxonomy codes are classifications for providers. The National Uniform Claim Committee (NUCC) maintains the Health Care Provider Taxonomy list. The most commonly used code for chiropractic providers is 111N00000X, however, there are taxonomy codes for specialists such as a pediatric chiropractor. Be sure to check the official taxonomy list to ensure proper taxonomy code selection.

> See Resource 197 for additional provider types and a complete taxonomy list with definitions.

Alert: Be aware that some providers have found that their taxonomy codes were not correct in the NPI database and because of that error, they were paid incorrectly. Since taxonomy codes have changed over the years, it is advisable to check the taxonomy code list, select the one that most closely matches you and then see Resource 289 to view or update your NPI data.

New Identifiers

In September 2012, two new HIPAA Identifiers were announced, the Health Plan Identifier (HPID) and the Other Entity Identifier (OEID). The OEID will be used to uniquely identify entities that are not health plans, health care providers, or individuals. Both these identifiers were created in order to reduce problems such as misrouting of transactions, problems with patient eligibility verification, and transaction rejections due to insurance identification errors.

The application process for these new identifiers is currently underway. Providers need to be aware of notifications from these entities because Covered Entities will be required to use these new identifiers on transactions beginning November 7, 2016.

Additional Help with HIPAA

> See Resource 313 or ACAtoday.org/HIPAA for FAQs, website links, and other helps with HIPAA.

Review: HIPAA Compliance

- Privacy is one of the main HIPAA components. What are the other four? *F-14*
- What are the exceptions to the HIPAA requirements? *F-15*
- What are the code sets required under HIPAA regulations? *F-17*
- What is is called when a payer sends payments directly to the provider's bank account? *F-19*
- If your practice has a website, what information are you required to post on it? *F-21*

3. Medicare Compliance

Because the Medicare eligible population is growing and is projected to continue to grow for another decade and a half, providers stand to lose a significant patient base if they do not accept Medicare. This section is intended to guide you in your Medicare compliance.

Years ago, Medicare implemented several different programs in order to address the problem of improper claim payments. According to the July 2014 report to Congress, compared to 2012, the Medicare Improper Payment Rate increased from 8.5% to 10.1% in 2013, at an estimated cost of $6.4 billion.

Medicare has the right to review any claim at any time for any reason. There are several different Medicare claim review programs. Some happen before a claim is paid (NCCI, MEU, or local review) and some happen after (CERT, RAC, etc.).

There are three entities that can initiate reviews of Medicare cases:

1. The Office of Inspector General of the U.S. Department of Health & Human Services (OIG)
2. The Centers for Medicare and Medicaid Services (CMS) and their contractors
3. Medicare Administrative Contractors (MACs) – previously known as carriers or intermediaries

There are three types of reviews that these entities can perform:

1. Automated reviews performed by the computer
2. Routine reviews performed by non-medical staff
3. Complex reviews performed by licensed professionals

Alert: Automated and routine reviews **do not** usually involve record requests. However, complex reviews do involve records requests. The most important point to remember is that if a Medicare-related entity is requesting medical records, you are under review.

See Resource 210 for the latest information and webinars.

ACA Medicare/OIG Portion Disclaimer; At the time of printing, the federal government had not yet released its changes for 2015. Every effort was made to update the information in the 2015 DeskBook with information available at the time of review. Ongoing updates on CMS-related topics will be posted on the ACA website at (ACAtoday.org/Medicare) and through its articles and publications.

Automated Reviews

National Correct Coding Initiative (NCCI) Edits

This claim editing program was created by CMS to identify coding errors which could lead to inappropriate payment of Medicare claims. CMS developed its coding policies based on coding conventions defined in the American Medical Association's CPT manual, national and local policies (NCD, LCD) and edits, coding guidelines developed by national societies, analysis of standard medical and surgical practices, and a review of current coding practices. These edits are updated quarterly.

The purpose of the NCCI edits is to prevent improper payment when incorrect code combinations are reported. As such, they are an excellent resource for catching potential problems before they are billed.

> "HCPCS/CPT codes representing services denied based on NCCI edits may not be billed to Medicare beneficiaries. Since these denials are based on incorrect coding rather than medical necessity, the provider cannot utilize an "Advanced Beneficiary Notice" (ABN) form to seek payment from a Medicare beneficiary. Furthermore, since the denials are based on incorrect coding rather than a legislated Medicare benefit exclusion, the provider cannot seek payment from the beneficiary." - *Medicare Claim Review Programs: MR, NCCI Edits, MUEs, CERT, and Recovery Audit Program*

Alert: Be aware that even though NCCI edits are meant only for use in Medicare because they are based on Medicare coverage policies, they are sometimes used by third-party payers. Be aware of individual payer policies.

See *Section H–Procedure Codes* for more about NCCI edits, real life examples and problematic edits.

Medically Unlikely Edits (MUE)

Like the NCCI edits, Medically Unlikely Edits (MUEs) are also a pre-payment edit established by CMS to reduce claim payment errors. An MUE for a HCPCS/CPT code is the maximum number of units of service a provider would report, under most circumstances, for a single patient on a single date of service.

In medically reasonable and necessary cases where the number of units exceeds the MUE, the code can sometimes be billed with the appropriate use of modifiers. Most commonly, these will be modifiers 76, 77, 91 and 59 (use 59 only if no other more appropriate modifier is available). Additionally, modifier GD has been established for use with HCPCS codes; however, please note that this modifier is "informational only."

There is not an MUE for every HCPCS/CPT code. Although CMS publishes most MUE values on its website, some MUE values are confidential and are for CMS and CMS contractors' use only.

OIG Reviews

The Office of the Inspector General (OIG) of the Department of Health & Human Services (HHS) is responsible for prosecuting and preventing fraud in government healthcare programs. They have their own inspectors and auditors and they can enter your office and inspect your files without a warrant. They can also go back to the first day of your practice if they want to.

The OIG can also levy Civil Money Penalties (CMP) and refer cases to the Department of Justice (DOJ) for prosecution. In 2013, they collected $2.6 billion.

Therefore, it is recommended that providers who bill Medicare and/or Medicaid services create and maintain an OIG recommended compliance plan.

> See Chapter 4–OIG Compliance Program in this section for more information on OIG Reviews and implementing a compliance plan.

CMS Reviews

CMS (Centers for Medicare and Medicaid Services) is concerned with waste, fraud, and abuse. During their reviews, if they find evidence of fraud, they turn the case over to the OIG for further action. They use contractors and subcontractors to perform reviews. There are three review entities, besides the claims contractors (MACs) that might review your Medicare documentation or claims:

- Comprehensive Error Rate Testing (CERT)
- Zone Program Integrity Contractors (ZPIC) – formerly known as Program Safeguard Contractors (PSCs)
- Recovery Audit Contractors (RAC)

Comprehensive Error Rate Testing (CERT)

The CERT program was developed to measure improper payments in the Medicare Fee-For-Service programs. To accomplish this task, the CERT contractor selects a stratified random sample of approximately 40,000 claims submitted to Parts A/B and DME during each reporting period. A request for records from the submitting health-care provider is sent and a formal review of records by the contractor takes place. When the review is completed, letters of any overpayments or underpayments are sent to the provider.

Any suspected abuse or fraud cases are turned over to the appropriate entity for further action. Because random samples are utilized, patterns of billing are not identified and therefore, by definition, a CERT audited claim cannot be labeled fraudulent.

Zone Program Integrity Contractors (ZPIC)

ZPICs have replaced the Program Safeguard Contractors (PSCs) as part of the Medicare Modernization Act (MMA) of 2003. Their primary role is to investigate instances of suspected fraud, waste, and abuse in the Medicare program. ZPICs also support victims of Medicare identity theft. A provider or supplier who believes that he/she may have had their provider information stolen and used to submit Medicare claims can request that the ZPIC for their zone investigate the case. There are seven ZPIC zones.

Claims selected for postpayment review may be reopened within one year for any reason or within four years for good cause. Cost report determinations may be reopened within three years after the Notice of Program Reimbursement has been issued. If they find any evidence of fraud, the case is turned over to the OIG who has the authority to review claims clear back until the day the practice was opened.

There seems to be some controversy regarding the sampling methods utilized by ZPICs. Statistical sampling is used by CMS because a claim by claim review is time-consuming. Some providers have successfully argued against the penalties because faulty statistical sampling was used.

Recovery Audit Contractors (RAC)

The Medicare Recovery Audit Contractor (RAC) program was created to detect and correct **past** improper payments under the Medicare program. RACs have also begun to perform pre-payment reviews as well. Improper payments for claims can occur for the following reasons:

- Payments are made for services that do not meet Medicare's medical necessity criteria.
- Payments are made for services that are incorrectly coded.
- Providers fail to submit documentation when requested, or fail to submit enough documentation to support the claim.
- Other reasons, such as basing claim payments on outdated fee schedules, or the provider is paid twice because duplicate claims were submitted.

The RAC program uses both automated and complex reviews, and RAC auditors can go back as far as three years on your records. The appeals process is the same as for all other Medicare denials and reviews.

RAC auditors have a limit to the number of medical records that they can request:

- Solo practitioner: 10 medical records per 45 days per NPI
- Partnership (2-5 individuals): 20 medical records per 45 days per NPI
- Group (6-15 individuals): 30 medical records per 45 days per NPI

Claims are reviewed on a post-payment basis using the same policies used by Medicare carriers: National Coverage Determinations (NCDs), Local Coverage Determinations (LCDs), and Medicare manuals. Generally, they do not review claims previously reviewed by other entities.

Two high-risk areas have been identified:

1. Provider non-compliance with timely submission of requested medical documentation;
2. Insufficient documentation that did not justify that the services billed were covered, medically necessary, or correctly coded.

RAC Appeals

The appeal process for RAC denials is the same as for MAC denials. Appeals must be filed before the 120th day after the Demand Letter. You do have the right to disagree with the RAC determination. Be aware that there have been cases where RACs did not abide by the rules. In cases such as these, it is very important to contact a healthcare attorney.

> The RAC appeals process is the same as for other Medicare appeals. See *Section C–Medicare* for additional guidance on appeals.

> Be proactive and contact your RAC auditor to inform them of the correct contact person and address to use when sending their Medical Record Request Letters. This serves two purposes:
> 1. They know your office is serious about compliance, and
> 2. Their requests do not get lost or misplaced in your office. Appeals are on a limited time frame and every day counts.

MAC Reviews

The focus of MAC reviews is generally for coverage and/or coding determinations. They perform both pre and post-payment reviews which can go back up to two years.

Other Review Considerations

Progressive Corrective Action (PCA)

PCA is an operational principle utilized by medical review activities in order to best allocate resources in the review process. It generally starts with data review and analysis, which can lead to "Probe" reviews which utilize a small sampling of records. Should the probe reveal significant problems, more extensive reviews may be conducted.

How to Respond to a Request for Records

Just like testifying in court, not enough information is bad and too much information is bad. You need to demonstrate that the services in question were medically necessary without causing Medicare to want to review further. When you receive a request for records, you need to consider the following:

- Most importantly, do **not** ignore the request for records.
- Note what they are requesting. **Read carefully** and don't make assumptions. If you are unclear about the request, call them and ask questions.
- Pay close attention to their requested time frame. You only need to submit records for that specific time period. However, be sure to provide all information pertinent to that time period which may include the initial examination or re-examinations which should establish medical necessity for the treatment visits being reviewed.
- Note the deadline. Make sure there is plenty of time for the records to reach the requestor by their deadline.
- Any correspondence or communication should be clearly logged. Document who you spoke to, the date and time, topic, purpose of disclosure, and outcome of discussion, etc.
- Make sure that you have a copy of all records submitted.
- Send the requested information in a manner that requires a signature upon receipt. Save the tracking information.
- Log the date sent and other helpful information.

Tip: It is essential to regularly monitor and effectively manage record requests as explained above. This information should be recorded where it can be easily maintained. Some providers maintain a separate manual specifically for payer record requests.

Review: Medicare Reviews

- When can Medicare review claims? *F-30*
- What are NCCI edits? *F-31*
- What is the main purpose of the OIG? *F-31*
- Which three review entities does CMS use? *F-32*
- How many years can RAC go back looking through records? *F-33*
- Why is it important to pay close attention to the time frame when responding to a request for records? *F-34*

4. OIG Compliance Program Guidance

The Office of the Inspector General (OIG) is the enforcement division of the Department of Health and Human Services (HHS) and their mission is to fight waste, fraud, and abuse in Medicare, Medicaid, and more than 300 other HHS programs. They do this through a nationwide network of audits, investigations, and evaluations which result in cost-saving or policy recommendations for decision-makers and the public. That network also assists in the development of cases for criminal, civil, and administrative enforcement.

Each year, the OIG conducts statistical analysis on claims received. They report on their finding and develop an official Work Plan which is the basis for RAC and many MAC reviews. In addition to the Work Plan, they also monitor the Affordable Care Act's "Ethics and Compliance Program."

Another responsibility of the OIG is the creation of compliance program guidance in an effort to involve healthcare providers in preventing the submission of erroneous claims and combating fraud. This chapter explains the published guidelines of this currently voluntary compliance program and also includes some key topics of the 2014 Work Plan relevant to Chiropractic physicians. Be aware that the 2015 Work Plan will not be made available until January 2015.

- See Resource 290 to review the entire OIG Work Plan which is updated annually.
- See Resource 298 for the latest articles and webinars.

See *OCCM Practice Compliance Manual* (Resource 291) for comprehensive compliance manual assistance.

OIG Compliance Program Guidance

In 2000, the OIG published guidance on a voluntary compliance program for individuals and small group physician practices. The Patient Protection and Affordable Care Act of 2010 (PPACA) mandated that a compliance program become compulsory as of a future date to be determined by the Secretary of HHS. As of the date of this publication, no announcement has been made by HHS or OIG regarding the details of what exactly must be included in such a program. Some industry experts had anticipated an announcement in 2014, but at the time of publication, no announcement had been made.

Once the final compliance dates and details have been set, this program will be required for all providers who bill Federal healthcare programs (e.g., Medicare, Medicaid, etc.) If you do not

---

ACA Medicare/OIG Portion Disclaimer; At the time of printing, the federal government had not yet released its changes for 2015. Every effort was made to update the information in the 2015 DeskBook with information available at the time of review. Ongoing updates on CMS-related topics will be posted on the ACA website at (ACAtoday.org/Medicare) and through its articles and publications.

participate in Federal healthcare programs, this plan is not required, however, every office should carefully review the components of the OIG compliance program guidance and voluntarily implement steps to further ensure the safety and protection of their patients. It is likely that other payers will eventually require a formal compliance program in the future.

Even though this is currently a **voluntary** program for **most** providers, it should be noted that the following organizations are **required** to implement this program:

- Skilled Nursing Facilities and Nursing Facilities as of March 23, 2013 (although CMS has indicated that they will not yet be enforcing that deadline), and
- Organizations which are part of the Corporate Identity Agreements program—usually as a result of prior compliance problem(s).

Creating an OIG compliance program is similar to creating a HIPAA compliance plan in that organizations need to appoint a compliance officer and create a working notebook containing the currently recommended components. Highly sensitive information such as contracts should be kept in a separate, secure place and only be referenced in the Compliance Manual.

A good compliance program should identify areas of risk and create an effective program to mitigate that risk. In addition, the plan should also be periodically reviewed for accuracy. There is no "one size fits all," so use common sense and a reasonable approach when developing a plan to fit your practice. The OIG compliance program guidance for individual and small group physician practices suggests seven components, some of which sound very similar to HIPAA requirements. Although all seven may not be necessary, the voluntary implementation of all can be helpful should your office be audited or investigated.

1. Conduct internal monitoring and auditing through periodic internal audits.

   > **Note:** Monitor and review your plan on a regular basis–at least annually. The plan may also need to be modified at other times as you discover problems.

2. Implement written compliance and practice standards. This should not be just an outline, but should be detailed and available to all employees.
3. Designate a compliance officer or contact to monitor compliance efforts and enforce practice standards.
4. Conduct appropriate training and education on your defined practice standards and procedures.
5. Respond appropriately to detected violations by investigating allegations and disclosure incidents and developing corrective action. This step may require coordination with the appropriate government entities.
6. Develop open lines of communication with employees, such as (1) discussions at staff meetings regarding how to avoid erroneous or fraudulent conduct and (2) community bulletin boards, to keep practice employees updated regarding compliance activities.
7. Enforce disciplinary standards through well-publicized guidelines.

These seven tasks are further defined in the following "OIG Steps to Compliance" section.

Tip: Many offices find it easier to engage a professional compliance auditor to visit the practice, investigate and document the workflow, look for weak spots and suggest remediations, and to create the ongoing processes by which the office can continue with the compliance program thereafter.

See Resource 292 for in-house consulting options.

OIG Steps to Compliance

Step One: Auditing and Monitoring

An ongoing evaluation process is important to a successful compliance program. This ongoing evaluation includes not only whether the physician practice's standards and procedures are in fact current and accurate, but also whether the compliance program is working, i.e., whether individuals are properly carrying out their responsibilities and claims are submitted appropriately. This is an excellent way to ascertain what, if any, problem areas exist and focus on the risk areas associated with those problems.

Conduct a legal audit of your contracts, investments, referral arrangements and marketing practices to ensure compliance with the law. This may require the assistance of an attorney. Document the names/types of each legal document/arrangement but DO NOT include the actual contract in your Compliance Manual.

How to Perform an Internal Baseline Audit

When it comes to claims review, it is helpful to begin with your own internal audit called a baseline audit. This is just a start. Many sources recommend that you have an outsider review your records because we often miss our own mistakes when doing a self-audit. Sometimes another provider may have the same problems that you do. In this case, it is good to hire a certified auditor that is trained to catch your mistakes.

> See Resource 264 for assistance in selecting a certified auditor or certified compliance specialist.

Baseline Audit Process

Do your own random sampling of 20-30 records per provider. If you have billing software, most will have some sort of reporting function which allows you to find out the most commonly used codes in your practice. Identify patients which were billed using those codes and pull their records. Because these are the most commonly used, auditing these records will reveal the biggest problems you may encounter not only during an audit, but also during the ICD-10 transition.

Additionally, review some records which contain data that are established OIG target items. They are being targeted by the OIG because of known problems in documentation and billing.

When you find problems, address them immediately and record your corrective actions in your compliance log. Train providers on the solution/corrective action and then perform a re-audit AFTER a couple of weeks of practice with the new program. Like shampoo, repeat until records are clean.

It is recommended that this level of audit be performed at a minimum of once per year.

> Review the "OIG Work Plan" segment in this chapter for areas which need extra focus and attention.

> *Complete & Easy ICD-10 Coding for Chiropractic* (Resource 294) is available from the ChiroCode Store.

Medical Record Self-Audit Form

Using the Medical Record Self-Audit Form makes the baseline audit process easier. Some practices use a form like this on every chart before it is filed. This is only a sample—individual provider needs may vary by state.

Sample: *Medical Record Self-Audit Form*

See Resource 295 for a full-size version of this form, with instructions.

Go to ACAtoday.org/audits for additional resources to assist your clinic in performing self-audits.

What are You Looking For?

Begin by knowing what the auditors are looking for. For example, from 2001-2010, there was a 48% increase in level of E/M services billed. The states with the highest increases were California, New York, Florida and Texas. Therefore, it stands to reason that those codes and states are being carefully watched and flagged for audits. Be hyper-vigilant and fully aware of both the 1995 and 1997 guidelines for using E/M codes. You MUST meet all the criteria required for History, Exam and Medical Decision Making.

Recent audit and data mining efforts have revealed that the following codes are often billed incorrectly or not properly documented and thus down-coded or denied:

- Procedure codes: 99213, 99203, 99214, 99204
- Diagnosis code: 724.2 Lumbago

Review Chapter 3–Evaluation and Management in *Section H–Procedures* for more about E/M requirements.

Review of Systems Changes

One of the newest items that auditors are closely examining is the Review of Systems (ROS). If the ROS is not related to the Chief Complaint (CC), some auditors are saying it is not considered to be medically necessary. Make sure that the Chief Compliant justifies any additional ROS.

Scheduling

Auditors are also carefully reviewing practice schedules because physicians typically spend 45 minutes or more of face-to-face time on higher levels of Evaluation and Management services. Thus, your schedule should appropriately indicate that the provider was able to spend that much face-to-face time for all patient encounters on that particular day.

Review your Claims Errors

Carefully review each EOB and/or Remittance Advice (RA). You can be sure that these errors are the ones that will be audited. What is being kicked out and how can you keep them from being kicked out in the first place? What new safeguards can you set up in your practice to reduce error rates and ensure better payments?

Self-Disclosure Protocol (SDP)

Although it may seem counter-intuitive to voluntarily report to OIG that you have made a mistake, penalties may be less severe than if the problem is discovered by the OIG before you report it. You may be able to avoid civil and administrative litigation, both of which are time-consuming and expensive. The key to this process is to closely follow the SDP guidelines, be cooperative, forthcoming, thorough, and transparent. Before opting for SDP, it is suggested that practices consult with a qualified healthcare attorney.

> See Resource 297 for detailed information on self-disclosure protocol.

Step Two: Establish Practice Standards and Procedures

After the internal audit identifies the practice's risk areas, the next step is to develop a method for dealing with those risk areas through the practice's standards and procedures. Written standards and procedures are a central component of any compliance program. Those standards and procedures help to reduce the prospect of erroneous claims and fraudulent activity by identifying risk areas for the practice and establishing tighter internal controls to counter those risks, while also helping to identify any aberrant billing practices. Many physician practices already have something similar to this called "practice standards" that include practice policy statements regarding patient care, personnel matters, and practice standards and procedures on complying with state and federal laws.

> **Tip:** These policies and procedures should be written in a user friendly manner using everyday terms instead of "legalese." Everyone on staff needs to be able to open the manual, read it, and understand what it says.

Step Three: Designation of a Compliance Officer

After the audits have been completed and the risk areas identified, ideally one member of the physician practice staff needs to accept the responsibility of developing a corrective action plan, if necessary, and oversee the practice's adherence to that plan. This person can either be in charge of all compliance activities for the practice or play a limited role merely to resolve the current issue. In a formalized institutional compliance program there is a compliance officer who is responsible for overseeing the implementation and day-to-day operations of the compliance program. However, the resource constraints of physician practices make it so that it is often impossible to designate one person to be in charge of compliance functions.

It is acceptable for a physician practice to designate more than one employee with compliance monitoring responsibility. Another possibility is that one individual could serve as compliance officer for more than one entity.

The Compliance Officer needs to be responsible for the following tasks:

- Maintain the OIG Compliance Manual. This includes logging requests for medical records. Log the date the request was received, when the records were mailed and signature for proof of delivery. This log could be a spreadsheet on a computer which is periodically printed and added to the Compliance Manual.
- Implement employee training which is also logged in the Compliance Manual.

Step Four: Conducting Appropriate Training and Education

Education is an important part of any compliance program and is the logical next step after problems have been identified and the practice has designated a person to oversee educational training. Ideally, education programs will be tailored to the physician practice's needs, specialty and size and will include both compliance and specific training.

There are three basic steps for setting up educational objectives:

1. Determining who needs training (both in coding and billing and in compliance);
2. Determining the type of training that best suits the practice's needs (e.g., seminars, in-service training, self-study, or other programs); and
3. Determining when and how often education is needed and how much each person should receive.

Training may be accomplished through a variety of means, including in-person training sessions (i.e., either on site or at outside seminars), distribution of newsletters, or even a readily accessible office bulletin board. Regardless of the training modality used, a physician practice should ensure that the necessary education is communicated effectively and that the practice's employees come away from the training with a better understanding of the issues covered.

Don't forget about employee feedback. Are there areas they are concerned about? Find out which procedures or functions they feel like they need more training in and then work with them to make sure that it happens.

Finally, document this training in your compliance log.

Step Five: Responding To Detected Offenses and Developing Corrective Action Initiatives

When a practice determines it has detected a possible violation, the next step is to develop a corrective action plan and determine how to respond to the problem. Violations of a physician practice's compliance program, significant failures to comply with applicable state and federal laws, and other types of misconduct threaten a practice's status as a reliable, honest, and trustworthy provider of health care.

Consequently, upon receipt of reports or reasonable indications of suspected noncompliance, it is important that the compliance contact or other practice employee look into the allegations to determine whether a significant violation of applicable law or the requirements of the compliance program has indeed occurred, and, if so, take decisive steps to correct the problem. As appropriate, such steps may involve a corrective action plan, the return of any overpayments, a report to the government, and/or a referral to law enforcement authorities.

> **Settlements:** Medicare does not and will not negotiate settlement amounts. However, since the audit program for Medicaid is just beginning, according to one healthcare attorney, Medicaid auditors have been more willing to work out a settlement agreement.

Overpayments

Some providers have expressed concern that sending a refund check will initiate a further review and "flag" them as a target. Since providers only have 60 days to return the money or face "false claim" charges, it is legally in your best interest to quickly return over-payments. One healthcare attorney stated that in the cases he has been involved in, it is actually **in the provider's favor** to show that they are trying to remain in compliance.

It is prudent to include a special cover letter which includes phrases such as:

- While performing a self-audit, we discovered an error.
- We have taken the following corrective actions to ensure that this does not happen again.
- Enclosed is a check to return this overpayment.

See Resource 195 for more about voluntary overpayment refunds.

Step Six: Developing Open Lines of Communication

In order to prevent problems from occurring and to have a frank discussion of why the problem happened in the first place, physician practices need to have open lines of communication. Especially in a smaller practice, an open line of communication is an integral part of implementing a compliance program. Guidance previously issued by the OIG has encouraged the use of several forms of communication between the compliance officer/ committee and provider personnel, many of which focus on formal processes and are more costly to implement (e.g., hotlines and e-mail). However, the OIG recognizes that the nature of some practices is not as conducive to implementing these types of measures. In the small physician practice setting, the communication element may be met by implementing a clear "open door" policy between the physicians and compliance personnel and practice employees. This policy can be implemented in conjunction with less formal communication techniques, such as conspicuous notices posted in common areas and/or the development and placement of a compliance bulletin board where everyone in the practice can receive up-to-date compliance information.

Step Seven: Enforcing Disciplinary Standards Through Well-Publicized Guidelines

The last step that a physician practice may wish to take is to incorporate measures into its practice to ensure that practice employees understand the consequences if they behave in a non-compliant manner. An effective physician practice compliance program includes procedures for enforcing and disciplining individuals who violate the practice's compliance or other practice standards. Enforcement and disciplinary provisions are necessary to add credibility and integrity to a compliance program.

The OIG recommends that a physician practice's enforcement and disciplinary mechanisms ensure that violations of the practice's compliance policies will result in consistent and appropriate sanctions, including the possibility of termination, against the offending individual. At the same time, it is advisable that the practice's enforcement and disciplinary procedures be flexible enough to account for mitigating or aggravating circumstances. The procedures might also stipulate that individuals who fail to detect or report violations of the compliance program may also be subject to discipline.

Disciplinary actions could include:

- Warnings (oral)
- Reprimands (written)
- Probation
- Demotion
- Temporary suspension
- Termination
- Restitution of damages
- Referral for criminal prosecution

Inclusion of disciplinary guidelines in procedure manuals and in-house training is sufficient to meet the "well publicized" standard of this element. It is suggested that any communication resulting in the finding of non-compliant conduct be documented in the compliance folder by including the date of incident, name of the reporting party, name of the person responsible for taking action, and the follow-up action taken.

Exclusions Database Reviews

One very important task is to conduct background checks on providers in addition to ALL clinical and administrative staff. Print the results and include a copy in the individuals employment record. Document the completion of this task in your OIG Compliance Manual log. It is recommended that this task be completed quarterly because the exclusions database is updated monthly.

> Go to exclusions.oig.hhs.gov to quickly and easily check the list of sanctioned individuals.

High Risk Areas

There are several areas targeted for review by the OIG because of their high potential for committing fraud. Be sure to carefully review the segment "OIG Work Plan" for other areas under review.

- Upcoding. Watch your documented time, especially on E/M Services.
- Billing unnecessary services, or those considered unreasonable or NOT medically necessary.
- Duplicate billing.
- Overpayments.
- Billing "incident to" services. This has to do with supervision of lower-level provider services which should be non-covered.
- Violating assignment billing rules.
- Improper inducements, kickbacks and self-referrals.

OIG Work Plan

The OIG has announced that the following reviews are either currently a work in progress, or are being planned for the future. Current items should be addressed immediately as part of your OIG compliance program Items with a date in the future should also be addressed to ensure early compliance. This is not a comprehensive list of the complete work plan. An updated work plan should be available sometime in January 2015.

> - See Resource 298 for reports on OIG findings.
> - See Resource 290 to review the entire Work Plan.

- **Part B Payments for Noncovered Services.** Medicare Part B payments for chiropractic services will be reviewed to determine whether such payments were in accordance with Medicare requirements. Previous OIG work identified inappropriate payments for chiropractic services and so these services will now be more closely monitored.
- **Questionable Billing and Maintenance Therapy.** The 2014 OIG Work Plan stated that "We will determine the extent of questionable billing for chiropractic services. We will also identify trends suggestive of maintenance therapy billing." This is considered a work in progress for 2015, so providers need to pay close attention to their Medicare billing and documentation recommendations.

> See *Section C–Medicare* for important information regarding the appropriate billing of chiropractic manipulations.

- **Error Prone Providers.** If you consistently have errors on claims submitted to Medicare, you could be on their list. Document the most commonly made errors in your office by reviewing Remittance Advice statements. Implement an action plan to stop these errors from being repeated which increases your clean claim submission rate. Understanding medical necessity rules is also helpful.
- **Medicare Secondary Payer Recovery.** In 2006 Medicare began reviewing claims they paid as the Primary payer which should have been paid as the secondary. To prevent incorrect billing, your Patient Coverage process MUST include verification of payer status. DO NOT bill Medicare as Primary if they are really the secondary payer.
- **Zone Program Integrity Contractors' (ZPIC).** Identification of potential fraud and abuse (current). This program replaces the program safeguard contractors (PSCs) to consolidate fraud and abuse activities by CMS. Know and understand what the ZPICs are reviewing to ensure program compliance.
- **Coding of Evaluation and Management Services.** Providers are responsible for ensuring that the codes they submit accurately reflect the services they provide. Upbilling E/M services is a common practice. If you use an EHR, watch carefully to ensure that it is not inappropriately upbilling or using a higher E/M service rate than it should. Documentation must support all components of the E/M Service.
- **Place of Service (POS) Errors.** Never bill using an inappropriate Place of Service code in order to be paid at a higher rate. If you see the patient in a facility setting, use the appropriate facility code and vice versa.
- **Other Insurance Coverage.** In addition to the Secondary Payer edit, OIG will check beneficiary coverage to see if there is other insurance. The Insurance Coverage Verification form (Resource 148) is critical to your OIG compliance program. You must re-verify coverage at least annually, and you are responsible to ask if there is other insurance.
- **Payments on Claims with Modifiers GA and GZ.** Claims billed using modifiers GA (waiver of liability statement issued) and GZ (service not reasonable and necessary) will be reviewed. Many claims using these modifiers were inappropriately paid by Medicare, so check your claims billed with these modifiers. If Medicare paid for any services with the GZ modifier, then refund it immediately. For any services using the GA modifier, make sure they were billed correctly.
- **Comprehensive Outpatient Rehabilitation Facilities.** A study revealed that many CORF services did not meet Medicare reimbursement standards because they were not medically necessary or lacked documentation that such services were provided. Review CORF requirements and ensure documentation supports all requirements.
- **Modifier GY Usage.** Modifier GY is used for coding services that are statutorily excluded or do not meet the definition of a Medicare covered service. Beneficiaries are liable, either personally or through other insurance, for all charges associated with the provision of these services. Although not required to give advance notice to the beneficiary, these claims are now being more carefully reviewed.
- **Providers' Compliance With Assignment Rules.** Records will be reviewed to determine if the provider is over-charging the patient when they accept assignment. You cannot bill the patient beyond the Medicare allowed amount. A program is being implemented to teach beneficiaries their rights and responsibilities.

Additional Help and Information on OIG

Professional Help

Although there are many self-help programs and important basics included in this book, you may need professional assistance. If you seek out professional assistance on completing a compliance program, choose a professional with a credible certification in healthcare compliance such as a Certified Medical Compliance Specialist (MCS-P) or Certified Healthcare Compliance Consultant (CHCC). They can also assist with other forms of compliance such as OSHA and HIPAA as well.

See Resource 264 for information on certified compliance specialists.

Other Help

- See Resource 299 for OIG's booklet "Avoiding Medicare and Medicaid Fraud and Abuse"
- See Resource 298 for additional information and helpful resources.

Review: OIG Compliance Program Guidance
■ How often should you monitor and review your OIG compliance plan? F-36
■ What is your own internal audit called? F-37
■ Why would you want to self report mistakes to the OIG? F-39
■ Who on your staff is responsible to maintain your OIG Compliance Manual? F-39
■ What are some of the areas being targeted by the OIG? F-42

5. Audit Protection

Audits Are Here to Stay

It used to be that when you submitted a claim it was paid. This is no longer the case. With the current trend by payers to perform post-payment audits and refund demands, it's no longer about if you'll be audited, but when this will happen to you. Post-payment audits are here to stay.

Audits are a reality for practices; therefore, significant attention should be focused on audit protection. It has been said that a good offense is a good defense, and that certainly applies to audits. You need to be prepared to defend your standards. Be sure to review and understand state and federal fraud and abuse laws and compliance regulations.

One excellent defense against audits is your documentation. As you consider the audit-protection tips in this chapter, also review the standards set forth in *Section D–Documentation* of this book.

Healthcare providers today face greater scrutiny of their billing, coding and documentation than ever before. Practices can lose large sums of money due to errors in these areas. Profiling of practices by payers is a common occurrence. Denial of payments and post payment audits due to lack of medical necessity in the documentation is a reality across the country. Do not be deluded into thinking this cannot or will not happen to your office.

- See Resource 302 for the latest information, articles and webinars on protecting your practice from audits.
- See Resource 264 for help in finding specialist.

- See *Section: D–Documentation* for guidelines about using your documentation as preventative measures against an audit.

- See *Clinical Documentation Manual,* (Resource 151) by the ACA, for helpful documentation examples.

Who is Watching?

There are several federal programs designed to alert appropriate agencies of potential problems.

- The False Claims Act rewards whistle-blowers up to 25%-30% of recovered funds. Quite often the whistle-blower is a disgruntled employee or business associate.
- The OIG encourages beneficiaries (your patients) to be involved in indentifying fraudulent charges. They send out newsletters with hot-line numbers to call. The OIG reports that these hotlines receive a high volume of calls.
- FBI funding for healthcare investigation was $128.1 million in 2013.

- Both Medicare Adminstrative Contractors (MACs) and Recovery Audit Contractors (RACs) are reviewing previously paid claims for potential problems. When inconsistencies are identified, the audit process is initiated. See Key Points of the OIG Work Plan in the previous section for key areas under review.
- The OIG is initiating programs with medical students on how to spot and report fraud as they enter the workplace.

Why Be Concerned?

A seemingly innocent mistake can lead to thousands of dollars in payment demands that are difficult to fight. It begins innocently enough; for example, your office receives a "Preliminary Audit Report" which states that a random sampling of claims over a specified time period (usually several years) indicated an error rate of $1.81 per claim. That may not sound so bad.

The next part of the letter is where math and random sampling become troublesome. They apply that calculated error rate to every single claim filed during that time period, use a statistical formula for cluster sampling and, that $1.81 turns into more than $20,000 due in 15 days. To top it off, that amount does not include the charges for all investigative, legal and expert witnesses for which they are entitled to by law. Additionally, there could be a fine of up to $10,000 for each claim determined to be a "false claim."

How to Prepare for an Audit

Staff Training and Education

Does your staff know what to do when they receive a request for records? Are they confident in their understanding of HIPAA requirements? HIPAA requires that security and privacy training be performed on a regular basis and well documented. This minimizes the chances for HIPAA violations in addition to other documentation requirements. Often during one audit, violations will be found in other compliance areas such as OSHA. Training gives your staff confidence in compliance procedures and reduces stress about being audited.

Provider Communication

Providers need to properly document patient encounters. Insufficient documentation is one of the most frequent reasons for down-coded claims. According to the 2013 Medicare Improper Payment Report, 51.7 percent of chiropractic claims were paid improperly and 92.5% of those were due to insufficient documentation. Training and review of records is very important. Refer to the documentation section for help.

Your Best Defense: An Effective, Current Compliance Plan

Carefully constructing and following a compliance plan is the best thing you can do. This plan includes an annual internal audit (it is even better if that audit is done by a Certified Compliance Specialist.) The OIG stated that, among other things, an effective compliance plan can be used as a mitigating factor against fines and jail time.

- See Resource 264 for help in finding a specialist.
- See Resource 303 for more about mitigating factors used by the federal government in determining penalties.

Implement Claims Tracking and Review Program

Every practice should have a tracking program which actively reviews denials and underpayments. Once problem areas are established, how do you analyze the data to reduce future problems? Is this communicated to your staff through training programs?

This program should include an effective appeals policy and procedure. Are you monitoring unpaid claims? Do you quickly respond to requests for records and is that information logged, i.e. when the request was received, who received it and when were the records submitted?

> See *Section B–Insurance and Reimbursement* for more about monitoring unpaid claims.

Implement a Compliance Program

Refer to Chapter 4–OIG Compliance Plan Program in this *Compliance and Audit Protection* section for details on how to implement this type of program. Once it is implemented, it is very important to review and re-evaluate it on a regular basis. This includes monitoring billing, documentation and other procedures as they relate to all compliance programs such as HIPAA. Getting input from your staff can also be helpful to learn what works about the program and what doesn't. Having this information documented is very helpful in an audit to demonstrate compliance.

One very important component of this program is the self-audit. Self-audits help identify problems before the auditors send their letters. This gives you a chance to fix your problems and demonstrate your compliance efforts as well. Providers can minimize the incidence of payer audits and recoupments by performing self-audits which are an inexpensive way to determine whether services have been properly documented and billed. Self-audits can also help demonstrate compliance if a carrier states that your treatment patterns are inappropriate. Many payers have general guidelines regarding the percentage of manipulative treatments that should be performed at each coding level. While it may be helpful to compare the results of your self audit against a payer's benchmarks, providers should always treat according to medical necessity and fully document the need for the level(s) of manipulative treatment and other care.

> Go to ACAtoday.org/audits for some examples of self-audit tools and provider information.

GENERAL AUDIT PROTECTION

Seven Everyday Steps

Auditors have to move quickly; they won't spend hours poring through all your notes. With standard insurance, when auditors look at claims they often use a software tool that utilizes 16-20 criteria points. You usually need about a 80-90% score to pass, so you can only miss about three questions. All payers use similar tools, so make sure you are meeting the criteria. Here are seven simple steps that you should follow with every patient because not doing them can cause you to score poorly on an audit.

1. **Doctor/staff entry.** Have the doctor sign every treatment note or record.

    > See the "Signatures" segment in *Section D–Documentation* for more about acceptable signature requirements.

2. **Legibility.** It doesn't matter if you can read your notes. Are they legible to a third party? No auditor will ask you to translate them. If the notes are not legible they don't meet current documentation standards.
3. **Abbreviations.** Most auditors are not doctors of chiropractic, so they may not understand chiropractic-specific language like ASRA, PLS, etc. If you use abbreviations provide a legend to avoid problems.
4. **Past medical history.** Many doctors of chiropractic fail to document all components of the history level of the new patient exam. "If it's not documented it's not done." The auditor will assume that you failed to perform this.
5. **Allergies.** This is a tricky one that has caused doctors of chiropractic to fail audits because it is aimed at medical doctors. Doctors are required to screen for allergies before prescribing medications or supplements. Be sure to clearly document relevant allergies, especially if you sell supplements.
6. **X-rays.** A written x-ray report is necessary and checklist reports are not acceptable. Do your x-rays contain standard criteria? Such criteria are:
   - **Demographics.** Patient name, birthdate, clinic name, etc.
   - **Markers.** Left, right, etc.
   - **Collimation.** Is there demonstration of adequate collimation attempted?
   - **Shielding.** Is appropriate gonadal shielding used where indicated?
   - **Artifacts.** Are metal, piercings or other artifacts present on the films? Piercings are a big problem as some cannot be removed. Document any patient refusals to remove piercings.
7. **Referrals.** All referrals need to be documented in your chart notes. That includes referrals made to other providers and from other providers.

Clinical Documentation Manual, (Resource 151) by the ACA, is an excellent guide to documentation standards.

General Compliance Benchmarks

Be proactive; establish compliance benchmarks that will help you monitor your practice in a meaningful way.

- **Use claim scrubbing software**, which is a feature of many billing systems and electronic clearinghouses. This allows you to detect claims errors before they are submitted.
- **Assess risk.** Use the data from your billing reports to assess your risk and then make a plan for correction. Example: Are you billing a high number of 98942s or high level exams? Make sure these services are appropriately documented, coded and billed.
- **Self audit.** You need to figure out, by auditing your own claims, where errors lie. If you never audit your own claims, you may never know you have problems or errors and will continue to make them in the future.
- **Current code book.** Using outdated codes or unofficial terminology creates confusion on the part of an auditor. It can also indicate that you are not up-to-date with other things like documentation and thus make your office appear less than fully compliant.

What to Do If You Are Audited

When a payer audits you the first thing to do is respond to the audit in a timely manner. Do not ignore it; it won't go away. In the initial stage of the audit, they will probably ask you to send them your notes on approximately 5-10 patients. Either have a healthcare attorney or yourself send exactly what they are requesting. Keep the following in mind:

- Do not add or alter your notes or records in any way.
- Never send originals. Remember, the carrier has a legal right to review copies of the notes, not the originals, unless your contract states otherwise.
- Send your notes by certified mail, return receipt requested, to ensure that the carrier has received it and to prove that you sent it.
- Once you have sent the requested notes, there is nothing more to do but go back to practicing.

AVOIDING AN AUDIT

While everyone wants to avoid an audit, there is no silver-bullet methodology to guarantee that it will never happen to you. There are far too many triggers which raise audit red flags. However, knowing these high risk areas and taking preventive measures, are the biggest helps.

See Resource 302 for additional information, help, articles and webinars.

Managing risk in the following areas will yield the most effective results:

1. Disgruntled people
2. Billing patterns
3. Modifiers
4. Documentation
5. E/M billing
6. Chiropractic specific services
7. Not medically necessary

Some of these problems overlap. For example, much of the E/M down-coding occurs because of documentation problems.

1. Disgruntled People

This is one of the biggest triggers. All it takes is a phone call and the auditors are on their way. It doesn't matter where the complaint comes from, if there is a complaint, it is quickly investigated whether or not it is true. Complaints usually are initiated by one of the following:

- **Disgruntled employees.** A disgruntled employee is more likely to turn a doctor in for an audit than anyone else. If you have an employee who thinks you are not doing something right, it is very important to get it cleared up with them. Sit down and make sure that everyone understands. Get a second opinion if necessary. It is NOT worth having a disgruntled employee lodge a complaint.

- **Disgruntled patients.** Sometimes a chiropractic patient becomes disgruntled if they receive an unexpected bill. To mitigate this risk, it is important to clearly emphasize patient financial responsibilities with all the necessary paperwork.

  See "Establish Patient Financial Responsibility" in *Section B–Insurance and Reimbursement* for more information.

- **Disgruntled competitors.** What is becoming more common is having a competitor lodge a complaint in order to "even the score". There is not much that you can do about this problem. Your compliance efforts will show auditors the real story.

2. Billing Patterns

The information on actual claims is the basis for this section. It is not only how, when and what is billed. Although not mentioned specifically below, carefully review the OIG Work Plan for additional triggers. Below are some specific examples.

- **Diagnosis determines treatment.** Cervicalgia (neck pain) and Lumbalgia (low back pain) are short-term diagnoses and need to be carefully documented. Whatever diagnosis is chosen, it should be fully supported by appropriate documentation.

- **Routine waiving of co-pays and deductibles.** Do not waive these financial responsibilities of the patient. "Any supplier (or provider) who routinely waives co-payments or deductibles can be criminally prosecuted and excluded from participating in the Federal health care programs" per Medicare Transmittal #B0069 (Resource 311). Other payers have similar policies.

    See *Section B–Insurance* for instructions on how to implement a "Financial Hardship Policy" in your practice.

- **Clustering.** The practice of coding/charging one or two middle levels of service codes exclusively, under the philosophy that some will be higher, some lower, and the charges will average out over an extended period (in reality, this overcharges some patients while undercharging others).

- **Upcoding by a staff member or a billing company.** A staff member may do this to help you make more money. A billing company could do this to help increase their own commissions. Either scenario can easily trigger an audit.

- **Double billing.** Although duplicate billing can occur due to simple error, knowingly submitting duplicate claims—which is sometimes evidenced by systematic or repeated double billing—can create liability under criminal, civil, and/or administrative law.

- **Misuse of provider identification numbers.** This is improper billing.

- **Unbundling.** Billing for each component of the service instead of billing or using an all-inclusive code.

- **Improper ICD-9 coding.** On submitted claims any of the following could be considered improper: 1) high usage of general non-specific codes, 2) not using highest level of specificity, and 3) selecting a diagnosis that is not supported by the documentation.

- **Inconsistent coding among partners in a practice.** When different partners in a practice code and treat for varying levels of care it sends up red flags.

3. Modifiers

- **Separating the professional component (modifier 26) from the technical component (modifier TC) on X-rays.** Separating the global fee into technical (TC) and professional allows for a higher reimbursement. Remember that any time something is done for financial intent it could be construed as fraud.

- **Improper use of modifiers.** This can trigger a review if you use the wrong modifiers, use a modifier too much, or use certain ones more than other doctors of chiropractic in your area.

    See Chapter 6–Procedure Modifers of *Section H–Procedure Codes* for for details on how to properly use modifiers.

4. Documentation

Documentation problems such as missing treatment plans, poorly documented visits, cloned records and other such issues tend to be the biggest problem facing providers when it comes to audits. Properly documented visits help you avoid audits and defend against them as well.

> See *Section D–Documentation* for information about excellent documentation standards.

5. Evaluation and Management Billing

The biggest problem is the over use of high level E/M codes. The exam level should be appropriate for the condition and properly coded in the documentation.

- **99204 (new patient) 99214 (established patient).** These are comprehensive examinations that carry the requirement of an extended clinical history, and extended review of systems, family and social history, and a comprehensive exam which finds multiple diagnoses with a moderate complexity of decision-making.
- **99205 (new patient) 99215 (established patient).** These are comprehensive examination codes. This level of service requires comprehensive histories, examination and a highly complex level of clinical decision-making, where there is a high risk of mortality. These cases are not common in an ambulatory setting.
- **99211.** Often called the "Nurses Code", it does not typically describe doctor services.
- **Billing new patient codes for established patients.** Internal data mining makes it easy to identify this practice. Carefully review the official definition of "new patient" in the procedure code section of this book. Existing patients who have a new payer due to a new injury, such as a car accident, should still be billed as an established patient.
- **Billing an E/M code in place of CMT.** Many doctors use an E/M code in place of the CMT because chiropractic visits are not covered or were exhausted. Again the doctor always has to select the code that accurately describes the service preformed.

> See Chapter 3–Evaluation and Management in *Section H–Procedure Codes* for details on proper E/M coding.

6. Chiropractic Specific Services

- **Treatment Date (Item 14 of the 1500 claim form).** Monitor this date and update when appropriate. A date over two months old may start to look like maintenance care.
- **97140 and Diagnosis.** Claims and documentation must include the proper diagnosis code/pointer. If that pointer is not there, it tells the auditor that you don't know how to use the code properly.
- **97112 Usage.** Pay attention to the official CPT definition and make sure the documentation fits the code description.
- **Routine billing.** Routine use of 98941 (3-4 Regions) or 98942(5 Regions) on every patient will trigger a flag since it is outside statistical norms.
- **Billing a 97140-59 Manual Therapy with a 98942 or a 98941.** The likelihood of performing 97140 in a separate and distinct region other than the 3-4 or 5 areas adjusted is rather low. Remember you have to have a diagnosis for every area you treat. Some payers have begun to require documentation upon submission of this code, even with the modifier.

See Resource 304, 305 and 306 for additional information.

- Go to ACAtoday.org/appeals to be linked to ACA information.
- See also ACAtoday.org/level2_css.cfm?T1ID=15&T2ID=364 for information.

- **Incorrect usage of 97032.** Carefully review official descriptions – was the service truly attended or not attended? Just being in the room does not fall under the definition of attendance. Documentation must support the proper usage of this code.
- **Routine use of x-rays.** Everyone, regardless of diagnosis, receives full spine x-rays or repeat x-rays to evaluate how they are doing. Insurance companies frown upon re-x-raying a patient to monitor improvement.
- **98940-98942 Coding Patterns.** Many payers utilize data mining programs which mathematically estimate coding norms based on claims billed. When a provider falls outside what the payer considers their normal coding pattern, the provider may be considered an 'outlier' and thus be flagged for an audit.

> **Warning:** Never attempt to 'fly under the radar' of the auditors by coding an inappropriate level of service. Always bill and properly document every visit with supportive notes. Then, if your practice is ever identified as an 'outlier', your records will support your claims. Down-coding has the potential to negatively alter any future payer calculations of coding patterns based on submitted claims. More importantly, under-coding could be considered fraud because it is making a false statement about the treatment provided.

See Resource 310 for additional information.

- **Billing a manual therapy in place of the CMT.** The doctor must always select the code that accurately describes the service preformed. Manual therapy is a timed code. Adjustment codes are not timed. The code for a chiropractic adjustment is 9894x, not 97140.
- **Static treatment plans.** This is when, no matter what the diagnosis, every patient gets the same treatment with the same duration and frequency. Care should be individualized.
- **Excessive sales of high end DME.** If the mark-up is above the usual and customary fees this could trigger a red flag.
- **Excessive use of passive therapies.** Passive care for extended periods of time without proper justification are often viewed as palliative and thought to foster chronicity. Typically, as treatment progresses, passive care should be decreased and active care should be increased. Active care (e.g. therapeutic exercise) prescribed as part of a treatment plan, can be used in conjunction with passive care as long as the provider is clear to document the rationale and necessity of such a program.

7. Not Medically Necessary

One of biggest problems is that many services are deemed not medically necessary and much of the proof falls back on the medical record. However, such services are routinely denied. Here are some specific situations as they relate to audits.

- **Irrelevant physical examinations.** The exam must pertain to the patient's presenting problems or complaints and their history. It may be appropriate to manipulate/adjust a segment(s) that may not be symptomatic and/or located in the same spinal region as the area of chief complaint, but is contributing to the patient's overall condition. The need for treatment to these segments should be established through clinical measures and have a direct therapeutic effect and be well documented.

Objective findings could necessitate a more comprehensive exam. It is essential that such findings are clearly indicated in the documentation to support the clinical need for this extended examination.

> See Resource 307 for additional information.

- **Unnecessary Durable Medical Equipment (DME).** There must be clinical rationale for the DME and proof that it supports the healing process. Proper coding for all DME billed must have the correct HCPCS (pronounced "hick-picks") code. These codes must be present for each item. The 1500 claim form must point to the associated and correct ICD code.

- **Unnecessary diagnostic testing.** The need for any diagnostic testing must be substantiated in the patient's record. The rationale for ordering the test should be based on the provider's inability to establish a diagnosis to a reasonable degree of clinical certainty without the test results and/or to rule out pathologies, etc. Results of the test should be reviewed and considered in the overall management of the patient's condition.

- **Unnecessary services.** Billing procedures for parts of the body that are not associated with the patient complaint, presenting problem or those found through objective measures. However, be aware that payer policy may have specific requirements on this issue, so be sure to check with the insurer.

- **Unjustified frequency of re-examinations and re-x-rays.** Often there is little or no documented clinical assessment of the patient's progress that would require the billing for such services. Essential and required information should be in the daily notes. If progress has not been noticed, there should be a referral or further testing and evaluation.

REFUND REQUESTS AND DEMANDS

There is a growing trend of post-payment audits by payers and their claim recovery contractors in the form of either a refund request or demand. Providers need to carefully examine the exact wording in the letter. Is this a polite request or is it a demand which has severe implications? In many cases, providers are experiencing forced paybacks where the payer simply "takes" money that they feel they are owed and are calling it a "payment offset". Providers need to examine each payer request/demand carefully and determine the validity of the claim and then respond accordingly.

> Carefully watch EOBs and RA's for lost revenue due to payment offsets.

Providers can and should refuse to pay inappropriate demands for refunds in many situations such as those listed below. In situations such as these where it is not an ERISA claim in which your written contract prohibits such action, the "Response Letter to Refund Demands" (Resource 309) could be of great value:

- A review of your records indicates that their request is wrong. You have properly billed, documented, and rendered the services.

- Your contract with that payer specifically states that they are contractually bound to honor your payment because you met its policy requirements. You did what you were asked, met their requirements at that time and thus qualify to be paid.
- The payer incorrectly covered a service that it now says is not covered. The letter will often say that this was a mistake on their part and now they want the money back.

If you do not have a written contract with the insurance payer that allows them to ask for refunds, the following response letter could be of great value for non-ERISA claims.

Response Letter to Refund Demands For Insurance Payment Errors

This response letter to refund demands for payer payment errors is ideal for most events wherein the claim was submitted in good faith and paid in good faith. Additionally, if you had recorded the verification of coverage with the payer, they could be held guilty of misrepresentation.

> This letter is for commercial payers only and is not appropriate for Medicare, workers' compensation, etc., wherein federal or state law might apply. Also, if you have a contract with a private payer, your contract agreement could require the repayment or recoupment of funds, even if they make an error. Such matters require legal counsel.

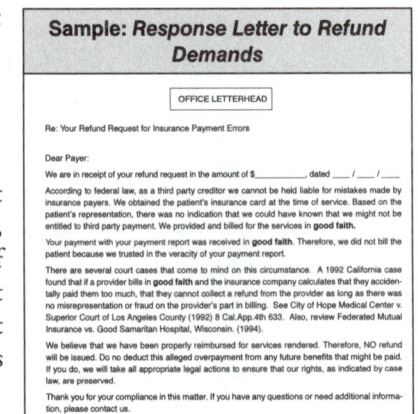

See Resource 309 for a full-size version of this form, with instructions.

Third-Party Refund Demands

> Some payers have begun to use third-party companies to request recoupment of fees. This can be confusing as to where the payment should really go. Carefully review your contract to see if this practice is specifically mentioned. If not, you may be able to use the following letter which tells them that you will only pay any fees directly to the contracted party and ONLY them.

See Resource 308 for a full-size version of this form, with instructions

Fighting Payment Offsets

Payment offsets are placing a financial burden on healthcare providers. The problem is that the situation is not as black and white as we would like it to be. To effectively fight payment offsets, providers need to understand the requirements of their state prompt pay laws, as well as audit and recoupment laws, and also the insurance company's internal claim and dispute appeals process.

Just as prompt pay laws assist in getting claims paid, they also outline the time limits in which payers can request refunds. If their request occurs after those deadlines, then they **cannot** take the money. Immediately begin an appeals process and specifically quote the language of the prompt pay/audit and recoupment law in your appeal. They might still take the money, but you have the law on your side. Consult an attorney if necessary.

Every insurance payer has clearly defined procedures for claim disputes and this includes refunds. Read your contract or contact the provider relations department to obtain the specific rules regarding disputes. If you do not meet their time lines for an appeal, you may be waiving your right to dispute a payment offset.

> See Chapter 3–Guidelines for Unpaid Claims in *Section E–Claims and Appeals* for more about prompt pay laws.

Review: OIG Compliance Program Guidance

- What are the seven simple steps to follow with every patient to score well on audits? *F-47 to F-48*
- What is the first thing that needs to be done when a payer audits you? *F-48*
- How are having disgruntled employees a risk for being audited? *F-49*
- Does upcoding really help you make more money? *F-50*
- For many carriers, 99205 should only be used when your patient presents with what? *F-51*
- What is a "payment offset"? *F-53*

Notes

1. Diagnosis Coding
Page G-3

2. Commonly Used ICD-9-CM Codes (Anatomic List)
Page G-12

3. Commonly Used ICD-10-CM Codes (Anatomic List)
Page G-21

4. Numeric ICD-9-CM (Tabular) List
Page G-33

5. Alphabetic List (ICD-9-CM)
Page G-111

G DIAGNOSIS CODES

DIAGNOSIS CODES

OBJECTIVES

ICD-9-CM codes are the HIPAA required code set for diagnostic coding on claim forms. As such, it is important to understand which codes should be used for proper billing. This section contains just the excerpts which are of primary importance to chiropractic.

OUTLINE

1. Diagnosis Coding *G-3*
   - Overview of ICD-9-CM *G-3*
   - ICD-9-CM Code Usage *G-4*
   - Billing with ICD-9-CM *G-5*
   - ICD-10-CM Is Here *G-7*
   - Review *G-11*

2. Commonly Used ICD-9-CM Diagnosis Codes (Anatomic List) *G-12*
   - Anatomic List *G-12*
   - Cervical and Head Diagnoses *G-13*
   - Thoracic Diagnoses *G-14*
   - Lumbar Diagnoses *G-15*
   - Sacral Diagnoses *G-17*
   - Upper Extremity Diagnoses (non-spinal) *G-18*
   - Lower Extremity Diagnoses (non-spinal) *G-19*
   - Abdomen (non-spinal) *G-20*
   - Review *G-20*

3. Commonly Used ICD-10-CM Diagnosis Codes (Anatomic List) *G-21*
   - Anatomic List *G-21*
   - Cervical and Head Diagnoses *G-23*
   - Thoracic Diagnoses *G-24*
   - Lumbar Diagnoses *G-26*
   - Sacral Diagnoses *G-27*
   - Upper Extremity Diagnoses (extra-spinal) *G-28*
   - Lower Extremity Diagnoses (extra-spinal) *G-30*
   - Other Conditions (Alphabetical) *G-31*

4. Numeric ICD-9-CM (Tabular) List *G-33*
   - Coding Conventions *G-34*
   - Infectious and Parasitic Diseases (001-139) *G-35*
   - Endocrine, Nutritional and Metabolic Diseases, and Immunity Disorders (240-279) *G-35*
   - Mental Disorders (290-319) *G-37*
   - Diseases of the Nervous System and Sense Organs (320-389) *G-38*
   - Diseases of the Circulatory System (390-459) *G-45*
   - Diseases of the Digestive System (520-579) *G-45*
   - Diseases of the Genitourinary System (580-629) *G-46*
   - Diseases of the Musculoskeletal System and Connective Tissue (710-739) *G-46*
   - Congenital Anomalies (740-759) *G-66*
   - Symptoms, Signs, and Ill-Defined Conditions (780-799) *G-69*
   - Injury and Poisoning (800-999) *G-72*
   - Supplementary Classification of Factors Influencing Health Status and Contact with Health Services (V01 - V91) *G-85*
   - Supplemental Classification of External Causes of Injury and Poisoning (E000 to E999) *G-92*

5. Alphabetic List (ICD-9-CM) *pg G-111*

1. Diagnosis Coding

OVERVIEW OF ICD-9-CM

ICD-9-CM is the International Classification of Diseases 9th Revision, Clinical Modification, and is used in the United States to code signs, symptoms, injuries, diseases, and conditions. It is the HIPAA required code set for diagnosis coding until October 1, 2015 when ICD-10-CM becomes the new standard.

> See Resource 344 for additional information, articles and webinars about diagnosis coding.

Code Sections in This Book

Anatomic Index

The **Anatomic Index**, created by the ChiroCode Institute, is a quick and easy anatomic reference for diagnostic codes. The code descriptions are listed alphabetically within each anatomic region by subluxation, associated diagnoses, and symptoms. After identifying the disorder or ailment, always go to the Numeric List for full code information.

Numeric List

The **Numeric List**, also called the Tabular List, includes codes that might be reported by chiropractic physicians. This is not a limitation on the use of codes but rather a listing of the most commonly used ICD-9-CM codes within the chiropractic profession. The Highest Specificity Column shows codes in **bold** that are relevant for billing. They are the most specific codes

---

ACC Position Statement on Diagnosis

Concerning diagnosis as taught in chiropractic schools:

> "A diagnosis is an expert opinion identifying the nature and cause of a patient's concern or complaint, and/or abnormal finding(s). It is essential to the ongoing process of reasoning used by the doctor of chiropractic in cooperation with the patient to direct, manage, and optimize the patient's health and well-being.

> "The process of arriving at a diagnosis by a doctor of chiropractic includes: obtaining pertinent patient history; conducting physical, neurological, orthopedic, and other appropriate examination procedures; ordering and interpreting specialized diagnostic imaging and/or laboratory tests as indicated by symptoms and/or clinical findings; and performing postural and functional biomechanical analysis to determine the presence of articular dysfunction and/or subluxation."

-July 2003 Position Statement by the Association of Chiropractic Colleges (ACC)

available for the diagnosis. It is essential that you use this column in order to be reimbursed properly. Always check this section after looking in the Anatomic Index or Alphabetic List. Also check here for any *includes*, *excludes* and other notes on code usage. See page G-34 for a list of coding conventions.

"V" Codes

Supplementary Classification of Factors Influencing Health Status and Contact with Health Services (V01 - V86). These deal with occasions and circumstances **other than a disease or injury.** They include well patient services (e.g., routine checkup), ongoing services (e.g., cast changes), and circumstances influencing health (e.g., smoking).

"E" Codes

Supplemental Classification of External Causes of Injury and Poisoning (E800 to E999). These are used to identify **external causes** of accidents, injury, or poisoning.

Alphabetic List

The **Alphabetic List** was created by the ChiroCode Institute. This is only the first step to selecting an appropriate diagnostic code. After identifying the disease or ailment, always go to the Numeric List for highest specificity and other important code information.

ICD-9-CM Code Usage

Highest Specificity Coding

Diagnosis codes are to be used with the highest number of digits available. ICD-9-CM diagnosis codes are composed of codes with 3, 4, or 5 digits. Codes with three digits are included in ICD-9-CM as the heading of a category of codes that may be further subdivided by the use of fourth and/or fifth digits, which provide greater specificity.

A three-digit code is to be used only if it is not further subdivided (for example, 734 Flat foot). Where fourth-digit subcategories and/or fifth-digit subclassifications are provided, they must be used. A code is invalid if it has not been coded to the full number of digits required for that code. For example, Curvature of spine, code 737, has fourth digits that describe the types of curvature (eg, 737.1 Kyphosis (acquired)), and fifth digits that provide further clarification (eg, 737.12 Kyphosis, postlaminectomy). It would be incorrect to report a code in category 737 without a fourth and fifth digit.

On occasion, a payer will request a 5-digit ICD-9 code when you are already coding at the highest level of specificity with 3 or 4 digits. In this case it would be impossible (and a violation of HIPAA code set rules) to have a 5-digit code.

Always code from the Numeric List, which lists the ICD-9 codes at their highest level of specificity in the bold, indented Highest Specificity Column.

ICD-9-CM Code Updates

Updates to the ICD-9-CM code set are released annually and are effective on October 1st of each year. There is a partial code freeze for both the ICD-9-CM codes and the ICD-10-CM code sets prior to the implementation of the ICD-10 which is set for October 1, 2015. As of October 1, 2016 (one year after the implementation of ICD-10), regular updates to ICD-10 will resume.

ICD-9-CM Linkage to CPT

ICD-9-CM codes form a crucial partnership with CPT procedural codes. The ICD-9-CM codes indicate the reason **why** the CPT procedure or service was performed.

Most third party payers employ claims edits or automatic review commands within the computer software used to review claims. "Diagnosis to procedure" edits are among the most common type of edits applied to claims. These edits ensure that payment is only made for specific procedure codes when provided for a patient with a specific diagnosis code or predetermined range of ICD-9-CM codes. All Medicare claims are required to contain a relationship between the CPT procedure code and the ICD-9-CM diagnostic code, and most insurance companies use similar edits.

The diagnosis you select must be as specific as possible when translating the physician's written narrative statements into ICD-9-CM codes, and must also be validated in the patient's record. The selection of the primary diagnosis for a patient encounter is usually "the reason the physician saw the patient that day," not necessarily the patient's most serious condition. However, in Medicare the subluxation is almost always listed as the **primary code.** See the Anatomic List on page G-12 for examples. You should also code any condition the physician actively manages during the face-to-face physician-patient encounter, and any condition that impacts the overall management or treatment of that patient.

> **Tip:** To assign an accurate code:
> - Go first to the anatomic or alphabetic section to look up the condition, disease, or injury.
> - Secondly, confirm the propriety of the code in the Numeric (Tabular) List, which has detailed information such as 'includes' and 'excludes'.

BILLING WITH ICD-9-CM

The existence or use of a code does not necessarily mean that it will meet the requirements established by a third party payer. The required codes may vary between payers. For example, some carriers require the 839 series for subluxation, while others might require the 739 series.

Generally, codes with higher numbers (739-subluxations or 800-injuries) should be listed first as primary on insurance claim forms. Secondary codes are used for associated or complicating factors.

It is helpful to remember that procedure codes express **what** is done, but the diagnostic codes express **why** it is done. Diagnostic codes are generally used to determine whether payment should be made for a claim, not how much. It is important with chiropractic claims to list the primary and secondary diagnoses that indicate the need for chiropractic services. Typically, the reason the patient sought treatment was due to a subluxation, and the subluxation should be listed first.

> **Tip:** The primary diagnosis on a claim is the one listed first and should be the most serious reason/condition for the patient encounter. However, be aware of individual payer differences, such as Medicare, which might require that subluxation be listed as the primary diagnosis for chiropractic services. See *Section E–Claims and Denials* for more information on how to properly indicate diagnosis codes on the claim form.

Diagnoses for Motor Vehicle Accidents

From a motor vehicle accident (MVA) perspective, such a simplistic protocol for claims could be financially devastating to the patient. Settlement offers are determined by all of the diagnoses and their associated values. Hence, comprehensive reporting of all ICD-9 codes associated with the accident/collision are critical for proper MVA payments (e.g., contusions, abrasions, etc.).

Basic Coding Principles

To code accurately, it is necessary to have a working knowledge of medical terminology and to understand the complexity of transforming descriptions of diseases, conditions, and injuries into their ICD-9-CM numerical designations. Accurate coding describes the medical necessity of a procedure and expedites the payment process. Incorrect coding can lead to allegations of, and investigations for, fraud and abuse.

- **Never rely solely upon the short descriptors** in the Anatomic Index or the Alphabetic Index. Always select a code from the Numeric List. Code to the highest specificity.

- **Take the necessary time** to code from the physician's diagnostic statements in the patient's chart or clinical records. Careful attention to symptoms, conditions, and etiology can help ensure diagnostic accuracy and maximum reimbursement. The ICD-9-CM code gives the reason why the procedure or service was rendered. The code(s) should relate to the procedure code being billed.

- **Code by subluxation first** for Medicare and other payers, as may be mandated. In most instances, subluxation is the reason for the encounter in a chiropractic practice. If a patient presents with a headache, what are the options for treatment of a headache? A doctor of chiropractic typically treats one of the **causes** of the headache: the subluxation. Therefore, for some payers, it is the requested principle diagnosis for treatment with the secondary diagnosis being the headache. The coding hierarchy may vary by payer.

- **Symptoms and ill-defined** conditions can be used, but **only** in the absence of a definitive primary diagnosis. Use codes for the presenting symptoms sequenced by the highest level of severity or the main focus of treatment delivered.

- **Coexisting conditions:** List additional codes to describe any coexisting conditions managed by the physician that day.

- **Chronic conditions:** Codes for chronic diseases may be coded as often as the patient receives treatment for the condition. Do not code a diagnosis that is not influencing the patient's care for each service and/or procedure.

- **Injuries:** Review all coding principles when coding for injuries and fractures. When coding an injury, reference the condition, not just the anatomical site. Identify multiple diagnoses when applicable (e.g., injuries, disease, etc.). List the major problem first, with no more than 2-3 associated diagnostic codes. Make sure that the codes listed are consistent with areas treated.

- **Choose specific diagnoses.** Avoid codes for diseases or diagnoses that include the words rule-out, possible, probable, or suspected.

- **Select codes to their highest level of specificity.** Use the fourth and fifth-digit subclassifications whenever available.

- **When possible, avoid codes with a .8 or .9 in the last digit.** They are known as "dump" codes because of vague descriptions (e.g., other, unlisted). Always look for a more specific code in the lower range of numbers, provided sufficient documentation is available.

- **Non-relevant conditions:** Do not code conditions which are not related to the current reason for the patient encounter.

- **Codes V01.0-V89** deal with occasions when circumstances other than a disease or injury are recorded as diagnoses or problems.
- **Report all relevant codes, especially on auto/PI cases:** Many other conditions often exist, even though not treated (e.g., bruises, contusions, etc). Complete reporting impacts a proper settlement.
- **Late effects (sequela):** Code when a treated condition is a late effect of an earlier injury or disease. A late effect is the residual effect that remains after the termination of the acute phase of an illness or injury.
- **Modifiers** for ICD-9 codes do not exist.
- **HHS Guidelines:** Study and reference the official ICD-9-CM and ICD-10-CM Guidelines for Coding and Reporting. These national standards explain basic principles and habits for correct ICD coding.

- See Resource 356 for the official ICD-9-CM coding guidelines.
- See Resource 357 for the official ICD-10-CM coding guidelines.

ICD-10-CM Is Here

The current ICD-9-CM system is 30 years old, uses outdated and obsolete terminology, and contains outdated codes that produce inaccurate and limited data that is inconsistent with current medical practice. ICD-9-CM cannot accurately describe the diagnoses of the 21st century. The ICD-10-CM code set will facilitate more accurate and relevant evaluation of medical processes and outcomes. It will also upgrade administrative transcriptions, e-prescribing, and Health Information Technology (HIT) adoption.

The compliance date for ICD-10-CM is October 1, 2015. All HIPAA covered entities must implement the new code set for all services that occur on or after that date. This is the year of the transition.

A complete list of ICD-10-CM codes for chiropractic, overviews, reference guides and translation tables are included in ChiroCode's *Complete & Easy Coding for Chiropractic* (Resource 294) and available in the ChiroCode Store.

Complete & Easy ICD-10 Coding for Chiropractic (Resource 294) is available in both the ChiroCode online store and the ACA store.

See Chapter 3–Commonly Used ICD-10-CM Diagnosis Codes (Anatomic List) for additional information and links to other resources.

Go to ACAtoday.org/ICD10 for information by the ACA about ICD-10.

Differences Between ICD-9-CM and ICD-10-CM

There are notable differences between the two coding systems. Figure 7.1 shows an overview of these changes.

ICD-10-CM has twice the number of categories as ICD-9-CM. ICD-10-CM has new chapters, categories, titles and regrouped conditions. Other notable improvements include:

- Additional information relevant to ambulatory and managed care encounters;
- Expanded injury codes;
- Combination diagnosis/symptom codes, which reduce the number of codes needed to fully describe a condition;
- Greater specificity in code assignment.

The ChiroCode Institute has produced the *ChiroCode Complete & Easy ICD-10 Coding for Chiropractic*, which provides a comprehensive overview of ICD-10-CM and helps to make the transition. Figures 7.2 and 7.3 show sample pages from this book.

See Chapter 3–Commonly Used ICD-10-CM Codes for Chiropractic of this *Diagnosis Codes* section for codes and more information on this code set.

FIGURE 7.1
Differences between ICD-9-CM and ICD-10-CM

Feature	ICD-9-CM	ICD-10-CM
Number of Codes	About 13,000 codes	About 68,000 codes
Number of Characters	• 3-5 characters in length • In chapters 1-17, all characters (1-5) are numeric • In supplemental chapters (E and V codes), character 1 is alpha and characters 2-5 are numeric • A decimal is used after 3 characters	• 3-7 characters in length • Character 1 is alpha • Character 2 is numeric • Characters 3-7 are alpha or numeric • A decimal is used after 3 characters • Some codes use "x" as a place holder for characters 4-6 when needed • A 7th character used in certain chapters (obstetrics, musculoskeletal, injuries, and external causes of injury)
Code Structure	Category . Etiology, anatomic site, manifestation	Category . Etiology, anatomic site, severity Extension
Code Examples	725 350.1 922.31 V 69.0	M35.3 G50.0 S30.0xxA Z72.3
Number of Chapters	17 chapters E codes and V codes are in supplemental chapters	21 chapters E codes and V codes are now chapters 20 and 21
Start Dates	1975 (1979 in the United States)	1994 (2015 in the United States)
Expansion	Expansion ability is limited	Has significant ability to expand without a structural change
Detail	Lacks detail	Very specific
Laterality	Lacks laterality (codes identifying right and left sides)	Includes laterality where appropriate
Encounters	Initial and subsequent encounters are not defined	Initial and subsequent encounters are defined
Combination Codes	Combination codes are limited	Combination codes are frequent

FIGURE 7.2

Code Map Sample Page from *ChiroCode Complete & Easy ICD-10 Coding for Chiropractic*

ICD-9-CM CODE			ICD-10-CM Equivalent Codes*	
17. Injury and Poisoning (800-999)				
FRACTURE OF NECK AND TRUNK (805-809)				
805	FRACTURE OF VERTEBRAL COLUMN WITHOUT MENTION OF SPINAL CORD INJURY			
805.0	Cervical, closed			
	805.00	Cervical vertebra, unspecified level	S12.9xx_	Fracture of neck, unspecified
	805.01	First cervical vertebra	S12.000_	Unspecified displaced fracture of first cervical vertebra
			S12.001_	Unspecified nondisplaced fracture of first cervical vertebra
	805.02	Second cervical vertebra	S12.100_	Unspecified displaced fracture of second cervical vertebra
			S12.101_	Unspecified nondisplaced fracture of second cervical vertebra
	805.03	Third cervical vertebra	S12.200_	Unspecified displaced fracture of third cervical vertebra
			S12.201_	Unspecified nondisplaced fracture of third cervical vertebra
	805.04	Fourth cervical vertebra	S12.300_	Unspecified displaced fracture of fourth cervical vertebra
			S12.301_	Unspecified nondisplaced fracture of fourth cervical vertebra
	805.05	Fifth cervical vertebra	S12.400_	Unspecified displaced fracture of fifth cervical vertebra
			S12.401_	Unspecified nondisplaced fracture of fifth cervical vertebra
	805.06	Sixth cervical vertebra	S12.500_	Unspecified displaced fracture of sixth cervical vertebra
			S12.501_	Unspecified nondisplaced fracture of sixth cervical vertebra
	805.07	Seventh cervical vertebra	S12.600_	Unspecified displaced fracture of seventh cervical vertebra
			S12.601_	Unspecified nondisplaced fracture of seventh cervical vertebra
	805.08	Multiple cervical vertebrae	S12.9xx_	Fracture of neck, unspecified
805	Fracture of vertebral column without mention of spinal cord injury			
	805.2	Dorsal [thoracic], closed	S22.009_	Unspecified fracture of unspecified thoracic vertebra
	805.4	Lumbar, closed	S32.009_	Unspecified fracture of unspecified lumbar vertebra
	805.6	Sacrum and coccyx, closed	S32.10x_	Unspecified fracture of sacrum
	805.8	Unspecified, closed	S12.9xx_	Fracture of neck, unspecified

*A one-to-one match does not always exist between codes in ICD-9-CM and ICD-10-CM. This ICD-10-CM Code Map is excerpted from the General Equivalence Map by CMS to assist in finding an ICD-10-CM code that is equivalent to an ICD-9-CM code.

Do not code directly from this code map. After locating an ICD-10-CM code in this list, find the corresponding code in the the ICD-10-CM Tabular List and then determine whether that code or another code within that category is the best choice.

"_" indicates that the code has a seventh character (such as "A" for initial encounter).

"x" is a placeholder character (assigned when a code requires a 7th character and there are less than six characters in the code).

This sample Code Map page allows easy conversion between ICD-9-CM and ICD-10-CM codes.

FIGURE 7.3

Tabular List Sample Page from *ChiroCode Complete & Easy ICD-10 Coding for Chiropractic*

Code	Description
S06.897_	Other specified intracranial injury with loss of consciousness of any duration with death due to brain injury prior to regaining consciousness
S06.898_	Other specified intracranial injury with loss of consciousness of any duration with death due to other cause prior to regaining consciousness
S06.899_	Other specified intracranial injury with loss of consciousness of unspecified duration
S06.9	Unspecified intracranial injury Brain injury NOS Head injury NOS with loss of consciousness *Excludes1:* *head injury NOS (S09.90)*
S06.9x	Unspecified intracranial injury
S06.9x0_	Unspecified intracranial injury without loss of consciousness
S06.9x1_	Unspecified intracranial injury with loss of consciousness of 30 minutes or less
S06.9x2_	Unspecified intracranial injury with loss of consciousness of 31 minutes to 59minutes
S06.9x3_	Unspecified intracranial injury with loss of consciousness of 1 hour to 5 hours 59minutes
S06.9x4_	Unspecified intracranial injury with loss of consciousness of 6 hours to 24 hours
S06.9x5_	Unspecified intracranial injury with loss of consciousness greater than 24 hours with return to pre-existing conscious level
S06.9x6_	Unspecified intracranial injury with loss of consciousness greater than 24 hours without return to pre-existing conscious level with patient surviving
S06.9x7_	Unspecified intracranial injury with loss of consciousness of any duration with death due to brain injury prior to regaining consciousness
S06.9x8_	Unspecified intracranial injury with loss of consciousness of any duration with death due to other cause prior to regaining consciousness
S06.9x9_	Unspecified intracranial injury with loss of consciousness of unspecified duration

INJURIES TO THE NECK (S10-S19)

Includes:
  injuries of nape
  injuries of supraclavicular region
  injuries of throat
Excludes2:
  burns and corrosions (T20-T32)
  effects of foreign body in esophagus (T18.1)
  effects of foreign body in larynx (T17.3)
  effects of foreign body in pharynx (T17.2)
  effects of foreign body in trachea (T17.4)
  frostbite (T33-T34)
  insect bite or sting, venomous (T63.4)

Code	Description

S10	SUPERFICIAL INJURY OF NECK
	Add the appropriate 7th character to each code from category S10
	  A - initial encounter
	  D - subsequent encounter
	  S - sequela
	Example: S10.0xxA

S10.0xx_	Contusion of throat
	  Contusion of cervical esophagus
	  Contusion of larynx
	  Contusion of pharynx
	  Contusion of trachea

S10.1	Other and unspecified superficial injuries of throat
S10.10x_	Unspecified superficial injuries of throat
S10.11x_	Abrasion of throat
S10.12x_	Blister (nonthermal) of throat
S10.14x_	External constriction of part of throat
S10.15x_	Superficial foreign body of throat Splinter in the throat
S10.16x_	Insect bite (nonvenomous) of throat
S10.17x_	Other superficial bite of throat *Excludes1:* *open bite of throat (S11.85)*
S10.8	Superficial injury of other specified parts of neck
S10.80x_	Unspecified superficial injury of other specified part of neck
S10.81x_	Abrasion of other specified part of neck
S10.82x_	Blister (nonthermal) of other specified part of neck
S10.83x_	Contusion of other specified part of neck
S10.84x_	External constriction of other specified part of neck
S10.85x_	Superficial foreign body of other specified part of neck Splinter in other specified part of neck

↑ Highest Specificity Column (code from this column only)   ↑ Highest Specificity Column (code from this column only)

A "_" after a code indicates that a 7th character is needed

This sample Tabular List page shows both placeholder characters ("x"), which mark reserved spaces for future ICD-10-CM expansion, and underscore ("_") characters, which are to be selected from the 7th-character tables which are provided.

Review: Diagnosis Coding

- Where can you find a quick and easy anatomic reference for diagnostic codes? *G-3*
- In the numeric list, which codes are shown in bold? *G-3*
- What is the difference between the "V" codes and the "E" codes? *G-4*
- Why is it recommended that you code by the subluxation first? *G-6*
- Which codes are known as the "dump codes"? *G-6*
- What are some of the differences between the new ICD-10-CM codes and the current ICD-9-CM codes? *G-7 to G-8*

2. Commonly Used ICD-9-CM Diagnosis Codes (Anatomic List)

ANATOMIC LIST

This Anatomic List allows you to quickly locate commonly used ICD-9-CM diagnosis codes based on the common anatomic sites treated in chiropractic offices. The codes are categorized by subluxation, presenting problems, symptoms and ill-defined conditions. Since many payers follow Medicare as a standard, the categories also follow Medicare standards. Some of the codes also include Medicare screening/treatment levels. These levels signify short, moderate and long-term care and will help you determine your treatment plans.

There is no way to know when a Medicare contractor will request a beneficiary's records. Some types of medical review are based on the doctor's volume, some are based on coding patterns, some are based on other factors (e.g., diagnosis), and some are purely random.

Sometimes, a medical review is based on the number of visits within a specific time frame or for a particular diagnosis. Because details on these types of reviews can be considered "proprietary", there is not a single definitive answer on either the number of visits or a specific diagnosis code. However, some contractors publish "review guidelines" to help you know when you hit a point where your notes may be required to authorize further care. These can be found in your Local Coverage Determination (LCD).

Many of the claims contractors (A/B MACs) have divided their acceptable secondary diagnoses (found in your LCD) into categories such as "short-term," "moderate-term," and "long-term," indicating that the diagnoses in each successive section will probably get more visits prior to review. A generalized range for these categories might be:

- Short term (10-12 visits prior to possible review)
- Moderate term (18-24 visits prior to possible review)
- Long term (24-30 visits prior to possible review)

As for visits per month or per year, we have seen published numbers of 12 per month and 18/25/30 per year. When visits go beyond these various numbers, there is a chance you will need to provide your records before further care is approved.

However, never discount the fact that many reviews are entirely random and absolutely cannot be predicted. Remember that you are required to comply with the Medicare regulations on EVERY visit. If you do this, finding yourself under review should not be a problem. Remember that these are only guidelines and proving medical necessity of the treatment will be the primary consideration.

CERVICAL AND HEAD DIAGNOSES

SUBLUXATION

Subluxation, nonallopathic lesions, segmental dysfunction, somatic dysfunction

739.0	Head (not covered by Medicare)	
739.0	Occipitocervical	
739.1	Cervical Region: C1 to C7	

Subluxation, dislocation, displacement, due to injury

839.00	Cervical vertebra region, unspecified	
839.01	Cervical vertebra region, C1	
839.02	Cervical vertebra region, C2	
839.03	Cervical vertebra region, C3	
839.04	Cervical vertebra region, C4	
839.05	Cervical vertebra region, C5	
839.06	Cervical vertebra region, C6	
839.07	Cervical vertebra region, C7	
839.08	Cervical vertebra region, multiple cervical sites	

The 839 series is designated for use **with injuries**, but some carriers fail to follow this national ICD-9 standard and use the 739 code set.

PRESENTING PROBLEM

Code	Description	
307.81	Tension headache	[S]
339.11	Headache, tension type, episodic	[S]
339.12	Headache, tension type, chronic	[S]
346.0x	Headache, migraine, with aura	
346.2	Headache, variants of, not elsewhere classified, without intractable migraine	
346.21	Headache, variants of, not elsewhere classified, with intractable migraine	
353	Brachial plexus lesions	[M]
353.2	Cervical root lesions, NEC	[M]
354	Carpal tunnel syndrome	
627.2	Headache, menopausal	
720.1	Enthesopathy, spinal	[M]
721	Cervical spondylosis without myelopathy	[S]
721	Spondylosis, without myelopathy, cervical	[S]
721.1	Spondylosis, with myelopathy, cervical	[S]
721.7	Spondylopathy, traumatic	[L]
721.9	Spondylosis, without myelopathy, unspecified site	[S]
721.91	Spondylosis, with myelopathy, unspecified site	[S]
722	Displacement of cervical intervertebral disc without myelopathy	[L]
722.3	Schmorl's nodes	
722.4	Degeneration of cervical intervertebral disc	[L]
722.71	Cervical disc disorder with myelopathy	
722.81	Postlaminectomy syndrome, cervical region	[L]
722.91	Disc disorder, cervical region, other and unspecified	
723	Spinal stenosis in cervical region	[M]
723.1	Cervicalgia	[S]
723.2	Cervicocranial syndrome	[M]
723.3	Cervicobrachial syndrome (diffuse)	[M]
723.4	Brachial neuritis or radiculitis NOS	[M]
723.5	Torticollis, unspecified	[M]
723.7	Ossification of posterior/longitudinal ligament, cervical	
723.9	Cervical disorder NOS	
724.8	Other symptoms, referable to back (facet syndrome)	[M]
737.41	Kyphosis, cervical	
738.4	Spondylolisthesis, acquired	[M]
756.2	Cervical rib	
830	Dislocation of jaw (TMJ)	
847	Sprains and strains, neck	[M]
848.1	Sprain/strain, jaw (TMJ)	
951.9	Headache, cranial nerve(s) injury, unspecified	
307.81	Headache, tension (psychological factors)	
339.1	Headache, tension type	[S]
346.1x	Headache, migraine, without aura	
346.2	Headache, migraine variants of	
346.9x	Headache, migraine, unspecified	
524.6x	TMJ disorders	
625.4	Headache, premenstrual	
953.x	Injury, nerve root and spinal plexus	
953.4	Injury, brachial nerve root, brachial plexus	[M]

Never code from this Anatomic Index. It is only the first step to finding a probable code. For example, "supraspinatus" is not in the short description of the 726.10 code, but it is found in its expanded definition and notes within the numeric/tabular section.

> 726.1 Rotator cuff syndrome of shoulder and allied disorders
>> 726.10 Disorders of bursae and tendons in shoulder region, unspecified
>>> Rotator cuff syndrome NOS; Supraspinatus syndrome NOS

Do not code from this Anatomic List. Always check the Numeric List for highest specificity codes and instructions for code usage. An "x" indicates that another digit is needed.

CERVICAL AND HEAD DIAGNOSES, CONTINUED

SYMPTOMS AND ILL-DEFINED CONDITIONS

Use only in the absence of a definitive primary diagnosis. Use for the presenting symptoms, sequenced by the highest level of severity or the main focus of treatment delivered.

Code	Description
719.40	Pain in joint, site unspecified
719.41	Pain in joint, shoulder region
719.42	Pain in joint, upper arm
719.43	Pain in joint, forearm
719.44	Pain in joint, hand
719.45	Pain in joint, pelvic region and thigh
719.46	Pain in joint, lower leg
719.47	Pain in joint, ankle and foot
719.48	Pain in joint, other specified sites
719.49	Pain in joint, multiple sites
719.53	Stiffness of joint, NEC, forearm
719.54	Stiffness of joint, NEC, hand
719.58	Stiffness of joint, NEC, other specified sites
729.5	Pain in limb
780.4	Vertigo NOS
780.4	Dizziness and giddiness
780.50	Sleep disturbance, unspecified
780.51	Sleep disturbance, insomnia with sleep apnea, unspecified
780.52	Sleep disturbance, insomnia, unspecified
780.53	Sleep disturbance, hypersomnia with sleep apnea, unspecified
780.54	Sleep disturbance, hypersomnia, unspecified
780.55	Sleep disturbance, disruptions of 24-hour sleep-wake cycle, unspecified
780.56	Sleep disturbance, dysfunctions associated with sleep stages or arousal from sleep
780.57	Sleep apnea, unspecified
780.59	Sleep disturbance, other
780.7x	Malaise and fatigue
781.0	Facial twitch, involuntary spasm
782.0	Burning or prickling
782.0	Disturbance of skin sensation
782.0	Numbness or tingling
782.0	Paresthesia
782.3	Edema
784.0	Headache
784.92	Pain in jaw

THORACIC DIAGNOSES

SUBLUXATION

Subluxation, nonallopathic lesions, segmental dysfunction, somatic dysfunction

Code	Description
739.2	Thoracic region: T1 to T12

Subluxation, dislocation, displacement, due to injury

Code	Description
839.21	Thoracic vertebra region: T1 to T12

*The 839 series is designated for use **with injuries**, but some carriers do not follow this national ICD-9 standard*

PRESENTING PROBLEM

Code	Description	
353.0	Costoclavicular syndrome	
353.0	Lexus lesions, brachial	[S]
353.3	Root lesions, thoracic NEC	[M]
353.8	Nerve root and plexus disorders, other	
718.48	Contracture of joint, other specified sites	
720.1	Enthesopathy, spinal	[M]
721.7	Kummell's disease or spondylitis (kyphosis)	
722.11	Intervertebral disc disorder, thoracic, displacement of, without myelopathy	[M]
722.31	Schmorl's node, thoracic	
722.51	Intervertebral disc disorder, thoracic or thoracolumbar, degeneration of	[M]
722.72	Intervertebral disc disorder, thoracic region, with myelopathy	
722.82	Postlaminectomy syndrome, thoracic	
722.92	Intervertebral disc disorder, thoracic region, other and unspecified	[L]
723.3	Cervicobrachial syndrome (diffuse)	[L]
723.4	Neuritis or radiculitis, NOS, brachial	[M]
724.4	Neuritis or radiculitis, thoracic, unspecified	
724.5	Backache, unspecified	
724.8	Facet syndrome – see Other symptoms referable to back	
724.8	Other symptoms, referable to back (facet syndrome)	[M]

THORACIC DIAGNOSES, CONTINUED

724.9	Ankylosis of spine NOS			756.12	Spondylolisthesis, congenital	[M]
724.9	Compression of spinal nerve root NEC			721.7	Spondylopathy, traumatic	[L]
724.9	Other unspecified back disorders			721.41	Spondylosis, thoracic, with myelopathy	
724.9	Spinal disorders NOS	[M]		721.2	Spondylosis, thoracic, without myelopathy	[S]
731.0	Osteitis deformans			721.91	Spondylosis, with myelopathy, unspecified site,	[S]
733.13	Collapsed vertebra NOS	[L]		721.90	Spondylosis, without myelopathy, unspecified site,	[S]
738.4	Spondylolisthesis, acquired	[M]		847.1	Sprains and strains, thoracic	[M]
807.00	Fracture of rib(s), unspecified			848.3	Sprains and strains, ribs	
905.1	Late effect of fracture, spine			724.01	Stenosis, spinal, thoracic region	[M]
953.1	Nerve root and spinal plexus injury, dorsal root					
953.4	Nerve root and spinal plexus injury, brachial plexus	[M]				

SYMPTOMS AND ILL-DEFINED CONDITIONS

Use only in the absence of a definitive primary diagnosis. Use for the presenting symptoms, sequenced by the highest level of severity or the main focus of treatment delivered.

			719.7	Difficulty in walking	
			724.1	Pain in thoracic spine	
			781.3	Lack of coordination	
719.41	Pain in joint, shoulder region		781.92	Abnormal posture	
719.42	Pain in joint, upper arm (elbow)		782.0	Numbness or tingling	
719.44	Pain in joint, hand		782.0	Paresthesia	
719.48	Pain in joint, other specified sites		786.50	Pain, chest, unspecified	

LUMBAR DIAGNOSES

SUBLUXATION

Subluxation, nonallopathic lesions, segmental dysfunction, somatic dysfunction

739.3 Lumbar region: L1 to L5

Subluxation, dislocation, displacement, due to injury

839.20 Lumbar vertebra region: L1 to L5

*The 839 series is designated for use **with injuries**, but some carriers fail to follow this national ICD-9 standard and use the 739 code set.*

PRESENTING PROBLEM

353.1	Plexus lesions, lumbosacral	[M]		721.91	Spondylosis, with myelopathy, unspecified site	[S]
353.4	Root lesions, lumbosacral, NEC	[M]		722.10	Intervertebral disc disorder, lumbar, displacement of, without myelopathy	[L]
353.8	Nerve root and plexus disorders, other	[M]		722.32	Schmorl's node, lumbar	
718.48	Contracture of joint, other specified sites	[M]		722.52	Intervertebral disc disorder, lumbar or lumosacral, degeneration of	[L]
720.0	Ankylosing spondylitis			722.73	Intervertebral disc disorder, lumbar region, with myelopathy	
720.1	Enthesopathy, spinal	[M]		722.83	Postlaminectomy syndrome, lumbar region	[L]
721.3	Spondylosis, lumbosacral, without myelopathy	[S]		722.93	Calcification IVC or IVD, discitis, lumbar	
721.42	Spondylosis, lumbosacral, with myelopathy			722.93	Intervertebral disc disorder, lumbar region, other and unspecified	[M]
721.5	Kissing spine [Baastrup's Syndrome]					
721.6	Ankylosing vertebral hyperostosis					
721.7	Traumatic spondylopathy	[L]				
721.90	Spondylosis, without myelopathy, unspecified site	[S]				

Do not code from this Anatomic List. Always check the Numeric List for highest specificity codes and instructions for code usage. An "x" indicates that another digit is needed.

Lumbar Diagnoses, continued

Code	Description		Code	Description	
724.02	Stenosis, spinal, lumbar region, without neurogenic claudication	[M]	733.00	Osteoporosis, unspecified, wedging of vertebra NOS	
724.03	Stenosis, spinal, lumbar region, with neurogenic claudication	[M]	737.30	Scoliosis (and kyphoscoliosis), idiopathic	
724.2	Lumbago	[S]	738.4	Spondylolisthesis, acquired	[M]
724.4	Neuritis or radiculitis, lumbosacral, unspecified	[M]	756.10	Congenitial anomaly of spine, unspecified	
724.5	Backache, unspecified	[S]	756.12	Spondylolisthesis, congenital	[M]
724.6	Ankylosis or instability	[M]	756.15	Fusion of spine [vertebra], congenital	
724.8	Facet syndrome		805.4	Compression fracture, lumbar	
724.8	Ossification of posterior longitudinal ligament NOS		846.0	Sprains and strains, lumbosacral (joint) (ligament)	[M]
724.8	Other symptoms, referable to back (facet syndrome)	[M]	847.2	Sprains and strains, lumbar	[M]
			922.31	Contusion, Back	
724.9	Ankylosis of spine NOS		922.32	Contusion, Buttocks	
724.9	Compression of spinal nerve root NEC		922.33	Contusion, Interscapular region	
724.9	*Other unspecified back disorders* Caution: Some carriers may deny 724.9 due to non-specificity	[M]	953.2	Injury, lumbar nerve root	
			953.2	Nerve root and spinal plexus injury, lumbar root	[L]

SYMPTOMS AND ILL-DEFINED CONDITIONS

Use only in the absence of a definitive primary diagnosis. Use for the presenting symptoms, sequenced by the highest level of severity or the main focus of treatment delivered.

Code	Description
719.48	Pain in joint, other specified sites
719.49	Pain in joint, multiple sites
719.58	Stiffness of joint, other specified sites
719.59	Stiffness of joint, multiple sites
719.7	Difficulty in walking
724.2	Lumbago - lumbalgia (low back pain)
724.5	Backache, unspecified verebrogenic (pain) syndrome NOS
781.2	Abnormality of gait
782.0	Numbness or tingling
782.0	Paresthesia

Medicare Screens

Letters in brackets after indicate a maximum number of days for screening purposes:

[S] = Short Term Treatment, up to 10 treatments;

[M] = Moderate Term Treatment, up to 20 treatments;

[L] = Long Term Treatment, up to 30 treatments (or more)

These Medicare screening categories are by CMS. They are not pre-approved terms of care, and do not include complicating factors or other issues. Your local Medicare contractor could have different screens—consult them for specific code inclusion and visit screens. Remember that clinical need preempts any screens.

SACRAL DIAGNOSES

SUBLUXATION

Subluxation, nonallopathic lesions, segmental dysfunction, somatic dysfunction

739.4	Sacral region
	Sacrococcygeal region
	Sacroiliac region
739.5	Pelvic region
	Hip region
	Pubic region

Subluxation, dislocation, displacement, due to injury

839.41	Coccyx region
839.42	Sacrum region
	Sacroiliac joint

The 839 series is designated for use **with injuries**, but some carriers fail to follow this national ICD-9 standard and use the 739 code set.

Note: ICD-9 officially places the sacroilliac region in the code for the sacral region (739.4) The CPT description by the AMA places the sacrioliac joint in the pelvic region. See page H-80. for these codes. CMS defines pelvis as Ilium and Sacro-iliac.

PRESENTING PROBLEM

353.1	Plexus lesions, lumbosacral	
353.8	Nerve root and plexus disorders, other	[M]
718.48	Contracture of joint, other specified sites	[M]
720.1	Enthesopathy, spinal	[M]
720.2	Sacroilitis not elsewhere classified	
721.3	Spondylosis, lumbosacral without myelopathy	[S]
721.7	Traumatic spondylopathy	[L]
721.90	Spondylosis of unspecified site, without myelopathy	[S]
721.91	Spondylosis of unspecified site, with myelopathy	
724.3	Sciatica; neuralgia or neuritis of nerve	[L]
724.5	Backache, unspecified	[S]
724.6	Ankylosis or instability of sacroiliac	[M]
724.6	Ankylosis of sacrum	
724.71	Hypermobility of coccyx	
724.79	Coccygodynia, or other sacral disorders	[M]
724.8	Facet syndrome	
724.8	Other symptoms, referable to back (facet syndrome)	[M]
724.9	Ankylosis of spine NOS	

724.9	Other unspecified back disorders	
	Caution: Some carriers may deny 724.9 due to non-specificity	
726.5	Bursitis of hip	
726.5	Iliac crest spur, hip region	
726.5	Trochanteris tendinitis, hip region	
738.4	Spondylolisthesis, acquired	[M]
756.12	Spondylolisthesis, congenital	[M]
843.9	Sprains and strains, Hip and thigh	
846.1	Sprains and strains, Sacroiliac ligament	[M]
846.2	Sprains and strains, Sacrospinatus ligament	[M]
846.3	Sprains and strains, Sacrotuberous ligament	[M]
846.8	Sprains and strains, Other specified sites	[M]
847.3	Sprains and strains, sacrum	[M]
847.4	Sprains and strains, coccyx	[M]
848.5	Sprains and strains, Pelvis	
953.3	Nerve root and spinal plexus injury, sacral root	
953.5	Nerve root and spinal plexus injury, lumbosacral plexus	[M]

SYMPTOMS AND ILL-DEFINED CONDITIONS

Use only in the absence of a definitive primary diagnosis. Use for the presenting symptoms, sequenced by the highest level of severity or the main focus of treatment delivered.

719.40	Pain in joint, site unspecified
719.45	Pain in joint, pelvic region and thigh
719.46	Pain in joint, lower leg
719.47	Pain in joint, ankle and foot
719.48	Pain in joint, other specified sites
719.49	Pain in joint, multiple sites
719.55	Stiffness of joint, pelvic region and thigh (hip) NEC
719.7	Difficulty in walking
724.3	Sciatica; neuralgia or neuritis of nerve
729.5	Pain in limb (leg)
781.2	Abnormality of gait

UPPER EXTREMITY DIAGNOSES (NON-SPINAL)

SUBLUXATION

Subluxation, nonallopathic lesions, segmental dysfunction, somatic dysfunction

739.7 Upper extremities
 Acromioclavicular region
 Sternoclavicular region

Subluxation, dislocation, displacement, due to injury

831.00 Shoulder, unspecified
832.00 Elbow, unspecified
833.00 Wrist, unspecified

834.00 Finger, unspecified
839.8 Multiple and ill-defined
 Arm
 Back
 Hand
 Multiple locations except fingers or toes alone
 Unspecified location

*The 839 series is designated for use **with injuries**, but some carriers fail to follow this national ICD-9 standard and use the 739 code set.*

PRESENTING PROBLEM

Shoulder

718.48 Contracture of joint, other specified sites
726.0 Adhesive capsulitis of shoulder
726.10 Rotator cuff syndrome, shoulder
726.11 Calcifying tendinitis, of shoulder
726.2 Periarthritis of shoulder
726.2 Scapulohumeral fibrositis
840.0 Sprains and strains, acromioclavicular
840.3 Sprains and strains, infraspinatus
840.4 Sprains and strains, rotator cuff
840.5 Sprains and strains, subscapularis (muscle)
840.6 Sprains and strains, supras pinatus (muscle) (tendon)
840.8 Sprains and strains, other specified sites of shoulder and upper arm
840.9 Sprains and strains, shoulder, upper arm, unspecified
923.00 Contusion, shoulder

Arm, Elbow

726.31 Medial epicondylitis, elbow
726.32 Lateral epicondylitis, golfer's elbow
726.33 Bursitis of elbow
726.33 Olecranon bursitis, elbow
726.90 Capsulitis NOS
726.90 Periarthritis NOS
726.90 Tendonitis NOS
726.91 Exostosis of elbow
832.00 Dislocation closed, elbow, unspecified
840.2 Sprains and strains, coracohumeral (ligament)
840.3 Sprains and strains, infraspinatus (muscle) (tendon)
840.5 Sprains and strains, subscapularis (muscle)

841.0 Sprains and strains, radial collateral ligament
841.1 Sprains and strains, ulnar collateral ligament
841.2 Sprains and strains, radiohumeral (joint)
841.2 Sprains and strains, radiohumeral (joint)
841.3 Sprains and strains, ulnohumeral joint
841.8 Sprains and strains, other specified sites of elbow and forearm
841.9 Sprains and strains, unspecified site of elbow and forearm
923.03 Contusion, upper arm
923.10 Contusion, forearm
923.11 Contusion, elbow

Wrist, Hand, Fingers

354.0 Carpel tunnel syndrome
726.4 Bursitis of wrist or hand
726.4 Periarthritis of wrist
726.91 Bone spur NOS
726.91 Exostosis of wrist
842.00 Sprains and strains, wrist, unspecified site
842.01 Sprains and strains, carpal (joint)
842.02 Sprains and strains, radiocarpal (joint) (ligament)
842.09 Sprains and strains, wrist, other
842.10 Sprains and strains, hand, unspecified
842.11 Sprains and strains, carpometacarpal (joint)
842.12 Sprains and strains, metacarpophalangeal (joint)
842.13 Sprains and strains, interphalangeal (joint)
842.19 Sprains and strains, hand, other

UPPER EXTREMITY DIAGNOSES (NON-SPINAL), CONTINUED

SYMPTOMS AND ILL-DEFINED CONDITIONS

Use only in the absence of a definitive primary diagnosis. Use for the presenting symptoms, sequenced by the highest level of severity or the main focus of treatment delivered

Shoulder

719.41	Pain in joint, shoulder
719.51	Stiffness of joint, shoulder

Arm, Elbow

719.42	Pain in joint, elbow (upper arm)
719.43	Pain in joint, forearm

719.52	Stiffness of joint NEC, upper arm
719.53	Stiffness of joint NEC, forearm
729.5	Pain in limb

Wrist, Hand, Fingers

719.44	Pain in joint, hand
719.54	Stiffness of joint, NEC, hand
729.5	Hand pain

LOWER EXTREMITY DIAGNOSES (NON-SPINAL)

SUBLUXATION

Subluxation, nonallopathic lesions, segmental dysfunction, somatic dysfunction

739.6	Lower extremities

Subluxation, dislocation, displacement, due to injury

836.3	Knee (patella)
837.0	Ankle
838.00	Foot, unspecified

838.06	Foot, interphalangeal (joint), foot
838.04	Foot, metatarsal (bone), joint unspecified
838.05	Foot, metatarsophalangeal (joint)
838.02	Foot, midtarsal (joint)
838.09	Foot, other
838.01	Foot, tarsal (bone), joint unspecified
838.03	Foot, tarsometatarsal (joint)

PRESENTING PROBLEM

Pelvic Region and Thigh

719.45	Pain in joint, pelvic region and thigh

Leg and Knee

716.96	Arthritis
718.56	Ankylosis
726.60	Bursitis of knee NOS
736.6	Deformity of knee (acquired) NOS
736.81	Deformities, unequal leg length (acquired)
729.1	Fibromyalgia

715.16	Osteoarthrosis, lower leg
717.6	Joint mice
732.4	Osgood-Schlatter
844.9	Sprains and strains, knee or leg NOS

Ankle, Foot and Toes

845.00	Sprains and strains, ankle, unspecified site
845.10	Sprains and strains, foot, unspecified site
845.13	Sprains and strains, toe

Extremities

Medicare does not currently cover extremity manipulation for doctors of chiropractic. However, the same sequence for a subluxation being in the first position is suggested for consistency and uniformity. Consult your local and private payers for their policy regarding diagnostic positions on the 1500 health insurance claim form.

The CPT® uses the term "extra-spinal" for non-spinal regions or regions beyond the spine. These ICD-9 codes relate to these regions and to the 98943 code.

Do not code from this Anatomic List. Always check the Numeric List for highest specificity codes and instructions for code usage. An "x" indicates that another digit is needed.

Lower Extremity Diagnoses (non-spinal), continued

Symptoms and Ill-Defined Conditions

Use only in the absence of a definitive primary diagnosis. Use for the presenting symptoms, sequenced by the highest level of severity or the main focus of treatment delivered.

Leg and Knee

719.46	Pain in joint, lower leg
719.56	Stiffness of joint, NEC, lower leg
719.59	Stiffness of joint, NEC, multiple sites
719.86	Calcium deposits

716.96	Inflammation of joint NOS

Ankle, Foot and Toes

719.47	Pain in joint, ankle and foot
719.57	Stiffness of joint, ankle and foot

Abdomen (non-spinal)

Symptoms and Ill-Defined Conditions

Use only in the absence of a definitive primary diagnosis. Use for the presenting symptoms, sequenced by the highest level of severity or the main focus of treatment delivered

787.02	Nausea alone
787.01	Nausea with vomiting
787.03	Vomiting alone
789.06	Pain, abdominal, epigastric
789.07	Pain, abdominal, generalized
789.04	Pain, abdominal, left lower quadrant
789.02	Pain, abdominal, left upper quadrant
789.09	Pain, abdominal, other specified sites

789.05	Pain, abdominal, periumbilic
789.03	Pain, abdominal, right lower quadrant
789.01	Pain, abdominal, right upper quadrant
789.00	Pain, abdominal, unspecified site

Review: Commonly Used ICD-9-CM Codes

- When should you code from the ICD-9-CM anatomic list? *G-12*
- Where can I find Medicare's acceptable secondary diagnoses codes? *G-12*

3. Commonly Used ICD-10-CM Diagnosis Codes (Anatomic List)

ANATOMIC LIST

This Anatomic List allows you to quickly locate commonly used ICD-10-CM diagnosis codes based on the common anatomic sites treated in chiropractic offices. The codes are categorized by subluxation, presenting problems, symptoms, ill-defined and other conditions.

Guidelines and Conventions

This *Commonly Used ICD-10-CM Codes* chapter is intended to help you get familiar with this new code set. This is a unique year in that two different code sets will be used during 2015 (ICD-9-CM through September and ICD-10-CM thereafter). Due to the size of the ICD-10-CM code sets, only the ICD-9-CM Tabular listing is included in this edition of the *ChiroCode DeskBook*. For the tabular listings, refer to the publication *Complete & Easy ICD-10 Coding for Chiropractic* (Resource 294) which is a comprehensive ICD-10 coding resource for chiropractic services.

You are **strongly** advised not to code just from this commonly used code list, but to use it as a starting point. A complete tabular list will guide you to the correct code and include other necessary information for you to ensure proper code selection.

> *Complete & Easy ICD-10 Coding for Chiropractic* (Resource 294) is available in both the ChiroCode online store and from the ACA store.

> - See Resource 359 to search ICD-10-CM codes and descriptions.
> - See Resource 360 to see information by the CDC on ICD-10-CM.

> For additional ICD-10-CM information see the following resources:
> - Go to ACAtoday.org/ICD10 to download the ACA's ICD-10 Toolkit.
> - Go to FindaCode.com/icd-10-cm to review and search ICD-10-CM codes. To download the free Find-A-Code app for ICD-10 go to the Google Play Store or the Apple App Store from your Smart Phone, iPad, Tablet or Device.

Additional Characters

Most of the codes in this Commonly Used Codes list end in the fifth- or sixth-character. Start your search in the "ICD-10-CM Tabular List for Chiropractic" section of the *Complete and Easy ICD-10 Coding for Chiropractic* book at that code number.

Some of the codes end with an underscore, "_". (For example, S13.180_ Subluxation of C7/T1 cervical vertebrae.) The underscore indicates that a seventh character is required. Select it by looking at the choices for the code (S13.180_) in the "ICD-10-CM Tabular List for Chiropractic" section of the *Complete & Easy ICD-10 Coding for Chiropractic* book (Resource 294).

Placeholder X's

Some of the codes contain an "x" in the fifth- or sixth-character. (For example, S03.0xx Dislocation of jaw.) The x is a placeholder that holds the code open at that level for future expansion. Any x characters must be observed and preserved as if they were the future, permanent code designation for the diagnosis.

CERVICAL AND HEAD DIAGNOSES

SUBLUXATION

M99.00	Segmental and somatic dysfunction of head region	S13.110_	Subluxation of C0/C1 cervical vertebrae
M99.01	Segmental and somatic dysfunction of cervical region	S13.120_	Subluxation of C1/C2 cervical vertebrae
		S13.130_	Subluxation of C2/C3 cervical vertebrae
		S13.140_	Subluxation of C3/C4 cervical vertebrae
M99.10	Subluxation complex (vertebral) of head region	S13.150_	Subluxation of C4/C5 cervical vertebrae
M99.11	Subluxation complex (vertebral) of cervical region	S13.160_	Subluxation of C5/C6 cervical vertebrae
		S13.170_	Subluxation of C6/C7 cervical vertebrae
S13.100_	Subluxation of unspecified cervical vertebrae	S13.180_	Subluxation of C7/T1 cervical vertebrae

OTHER CONDITIONS

	Migraine without aura, not intractable		Ankylosing spondylitis of
G43.001	with status migrainosus	M45.1	occipito-atlanto-axial region
G43.009	without status migrainosus	M45.2	cervical region
	Migraine with aura, not intractable	M45.3	cervicothoracic region
G43.101	with status migrainosus		Other spondylosis with myelopathy
G43.109	without status migrainosus	M47.11	occipito-atlanto-axial region
G44.209	Tension-type headache, unspecified, not intractable	M47.12	cervical region
		M47.13	cervicothoracic region
G44.219	Episodic tension-type headache, not intractable		Spondylosis without myelopathy or radiculopathy,
	Chronic tension-type headache,		
G44.221	intractable	M47.811	occipito-atlanto-axial region
G44.229	not intractable	M47.812	cervical region
G54.0	Brachial plexus disorders	M47.813	cervicothoracic region
G54.2	Cervical root disorders, not elsewhere classified		Spinal stenosis,
M26.61	Adhesions and ankylosis of temporomandibular joint	M48.01	occipito-atlanto-axial region
		M48.02	cervical region
M26.62	Arthralgia of temporomandibular joint	M48.03	cervicothoracic region
M26.63	Articular disc disorder of temporomandibular joint		Cervical disc disorder with myelopathy,
		M50.01	occipito-atlanto-axial region
M26.69	Other specified disorders of temporomandibular joint	M50.02	mid-cervical region
		M50.03	cervicothoracic region
M40.03	Postural kyphosis, cervicothoracic region		Cervical disc disorder with radiculopathy,
	Other kyphosis,	M50.11	occipito-atlanto-axial region
M40.292	cervical region	M50.12	mid-cervical region
M40.293	cervicothoracic region	M50.13	cervicothoracic region
	Neuromuscular scoliosis		Other cervical disc displacement,
M41.41	occipito-atlanto-axial region	M50.21	occipito-atlanto-axial region
M41.42	cervical region	M50.22	mid-cervical region
M41.43	cervicothoracic region	M50.23	cervicothoracic region

Never code from this Anatomic Index. It is only the first step to finding a probable code. Refer to the tabular listing for additional required digits and other pertinent coding information.

CERVICAL AND HEAD DIAGNOSES - CONTINUED

OTHER CONDITIONS - CONT.

	Other cervical disc degeneration,	M60.9	Myositis, unspecified
M50.31	occipito-atlanto-axial region	M79.1	Myalgia
M50.32	mid-cervical region	M79.3	Panniculitis, unspecified
M50.33	cervicothoracic region	M79.7	Fibromyalgia
	Other cervical disc disorders,	N94.3	Premenstrual tension syndrome
M50.81	occipito-atlanto-axial region	N95.1	Menopausal and female climacteric states
M50.82	mid-cervical region	Q05.5	Cervical spina bifida without hydrocephalus
M50.83	cervicothoracic region	R51	Headache
	Cervical disc disorder, unspecified,	S03.4xx_	Sprain of jaw
M50.91	occipito-atlanto-axial region	S12._ _ _ _	Fracture of cervical vertebra and other parts of neck
M50.92	mid-cervical region		
M50.93	cervicothoracic region	S13.4xx_	Sprain of ligaments of cervical spine
M53.0	Cervicocranial syndrome	S13.8xx_	Sprain of joints and ligaments of other parts of neck
M53.1	Cervicobrachial syndrome		
M53.82	Other specified dorsopathies, cervical region		
	Radiculopathy,		
M54.11	occipito-atlanto-axial region		
M54.12	cervical region		
M54.13	cervicothoracic region		
M54.2	Cervicalgia		

THORACIC DIAGNOSES

SUBLUXATION

M99.02	Segmental and somatic dysfunction of thoracic region	S23.132_	Subluxation of T5/T6 thoracic vertebra
		S23.140_	Subluxation of T6/T7 thoracic vertebra
M99.12	Subluxation complex (vertebral) of thoracic region	S23.142_	Subluxation of T7/T8 thoracic vertebra
		S23.150_	Subluxation of T8/T9 thoracic vertebra
S23.100_	Subluxation of unspecified thoracic vertebra	S23.152_	Subluxation of T9/T10 thoracic vertebra
S23.110_	Subluxation of T1/T2 thoracic vertebra	S23.160_	Subluxation of T10/T11 thoracic vertebra
S23.120_	Subluxation of T2/T3 thoracic vertebra	S23.162_	Subluxation of T11/T12 thoracic vertebra
S23.122_	Subluxation of T3/T4 thoracic vertebra	S23.170_	Subluxation of T12/L1 thoracic vertebra
S23.130_	Subluxation of T4/T5 thoracic vertebra		

THORACIC DIAGNOSES - CONTINUED

OTHER CONDITIONS

Code	Description
G54.0	Brachial plexus disorders
G54.3	Thoracic root disorders, not elsewhere classified
	Postural kyphosis,
M40.04	thoracic region
M40.05	thoracolumbar region
	Other secondary kyphosis,
M40.14	thoracic region
M40.15	thoracolumbar region
	Unspecified kyphosis,
M40.204	thoracic region
M40.205	thoracolumbar region
	Other kyphosis,
M40.294	thoracic region
M40.295	thoracolumbar region
M40.35	Flatback syndrome, thoracolumbar region
M40.45	Postural lordosis, thoracolumbar region
M40.55	Lordosis, unspecified, thoracolumbar region
	Infantile idiopathic scoliosis,
M41.04	thoracic region
M41.05	thoracolumbar region
	Juvenile idiopathic scoliosis,
M41.114	thoracic region
M41.115	thoracolumbar region
	Adolescent idiopathic scoliosis,
M41.124	thoracic region
M41.125	thoracolumbar region
	Other idiopathic scoliosis,
M41.24	thoracic region
M41.25	thoracolumbar region
	Thoracogenic scoliosis,
M41.34	thoracic region
M41.35	thoracolumbar region
	Neuromuscular scoliosis,
M41.44	thoracic region
M41.45	thoracolumbar region
	Spondylolysis,
M43.04	thoracic region
M43.05	thoracolumbar region
M43.8x9	Other specified deforming dorsopathies, site unspecified
	Ankylosing spondylitis of
M45.4	thoracic region
M45.5	thoracolumbar region
M46.45	Discitis, unspecified, thoracolumbar region
M47.14	Other spondylosis with myelopathy, thoracic region
M47.814	Spondylosis without myelopathy or radiculopathy, thoracic region
	Spinal stenosis,
M48.04	thoracic region
M48.05	thoracolumbar region
	Kissing spine,
M48.24	thoracic region
M48.25	thoracolumbar region
	Intervertebral disc disorders with myelopathy,
M51.04	thoracic region
M51.05	thoracolumbar region
	Intervertebral disc disorders with myelopathy,
M51.04	thoracic region
M51.05	thoracolumbar region
	Other intervertebral disc displacement,
M51.24	thoracic region
M51.25	thoracolumbar region
	Other intervertebral disc degeneration,
M51.34	thoracic region
M51.35	thoracolumbar region
	Schmorl's nodes,
M51.44	thoracic region
M51.45	thoracolumbar region
	Other intervertebral disc disorders,
M51.84	thoracic region
M51.85	thoracolumbar region
M53.1	Cervicobrachial syndrome
M53.9	Dorsopathy, unspecified
M54.08	Panniculitis affecting regions of neck and back, sacral and sacrococcygeal region
	Radiculopathy,
M54.14	thoracic region
M54.15	thoracolumbar region
M54.6	Pain in thoracic spine
M60.9	Myositis, unspecified
M79.1	Myalgia
M79.7	Fibromyalgia

Never code from this Anatomic Index. It is only the first step to finding a probable code. Refer to the tabular listing for additional required digits and other pertinent coding information.

THORACIC DIAGNOSES - CONTINUED

OTHER CONDITIONS - CONT.

M96.1	Postlaminectomy syndrome, not elsewhere classified	S23.41x_	Sprain of ribs
R29.3	Abnormal posture	S23.8xx	Sprain of other specified parts of thorax
S22._ _ _ _	Fracture of rib(s), sternum and thoracic spine		
S23.3xx_	Sprain of ligaments of thoracic spine		

LUMBAR DIAGNOSES

SUBLUXATION

M99.03	Segmental and somatic dysfunction of lumbar region	S33.120_	Subluxation of L2/L3 lumbar vertebra
M99.13	Subluxation complex (vertebral) of lumbar region	S33.130_	Subluxation of L3/L4 lumbar vertebra
S33.100_	Subluxation of unspecified lumbar vertebra	S33.140_	Subluxation of L4/L5 lumbar vertebra
S33.110_	Subluxation of L1/L2 lumbar vertebra		

OTHER CONDITIONS

G54.1	Lumbosacral plexus disorders	M47.817	Spondylosis without myelopathy or radiculopathy, lumbosacral region
G54.4	Lumbosacral root disorders, not elsewhere classified		Spinal stenosis,
G54.8	Other nerve root and plexus disorders	M48.06	lumbar region
M24.50	Contracture, unspecified joint	M48.07	lumbosacral region
M25.60	Stiffness of unspecified joint, not elsewhere classified		Ankylosing hyperostosis [Forestier],
		M48.16	lumbar region
	Neuromuscular scoliosis,	M48.17	lumbosacral region
M41.46	lumbar region		Intervertebral disc disorders with myelopathy,
M41.47	lumbosacral region	M51.06	lumbar region
	Spondylolysis,	M51.07	lumbosacral region
M43.06	lumbar region		Other intervertebral disc displacement,
M43.07	lumbosacral region	M51.26	lumbar region
	Spondylolisthesis,	M51.27	lumbosacral region
M43.16	lumbar region		Other intervertebral disc degeneration,
M43.17	lumbosacral region	M51.36	lumbar region
	Ankylosing spondylitis	M51.37	lumbosacral region
M45.6	lumbar region		Other intervertebral disc disorders,
M45.7	of lumbosacral region	M51.86	lumbar region
	Discitis, unspecified,	M51.87	lumbosacral region
M46.46	lumbar region	M51.27	Other intervertebral disc displacement, lumbosacral region
M46.47	lumbosacral region		
M47.16	Other spondylosis with myelopathy, lumbar region		Radiculopathy,
		M54.15	thoracolumbar region

LUMBAR DIAGNOSES - CONTINUED

Code	Description
M54.16	lumbar region
M54.17	lumbosacral region
M54.5	Low back pain
M54.89	Other dorsalgia
Q05.7	Lumbar spina bifida without hydrocephalus
R26.0	Ataxic gait
R26.1	Paralytic gait
R26.2	Difficulty in walking, not elsewhere classified
R26.89	Other abnormalities of gait and mobility
S32.0_ _ _	Fracture of lumbar vertebra
S33.5xx_	Sprain of ligaments of lumbar spine
S33.8xx_	Sprain of other parts of lumbar spine and pelvis

SACRAL / PELVIC DIAGNOSES

SUBLUXATION

Code	Description
M99.04	Segmental and somatic dysfunction of sacral region
M99.05	Segmental and somatic dysfunction of pelvic region
M99.14	Subluxation complex (vertebral) of sacral region
M99.15	Subluxation complex (vertebral) of pelvic region
S33.8xx_	Sprain of other parts of lumbar spine and pelvis

OTHER CONDITIONS

Code	Description
	Stiffness of
M25.651	right hip, not elsewhere classified
M25.652	left hip, not elsewhere classified
M43.08	Spondylolysis, sacral and sacrococcygeal region
	Fusion of spine,
M43.27	lumbosacral region
M43.28	sacral and sacrococcygeal region
M45.8	Ankylosing spondylitis sacral and sacrococcygeal region
M46.1	Sacroiliitis, not elsewhere classified
M47.817	Spondylosis without myelopathy or radiculopathy, lumbosacral region
M48.08	Spinal stenosis, sacral and sacrococcygeal region
M48.18	Ankylosing hyperostosis [Forestier], sacral and sacrococcygeal region
M53.2x7	Spinal instabilities, lumbosacral region
M53.3	Sacrococcygeal disorders, not elsewhere classified
M54.18	Radiculopathy, sacral and sacrococcygeal region
	Sciatica,
M54.31	right side
M54.32	left side
	Lumbago with sciatica,
M54.41	right side
M54.42	left side
	Trochanteric bursitis,
M70.61	right side
M70.62	left side
	Other bursitis of hip,
M70.71	right side
M70.72	left side
	Psoas tendinitis,
M76.11	right side
M76.12	left side
	Iliac crest spur,
M76.21	right side
M76.22	left side

Never code from this Anatomic Index. It is only the first step to finding a probable code. Refer to the tabular listing for additional required digits and other pertinent coding information.

Sacral / Pelvic Diagnoses - continued

Q05.8	Sacral spina bifida without hydrocephalus		Unspecified sprain of
Q76.2	Congenital spondylolisthesis	S73.101_	right hip
R26.0	Ataxic gait	S73.102_	left hip
R26.1	Paralytic gait		Strain of unspecified muscles, fascia and tendons at thigh level,
R26.2	Difficulty in walking, not elsewhere classified		
R26.89	Other abnormalities of gait and mobility	S76.911_	right thigh
S32.1___	Fracture of sacrum	S76.912_	left thigh
	Sprain of		
S33.6xx_	sacroiliac joint		
S33.8xx_	other parts of lumbar spine and pelvis		

Upper Extremity Diagnoses (extra-spinal)

SUBLUXATION

M99.07	Segmental and somatic dysfunction of upper extremity	S43.2___	sternoclavicular joint
		S43.3___	other and unspecified parts of shoulder girdle
M99.17	Subluxation complex (vertebral) of upper extremity	S53.0___	radial head
		S53.1___	ulnohumeral joint
	Subluxation and dislocation of	S63.0___	wrist and hand joints
S43.0___	shoulder joint	S63.1___	thumb
S43.1___	acromioclavicular joint	S63.2___	other finger(s)

OTHER CONDITIONS

	Carpal tunnel syndrome,	M70.___	Soft tissue disorders related to use, overuse, and pressure
G56.01	right upper limb		
G56.02	left upper limb		Olecranon bursitis,
	Pain in	M70.21	right elbow
M25.511	right shoulder	M70.22	left elbow
M25.512	left shoulder		Adhesive capsulitis of
M25.521	right elbow	M75.01	right shoulder
M25.522	left elbow	M75.02	left shoulder
M25.531	right wrist		Rotator cuff syndrome,
M25.532	left wrist	M75.11	right shoulder
	Stiffness of	M75.12	left shoulder
M25.611	right shoulder, not elsewhere classified		Calcific tendinitis of
M25.612	left shoulder, not elsewhere classified	M75.31	right shoulder
M25.621	right elbow, not elsewhere classified	M75.32	left shoulder
M25.622	left elbow, not elsewhere classified		Bursitis of
M25.631	right wrist, not elsewhere classified	M75.51	right shoulder
M25.632	left wrist, not elsewhere classified	M75.52	left shoulder
M25.641	right hand, not elsewhere classified		
M25.642	left hand, not elsewhere classified		

UPPER EXTREMITY DIAGNOSES (EXTRA-SPINAL) - CONTINUED

OTHER CONDITIONS

	Other shoulder lesions,			Injury of
M75.81	right shoulder		S44._ _ _ _	nerves at shoulder and upper arm level
M75.82	left shoulder		S46._ _ _ _	muscle, fascia and tendon at shoulder and upper arm level
	Medial epicondylitis,		S53.4_ _ _	Sprain of elbow
M77.01	right elbow			Traumatic rupture of
M77.02	left elbow		S63.321_	right radiocarpal ligament
	Lateral epicondylitis,		S63.322_	left radiocarpal ligament
M77.11	right elbow		S63.5_ _ _	Other and unspecified sprain of wrist
M77.12	left elbow			Sprain of other part of
M77.9	Enthesopathy, unspecified		S63.8x1_	right wrist and hand
	Pain in		S63.8x2_	left wrist and hand
M79.641	right hand			
M79.642	left hand			
M79.644	right finger(s)			
M79.645	left finger(s)			
	Sprain of			
S43.4_ _ _	shoulder joint			
S43.5_ _ _	acromioclavicular joint			
S43.6_ _ _	sternoclavicular joint			

Never code from this Anatomic Index. It is only the first step to finding a probable code. Refer to the tabular listing for additional required digits and other pertinent coding information.

Lower Extremity Diagnoses (extra-spinal)

SUBLUXATION

M99.06	Segmental and somatic dysfunction of lower extremity		Subluxation and dislocation of
		S73.0_ _ _	hip
M99.16	Subluxation complex (vertebral) of lower extremity	S83.0_ _ _	patella
		S83.1_ _ _	knee
		S93.0_ _ _	ankle joint
		S93.1_ _ _	toe
		S93.3_ _ _	foot

OTHER CONDITIONS

	Unilateral primary osteoarthritis,	S74._ _ _ _	nerves at hip and thigh level
M17.11	right knee	S76._ _ _ _	muscle, fascia and tendon at hip and thigh level
M17.12	left knee		
	Other specified acquired deformities of		Sprain of
M21.861	right lower leg	S83.4_ _ _	collateral ligament of knee
M21.862	left lower leg	S83.5_ _ _	cruciate ligament of knee
	Ankylosis,	S83.6_ _ _	the superior tibiofibular joint and ligament
M24.661	right knee	S83.9_ _ _	unspecified site of knee
M24.662	left knee		Injury of
M25.5_ _	Pain in joint	S84._ _ _ _	nerves at lower leg level
M25.6_ _	Stiffness of joint, not elsewhere classified	S86._ _ _ _	muscle, fascia and tendon at lower leg level
	Other specified joint disorders,	S93.4_ _ _	Sprain of ankle
M25.861	right knee		Injury of
M25.862	left knee	S94._ _ _ _	nerves at ankle and foot level
M70._ _ _	Soft tissue disorders related to use, overuse, and pressure	S96._ _ _ _	muscle and tendon at ankle and foot level
S73.1_ _ _	Sprain of hip		
	Injury of		

OTHER CONDITIONS (ALPHABETIC)

This section is an alphabetical listing of other conditions which might also be used in a chiropractic setting. This is not an exhaustive list of all ICD-10-CM coding possibilities, but rather some commonly used diagnosis. ICD-10 CM is extensive and many single codes in ICD-9 will map to several different possibilities, therefore this list is only a starting point. In order to review a more comprehensive ICD-10-CM code resource, we suggest the *ICD-10 Coding for Chiropractic* book (Resource 294) or 🖱 FindACode.com.

Code	Description
D50.8	Anemias; other iron deficiency
J20._	Bronchitis; acute
G54.0	Brachial plexus disorders
J68.0	Bronchitis and pneumonitis due to chemicals, gases, fumes and vapors
G56.0_	Carpal tunnel syndrome
G83.4	Cauda equina syndrome
G56.4_	Causalgia of upper limb
G54.2	Cervical root disorders, not elsewhere classified
G90.5_ _	Complex regional pain syndrome I (CRPS I)
G43.A_	Cyclical vomiting
	Diabaetes mellitus
E08._ _	due to underlying condition
E09._ _	drug or chemical induced
E13._ _	Other specified
E10._ _	Type 1
E11._ _	Type 2
D50.1	Dysphagia; sideropenic
N40._	Enlarged prostate
M10.00	Gout; idiopathic, unspecified site
R51	Headache
G44.0_ _ _	cluster headaches and other trigeminal autonomic cephalgias (TAC)
G44.5_ _	complicated headache syndromes
G44.4_ _	drug-induced headache, NEC
G44.8_ _	other specified headache syndromes
G43.C_	periodic headache syndromes in child or adult
G44.3_ _ _	post-traumatic
G44.1	vascular, not elsewhere classified
G44.2_ _ _	tension-type
K64._	Hemorrhoids and perianal venous thrombosis
E78.0	Hypercholesterolemia; pure
K38.0	Hyperplasia of appendix
I10	Hypertension; essential (primary)
E16.2	Hypoglycemia, unspecified
E20._	Hypoparathyroidism
D50.8	Iron deficiency anemias; other
H83.0_	Labyrinthitis
	Lesion(s)
G56.1_	other lesions of median nerve;
G56.3_	radial nerve
G56.2_	ulnar nerve
G54.1	Lumbosacral plexus disorders
G54.4	Lumbosacral root disorders, NEC
H81.0_	Meniere's disease
	Migraine
G43.D_	abdominal
G43.7_ _	chronic, without aura
G43.4_ _	hemiplegic
G43.B_	ophalmoplegic
G43.8_ _	other
G43.6_ _	persistent migraine aura with cerebral infarction
G43.5_ _	persistent migraine aura without cerebral infarction
G43.1_ _	with aura
G43.0_ _	without aura
G43.9_ _	unspecified
G58.7	Mononeuritis multiplex
G56.8_	Mononeuropathies of upper limb; other specified
	Mononeuropathy
G59	in diseases classified elsewhere
G56.9_	of upper limb; unspecified

Do not code from this Alphabetic List. It is only the first step to finding a probable code. Refer to the tabular listing for additional required digits and other pertinent coding information.

Other Conditions (Alphabetic) - continued

	Nerve root and plexus disorder		Sinusitis
G54.9	unspecified	J01.9_	acute
G54.8	other	J01.1_	acute frontal
G54.5	Neuralgic amyotrophy	J01.0_	acute maxillary
H65.9_	Nonsuppurative otitis media; unspecified	J32._	chronic
		G47.3_	Sleep apnea
	Obesity	M06.1	Still's disease; adult-onset
E66.01	morbid (severe), due to excess calories	M26.6_	Temporomandibular joint disorders
E66.9	unspecified	G54.3	Thoracic root disorders, not elsewhere classified
E66.3	Overweight		
		H93.1_ _	Tinnitus
	Phantom limb syndrome		
G54.6	with pain	I83._ _ _	Varicose veins of lower extremities
G54.7	without pain	H81.13	Vertigo; benign paroxysmal, bilateral
J02.9	Pharyngitis; acute	E55.9	Vitamin D deficiency, unspecified
M06.4	Polyarthropathy; inflammatory		
E20.1	Pseudohypoparathyroidism	B02.2_	Zoster with other nervous system involvement
	Rheumatoid		
M05._ _ _	arthritis with rheumatoid factor		
M06.0_ _	arthritis without rheumatoid factor		
M06.9	arthritis, unspecified		
M06.8_ _	arthritis; other specified		
M06.2_ _	bursitis		
M06.3_ _	nodule		

Review: Commonly Used ICD-10-CM Codes

- When should you code from the ICD-10-CM anatomic list? *G-21*
- What does the underscore "_" mean in the ICD-10-CM anatomic list? *G-22*

4. Numeric ICD-9-CM (Tabular) List

This section contains code excerpts from the Numeric ICD-9-CM (Tabular) List of ICD-9-CM codes that pertain to chiropractic. Always code from this Numeric (Tabular) List, which provides the full code descriptions with essential includes and excludes. Use only codes from the Highest Specificity column for coding and claims.

For a complete listing of ICD-9-CM codes see Resource 359.

Numeric Chapters

The complete Numeric List has the following 17 chapters. Code excerpts from selected chapters are included herein:

1. Infectious and Parasitic Diseases (001-139)
2. Neoplasms (140-239) (not included in this book)
3. Endocrine, Nutritional and Metabolic Diseases, and Immunity Disorders (240-279)
4. Diseases of the Blood and Blood-Forming Organs (280-289)
5. Mental Disorders (290-319)
6. Diseases of the Nervous System and Sense Organs (320-389)
7. Diseases of the Circulatory System (390-459)
8. Diseases of the Respiratory System (460-519)
9. Diseases of the Digestive System (520-579)
10. Diseases of the Genitourinary System (580-629)
11. Complications of Pregnancy, Childbirth, and the Puerperium (630-677)
12. Diseases of the Skin and Subcutaneous Tissue (680-709)
13. Diseases of the Musculoskeletal System and Connective Tissue (710-739)
14. Congenital Anomalies (740-759)
15. Certain Conditions Originating in the Perinatal Period (760-779)
16. Symptoms, Signs, and Ill-Defined Conditions (780-799)
17. Injury and Poisoning (800-999)

Coding Conventions

The following coding conventions are used in the Numeric (Tabular) List:

Highest specificity codes are in bold type, in the second column.

Codes of highest specificity, whether they be 3, 4, or 5 digits, always appear in the second column. This column which is indicated with an arrow ↑ at the bottom of the page. Choose codes from this column to report on insurance claim forms.

> Inclusion terms are listed below the code with indentation like this example. These terms may be either be synonyms of the code title or a list of the various conditions assigned to that code. The inclusion terms are not necessarily exhaustive.

NOTES IN SMALL CAPS ARE ADDED BY THE CHIROCODE INSTITUTE

Includes	This note further defines, or gives examples of, the content of the category.
Excludes	The terms following the word "excludes" are to be coded elsewhere as indicated in each instance.
Note	Notes are used to define terms and give coding instructions.
Code first	This note is used for those codes not intended to be used as a principal diagnosis. It requires that the underlying disease (etiology) be coded first, with the code the note is applied to being coded second.
Use additional code	This instruction is placed in those categories where an additional code would give a more complete picture of the diagnosis.
:	Colons are used after an incomplete term which needs one or more of the modifiers following the colon to make it assignable to a given category.
;	A semicolon separates multiple inclusion terms.
( )	Parentheses enclose supplementary words. The terms within the parentheses are referred to as nonessential modifiers.
[ ]	Square brackets enclose synonyms, alternate wordings or explanatory phrases.
italics	Italicized code entries (other than "notes," "includes," and "excludes") cannot be used to identify a principal diagnosis.
NEC	"Not Elsewhere Classifiable." This abbreviation is used when the ICD-9-CM system does not provide a specific code for the patient's condition.
NOS	"Not Otherwise Specified." This abbreviation is the equivalent of 'unspecified' and is used only when the coder lacks the information necessary to code to a more specific four-digit subcategory.
●	Identifies a new diagnosis code added for 2015.
▲	Identifies a revised diagnosis code or subterm for 2015.

5-Digit ICD-9 codes

Q. *Our patient's insurance company is not paying our patient because our diagnostic code is not 5 digits. What can we do?*

A. Determine if a fifth digit exists for the diagnosis code set. If it does, you must use the appropriate five digit code. If it does not, they are not following ICD-9 standards. They are also violating HIPAA transaction standards. Not all ICD-9 codes extend to the 5th digit. Some end at the 3rd digit or the 4th digit. Make sure your coding is at the highest level of specificity. Is there a 5th digit for your diagnosis? Check the Numeric List, if the highest level of ICD-9 specificity is a 3rd or 4th digit only, you are coding correctly. See page G-4: highest specificity coding.

1. INFECTIOUS AND PARASITIC DISEASES (001-139)

Note:
Categories for "late effects" of infections and parasitic diseases are to be found at 137-139.

Includes:
diseases generally recognized as communicable or transmissible as well as a few diseases of unknown but possibly infectious origin

Excludes:
acute respiratory infections (460-466); carrier or suspected carrier of infectious organism (V02.0-V02.9); certain localized infections; influenza (487.0-487.8, 488.0-488.1).

NOTE: SEE ALSO PERSONAL HISTORY OF INFECTIOUS AND PARASITIC DISEASE (V12.0)

VIRAL DISEASES ACCOMPANIED BY EXANTHEM (050-059)

Excludes:
arthropod-borne viral diseases (060.0-066.9); Boston exanthem (048)

- 053 **HERPES ZOSTER**
  Includes:
  shingles; zona
- 053.1 With other nervous system complications
  - 053.10 **With unspecified nervous system complication**
  - 053.12 **Postherpetic trigeminal neuralgia**
  - 053.13 **Postherpetic polyneuropathy**
  - 053.14 **Herpes zoster myelitis**
  - 053.19 **Other**
- 053 Herpes zoster
  - 053.9 **Herpes zoster without mention of complication**
    Herpes zoster NOS

LATE EFFECTS OF INFECTIOUS AND PARASITIC DISEASES (137-139)

- 138 LATE EFFECTS OF ACUTE POLIOMYELITIS
  - 138 **Late effects of acute poliomyelitis**
    Note:
    This category is to be used to indicate conditions classifiable to 045 as the cause of late effects, which are themselves classified elsewhere. The "late effects" include conditions specified as such, or as sequelae, or as due to old or inactive poliomyelitis, without evidence of active disease.

3. ENDOCRINE, NUTRITIONAL AND METABOLIC DISEASES, AND IMMUNITY DISORDERS (240-279)

Excludes:
endocrine and metabolic disturbances specific to the fetus and newborn. (775.0-775.9)

DISORDER OF THE THYROID GLAND (240-246)

- 244 ACQUIRED HYPOTHYRODISM
  Includes:
  athyroidism (acquired); hypothyroidism (acquired); myxedema (adult) (juvenile); thyroid (gland) insufficiency (acquired)
  - 244.9 **Unspecified hypothyrodism**
    Hypothyrodism, primary or NOS; Myxedema, primary or NOS

DISEASES OF OTHER ENDOCRINE GLANDS (249-259)

- 250 DIABETES MELLITUS
  Excludes:
  gestational diabetes (648.8); hyperglycemia NOS (790.29); neonatal diabetes mellitus (775.1); nonclinical diabetes (790.29); secondary diabetes (249.0-249.9)

250.0 Diabetes mellitus without mention of complication

> Diabetes mellitus without mention of complication or manifestation classifiable to 250.1-250.9; Diabetes (mellitus) NOS

- **250.00** type II or unspecified type, not stated as uncontrolled

  Fifth-digit 0 is for use with type II patients, even if the patient requires insulin

  Use additional code, if applicable, for associated long-term (current) insulin use (V58.67)

- **250.01** type I [juvenile type], not stated as uncontrolled

- **250.02** type II or unspecified type, uncontrolled

  Fifth-digit 2 is for use with type II patients, even if the patient requires insulin

  Use additional code, if applicable, for associated long-term (current) insulin use (V58.67)

- **250.03** type I [juvenile type], uncontrolled

250.6 Diabetes with neurological manifestations

Use additional code to identify manifestation, as: diabetic: amyotrophy (353.5); gastroparalysis (536.3); gastroparesis (536.3); mononeuropathy (354.0-355.9); neurogenic arthropathy (713.5); peripheral autonomic neuropathy (337.1); polyneuropathy (357.2)

- **250.60** type II or unspecified type, not stated as uncontrolled

  Fifth-digit 0 is for use with type II patients, even if the patient requires insulin

  Use additional code, if applicable, for associated long-term (current) insulin use (V58.67)

- **250.61** type I [juvenile type], not stated as uncontrolled

- **250.62** type II or unspecified type, uncontrolled

  Fifth-digit 2 is for use with type II patients, even if the patient requires insulin

  Use additional code, if applicable, for associated long-term (current) insulin use (V58.67)

- **250.63** type I [juvenile type], uncontrolled

OTHER METABOLIC AND IMMUNITY DISORDERS (270-279)

Use additional code to identify any associated intellectual disabilities

274 GOUT

> Excludes:
> lead gout (984.0-984.9)

274.0 Gouty arthropathy

- **274.00** Gouty arthropathy, unspecified
- **274.01** Acute gouty arthropathy

  > Acute gout; Gout attack; Gout flare; Podagra

- **274.02** Chronic gouty arthropathy without mention of tophus (tophi)

  > Chronic gout

- **274.03** Chronic gouty arthropathy with tophus (tophi)

  > Chronic tophaceous gout; Gout with tophi NOS

274 Gout

- **274.9** Gout, unspecified

278 OVERWEIGHT, OBESITY AND OTHER HYPERALIMENTATION

> Excludes:
> hyperalimentation NOS (783.6); poisoning by vitamins NOS (963.5); polyphagia (783.6)

278.0 Overweight and obesity

Use additional code to identify Body Mass Index (BMI), if known (V85.0-V85.54)

> Excludes:
> adiposogenital dystrophy (253.8); obesity of endocrine origin NOS (259.9)

- **278.00** Obesity, unspecified

  > Obesity NOS

- **278.01** Morbid obesity

  > Severe obesity

- **278.02** Overweight

5. MENTAL DISORDERS (290-319)

NEUROTIC DISORDERS, PERSONALITY DISORDERS, AND OTHER NONPSYCHOTIC MENTAL DISORDERS (300-316)

NOTE: SEE ALSO PERSONAL HISTORY OF NEUROSIS (V11.2)

300 ANXIETY, DISSOCIATIVE AND SOMATOFORM DISORDERS

- **300.4** **Dysthymic disorder**
  Anxiety depression;
  Depression with anxiety;
  Depressive reaction;
  Neurotic depressive state;
  Reactive depression

  Excludes:
  adjustment reaction with depressive symptoms (309.0-309.1); depression NOS (311); manic-depressive psychosis, depressed type (296.2-296.3); reactive depressive psychosis (298.0)

306 PHYSIOLOGICAL MALFUNCTION ARISING FROM MENTAL FACTORS

NOTE: SEE UNABRIDGED ICD-9 FOR INCLUDES AND EXCLUDES.

- **306.0** **Musculoskeletal**
  Psychogenic paralysis;
  Psychogenic torticollis

  Excludes:
  Gilles de la Tourette's syndrome (307.23); paralysis as hysterical or conversion reaction (300.11); tics (307.20-307.22)

307 SPECIAL SYMPTOMS OR SYNDROMES, NOT ELSEWHERE CLASSIFIED

Note:
This category is intended for use if the psychopathology is manifested by a single specific symptom or group of symptoms which is not part of an organic illness or other mental disorder classifiable elsewhere.

Excludes:
those due to mental disorders classified elsewhere; those of organic origin

- **307.1** **Anorexia nervosa**

  Excludes:
  eating disturbance NOS (307.50);
  feeding problem (783.3)
  of nonorganic origin (307.59);
  loss of appetite (783.0);
  of nonorganic origin (307.59)

- **307.8** Pain disorders related to psychological factors

  - **307.80** **Psychogenic pain, site unspecified**
  - **307.81** **Tension headache**

    Excludes:
    headache: NOS (784.0);
    migraine (346.0-346.9);
    syndromes (339.00-339.89);
    tension type (339.10-339.12)

  - **307.89** **Other**

    <u>Code first</u> to type or site of pain

    Excludes:
    pain disorder exclusively attributed to psychological factors (307.80);
    psychogenic pain (307.80)

310 SPECIFIC NONPSYCHOTIC MENTAL DISORDERS DUE TO BRAIN DAMAGE

Excludes:
neuroses; personality disorders; or other nonpsychotic conditions occurring in a form similar to that seen with functional disorders but in association with a physical condition (300.0-300.9, 301.0-301.9)

NOTE: SEE ALSO PERSONAL HISTORY OF UNSPECIFIED MENTAL DISORDER (V11.9)

- **310.2** **Postconcussion syndrome**
  Postcontusion syndrome or encephalopathy;
  Posttraumatic brain syndrome, nonpsychotic;
  Status postcommotio cerebri

  <u>Use additional code</u> to identify associated post-traumatic headache, if applicable (339.20-339.22)

↑ Highest Specificity Column   ↑ Highest Specificity Column
NOTES IN SMALL CAPS are added by ChiroCode Institute

Excludes:
> frontal lobe syndrome (310.0); postencephalitic syndrome (310.89); any organic psychotic conditions following head injury (293.0-294.0)

6. Diseases of the Nervous System and Sense Organs (320-389)

NOTE: SEE ALSO PERSONAL HISTORY OF DISORDERS OF NERVOUS SYSTEM AND SENSE ORGANS (V12.4)

HEREDITARY AND DEGENERATIVE DISEASES OF THE CENTRAL NERVOUS SYSTEM (330-337)

Excludes:
> hepatolenticular degeneration (275.1); multiple sclerosis (340); other demyelinating diseases of central nervous system (341.0-341.9)

333 OTHER EXTRAPYRAMIDAL DISEASE AND ABNORMAL MOVEMENT DISORDERS

Includes:
> other forms of extrapyramidal, basal ganglia, or striatopallidal disease

Excludes:
> abnormal movements of head NOS (781.0); sleep related movement diorders (327.51-327.59)

NOTE: SEE ALSO PERSONAL HISTORY OF OTHER DISORDERS OF NERVOUS SYSTEM AND SENSE ORGANS (V12.49)

333.8 Fragments of torsion dystonia

Use additional E code, if desired, to identify drug, if drug-induced

333.83 Spasmodic torticollis

Excludes:
> torticollis: NOS (723.5); hysterical (300.11); psychogenic (306.0)

335 ANTERIOR HORN CELL DISEASE

335.1 Spinal muscular atrophy

335.10 Spinal muscular atrophy, unspecified

335.11 Kugelberg-Welander disease
> Spinal muscular atrophy: familial; juvenile

335.19 Other
> Adult spinal muscular atrophy

337 DISORDERS OF THE AUTONOMIC NERVOUS SYSTEM

Includes:
> disorders of peripheral autonomic, sympathetic, parasympathetic, or vegetative system

Excludes:
> familial dysautonomia [Riley-Day syndrome] (742.8)

337.0 Idiopathic peripheral autonomic neuropathy

337.00 Idiopathic peripheral autonomic neuropathy, unspecified

337.01 Carotid sinus syndrome
> Carotid sinus syncope

337.09 Other idiopathic peripheral autonomic neuropathy
> Cervical sympathetic dystrophy or paralysis

337 Disorders of the autonomic nervous system

337.2 Reflex sympathetic dystrophy

337.20 Reflex sympathetic dystrophy, unspecified
> Complex regional pain syndrome type I, unspecified

337.21 Reflex sympathetic dystrophy of the upper limb
> Complex regional pain syndrome type I of the upper limb

337.22 Reflex sympathetic dystrophy of the lower limb
> Complex regional pain syndrome type I of the lower limb

337.29 Reflex sympathetic dystrophy of other specified site
> Complex regional pain syndrome type I of other specified site

PAIN (338)

NOTE: CODES IN CATEGORY 338 MAY BE USED IN CONJUNCTION WITH CODES FROM OTHER CATEGORIES AND CHAPTERS TO PROVIDE MORE DETAIL ABOUT ACUTE OR CHRONIC PAIN AND NEOPLASM-RELATED PAIN UNLESS OTHERWISE INDICATED.

338   PAIN, NOT ELSEWHERE CLASSIFIED

Use additional code to identify: pain associated with psychological factors (307.89)

Excludes:
generalized pain (780.96); headache syndromes (339.00-339.89); localized pain, unspecified type – code to pain by site; migraines (346.0-346.9); pain disorder exclusively attributed to psychological factors (307.80); vulvar vestibulitis (625.71); vulvodynia (625.70-625.79)

338.0   Central pain syndrome
Déjérine-Roussy syndrome; Myelopathic syndrome; Thalamic pain syndrome (hyperesthetic)

338.1   Acute pain

338.11   Acute pain due to trauma

338.18   Other acute postoperative pain
Postoperative pain NOS

338.19   Other acute pain
Excludes:
neoplasm related acute pain (338.3)

338.2   Chronic pain
Excludes:
causalgia (355.9): lower limb (355.71); causalgia (355.9): upper limb (354.4); chronic pain syndrome (338.4); myofascial pain syndrome (729.1); neoplasm related chronic pain (338.3); reflex sympathetic dystrophy (337.20-337.29)

NOTE: CHRONIC PAIN IS CLASSIFIED TO THIS SUBCATEGORY. THERE IS NO TIME FRAME DEFINING WHEN PAIN BECOMES CHRONIC PAIN. THE PROVIDER'S DOCUMENTATION SHOULD BE USED TO GUIDE USE OF THESE CODES.

338.21   Chronic pain due to trauma

338.28   Other chronic postoperative pain

338.29   Other chronic pain

338   Pain, not elsewhere classified

338.4   Chronic pain syndrome
Chronic pain associated with significant psychosocial dysfunction

OTHER HEADACHE SYNDROMES (339)

See Resource 399 for more about using headache and syndrome codes.

339   OTHER HEADACHE SYNDROMES
Excludes:
headache: NOS (784.0); due to lumbar puncture (349.0); migraine (346.0-346.9)

339.0   Cluster headaches and other trigeminal autonomic cephalgias
TACS

339.00   Cluster headache syndrome, unspecified
Ciliary neuralgia; Cluster headache NOS; Histamine cephalgia; Lower half migraine; Migrainous neuralgia

339.01   Episodic cluster headache

339.02   Chronic cluster headache

339.03   Episodic paroxysmal hemicrania
Paroxysmal hemicrania NOS

339.04   Chronic paroxysmal hemicrania

339.05   Short lasting unilateral neuralgiform headache with conjunctival injection and tearing
SUNCT

339.09   Other trigeminal autonomic cephalgias

339.1   Tension type headache
Excludes:
tension headache NOS (307.81); tension headache related to psychological factors (307.81)

339.10   Tension type headache, unspecified

339.11   Episodic tension type headache

339.12   Chronic tension type headache

339.2 Post-traumatic headache
- **339.20** Post-traumatic headache, unspecified
- **339.21** Acute post-traumatic headache
- **339.22** Chronic post-traumatic headache

339 Other headache syndromes
- **339.3** Drug induced headache, not elsewhere classified

  Medication overuse headache; Rebound headache

- **339.4** Complicated headache syndromes
  - **339.41** Hemicrania continua
  - **339.42** New daily persistent headache

    NDPH
  - **339.43** Primary thunderclap headache
  - **339.44** Other complicated headache syndrome

- **339.8** Other specified headache syndromes
  - **339.81** Hypnic headache
  - **339.82** Headache associated with sexual activity

    Orgasmic headache; Preorgasmic headache
  - **339.83** Primary cough headache
  - **339.84** Primary exertional headache
  - **339.85** Primary stabbing headache
  - **339.89** Other specified headache syndromes

OTHER DISORDERS OF THE CENTRAL NERVOUS SYSTEM (340-349)

344 OTHER PARALYTIC SYNDROMES

Includes:

paralysis (complete) (incomplete), except as classifiable to 342 and 343

Excludes:

congenital or infantile cerebral palsy (343.0-343.9), hemiplegia (342.0-342.9), congenital or infantile (343.1, 343.4)

Note: This category is to be used when the listed conditions are reported without further specification or are stated to be old or long-standing but of unspecified cause. The category is also for use in multiple coding to identify these conditions resulting from any cause.

344.6 Cauda equina syndrome
- **344.60** Without mention of neurogenic bladder
- **344.61** With neurogenic bladder

  Cord bladder

  Detrusor hyperreflexia

346 MIGRAINE

NOTE: SEE ALSO 307.81 AND 349.0 FOR OTHER RELATED HEADACHES.

Excludes:

headache: NOS (784.0); syndromes (339.00-339.89)

346.0 Migraine with aura

Basilar migraine; Classic migraine; Migraine preceded or accompanied by transient focal neurological phenomena; Migraine triggered seizures; Migraine with acute-onset aura; Migraine with aura without headache (migraine equivalents); Migraine with prolonged aura; Migraine with typical aura; Retinal migraine

Excludes:

persistent migraine aura (346.5, 346.6)

- **346.00** without mention of intractable migraine without mention of status migrainosus without mention of refractory migraine without mention of status migrainosus
- **346.01** With intractable migraine, so stated, without mention of status migrainosus with refractory migraine, so stated, without mention of status migrainosus
- **346.02** Without mention of intractable migraine with status migrainosus without mention of refractory migraine with status migrainosus
- **346.03** With intractable migraine, so stated, with status migrainosus with refractory migraine, so stated, with status migrainosus

346.1 Migraine without aura

Common migraine

- **346.10** Without mention of intractable migraine without mention of status migrainosus without mention

- **346.11** With intractable migraine, so stated, without mention of status migrainosus with refractory migraine, so stated, without mention of status migrainosus
- **346.12** Without mention of intractable migraine with status migrainosus without mention of refractory migraine with status migrainosus
- **346.13** With intractable migraine, so stated, with status migrainosus with refractory migraine, so stated, with status migrainosus

346.2 Variants of migraine, not elsewhere classified

Abdominal migraine; Cyclical vomiting associated with migraine; Ophthalmoplegic migraine; Periodic headache syndromes in child or adolescent

Excludes:
cyclical vomiting NOS (536.2); psychogenic cyclical vomiting (306.4)

- **346.20** Without mention of intractable migraine without mention of status migrainosus without mention of refractory migraine without mention of status migrainosus
- **346.21** With intractable migraine, so stated, without mention of status migrainosus with refractory migraine, so stated, without mention of status migrainosus
- **346.22** Without mention of intractable migraine with status migrainosus without mention of refractory migraine with status migrainosus
- **346.23** With intractable migraine, so stated, with status migrainosus with refractory migraine, so stated, with status migrainosus

346.3 Hemiplegic migraine

Familial migraine; Sporadic migraine

- **346.30** Without mention of intractable migraine without mention of status migrainosus without mention of refractory migraine without mention of status migrainosus
- **346.31** With intractable migraine, so stated, without mention of status migrainosus with refractory migraine, so stated, without mention of status migrainosus
- **346.32** Without mention of intractable migraine with status migrainosus without mention of refractory migraine with status migrainosus
- **346.33** With intractable migraine, so stated, with status migrainosus with refractory migraine, so stated, with status migrainosus

346.4 Menstrual migraine

Menstrual headache; Menstrually related migraine; Premenstrual headache; Premenstrual migraine; Pure menstrual migraine

- **346.40** Without mention of intractable migraine without mention of status migrainosus without mention of refractory migraine without mention of status migrainosus
- **346.41** With intractable migraine, so stated, without mention of status migrainosus with refractory migraine, so stated, without mention of status migrainosus
- **346.42** Without mention of intractable migraine with status migrainosus without mention of refractory migraine with status migrainosus
- **346.43** With intractable migraine, so stated, with status migrainosus with refractory migraine, so stated, with status migrainosus

346.5 Persistent migraine aura without cerebral infarction

Persistent migraine aura NOS

- 346.50 Without mention of intractable migraine without mention of status migrainosus without mention of refractory migraine without mention of status migrainosus
- 346.51 With intractable migraine, so stated, without mention of status migrainosus with refractory migraine, so stated, without mention of status migrainosus
- 346.52 Without mention of intractable migraine with status migrainosus without mention of refractory migraine with status migrainosus
- 346.53 With intractable migraine, so stated, with status migrainosus with refractory migraine, so stated, with status migrainosus

346.6 Persistent migraine aura with cerebral infarction
- 346.60 Without mention of intractable migraine without mention of status migrainosus without mention of refractory migraine without mention of status migrainosus
- 346.61 With intractable migraine, so stated, without mention of status migrainosus with refractory migraine, so stated, without mention of status migrainosus
- 346.62 Without mention of intractable migraine with status migrainosus without mention of refractory migraine with status migrainosus
- 346.63 With intractable migraine, so stated, with status migrainosus with refractory migraine, so stated, with status migrainosus

346.7 Chronic migraine without aura
  Transformed migraine without aura
- 346.70 Without mention of intractable migraine without mention of status migrainosus without mention of refractory migraine without mention of status migrainosus
- 346.71 With intractable migraine, so stated, without mention of status migrainosus with refractory migraine, so stated, without mention of status migrainosus
- 346.72 Without mention of intractable migraine with status migrainosus without mention of refractory migraine with status migrainosus
- 346.73 With intractable migraine, so stated, with status migrainosus with refractory migraine, so stated, with status migrainosus

346.8 Other forms of migraine
- 346.80 Without mention of intractable migraine without mention of status migrainosus without mention of refractory migraine without mention of status migrainosus
- 346.81 With intractable migraine, so stated, without mention of status migrainosus with refractory migraine, so stated, without mention of status migrainosus
- 346.82 Without mention of intractable migraine with status migrainosus without mention of refractory migraine with status migrainosus
- 346.83 With intractable migraine, so stated, with status migrainosus with refractory migraine, so stated, with status migrainosus

346.9 Migraine, unspecified
  NOTE: USE THIS CODE WHEN THE DIAGNOSIS IS IDENTIFIED AS A "MIGRAINE," BUT IS NOT LISTED ABOVE.
- 346.90 Without mention of intractable migraine without mention of status migrainosus without mention of refractory migraine without mention of status migrainosus
- 346.91 With intractable migraine, so stated, without mention of status migrainosus with refractory migraine, so stated, without mention of status migrainosus

346.92 Without mention of intractable migraine with status migrainosus without mention of refractory migraine with status migrainosus

346.93 With intractable migraine, so stated, with status migrainosus with refractory migraine, so stated, with status migrainosus

DISORDERS OF THE PERIPHERAL NERVOUS SYSTEM (350-359)

Excludes:
diseases of: acoustic [8th] nerve (388.5); oculomotor [3rd, 4th, 6th] nerves (378.0-378.9); optic [2nd] nerve (377.0-377.9); peripheral autonomic nerves (337.0-337.9); neuralgia NOS or "rheumatic" (729.2); neuritis NOS or "rheumatic" (729.2); radiculitis NOS or "rheumatic" (729.2); peripheral neuritis in pregnancy (646.4)

350 TRIGEMINAL NERVE DISORDERS

Includes:
disorders of 5th cranial nerve

350.1 Trigeminal neuralgia
Tic douloureux; Trifacial neuralgia; Trigeminal neuralgia NOS

Excludes:
postherpetic (053.12)

350.2 Atypical face pain

350.8 Other specified trigeminal nerve disorders

350.9 Trigeminal nerve disorders, unspecified

351 FACIAL NERVE DISORDERS

Includes:
disorders of 7th cranial nerve

Excludes:
that in newborn (767.5)

351.0 Bell's palsy
Facial palsy

351.8 Other facial nerve disorders
Facial myokymia; Melkersson's syndrome

352 DISORDERS OF OTHER CRANIAL NERVES

352.0 Disorders of olfactory [1st] nerve

352.1 Glossopharyngeal neuralgia

352.2 Other disorders of glossopharyngeal [9th] nerve

352.3 Disorders of pneumogastric [10th] nerve
Disorders of vagal nerve

Excludes:
paralysis of vocal cords or larynx (478.30-478.34)

352.4 Disorders of accessory [11th] nerve

352.5 Disorders of hypoglossal [12th] nerve

352.6 Multiple cranial nerve palsies
Collet-Sicard syndrome; Polyneuritis cranialis

352.9 Unspecified disorder of cranial nerves

353 NERVE ROOT AND PLEXUS DISORDERS

Excludes:
conditions due to: intervertebral disc disorders (722.0-722.9); spondylosis (720.0-721.9); vertebrogenic disorders (723.0-724.9)

353.0 Brachial plexus lesions
Cervical rib syndrome; Costoclavicular syndrome; Scalenus anticus syndrome; Thoracic outlet syndrome

Excludes:
brachial neuritis or radiculitis NOS (723.4); that in newborn (767.6)

353.1 Lumbosacral plexus lesions

353.2 Cervical root lesions, not elsewhere classified

353.3 Thoracic root lesions, not elsewhere classified

353.4 Lumbosacral root lesions, not elsewhere classified

353.8 Other nerve root and plexus disorders

353.9 Unspecified nerve root and plexus disorder

354 MONONEURITIS OF UPPER LIMB AND MONONEURITIS MULTIPLEX

354.0 Carpal tunnel syndrome
Median nerve entrapment; Partial thenar atrophy

354.1 Other lesion of median nerve
Median nerve neuritis

354.2 Lesion of ulnar nerve
Cubital tunnel syndrome; Tardy ulnar nerve palsy

- **354.3 Lesion of radial nerve**
  Acute radial nerve palsy
- **354.4 Causalgia of upper limb**
  Complex regional pain syndrome type II of the upper limb
  Excludes:
  causalgia: NOS (355.9); lower limb (355.71)
  complex regional pain syndrome type II of the lower limb (355.71)
- **354.5 Mononeuritis multiplex**
  NOTE: SEE ALSO GUILLAIN-BARRE' SYNDROME OR CIDP (CHRONIC INFLAMMATORY DEMYELINATING POLYNEUROPATHY-357.0).
  SEE ALSO DIABETES MELLITUS AND COLLAGEN VASCULAR DISEASE. (COMBINATION OF SINGLE CONDITIONS CLASSIFIABLE TO 354 OR 355).
  Combinations of single conditions classifiable to 354 or 355
- **354.8 Other mononeuritis of upper limb**
- **354.9 Mononeuritis of upper limb, unspecified**

355 MONONEURITIS OF LOWER LIMB AND UNSPECIFIED SITE

- **355.0 Lesion of sciatic nerve**
  Excludes:
  sciatica NOS (724.3)
- **355.1 Meralgia paresthetica**
  Lateral cutaneous femoral nerve of thigh compression or syndrome
- **355.2 Other lesion of femoral nerve**
- **355.3 Lesion of lateral popliteal nerve**
  Lesion of common peroneal nerve
- **355.4 Lesion of medial popliteal nerve**
- **355.5 Tarsal tunnel syndrome**
- **355.6 Lesion of plantar nerve**
  Morton's metatarsalgia, neuralgia, or neuroma
- **355.7 Other mononeuritis of lower limb**
  - **355.71 Causalgia of lower limb**
    Excludes:
    causalgia: NOS (355.9); upper limb (354.4)
    complex regional pain syndrome of upper limb (354.4)
  - **355.79 Other mononeuritis of lower limb**
- **355.8 Mononeuritis of lower limb, unspecified**
- **355.9 Mononeuritis of unspecified site**
  Causalgia NOS; Complex regional pain syndrome NOS
  Excludes:
  causalgia: lower limb (355.71); upper limb (354.4)
  complex regional pain syndrome: lower limb (355.71); upper limb (354.4)

356 HEREDITARY AND IDIOPATHIC PERIPHERAL NEUROPATHY

- **356.0 Hereditary peripheral neuropathy**
  Déjérine-Sottas disease
- **356.1 Peroneal muscular atrophy**
  Charcot-Marie-Tooth disease; Neuropathic muscular atrophy
- **356.4 Idiopathic progressive polyneuropathy**
- **356.8 Other specified idiopathic peripheral neuropathy**
  Supranuclear paralysis
- **356.9 Unspecified**

DISEASES OF THE EAR AND MASTOID PROCESS (380-389)

Use additional external cause code, if applicable, to identify the cause of the ear condition

381 NONSUPPURATIVE OTITIS MEDIA AND EUSTACHIAN TUBE DISORDERS

- **381.4 Nonsuppurative otitis media, not specified as acute or chronic**
  Otitis media: allergic; catarrhal; exudative; mucoid; secretory; seromucinous; serous; transudative; with effusion

386	VERTIGINOUS SYNDROMES AND OTHER DISORDERS OF VESTIBULAR SYSTEM			

386   **VERTIGINOUS SYNDROMES AND OTHER DISORDERS OF VESTIBULAR SYSTEM**

Excludes:
     vertigo NOS (780.4)

386.0   Ménière's disease
     Endolymphatic hydrops; Lermoyez's syndrome; Ménière's syndrome or vertigo

     386.00   **Ménière's disease, unspecified**
         Ménière's disease (active)

     386.01   **Active Ménière's disease, cochleovestibular**

     386.02   **Active Ménière's disease, cochlear**

     386.03   **Active Ménière's disease, vestibular**

386.1   Other and unspecified peripheral vertigo

Excludes:
     epidemic vertigo (078.81)

     386.10   **Peripheral vertigo, unspecified**

     386.11   **Benign paroxysmal positional vertigo**
         Benign paroxysmal positional nystagmus

     386.19   **Other**
         Aural vertigo; Otogenic vertigo

386   Vertiginous syndromes and other disorders of vestibular system

     386.2   **Vertigo of central origin**
         Central positional nystagmus; Malignant positional vertigo

386.3   Labyrinthitis

     386.30   **Labyrinthitis, unspecified**

386   Vertiginous syndromes and other disorders of vestibular system

     386.9   **Unspecified vertiginous syndromes and labyrinthine disorders**

388   OTHER DISORDERS OF EAR

NOTE: SEE ALSO PERSONAL HISTORY OF OTHER DISORDERS OF NERVOUS SYSTEM AND SENSE ORGANS (V12.49).

388.3   Tinnitus

     388.30   **Tinnitus, unspecified**
     388.31   **Subjective tinnitus**
     388.32   **Objective tinnitus**

7. DISEASES OF THE CIRCULATORY SYSTEM (390-459)

HYPERTENSIVE DISEASE (401-405

401   ESSENTIAL HYPERTENSION

Includes:
     high blood pressure; hyperpiesia; hyperpiesis; hypertension (arterial) (essential) (primary) (systemic);
     hypertensive vascular: degeneration; disease

Excludes:
     elevated blood pressure without diagnosis of hypertension (796.2); pulmonary hypertension (416.0-416.9)
     that involving vessels of: brain (430-438); eye (362.11)

     401.0   **Malignant**
     401.1   **Benign**
     401.9   **Unspecified**

9. DISEASES OF THE DIGESTIVE SYSTEM (520-579)

NOTE: SEE ALSO PERSONAL HISTORY OF DIGESTIVE DISEASE (V12.7).

DISEASES OF ORAL CAVITY, SALIVARY GLANDS, AND JAWS (520-529)

524   DENTOFACIAL ANOMALIES, INCLUDING MALOCCLUSION

524.6   Temporomandibular joint disorders

Excludes:
     current temporomandibular joint: dislocation (830.0-830.1); strain (848.1)

     524.60   **Temporomandibular joint disorders, unspecified**
         Temporomandibular joint-pain-dysfunction syndrome [TMJ]

     524.61   **Adhesions and ankylosis (bony or fibrous)**

     524.62   **Arthralgia of temporomandibular joint**

     524.63   **Articular disc disorder (reducing or non-reducing)**

     524.64   **Temporomandibular joint sounds on opening and/or closing the jaw**

     524.69   **Other specified temporomandibular joint disorders**

↑ Highest Specificity Column
NOTES IN SMALL CAPS are added by ChiroCode Institute

↑ Highest Specificity Column

526 DISEASES OF THE JAWS
  526.9 Unspecified disease of the jaws

10. DISEASES OF THE GENITOURINARY SYSTEM (580-629)

OTHER DISORDERS OF FEMALE GENITAL TRACT (617-629)

625 PAIN AND OTHER SYMPTOMS ASSOCIATED WITH FEMALE GENITAL ORGANS
  625.4 **Premenstrual tension syndromes**
    Menstrual molimen; Premenstual dysphoric disorder; Premenstrual syndrome; Premenstrual tension NOS
    Excludes:
      menstrual migraine (346.4)

627 MENOPAUSAL AND POSTMENOPAUSAL DISORDERS
  Excludes:
    asymptomatic age-related (natural) postmenopausal status (V49.81)
  627.2 **Symptomatic menopausal or female climacteric states**
    Symptoms, such as flushing, sleeplessness, headache, lack of concentration, associated with the menopause

13. DISEASES OF THE MUSCULOSKELETAL SYSTEM AND CONNECTIVE TISSUE (710-739)

Use additional external cause code, if applicable, to identify the cause of the musculoskeletal condition

ARTHROPATHIES AND RELATED DISORDERS (710-719)

Excludes:
  disorders of spine (720.0-724.9)

710 DIFFUSE DISEASES OF CONNECTIVE TISSUE
  Includes:
    all collagen diseases whose effects are not mainly confined to a single system
  Excludes:
    those affecting mainly the cardiovascular system, i.e., polyarteritis nodosa and allied conditions (446.0-446.7)

  NOTE: SEE ALSO PERSONAL HISTORY OF ARTHRITIS (V13.4).

  710.0 **Systemic lupus erythematosus**
    Disseminated lupus erythematosus; Libman-Sacks disease

    Use additional code, if desired, to identify manifestation, as: endocarditis (424.91); nephritis (583.81); chronic (582.81); nephrotic syndrome (581.81)

    Excludes:
      lupus erythematosus (discoid) NOS (695.4)

  710.1 **Systemic sclerosis**
    Acrosclerosis; CRST syndrome; Progressive systemic sclerosis; Scleroderma

Use additional code, if desired, to identify manifestation, as: lung involvement (517.2); myopathy (359.6)

Excludes:
  circumscribed scleroderma (701.0)

710.4 Polymyositis

711 ARTHROPATHY ASSOCIATED WITH INFECTIONS

Includes:
  arthritis associated with conditions classifiable below; arthropathy associated with conditions classifiable below; polyarthritis associated with conditions classifiable below; polyarthropathy associated with conditions classifiable below

Excludes:
  rheumatic fever (390)

711.0 Pyogenic arthritis
  Arthritis or polyarthritis (due to): coliform (Escherichia coli); Hemophilus influenzae (H. influenzae); pneumococcal; Pseudomonas; staphylococcal; streptococcal
  Pyarthrosis

Use additional code, if desired, to identify infectious organism (041.0-041.8)

Code	Description
711.00	Site unspecified
711.01	Shoulder region
711.02	Upper arm
711.03	Forearm
711.04	Hand
711.05	Pelvic region and thigh
711.06	Lower leg
711.07	Ankle and foot
711.08	Other specified sites
711.09	Multiple sites

711.1 Arthropathy associated with Reiter's disease and nonspecific urethritis
Code first underlying disease as: nonspecific urethritis (099.4); Reiter's disease (099.3)

Code	Description
711.10	Site unspecified
711.11	Shoulder region
711.12	Upper arm
711.13	Forearm
711.14	Hand
711.15	Pelvic region and thigh
711.16	Lower leg
711.17	Ankle and foot
711.18	Other specified sites
711.19	Multiple sites

NOTE: CODES IN ITALICS CANNOT BE USED TO IDENTIFY A PRINCIPAL DIAGNOSIS

712 CRYSTAL ARTHROPATHIES

Includes:
  crystal-induced arthritis and synovitis

Excludes:
  gouty arthropathy (274.00-274.03)

712.1 Chondrocalcinosis due to dicalcium phosphate crystals
  Chondrocalcinosis due to dicalcium phosphate crystals (with other crystals)

Code first underlying disease (275.4)

Code	Description
712.10	Site unspecified
712.11	Shoulder region
712.12	Upper arm
712.13	Forearm
712.14	Hand
712.15	Pelvic region and thigh
712.16	Lower leg
712.17	Ankle and foot
712.18	Other specified sites
712.19	Multiple sites

NOTE: CODES IN ITALICS CANNOT BE USED TO IDENTIFY A PRINCIPAL DIAGNOSIS

712.2 Chondrocalcinosis due to pyrophosphate crystals
Code first underlying disease (275.4)

Code	Description
712.20	Site unspecified
712.21	Shoulder region
712.22	Upper arm
712.23	Forearm
712.24	Hand
712.25	Pelvic region and thigh
712.26	Lower leg
712.27	Ankle and foot
712.28	Other specified sites
712.29	Multiple sites

NOTE: CODES IN ITALICS CANNOT BE USED TO IDENTIFY A PRINCIPAL DIAGNOSIS

712.3 Chondrocalcinosis, unspecified
Code first underlying disease (275.4)

Code	Description
712.30	Site unspecified
712.31	Shoulder region
712.32	Upper arm
712.33	Forearm
712.34	Hand
712.35	Pelvic region and thigh
712.36	Lower leg

	712.37	**Ankle and foot**
	712.38	**Other specified sites**
	712.39	**Multiple sites**

NOTE: CODES IN ITALICS CANNOT BE USED TO IDENTIFY A PRINCIPAL DIAGNOSIS

714 RHEUMATOID ARTHRITIS AND OTHER INFLAMMATORY POLYARTHROPATHIES

Excludes:

rheumatic fever (390); rheumatoid arthritis of spine NOS (720.0)

714.0 Rheumatoid arthritis

Arthritis or polyarthritis: atrophic; rheumatic (chronic)

Use additional code, if desired, to identify manifestation, as: myopathy (359.6); polyneuropathy (357.1)

Excludes:

juvenile rheumatoid arthritis NOS (714.30)

714.2 Other rheumatoid arthritis with visceral or systemic involvement

Rheumatoid carditis

714.3 JUVENILE CHRONIC POLYARTHRITIS

714.30 Polyarticular juvenile rheumatoid arthritis, chronic or unspecified

Juvenile rheumatoid arthritis NOS; Still's disease

714.31 Polyarticular juvenile rheumatoid arthritis, acute

714.32 Pauciarticular juvenile rheumatoid arthritis

714.33 Monoarticular juvenile rheumatoid arthritis

714 Rheumatoid arthritis and other inflammatory polyarthropathies

714.4 Chronic postrheumatic arthropathy

Chronic rheumatoid nodular fibrositis; Jaccoud's syndrome

714.9 Unspecified inflammatory polyarthropathy

Inflammatory polyarthropathy or polyarthritis NOS

Excludes:

polyarthropathy NOS (716.5)

715 OSTEOARTHROSIS AND ALLIED DISORDERS

Note:

Localized, in the subcategories below, includes bilateral involvement of the same site

Includes:

arthritis or polyarthritis: degenerative; hypertrophic

degenerative joint disease; osteoarthritis

Excludes:

Marie-Strümpell spondylitis (720.0); osteoarthrosis [osteoarthritis] of spine (721.0-721.9)

715.0 Osteoarthrosis, generalized

Degenerative joint disease, involving multiple joints; Primary generalized hypertrophic osteoarthrosis

715.00	**Site unspecified**
715.04	**Hand**
715.09	**Multiple sites**

715.1 Osteoarthrosis, localized, primary

Localized osteoarthropathy; idiopathic

715.10	**Site unspecified**
715.11	**Shoulder region**
715.12	**Upper arm**
715.13	**Forearm**
715.14	**Hand**
715.15	**Pelvic region and thigh**
715.16	**Lower Leg**
715.17	**Ankle and foot**
715.18	**Other specified sites**

715.2 Osteoarthrosis, localized, secondary

Coxae malum senilis

715.20	**Site unspecified**
715.21	**Shoulder region**
715.22	**Upper arm**
715.23	**Forearm**
715.24	**Hand**
715.25	**Pelvic region and thigh**
715.26	**Lower leg**
715.27	**Ankle and foot**
715.28	**Other specified sites**

715.3 Osteoarthrosis, localized, not specified whether primary or secondary
> Otto's pelvis

- **715.30** Site unspecified
- **715.31** Shoulder region
- **715.32** Upper arm
- **715.33** Forearm
- **715.34** Hand
- **715.35** Pelvic region and thigh
- **715.36** Lower leg
- **715.37** Ankle and foot
- **715.38** Other specified sites

715.8 Osteoarthrosis involving, or with mention of more than one site, but not specified as generalized

- **715.80** Site unspecified
- **715.89** Multiple sites

715.9 Osteoarthrosis, unspecified whether generalized or localized

- **715.90** Site unspecified
- **715.91** Shoulder region
- **715.92** Upper arm
- **715.93** Forearm
- **715.94** Hand
- **715.95** Pelvic region and thigh
- **715.96** Lower leg
- **715.97** Ankle and foot
- **715.98** Other specified sites

716 OTHER AND UNSPECIFIED ARTHROPATHIES

Excludes:
> cricoarytenoid arthropathy (478.79)

NOTE: SEE ALSO PERSONAL HISTORY OF OTHER MUSCULOSKELETAL DISORDERS (V13.5).

716.1 Traumatic arthropathy

- **716.10** Site unspecified
- **716.11** Shoulder region
- **716.12** Upper arm
- **716.13** Forearm
- **716.14** Hand
- **716.15** Pelvic region and thigh
- **716.16** Lower leg
- **716.17** Ankle and foot
- **716.18** Other specified sites
- **716.19** Multiple sites

716.6 Unspecified monoarthritis
> Coxitis

- **716.60** Site unspecified
- **716.61** Shoulder region
- **716.62** Upper arm
- **716.63** Forearm
- **716.64** Hand
- **716.65** Pelvic region and thigh
- **716.66** Lower leg
- **716.67** Ankle and foot
- **716.68** Other specified sites

716.8 Other specified arthropathy

- **716.80** Site unspecified
- **716.81** Shoulder region
- **716.82** Upper arm
- **716.83** Forearm
- **716.84** Hand
- **716.85** Pelvic region and thigh
- **716.86** Lower leg
- **716.87** Ankle and foot
- **716.88** Other specified sites
- **716.89** Multiple sites

716.9 Arthropathy, unspecified
> Arthritis (acute) (chronic) (subacute); Arthropathy (acute) (chronic) (subacute); Articular rheumatism (chronic); Inflammation of joint NOS

- **716.90** Site unspecified
- **716.91** Shoulder region
- **716.92** Upper arm
- **716.93** Forearm
- **716.94** Hand
- **716.95** Pelvic region and thigh
- **716.96** Lower leg
- **716.97** Ankle and foot
- **716.98** Other specified sites
- **716.99** Multiple sites

717 INTERNAL DERANGEMENT OF KNEE

Includes:
> degeneration of articular cartilage or meniscus of knee; rupture, old of articular cartilage or meniscus of knee; tear, old of articular cartilage or meniscus of knee

Excludes:
> acute derangement of knee (836.0-836.6); ankylosis (718.5); contracture (718.4); current injury (836.0-836.6); deformity (736.4-736.6); recurrent dislocation (718.3)

	717.0	Old bucket handle tear of medial meniscus	717		Internal derangement of knee
		Old bucket handle tear of unspecified cartilage		717.9	Unspecified internal derangement of knee
	717.1	Derangement of anterior horn of medial meniscus			Derangement NOS of knee
	717.2	Derangement of posterior horn of medial meniscus	718		OTHER DERANGEMENT OF JOINT

717.3 **Other and unspecified derangement of medial meniscus**

    Degeneration of internal semilunar cartilage

717.4 Derangement of lateral meniscus

  717.40 **Derangement of lateral meniscus, unspecified**

  717.41 **Bucket handle tear of lateral meniscus**

  717.42 **Derangement of anterior horn of lateral meniscus**

  717.43 **Derangement of posterior horn of lateral meniscus**

  717.49 **Other**

717 Internal derangement of knee

  717.5 **Derangement of meniscus, not elsewhere classified**

    Congenital discoid meniscus; Cyst of semilunar cartilage; Derangement of semilunar cartilage NOS

  717.6 **Loose body in knee**

    Joint mice, knee; Rice bodies, knee (joint)

  717.7 **Chondromalacia of patella**

    Chondromalacia patellae; Degeneration [softening] of articular cartilage of patella

717.8 Other internal derangement of knee

  717.81 **Old disruption of lateral collateral ligament**

  717.82 **Old disruption of medial collateral ligament**

  717.83 **Old disruption of anterior cruciate ligament**

  717.84 **Old disruption of posterior cruciate ligament**

  717.85 **Old disruption of other ligaments of knee**

    Capsular ligament of knee

  717.89 **Other**

    Old disruption of ligaments of knee NOS

718 OTHER DERANGEMENT OF JOINT

Excludes:

  current injury (830.0-848.9); jaw (524.60-524.69)

NOTE: SEE ALSO PERSONAL HISTORY OF OTHER MUSCULOSKELETAL DISORDERS (V13.5).

718.0 Articular cartilage disorder

  Meniscus: disorder; rupture, old; tear, old;

  Old rupture of ligament(s) of joint NOS

Excludes:

  articular cartilage disorder: in ochronosis (270.2); knee (717.0-717.9);

  chondrocalcinosis (275.4); metastatic calcification (275.4)

  718.00 **Site unspecified**
  718.01 **Shoulder region**
  718.02 **Upper arm**
  718.03 **Forearm**
  718.04 **Hand**
  718.05 **Pelvic region and thigh**
  718.07 **Ankle and foot**
  718.08 **Other specified sites**
  718.09 **Multiple sites**

718.1 Loose body in joint

  Joint mice

Excludes:

  knee (717.6)

  718.10 **Site unspecified**
  718.11 **Shoulder region**
  718.12 **Upper arm**
  718.13 **Forearm**
  718.14 **Hand**
  718.15 **Pelvic region and thigh**
  718.17 **Ankle and foot**
  718.18 **Other specified sites**
  718.19 **Multiple sites**

718.3 Recurrent dislocation of joint

  718.30 **Site unspecified**
  718.31 **Shoulder region**
  718.32 **Upper arm**
  718.33 **Forearm**
  718.34 **Hand**

	718.35	Pelvic region and thigh
	718.36	Lower leg
	718.37	Ankle and foot
	718.38	Other specified sites
	718.39	Multiple sites
718.4	Contracture of joint	
	718.40	Site unspecified
	718.41	Shoulder region
	718.42	Upper arm
	718.43	Forearm
	718.44	Hand
	718.45	Pelvic region and thigh
	718.46	Lower leg
	718.47	Ankle and foot
	718.48	Other specified sites
	718.49	Multiple sites
718.5	Ankylosis of joint	

Ankylosis of joint (fibrous) (osseous)

Excludes:
spine (724.9); stiffness of joint without mention of ankylosis (719.5)

	718.50	Site unspecified
	718.51	Shoulder region
	718.52	Upper arm
	718.53	Forearm
	718.54	Hand
	718.55	Pelvic region and thigh
	718.56	Lower leg
	718.57	Ankle and foot
	718.58	Other specified sites
	718.59	Multiple sites
718.7	Developmental dislocation of joint	

Excludes:
congenital dislocation of joint (754.0-755.8); traumatic dislocation of joint (830-839)

	718.70	Site unspecified
	718.71	Shoulder region
	718.72	Upper arm
	718.73	Forearm
	718.74	Hand
	718.75	Pelvic region and thigh
	718.76	Lower leg
	718.77	Ankle and foot
	718.78	Other specified sites
	718.79	Multiple sites

718.8	Other joint derangement, not elsewhere classified

Flail joint (paralytic); Instability of joint

Excludes:
deformities classifiable to 736 (736.0-736.9)

	718.80	Site unspecified
	718.81	Shoulder region
	718.82	Upper arm
	718.83	Forearm
	718.84	Hand
	718.85	Pelvic region and thigh
	718.86	Lower leg
	718.87	Ankle and foot
	718.88	Other specified sites
	718.89	Multiple sites
719	OTHER AND UNSPECIFIED DISORDERS OF JOINT	

Excludes:
jaw (524.60-524.69)

NOTE: SEE ALSO PERSONAL HISTORY OF OTHER MUSCULOSKELETAL DISORDERS (V13.5).

719.0	Effusion of joint	

Hydrarthrosis; Swelling of joint, with or without pain

Excludes:
intermittent hydrarthrosis (719.3)

	719.00	Site unspecified
	719.01	Shoulder region
	719.02	Upper arm
	719.03	Forearm
	719.04	Hand
	719.05	Pelvic region and thigh
	719.06	Lower leg
	719.07	Ankle and foot
	719.08	Other specified sites
	719.09	Multiple sites
719.1	Hemarthrosis	

Excludes:
current injury (840.0-848.9)

	719.10	Site unspecified
	719.11	Shoulder region
	719.12	Upper arm
	719.13	Forearm
	719.14	Hand
	719.15	Pelvic region and thigh
	719.16	Lower leg
	719.17	Ankle and foot

	719.18	Other specified sites
	719.19	Multiple sites
719.3		Palindromic rheumatism

   Hench-Rosenberg syndrome; Intermittent hydrarthrosis

	719.30	Site unspecified
	719.31	Shoulder region
	719.32	Upper arm
	719.33	Forearm
	719.34	Hand
	719.35	Pelvic region and thigh
	719.36	Lower leg
	719.37	Ankle and foot
	719.38	Other specified sites
	719.39	Multiple sites
719.4		Pain in joint

   Arthralgia

	719.40	Site unspecified
	719.41	Shoulder region
	719.42	Upper arm
	719.43	Forearm
	719.44	Hand
	719.45	Pelvic region and thigh
	719.46	Lower leg
	719.47	Ankle and foot
	719.48	Other specified sites
	719.49	Multiple sites
719.5		Stiffness of joint, not elsewhere classified
	719.50	Site unspecified
	719.51	Shoulder region
	719.52	Upper arm
	719.53	Forearm
	719.54	Hand
	719.55	Pelvic region and thigh
	719.56	Lower leg
	719.57	Ankle and foot
	719.58	Other specified sites
	719.59	Multiple sites
719.6		Other symptoms referable to joint

   Joint crepitus; Snapping hip

	719.60	Site unspecified
	719.61	Shoulder region
	719.62	Upper arm
	719.63	Forearm
	719.64	Hand
	719.65	Pelvic region and thigh
	719.66	Lower leg
	719.67	Ankle and foot
	719.68	Other specified sites
	719.69	Multiple sites
719		Other and unspecified disorders of joint
	719.7	Difficulty in walking

Excludes:
   abnormality of gait (781.2)

719.8		Other specified disorders of joint

   Calcification of joint; Fistula of joint

Excludes:
   temporomandibular joint-pain-dysfunction syndrome [Costen's syndrome] (524.60)

	719.80	Site unspecified
	719.81	Shoulder region
	719.82	Upper arm
	719.83	Forearm
	719.84	Hand
	719.85	Pelvic region and thigh
	719.86	Lower leg
	719.87	Ankle and foot
	719.88	Other specified sites
	719.89	Multiple sites
719.9		Unspecified disorder of joint
	719.90	Site unspecified
	719.91	Shoulder region
	719.92	Upper arm
	719.93	Forearm
	719.94	Hand
	719.95	Pelvic region and thigh
	719.96	Lower leg
	719.97	Ankle and foot
	719.98	Other specified sites
	719.99	Multiple sites

DORSOPATHIES (720-724)

Excludes:

curvature of spine (737.0-737.9); osteochondrosis of spine (juvenile) (732.0); adult (732.8)

720		ANKYLOSING SPONDYLITIS AND OTHER INFLAMMATORY SPONDYLOPATHIES
	720.0	Ankylosing spondylitis

   Rheumatoid arthritis of spine NOS

   Spondylitis: Marie-Strümpell; rheumatoid

	720.1	Spinal enthesopathy

   Disorder of peripheral ligamentous or muscular attachments of spine;

Romanus lesion

720.2 Sacroiliitis, not elsewhere classified
Inflammation of sacroiliac joint NOS

720.8 Other inflammatory spondylopathies

720.81 Inflammatory spondylopathies in diseases classified elsewhere
Code first underlying disease, *as:* tuberculosis (015.0)
NOTE: CODES IN ITALICS CANNOT BE USED TO IDENTIFY A PRINCIPAL DIAGNOSIS

720.89 Other

720 Ankylosing spondylitis and other inflammatory spondylopathies

720.9 Unspecified inflammatory spondylopathy
Spondylitis NOS

721 SPONDYLOSIS AND ALLIED DISORDERS

721.0 Cervical spondylosis without myelopathy
Cervical or cervicodorsal: arthritis; osteoarthritis; spondylarthritis

721.1 Cervical spondylosis with myelopathy
Anterior spinal artery compression syndrome; Spondylogenic compression of cervical spinal cord; Vertebral artery compression syndrome

721.2 Thoracic spondylosis without myelopathy
Thoracic: arthritis; osteoarthritis; spondylarthritis

721.3 Lumbosacral spondylosis without myelopathy
Lumbar or lumbosacral: arthritis; osteoarthritis; spondylarthritis

721.4 Thoracic or lumbar spondylosis with myelopathy

721.41 Thoracic region
Spondylogenic compression of thoracic spinal cord

721.42 Lumbar region

721 Spondylosis and allied disorders

721.5 Kissing spine
Baastrup's syndrome

721.6 Ankylosing vertebral hyperostosis

721.7 Traumatic spondylopathy
Kümmell's disease or spondylitis

721.8 Other allied disorders of spine

721.9 Spondylosis of unspecified site

721.90 Without mention of myelopathy
Spinal: arthritis (deformans) (degenerative) (hypertrophic); osteoarthritis NOS
Spondylarthrosis NOS

721.91 With myelopathy
Spondylogenic compression of spinal cord NOS

722 INTERVERTEBRAL DISC DISORDERS

722.0 Displacement of cervical intervertebral disc without myelopathy
Neuritis (brachial) or radiculitis due to displacement or rupture of cervical intervertebral disc; Any condition classifiable to 722.2 of the cervical or cervicothoracic intervertebral disc

722.1 Displacement of thoracic or lumbar intervertebral disc without myelopathy

722.10 Lumbar intervertebral disc without myelopathy
Lumbago or sciatica due to displacement of intervertebral disc; Neuritis or radiculitis due to displacement or rupture of lumbar intervertebral disc; Any condition classifiable to 722.2 of the lumbar or lumbosacral intervertebral disc

722.11 Thoracic intervertebral disc without myelopathy
Any condition classifiable to 722.2 of thoracic intervertebral disc

722	Intervertebral disc disorders

- **722.2 Displacement of intervertebral disc, site unspecified, without myelopathy**

    Discogenic syndrome NOS; Herniation of nucleus pulposus NOS

    Intervertebral disc NOS: extrusion; prolapse; protrusion; rupture

    Neuritis or radiculitis due to displacement or rupture of intervertebral disc

- 722.3 Schmorl's nodes
    - **722.30 Unspecified region**
    - **722.31 Thoracic region**
    - **722.32 Lumbar region**
    - **722.39 Other**

722	Intervertebral disc disorders

- **722.4 Degeneration of cervical intervertebral disc**

    Degeneration of cervicothoracic intervertebral disc

- 722.5 Degeneration of thoracic or lumbar intervertebral disc
    - **722.51 Thoracic or thoracolumbar intervertebral disc**
    - **722.52 Lumbar or lumbosacral intervertebral disc**

722	Intervertebral disc disorders

- **722.6 Degeneration of intervertebral disc, site unspecified**

    Degenerative disc disease NOS; Narrowing of intervertebral disc or space NOS

- 722.7 Intervertebral disc disorder with myelopathy
    - **722.70 Unspecified region**
    - **722.71 Cervical region**
    - **722.72 Thoracic region**
    - **722.73 Lumbar region**
- 722.8 Postlaminectomy syndrome
    - **722.80 Unspecified region**
    - **722.81 Cervical region**
    - **722.82 Thoracic region**
    - **722.83 Lumbar region**

- 722.9 Other and unspecified disc disorder

    Calcification of intervertebral cartilage or disc; Discitis

    - **722.90 Unspecified region**
    - **722.91 Cervical region**
    - **722.92 Thoracic region**
    - **722.93 Lumbar region**

723	OTHER DISORDERS OF CERVICAL REGION

Excludes:

    conditions due to: intervertebral disc disorders (722.0-722.9); spondylosis (721.0-721.9)

NOTE: SEE ALSO PERSONAL HISTORY OF OTHER MUSCULOSKELETAL DISORDERS (V13.5).

- **723.0 Spinal stenosis in cervical region**
- **723.1 Cervicalgia**

    Pain in neck

- **723.2 Cervicocranial syndrome**

    Barré-Liéou syndrome; Posterior cervical sympathetic syndrome

    CAUTION: DO NOT USE IN PLACE OF COMMON HEAD AND NECK PAIN. THIS CONDITION COULD BE CONSIDERED AN ADVANCED NEUROLOGIC DISORDER.

- **723.3 Cervicobrachial syndrome (diffuse)**
- **723.4 Brachial neuritis or radiculitis NOS**

    Cervical radiculitis; Radicular syndrome of upper limbs

- **723.5 Torticollis, unspecified**

    Contracture of neck

    Excludes:

        congenital (754.1); due to birth injury (767.8); hysterical (300.11); ocular torticollis (781.93); psychogenic (306.0); spasmodic (333.83); traumatic, current (847.0)

- **723.6 Panniculitis specified as affecting neck**
- **723.7 Ossification of posterior longitudinal ligament in cervical region**

723.8 **Other syndromes affecting cervical region**
> Cervical syndrome NEC; Klippel's disease; Occipital neuralgia

723.9 **Unspecified musculoskeletal disorders and symptoms referable to neck**
> Cervical (region) disorder NOS

724 **OTHER AND UNSPECIFIED DISORDERS OF BACK**

Excludes:
> *collapsed vertebra (code to cause, eg, osteoporosis, 733.00-733.09)*
>
> *conditions due to: intervertebral disc disorders (722.0-722.9); spondylosis (721.0-721.9)*

NOTE: SEE ALSO PERSONAL HISTORY OF OTHER MUSCULOSKELETAL DISORDERS (V13.5).

724.0 Spinal stenosis, other than cervical
- **724.00** **Spinal stenosis, unspecified region**
- **724.01** **Thoracic region**
- **724.02** **Lumbar region without neurogenic claudication**
  > Lumbar region NOS
- **724.03** **Lumbar region, with neurogenic claudication**
- **724.09** **Other**

724 Other and unspecified disorders of back
- **724.1** **Pain in thoracic spine**
- **724.2** **Lumbago**
  > Low back pain; Low back syndrome; Lumbalgia
- **724.3** **Sciatica**
  > Neuralgia or neuritis of sciatic nerve
  >
  > *Excludes:*
  > *specified lesion of sciatic nerve (355.0)*
- **724.4** **Thoracic or lumbosacral neuritis or radiculitis, unspecified**
  > Radicular syndrome of lower limbs
- **724.5** **Backache, unspecified**
  > Vertebrogenic (pain) syndrome NOS
- **724.6** **Disorders of sacrum**
  > Ankylosis, lumbosacral or sacroiliac (joint); Instability, lumbosacral or sacroiliac (joint)

724.7 Disorders of coccyx
- **724.70** **Unspecified disorder of coccyx**
- **724.71** **Hypermobility of coccyx**
- **724.79** **Other**
  > Coccygodynia

724 Other and unspecified disorders of back
- **724.8** **Other symptoms referable to back**
  > Ossification of posterior longitudinal ligament NOS; Panniculitis specified as sacral or affecting back
- **724.9** **Other unspecified back disorders**
  > Ankylosis of spine NOS; Compression of spinal nerve root NEC; Spinal disorder NOS
  >
  > *Excludes:*
  > *sacroiliitis (720.2)*

RHEUMATISM, EXCLUDING THE BACK (725-729)

Includes:
disorders of muscles and tendons and their attachments, and of other soft tissues

725 POLYMYALGIA RHEUMATICA
- **725** **Polymyalgia rheumatica**

726 PERIPHERAL ENTHESOPATHIES AND ALLIED SYNDROMES

Note:
Enthesopathies are disorders of peripheral ligamentous or muscular attachments.

Excludes:
spinal enthesopathy (720.1)

- **726.0** **Adhesive capsulitis of shoulder**

726.1 Rotator cuff syndrome of shoulder and allied disorders
- **726.10** **Disorders of bursae and tendons in shoulder region, unspecified**
  > Rotator cuff syndrome NOS; Supraspinatus syndrome NOS
- **726.11** **Calcifying tendinitis of shoulder**
- **726.12** **Bicipital tenosynovitis**
- **726.13** **Partial tear of rotator cuff**
  > *Excludes:*
  > *complete rupture of rotator cuff, nontraumatic (727.61)*

726.19 Other specified disorders
Excludes:
complete rupture of rotator cuff, nontraumatic (727.61)

726 Peripheral enthesopathies and allied syndromes

726.2 Other affections of shoulder region, not elsewhere classified
Periarthritis of shoulder; Scapulohumeral fibrositis

726.3 Enthesopathy of elbow region

726.30 Enthesopathy of elbow, unspecified

726.31 Medial epicondylitis

726.32 Lateral epicondylitis
Epicondylitis NOS; Golfers' elbow; Tennis elbow

726.33 Olecranon bursitis
Bursitis of elbow

726.39 Other

726 Peripheral enthesopathies and allied syndromes

726.4 Enthesopathy of wrist and carpus
Bursitis of hand or wrist; Periarthritis of wrist

726.5 Enthesopathy of hip region
Bursitis of hip; Gluteal tendinitis; Iliac crest spur; Psoas tendinitis; Trochanteric tendinitis

726.6 Enthesopathy of knee

726.60 Enthesopathy of knee, unspecified
Bursitis of knee NOS

726.61 Pes anserinus tendinitis or bursitis

726.62 Tibial collateral ligament bursitis
Pellegrini-Stieda syndrome

726.63 Fibular collateral ligament bursitis

726.64 Patellar tendinitis

726.65 Prepatellar bursitis

726.69 Other
Bursitis: infrapatellar; subpatellar

726.7 Enthesopathy of ankle and tarsus

726.70 Enthesopathy of ankle and tarsus, unspecified
Metatarsalgia NOS
Excludes:
Morton's metatarsalgia (355.6)

726.71 Achilles bursitis or tendinitis

726.72 Tibialis tendinitis
Tibialis (anterior) (posterior) tendinitis

726.73 Calcaneal spur

726.79 Other
Peroneal tendinitis

726 Peripheral enthesopathies and allied syndromes

726.8 Other peripheral enthesopathies

726.9 Unspecified enthesopathy

726.90 Enthesopathy of unspecified site
Capsulitis NOS; Periarthritis NOS; Tendinitis NOS

726.91 Exostosis of unspecified site
Bone spur NOS

727 OTHER DISORDERS OF SYNOVIUM, TENDON, AND BURSA
NOTE: SEE ALSO PERSONAL HISTORY OF OTHER MUSCULOSKELETAL DISORDERS (V13.5).

727.0 Synovitis and tenosynovitis

727.00 Synovitis and tenosynovitis, unspecified
Synovitis NOS; Tenosynovitis NOS

727.01 *Synovitis and tenosynovitis in diseases classified elsewhere*
<u>Code first</u> underlying disease as: tuberculosis (015.0-015.9)
Excludes:
crystal-induced (275.4); gonococcal (098.51); gouty (274.00-274.03); syphilitic (095.7)
NOTE: CODES IN ITALICS CANNOT BE USED TO IDENTIFY A PRINCIPAL DIAGNOSIS

727.03 Trigger finger (acquired)

727.04 Radial styloid tenosynovitis
de Quervain's disease

727.05 Other tenosynovitis of hand and wrist

	727.06	Tenosynovitis of foot and ankle
	727.09	Other
727	Other disorders of synovium, tendon, and bursa	
	727.1	Bunion
	727.2	Specific bursitides often of occupational origin

        Beat: elbow; hand; knee

        Chronic crepitant synovitis of wrist

        Miners': elbow; knee

	727.3	Other bursitis

        Bursitis NOS

Excludes:

    bursitis:

        gonococcal (098.52);
        subacromial (726.19);
        subcoracoid (726.19);
        subdeltoid (726.19);
        syphilitic (095.7);"frozen shoulder"(726.0)

727.4	Ganglion and cyst of synovium, tendon, and bursa	
	727.40	Synovial cyst, unspecified

Excludes:

    that of popliteal space (727.51)

	727.41	Ganglion of joint
	727.42	Ganglion of tendon sheath
	727.43	Ganglion, unspecified
	727.49	Other

        Cyst of bursa

727.5	Rupture of synovium	
	727.50	Rupture of synovium, unspecified
	727.51	Synovial cyst of popliteal space

        Baker's cyst (knee)

	727.59	Other
727.8	Other disorders of synovium, tendon, and bursa	
	727.81	Contracture of tendon (sheath)

        Short Achilles tendon (acquired)

	727.82	Calcium deposits in tendon and bursa

        Calcification of tendon NOS; Calcific tendinitis NOS

Excludes:

    peripheral ligamentous or muscular attachments (726.0-726.9)

	727.83	Plica syndrome

        Plica knee

	727.89	Other

        Abscess of bursa or tendon

Excludes:

    xanthomatosis localized to tendons (272.7)

727	Other disorders of synovium, tendon, and bursa	
	727.9	Unspecified disorder of synovium, tendon, and bursa
728	DISORDERS OF MUSCLE, LIGAMENT, AND FASCIA	

Excludes:

    enthesopathies (726.0-726.9); muscular dystrophies (359.0-359.1); myoneural disorders (358.00-358.9); myopathies (359.2-359.9); nontraumatic hematoma of muscle (729.92); old disruption of ligaments of knee (717.81-717.89)

	728.0	Infective myositis

        Myositis: purulent; suppurative

Excludes:

    myositis: epidemic (074.1); interstitial (728.81); syphilitic (095.6); tropical (040.81)

728.1	Muscular calcification and ossification	
	728.10	Calcification and ossification, unspecified

        Massive calcification (paraplegic)

	728.11	Progressive myositis ossificans
	728.12	Traumatic myositis ossificans

        Myositis ossificans (circumscripta)

	728.19	Other

        Polymyositis ossificans

728 Disorders of muscle, ligament, and fascia

728.2 **Muscular wasting and disuse atrophy, not elsewhere classified**

Amyotrophia NOS; Myofibrosis

Excludes:

neuralgic amyotrophy (353.5); pelvic muscle wasting and disuse atrophy (618.83); progressive muscular atrophy (335.0-335.9)

728.3 **Other specific muscle disorders**

Arthrogryposis; Immobility syndrome (paraplegic)

Excludes:

arthrogryposis multiplex congenita (754.89); stiff-man syndrome (333.91)

728.4 **Laxity of ligament**

728.5 **Hypermobility syndrome**

728.6 **Contracture of palmar fascia**

Dupuytren's contracture

NOTE: SEE AND CODE ALSO GOUT, ARTHRITIS, DIABETES, EPILEPSY AND ALCOHOLISM WHEN FOUND.

728.7 Other fibromatoses

728.71 **Plantar fascial fibromatosis**

Contracture of plantar fascia; Plantar fasciitis (traumatic)

728.79 **Other**

Garrod's or knuckle pads; Nodular fasciitis; Pseudosarcomatous Fibromatosis (proliferative) (subcutaneous)

728.8 Other disorders of muscle, ligament, and fascia

728.81 **Interstital myositis**

728.83 **Rupture of muscle, nontraumatic**

728.85 **Spasm of muscle**

728.87 **Muscle weakness (generalized)**

Excludes:

generalized weakness (780.79)

728.88 **Rhabdomyolysis**

728.89 **Other**

Eosinophilic fasciitis

Use additional E code, if desired, to identify drug, if drug induced

728 Disorders of muscle, ligament, and fascia

728.9 **Unspecified disorder of muscle, ligament, and fascia**

729 OTHER DISORDERS OF SOFT TISSUES

Excludes:

acroparesthesia (443.89); carpal tunnel syndrome (354.0); disorders of the back (720.0-724.9); entrapment syndromes (354.0-355.9); palindromic rheumatism (719.3); periarthritis (726.0-726.9); psychogenic rheumatism (306.0)

NOTE: SEE ALSO PERSONAL HISTORY OF OTHER MUSCULOSKELETAL DISORDERS (V13.5).

729.0 **Rheumatism, unspecified and fibrositis**

729.1 **Myalgia and myositis, unspecified**

Fibromyositis NOS

729.2 **Neuralgia, neuritis, and radiculitis, unspecified**

Excludes:

brachial radiculitis (723.4); cervical radiculitis (723.4); lumbosacral radiculitis (724.4); mononeuritis (354.0-355.9); radiculitis due to intervertebral disc involvement (722.0-722.2,722.7); sciatica (724.3)

729.3 Panniculitis, unspecified

729.30 **Panniculitis, unspecified site**

Weber-Christian disease

729.31 **Hypertrophy of fat pad, knee**

Hypertrophy of infrapatellar fat pad

729.39 **Other site**

Excludes:

panniculitis specified as (affecting): back (724.8); neck (723.6); sacral (724.8)

729	Other disorders of soft tissues
729.4	**Fasciitis, unspecified**

Excludes:
    nodular fasciitis (728.79); necrotizing fasciitis (728.86)

729.5	**Pain in limb**
729.6	**Residual foreign body in soft tissue**

Excludes:
    foreign body granuloma: muscle (72z8.82); skin and subcutaneous tissue (709.4)

Use additional code to identify foreign body (V90.01-V90.9)

729.7 Nontraumatic compartment syndrome

Code first, if applicable, postprocedural complication (998.89)

Excludes:
    compartment syndrome NOS (958.90); traumatic compartment syndrome (958.90-958.99)

729.71	**Nontraumatic syndrome of upper extremity**
	Nontraumatic compartment syndrome of shoulder, arm, forearm, wrist, hand and fingers
729.72	**Nontraumatic syndrome of lower extremity**
	Nontraumatic compartment syndrome of hip, buttock, thigh, leg, foot and toes
729.73	**Nontraumatic compartment syndrome of abdomen**
729.79	**Nontraumatic compartment syndrome of other sites**

729.8 Other musculoskeletal symptoms referable to limbs

729.81	**Swelling of limb**
729.82	**Cramp**
729.89	**Other**

Excludes:
    abnormality of gait (781.2); tetany (781.7); transient paralysis of limb (781.4)

729.9 Other and unspecified disorders of soft tissue

729.90	**Disorders of soft tissue, unspecified**
729.91	**Post-traumatic seroma**

Excludes:
    seroma complicating a procedure (998.13)

729.92	**Nontraumatic hematoma of soft tissue**
	Nontraumatic hematoma of muscle
729.99	**Other disorders of soft tissue**
	Polyalgia

OSTEOPATHIES, CHONDROPATHIES, AND ACQUIRED MUSCULOSKELETAL DEFORMITIES (730-739)

730 OSTEOMYELITIS, PERIOSTITIS, AND OTHER INFECTIONS INVOLVING BONE

Excludes:
    jaw (526.4-526.5); petrous bone (383.2)

Use additional code, if desired, to identify organism, such as Staphylococcus (041.1)

730.0 Acute osteomyelitis

Abscess of any bone except accessory sinus, jaw, or mastoid; Acute or subacute osteomyelitis, with or without mention of periostitis

Use additional code to identify major osseous defect, if applicable (731.3)

730.00	**site unspecified**
730.01	**shoulder region**
730.02	**upper arm**
730.03	**forearm**
730.04	**hand**
730.05	**pelvic region and thigh**
730.06	**lower leg**
730.07	**ankle and foot**
730.08	**other specified sites**
730.09	**multiple sites**

730.1 Chronic osteomyelitis

Brodie's abscess; Chronic or old osteomyelitis, with or without mention of periostitis; Sequestrum of bone; Sclerosing osteomyelitis of Garré

Excludes:
    aseptic necrosis of bone (733.40-733.49)

Use additional code to identify major osseous defect, if applicable (731.3)

730.10	**site unspecified**
730.11	**shoulder region**

↑ Highest Specificity Column   ↑ Highest Specificity Column

NOTES IN SMALL CAPS are added by ChiroCode Institute

	730.12	upper arm
	730.13	forearm
	730.14	hand
	730.15	pelvic region and thigh
	730.16	lower leg
	730.17	ankle and foot
	730.18	other specified sites
	730.19	multiple sites

730.2 Unspecified osteomyelitis

> Osteitis or osteomyelitis NOS, with or without mention of periostitis

Use additional code to identify major osseous defect, if applicable (731.3)

	730.20	site unspecified
	730.21	shoulder region
	730.22	upper arm
	730.23	forearm
	730.24	hand
	730.25	pelvic region and thigh
	730.26	lower leg
	730.27	ankle and foot
	730.28	other specified sites
	730.29	multiple sites

731 OSTEITIS DEFORMANS AND OSTEOPATHIES ASSOCIATED WITH OTHER DISORDERS CLASSIFIED ELSEWHERE

731.0 Osteitis deformans without mention of bone tumor

> Paget's disease of bone

731.1 Osteitis deformans in diseases classified elsewhere

Code first underlying disease as: malignant neoplasm of bone (170.0-170.9)

731.2 Hypertrophic pulmonary osteoarthropathy

> Bamberger-Marie disease

731.3 Major osseous defects

Code first underlying disease, if known, such as: aseptic necrosis (733.40-733.49); malignant neoplasm of bone (170.0-170.9); osteomyelitis (730.00-730.29); osteoporosis (733.00-733.09); peri-prosthetic osteolysis (996.45)

731.8 Other bone involvement in diseases classified elsewhere

Code first underlying disease, as: diabetes mellitus (249.8, 250.8)

Use additional code to specify bone condition, such as: acute osteomyelitis (730.00-730.09)

NOTE: CODES IN ITALICS CANNOT BE USED TO IDENTIFY A PRINCIPAL DIAGNOSIS

732 OSTEOCHONDROPATHIES

732.0 **Juvenile osteochondrosis of spine**

> Juvenile osteochondrosis (of): marginal or vertebral epiphysis (of Scheuermann); spine NOS;
>
> Vertebral epiphysitis

Excludes:

> adolescent postural kyphosis (737.0)

732.1 **Juvenile osteochondrosis of hip and pelvis**

> Coxa plana; Ischiopubic synchondrosis (of van Neck)
>
> Osteochondrosis (juvenile) of: acetabulum; head of femur (of Legg-Calvé-Perthes); iliac crest (of Buchanan); symphysis pubis (of Pierson)
>
> Pseudocoxalgia

732.3 **Juvenile osteochondrosis of upper extremity**

> Osteochondrosis (juvenile) of: capitulum of humerus (of Panner); carpal lunate (of Kienbock); hand NOS; head of humerus (of Haas); heads of metacarpals (of Mauclaire); lower ulna (of Burns); radial head (of Brailsford); upper extremity NOS

732.4 Juvenile osteochondrosis of lower extremity, excluding foot

Osteochondrosis (juvenile) of: lower extremity NOS; primary patellar center (of Köhler); proximal tibia (of Blount); secondary patellar center (of Sinding-Larsen); tibial tubercle (of Osgood-Schlatter)

Tibia vara

732.5 Juvenile osteochondrosis of foot

Calcaneal apophysitis; Epiphysitis, os calcis

Osteochondrosis (juvenile) of: astragalus (of Diaz); calcaneum (of Sever); foot NOS; metatarsal: second (of Freiberg); metatarsal: fifth (of Iselin); os tibiale externum (Haglund); tarsal navicular (of Köhler)

732.6 Other juvenile osteochondrosis

Apophysitis specified as juvenile, of other site, or site NOS; Epiphysitis specified as juvenile, of other site, or site NOS; Osteochondritis specified as juvenile, of other site, or site NOS; Osteochondrosis specified as juvenile, of other site, or site NOS

732.7 Osteochondritis dissecans

732.8 Other specified forms of osteochondropathy

Adult osteochondrosis of spine

732.9 Unspecified osteochondropathy

Apophysitis: NOS; not specified as adult or juvenile, of unspecified site

Epiphysitis: NOS; not specified as adult or juvenile, of unspecified site

Osteochondritis: NOS; not specified as adult or juvenile, of unspecified site

Osteochondrosis: NOS; not specified as adult or juvenile, of unspecified site

733 OTHER DISORDERS OF BONE AND CARTILAGE

Excludes:

bone spur (726.91); cartilage of, or loose body in, joint (717.0-717.9, 718.0-718.9); giant cell granuloma of jaw (526.3); osteitis fibrosa cystica generalisata (252.01); osteomalacia (268.2); polyostotic fibrous dysplasia of bone (756.54); prognathism, retrognathism (524.1); xanthomatosis localized to bone (272.7)

NOTE: SEE ALSO PERSONAL HISTORY OF OTHER MUSCULOSKELETAL DISORDERS (V13.5).

733.0 Osteoporosis

Use additional code to identify major osseous defect, if applicable (731.3)

Use additional code to identify personal history of pathologic (healed) fracture (V13.51)

733.00 Osteoporosis, unspecified

Wedging of vertebra NOS

733.01 Senile osteoporosis

Postmenopausal osteoporosis

733.02 Idiopathic osteoporosis

733.03 Disuse osteoporosis

733.09 Other

Drug-induced osteoporosis

Use additional E code to identify drug

733.1 Pathologic fracture

Chronic fracture, Spontaneous fracture

Excludes:

traumatic fracture (800-829); stress fracture (733.93-733.95)

NOTE: SEE ALSO PERSONAL HISTORY OF PATHOLOGIC FRACTURE (V13.51).

733.10 Pathologic fracture, unspecified site

733.11 Pathologic fracture of humerus

733.12 Pathologic fracture of distal radius and ulna

Wrist NOS

733.13 Pathologic fracture of vertebrae

Collapse of vertebra NOS

NOTE: CODE ALSO ANY CANCER OR OSTEOPOROSIS.

733.2 Cyst of bone
- **733.20 Cyst of bone (localized), unspecified**
- **733.21 Solitary bone cyst**
  Unicameral bone cyst
- **733.22 Aneurysmal bone cyst**
- **733.29 Other**
  Fibrous dysplasia (monostotic)
  Excludes:
  cyst of jaw (526.0-526.2, 526.89); osteitis fibrosa cystica (252.01); polyostotic fibrous dysplasia of bone (756.54)

733.4 Aseptic necrosis of bone
Excludes:
osteochondropathies (732.0-732.9)

<u>Use additional code</u> to identify major osseous defect, if applicable (731.3)

- **733.40 Aseptic necrosis of bone, site unspecified**
- **733.41 Head of humerus**
- **733.42 Head and neck of femur**
  Femur NOS
  Excludes:
  Legg-Calvé-Perthes disease (732.1)
- **733.43 Medial femoral condyle**
- **733.44 Talus**
- **733.45 Jaw**
  <u>Use additional E code</u> to identify drug, if drug-induced
  Excludes:
  osteoradionecrosis of jaw (526.89)
- **733.49 Other**

733 Other disorders of bone and cartilage
- **733.5 Osteitis condensans**
  Piriform sclerosis of ilium
- **733.6 Tietze's disease**
  Costochondral junction syndrome; Costochondritis
- **733.7 Algoneurodystrophy**
  Disuse atrophy of bone; Sudeck's atrophy

733.8 Malunion and nonunion of fracture
- **733.81 Malunion of fracture**
- **733.82 Nonunion of fracture**
  Pseudoarthrosis (bone)

733.9 Other and unspecified disorders of bone and cartilage
NOTE: SEE ALSO PERSONAL HISTORY OF STRESS FRACTURE (V13.52).

- **733.90 Disorder of bone and cartilage, unspecified**
- **733.92 Chondromalacia**
  Chondromalacia: NOS; localized, except patella; systemic; tibial plateau
  Excludes:
  chondromalacia of patella (717.7)
- **733.93 Stress fracture of tibia or fibula**
  Stress reaction of tibia or fibula
  <u>Use additional</u> external cause code(s) to identify the cause of the stress fracture
- **733.94 Stress fracture of the metatarsals**
  Stress reaction of metatarsals
  <u>Use additional</u> external cause code(s) to identify the cause of the stress fracture
- **733.95 Stress fracture of other bone**
  Stress reaction of other bone
  <u>Use additional</u> external cause code(s) to identify the cause of the stress fracture
  Excludes:
  stress fracture of: femoral neck (733.96); fibula (733.93); metatarsals (733.94); pelvis (733.98); shaft of femur (733.97); tibia (733.93)
- **733.97 Stress fracture of shaft of femur**
  Stress reaction of shaft of femur
  <u>Use additional</u> external cause code(s) to identify the cause of the stress fracture

	733.99	Other
		Diaphysitis; Hypertrophy of bone; Relapsing polychondritis
734	FLAT FOOT	
	734	**Flat foot**
		Pes planus (acquired); Talipes planus (acquired)
		Excludes:
		congenital (754.61); rigid flat foot (754.61); spastic (everted) flat foot (754.61)
735	ACQUIRED DEFORMITIES OF TOE	
	735.0	**Hallux valgus (acquired)**
	735.1	**Hallux varus (acquired)**
	735.2	**Hallux rigidus**
	735.3	**Hallux malleus**
	735.4	**Other hammer toe (acquired)**
	735.5	**Claw toe (acquired)**
		NOTE: ALSO CODE/SEE RICKETS, LATE EFFECT (268.1).
	735.8	**Other acquired deformities of toe**
	735.9	**Unspecified acquired deformity of toe**
736	OTHER ACQUIRED DEFORMITIES OF LIMBS	
	Excludes:	
	congenital (754.3-755.9)	
	NOTE: SEE ALSO PERSONAL HISTORY OF OTHER MUSCULOSKELETAL DISORDERS (V13.5).	
736.0	Acquired deformities of forearm, excluding fingers	
	736.00	**Unspecified deformity**
		Deformity of elbow, forearm, hand, or wrist (acquired) NOS
	736.01	**Cubitus valgus (acquired)**
	736.02	**Cubitus varus (acquired)**
	736.03	**Valgus deformity of wrist (acquired)**
	736.04	**Varus deformity of wrist (acquired)**
	736.05	**Wrist drop (acquired)**
	736.06	**Claw hand (acquired)**
	736.07	**Club hand, acquired**
	736.09	**Other**
736.2	Other acquired deformities of finger	
	736.20	**Unspecified deformity**
		Deformity of finger (acquired) NOS
	736.21	**Boutonniere deformity**

	736.22	**Swan-neck deformity**
	736.29	**Other**
		Excludes:
		trigger finger (727.03)
736.3	Acquired deformities of hip	
	736.30	**Unspecified deformity**
		Deformity of hip (acquired) NOS
	736.31	**Coxa valga (acquired)**
	736.32	**Coxa vara (acquired)**
	736.39	**Other**
736.4	Genu valgum or varum (acquired)	
	736.41	**Genu valgum (acquired)**
	736.42	**Genu varum (acquired)**
736	Other acquired deformities of limbs	
	736.6	**Other acquired deformities of knee**
		Deformity of knee (acquired) NOS
736.7	Other acquired deformities of ankle and foot	
	Excludes:	
	deformities of toe (acquired) (735.0-735.9); pes planus (acquired) (734)	
	736.70	**Unspecified deformity of ankle and foot, acquired**
	736.71	**Acquired equinovarus deformity**
		Clubfoot, acquired
		Excludes:
		clubfoot not specified as acquired (754.5-754.7)
	736.72	**Equinus deformity of foot, acquired**
	736.73	**Cavus deformity of foot**
		Excludes:
		that with claw foot (736.74)
	736.74	**Claw foot, acquired**
	736.76	**Other calcaneus deformity**
	736.79	**Other**
		Acquired: pes not elsewhere classified; talipes not elsewhere classified
736.8	Acquired deformities of other parts of limbs	
	736.81	**Unequal leg length (acquired)**
	736.89	**Other**
		Deformity (acquired): arm or leg, not elsewhere classified; shoulder

736	Other acquired deformities of limbs
736.9	Acquired deformity of limb, site unspecified

737 **CURVATURE OF SPINE**

Excludes:
    congenital (754.2)

- **737.0 Adolescent postural kyphosis**
  Excludes:
      osteochondrosis of spine (juvenile) (732.0); adult (732.8)

- **737.1 Kyphosis (acquired)**
  - **737.10** Kyphosis (acquired) (postural)
  - **737.11** Kyphosis due to radiation
  - **737.12** Kyphosis, postlaminectomy
  - **737.19** Other
    Excludes:
        that associated with conditions classifiable elsewhere (737.41)

- **737.2 Lordosis (acquired)**
  - **737.20** Lordosis (acquired) (postural)
  - **737.21** Lordosis, postlaminectomy
  - **737.22** Other postsurgical lordosis
  - **737.29** Other
    Excludes:
        that associated with conditions classifiable elsewhere (737.42)

- **737.3 Kyphoscoliosis and scoliosis**
  - **737.30** Scoliosis [and kyphoscoliosis], idiopathic
  - **737.31** Resolving infantile idiopathic scoliosis
  - **737.32** Progressive infantile idiopathic scoliosis
  - **737.33** Scoliosis due to radiation
  - **737.34** Thoracogenic scoliosis
  - **737.39** Other
    Excludes:
        that associated with conditions classifiable elsewhere (737.43); that in kyphoscoliotic heart disease (416.1)

- **737.4 Curvature of spine associated with other conditions**
  <u>Code first</u> associated condition as: Charcot-Marie-Tooth disease (356.1); mucopolysaccharidosis (277.5); neurofibromatosis (237.70-237.79); osteitis deformans (731.0); osteitis fibrosa cystica (252.01); osteoporosis (733.00-733.09); poliomyelitis (138); tuberculosis [Pott's curvature] (015.0)
  - **737.40** Curvature of spine, unspecified
  - **737.41** Kyphosis
  - **737.42** Lordosis
  - **737.43** Scoliosis
    NOTE: CODES IN ITALICS CANNOT BE USED TO IDENTIFY A PRINCIPAL DIAGNOSIS

737 Curvature of spine
- **737.8 Other curvatures of spine**
- **737.9 Unspecified curvature of spine**
  Curvature of spine (acquired) (idiopathic) NOS; Hunchback, acquired
  Excludes:
      deformity of spine NOS (738.5)

738 **OTHER ACQUIRED DEFORMITY**

Excludes:
    congenital (754.0-756.9, 758.0-759.9); dentofacial anomalies (524.0-524.9)

NOTE: SEE ALSO PERSONAL HISTORY OF OTHER MUSCULOSKELETAL DISORDERS (V13.5).

- **738.2 Acquired deformity of neck**
- **738.3 Acquired deformity of chest and rib**
  Deformity: chest (acquired); rib (acquired)
  Pectus: carinatum, acquired; excavatum, acquired
- **738.4 Acquired spondylolisthesis**
  Degenerative spondylolisthesis; Spondylolysis, acquired
  Excludes:
      congenital (756.12)
  NOTE: SEE ALSO 756.11 FOR CONGENITAL SPONDYLOLYSYS (LUMBAR VERTEBRAE).

738.5 **Other acquired deformity of back or spine**
  Deformity of spine NOS
  Excludes:
    curvature of spine (737.0-737.9)

738.6 **Acquired deformity of pelvis**
  Pelvic obliquity
  Excludes:
    intrapelvic protrusion of acetabulum (718.6); that in relation to labor and delivery (653.0-653.4, 653.8-653.9)

738.8 **Acquired deformity of other specified site**
  Deformity of clavicle

738.9 **Acquired deformity of unspecified site**

739 **NONALLOPATHIC LESIONS, NOT ELSEWHERE CLASSIFIED**
  NOTE: INCLUDES SUBLUXATION OR DISPLACEMENT OF THE JOINT FROM ITS NORMAL POSITION, WHICH OCCURS WHEN THE ARTICULATING SURFACES LOSE PARTIAL CONTACT.
  IF DUE TO INJURY USE THE 839 SERIES.
  Includes:
    segmental dysfunction; somatic dysfunction

739.0 **Head region**
  Occipitocervical region

739.1 **Cervical region**
  Cervicothoracic region

739.2 **Thoracic region**
  Thoracolumbar region

739.3 **Lumbar region**
  Lumbosacral region

739.4 **Sacral region**
  Sacrococcygeal region; Sacroiliac region
  NOTE: ICD-9 OFFICIALLY PLACES THE SACROILIAC REGION IN THE CODE FOR THE SACRAL REGION (739.4) THE CPT DESCRIPTION BY THE AMA PLACES THE SACROILIAC JOINT IN THE PELVIC REGION.

739.5 **Pelvic region**
  Hip region; Pubic region

739.6 **Lower extremities**

739.7 **Upper extremities**
  Acromioclavicular region; Sternoclavicular region

739.8 **Rib cage**
  Costochondral region; Costovertebral region; Sternochondral region

739.9 **Abdomen and other**

Medicare and the 739/839 Codes

Medicare only pays for spinal Chiropractic Manipulative Treatment to correct subluxations. All Medicare carriers and MACs except for First Coast Service Options, which services Florida, Puerto Rico and the U.S. Virgin Islands, require that you use code 739.x as the primary diagnosis. A secondary diagnosis from the list provided in the carriers or MACs Local Coverage Determination must be used with each primary diagnosis.

Medicare considers "Acute arthropathies characterized by acute inflammation and ligamentous laxity and anatomic subluxation or dislocation, including acute rheumatoid arthritis and ankylosing spondylitis" to be an absolute contraindication to dynamic thrust. The use of the 839.x diagnosis indicates an anatomic (or medical) subluxation and should not be used with a Medicare patient.

The use of the 839.x diagnosis with a non-Medicare patient should be limited to those injury cases where you have loss of motion segment integrity as visualized on flexion and extension x-rays.

↑ Highest Specificity Column   ↑ Highest Specificity Column
NOTES IN SMALL CAPS are added by ChiroCode Institute

14. CONGENITAL ANOMALIES (740-759)

744   CONGENITAL ANOMALIES OF EAR, FACE, AND NECK

Excludes:
> *anomaly of: cervical spine (754.2, 756.10-756.19); larynx (748.2-748.3); nose (748.0-748.1); parathyroid gland (759.2); thyroid gland (759.2); cleft lip (749.10-749.25)*

744.9   Unspecified anomalies of face and neck
> Congenital: anomaly NOS of face [any part] or neck [any part]; deformity NOS of face [any part] or neck [any part]

754   CERTAIN CONGENITAL MUSCULOSKELETAL DEFORMITIES

Includes:
> *nonteratogenic deformities which are considered to be due to intrauterine malposition and pressure*

754.1   Of sternocleidomastoid muscle
> Congenital sternomastoid torticollis; Congenital wryneck; Contracture of sternocleidomastoid (muscle); Sternomastoid tumor

754.2   Of spine
> Congenital postural: lordosis; scoliosis

754.3   Congenital dislocation of hip

754.30   Congenital dislocation of hip, unilateral
> Congenital dislocation of hip NOS

754.32   Congenital subluxation of hip, unilateral
> Congenital flexion deformity, hip or thigh; Predislocation status of hip at birth; Preluxation of hip, congenital

754.33   Congenital subluxation of hip, bilateral

754.35   Congenital dislocation of one hip with subluxations of other hip

754.4   Congenital genu recurvatum and bowing of long bones of leg

754.40   Genu recurvatum

754.41   Congenital dislocation of knee (with genu recurvatum)

754.42   Congenital bowing of femur

754.43   Congenital bowing of tibia and fibula

754.44   Congenital bowing of unspecified long bones of leg

754.5   Varus deformities of feet

Excludes:
> *acquired (736.71, 736.75, 736.79)*

754.50   Talipes varus
> Congenital varus deformity of foot, unspecified; Pes varus

Subluxation - Nonallopathic Lesions and Segmental Dysfunction

Please note that the word "subluxation" does not appear in the ICD-9-CM terminology for this 739 code series. Historically, this 739 series has always been used to express a subluxation that is not due to an accident or injury. However, when there is a subluxation due to an accident or injury, refer to the 839 code series.

Segmental dysfunction, somatic dysfunction, and nonallopathic lesions are synonyms for subluxation.

Head Region

Please note that the Occipitocervical region of the spine is listed as a component of the "head region" within this ICD-9 context. Therefore, it is appropriate to use 739.0 for a diagnosis of a subluxation in the Occiptocervical region, which should also be documented in the chart/medical record.

754.51 Talipes equinovarus
Equinovarus (congenital)

754.52 Metatarsus primus varus

754.53 Metatarsus varus

754.59 Other
Talipes calcaneovarus

754.6 Valgas deformities of feet
Excludes:
valgus deformity of foot (acquired) (736.79)

754.60 Talipes valgus
Congenital valgus deformity of foot, unspecified

754.61 Congenital pes planus
Congenital rocker bottom flat foot; Flat foot, congenital
Excludes:
pes planus (acquired) (734)

754.62 Talipes calcaneovalgus

754.69 Other
Talipes: equinovalgus; planovalgus

754.7 Other deformities of feet
Excludes:
acquired (736.70-736.79)

754.70 Talipes, unspecified
Congenital deformity of foot NOS

754.71 Talipes cavus
Cavus foot (congenital)

754.79 Other
Asymmetric talipes; Talipes: calcaneus; equinus

755 OTHER CONGENITAL ANOMALIES OF LIMBS
Excludes:
those deformities classifiable to 754.0-754.8
NOTE: SEE ALSO PERSONAL HISTORY OF OTHER CONGENITAL MALFORMATIONS (V13.69).

755.2 Reduction deformities of upper limb

755.20 Unspecified reduction deformity of upper limb
Ectromelia NOS of upper limb; Hemimelia NOS of upper limb; Shortening or arm, congenital

755.3 Reduction deformities of lower limb

755.30 Unspecified reduction deformity of lower limb
Ectromelia NOS of lower limb; Hemimelia NOS of lower limb; Shortening of leg, congenital

755.31 Transverse deficiency of lower limb
Amelia of lower limb
Congenital absence of: foot; leg, including foot and toes; lower limb, complete; toes, all, complete
Transverse hemimelia of lower limb

755.32 Longitudinal deficiency of lower limb, not elsewhere classified
Phocomelia NOS of lower limb

755.33 Longitudinal deficiency, combined, involving femur, tibia, and fibula (complete or incomplete)
Congenital absence of thigh and (lower) leg (complete or incomplete) with or without metacarpal deficiency and/or phalangeal deficiency, incomplete; Phocomelia, complete, of lower limb

755.34 Longitudinal deficiency, femoral, complete or partial (with or without distal deficiencies, incomplete)
Congenital absence of femur (with or without absence of some [but not all] distal elements); Proximal phocomelia of lower limb

755.35 Longitudinal deficiency, tibiofibular, complete or partial (with or without distal deficiencies, incomplete)
Congenital absence of tibia and fibula (with or without absence of some [but not all] distal elements); Distal phocomelia of lower limb

↑ Highest Specificity Column ↑ Highest Specificity Column

755.36 Longitudinal deficiency, tibia, complete or partial (with or without distal deficiencies, incomplete)

> Agenesis of tibia; Congenital absence of tibia (with or without absence of some [but not all] distal elements)

755.37 Longitudinal deficiency, fibular, complete or partial (with or without distal deficiencies, incomplete)

> Agenesis of fibula; Congenital absence of fibula (with or without absence of some [but not all] distal elements)

755.38 Longitudinal deficiency, tarsals or metatarsals, complete or partial (with or without incomplete phalangeal deficiency)

755.39 Longitudinal deficiency, phalanges, complete or partial

> Absence of toe, congenital; Aphalangia of lower limb, terminal, complete or partial

Excludes:

> terminal deficiency of all five digits (755.31); transverse deficiency of phalanges (755.31)

755 Other congenital anomalies of limbs

755.4 Reduction deformities, unspecified limb

> Absence, congenital (complete or partial) of limb NOS; Amelia of unspecified limb; Ectromelia of unspecified limb; Hemimelia of unspecified limb; Phocomelia of unspecified limb

755.5 Other anomalies of upper limb, including shoulder girdle

755.50 Unspecified anomaly of upper limb

755.51 Congenital deformity of clavicle

755.52 Congenital elevation of scapula

> Sprengel's deformity

755.53 Radioulnar synostosis

755.54 Madelung's deformity

755.59 Other

> Cleidocranial dysostosis
> Cubitus: valgus, congenital; varus, congenital

Excludes:

> club hand (congenital) (754.89); congenital dislocation of elbow (754.89)

755.6 Other anomalies of lower limb, including pelvic girdle

755.60 Unspecified anomaly of lower limb

755.61 Coxa valga, congenital

755.62 Coxa vara, congenital

755.63 Other congenital deformity of hip (joint)

> Congenital anteversion of femur (neck)

Excludes:

> congenital dislocation of hip (754.30-754.35)

755.64 Congenital deformity of knee (joint)

> Congenital: absence of patella; genu valgum [knock-knee]; genu varum [bowleg]
> Rudimentary patella

755.66 Other anomalies of toes

> Congenital: hallux valgus; hallux varus; hammer toe

755.67 Anomalies of foot, not elsewhere classified

> Astragaloscaphoid synostosis; Calcaneonavicular bar; Coalition of calcaneus; Talonavicular synostosis; Tarsal coalitions

755.69 Other

> Congenital: angulation of tibia; deformity (of) ankle (joint); deformity (of) sacroiliac (joint); fusion of sacroiliac joint

755 Other congenital anomalies of limbs

755.8 Other specified anomalies of unspecified limb

| 756 | OTHER CONGENITAL MUSCULOSKELETAL ANOMALIES |

Excludes:
> congenital myotonic chondrodystrophy (359.23); those deformities classifiable to (754.0-754.8)

NOTE: SEE ALSO PERSONAL HISTORY OF OTHER CONGENITAL MALFORMATIONS (V13.69).

- **756.1** Anomalies of spine
  - **756.10** Anomaly of spine, unspecified
  - **756.11** Spondylolysis, lumbosacral region
    > Prespondylolisthesis (lumbosacral)
  - **756.12** Spondylolisthesis
  - **756.13** Absence of vertebra, congenital
  - **756.14** Hemivertebra
  - **756.15** Fusion of spine [vertebra], congenital
  - **756.16** Klippel-Feil syndrome
  - **756.17** Spina bifida occulta

    Excludes:
    > spina bifida (aperta) (741.0-741.9)
  - **756.19** Other
    > Platyspondylia; Supernumerary vertebra

| 756 | Other congenital musculoskeletal anomalies |

- **756.2** Cervical rib
  > Supernumerary rib in the cervical region
- **756.3** Other anomalies of ribs and sternum
  > Congenital absence of: rib; sternum
  > Congenital: fissure of sternum; fusion of ribs
  > Sternum bifidum

  Excludes:
  > nonteratogenic deformity of chest wall (754.81-754.89)
- **756.4** Chondrodystrophy
  > Achondroplasia; Chondrodystrophia (fetalis); Dyschondroplasia; Enchondromatosis; Ollier's disease

Excludes:
> congenital myotonic chondrodystrophy (359.23); lipochondrodystrophy [Hurler's syndrome] (277.5); Morquio's disease (277.5)

- **756.9** Other and unspecified anomalies of musculoskeletal system
  > Congenital: anomaly NOS of musculoskeletal system, NEC; deformity NOS of musculoskeletal system, NEC

16. SYMPTOMS, SIGNS, AND ILL-DEFINED CONDITIONS (780-799)

NOTE: SPECIAL INSTRUCTIONS APPLY TO THIS SECTION. SEE COMPLETE ICD-9-CM FOR FULL INFORMATION.

SYMPTOMS (780-789)

| 780 | GENERAL SYMPTOMS |

- **780.4** Dizziness and giddiness
  > Light-headedness; Vertigo NOS

  Excludes:
  > Ménière's disease and other specified vertiginous syndromes (386.0-386.9)
- **780.5** Sleep disturbances

  Excludes:
  > circadian rhythm sleep disorders (327.30-327.39); organic hypersomnia (327.10-327.19); organic insomnia (327.00-327.09); organic sleep apnea (327.20-327.29); organic sleep related movement disorders (327.51-327.59); parasomnias (327.40-327.49); that of nonorganic origin (307.40-307.49)
  - **780.50** Sleep disturbance, unspecified
  - **780.51** Insomnia with sleep apnea, unspecified
  - **780.52** Insomnia, unspecified
  - **780.53** Hypersomnia with sleep apnea, unspecified
  - **780.54** Hypersomnia, unspecified
  - **780.55** Disruptions of 24 hour sleep wake cycle, unspecified
  - **780.56** Dysfunctions associated with sleep stages or arousal from sleep

780.57	Unspecified sleep apnea	
780.58	Sleep related movement disorder, unspecified	

Excludes:
> restless legs syndrome (333.94)

780.59 Other

780.7 Malaise and fatigue

Excludes:
> debility, unspecified (799.3); fatigue (during): combat (308.0-308.9); heat (992.6); pregnancy (646.8); neurasthenia (300.5); senile asthenia (797.5)

780.71 Chronic fatigue syndrome

780.79 Other malaise and fatigue
> Asthenia NOS; Lethargy; Postviral (asthenic) syndrome; Tiredness

780 General symptoms

780.8 Generalized Hyperhidrosis
> Diaphoresis; Excessive sweating; Secondary hyperhidrosis

Excludes:
> focal (localized) (primary) (secondary) hyperhidrosis (705.21-705.22); Frey's syndrome (705.22)

780.9 Other general symptoms

Excludes:
> hypothermia: NOS (accidental) (991.6); due to anesthesia (995.89); of newborn (778.2-778.3)
>
> memory disturbance as part of a pattern of mental disorder

780.96 Generalized pain
> Pain NOS

781 SYMPTOMS INVOLVING NERVOUS AND MUSCULOSKELETAL SYSTEMS

Excludes:
> depression NOS (311); disorders specifically relating to: back (724.0-724.9); hearing (388.0-389.9); joint (718.0-719.9); limb (729.0-729.9); neck (723.0-723.9); vision (368.0-369.9); pain in limb (729.5)

781.0 Abnormal involuntary movements
> Abnormal head movements; Fasciculation; Spasms NOS; Tremor NOS

Excludes:
> abnormal reflex (796.1); chorea NOS (333.5); infantile spasms (345.60-345.61); spastic paralysis (342.1, 343.0-344.9); specified movement disorders classifiable to 333 (333.0-333.9); that of nonorganic origin (307.2-307.3)

781.2 Abnormality of gait
> Gait: ataxic; paralytic; spastic; staggering

Excludes:
> ataxia: NOS (781.3); locomotor (progressive) (094.0)
>
> difficulty in walking (719.7)

781.3 Lack of coordination
> Ataxia NOS; Muscular incoordination

Excludes:
> ataxic gait (781.2); cerebellar ataxia (334.0-334.9); difficulty in walking (719.7); vertigo NOS (780.4)

781.8 Neurologic neglect syndrome
> Asomatognosia; Hemi-akinesia; Hemi-inattention; Hemispatial neglect; Left-sided neglect; Sensory extinction; Sensory neglect; Visuospatial neglect

Excludes:
> visuospatial deficit (799.53)

781.9 Other symptoms involving nervous and musculoskeletal systems

781.91 Loss of height

Excludes:
> osteoporosis (733.00-733.09)

781.92 Abnormal posture

781.93 Ocular torticollis

781.94 Facial weakness
> Facial droop

Excludes:
facial weakness due to late effect of cerebrovascular accident (438.83)

781.99 Other systems involving nervous and musculoskeletal systems

782 SYMPTOMS INVOLVING SKIN AND OTHER INTEGUMENTARY TISSUE

Excludes:
symptoms relating to breast (611.71-611.79)

782.0 Disturbance of skin sensation
Anesthesia of skin; Burning or prickling sensation; Hyperesthesia; Hypoesthesia; Numbness; Paresthesia; Tingling

782.3 Edema
Anasarca; Dropsy; Localized edema NOS

Excludes:
ascites (789.51-789.59)
edema of: newborn NOS (778.5); pregnancy (642.0-642.9, 646.1);
fluid retention (276.69); hydrops fetalis (773.3, 778.0); hydrothorax (511.81- 511.89); nutritional edema (260, 262)

782.8 Changes in skin texture
Induration of skin; Thickening of skin

784 SYMPTOMS INVOLVING HEAD AND NECK

Excludes:
encephalopathy NOS (348.3); specific symptoms involving neck classifiable to 723 (723.0-723.9)

784.0 Headache
Facial pain; Pain in head NOS

Excludes:
atypical face pain (350.2); migraine (346.0-346.9); tension headache (307.81)

784.9 Other symptoms involving head and neck

784.92 Jaw pain
Mandibular pain; Maxilla pain

Excludes:
temporomandibular joint arthralgia (524.62)

786 SYMPTOMS INVOLVING RESPIRATORY SYSTEM AND OTHER CHEST SYMPTOMS

786.5 Chest pain

786.50 Chest pain, unspecified

787 SYMPTOMS INVOLVING DIGESTIVE SYSTEM

Excludes:
constipation (564.00-564.09); pylorospasm (537.81); congenital (750.5)

787.0 Nausea and vomiting
Emesis

Excludes:
hematemesis NOS (578.0)
vomiting: bilious, following gastrointestinal surgery (564.3)
vomiting: cyclical (536.2): associated with migraine (346.2); psychogenic (306.4)
vomiting: excessive, in pregnancy (643.0-643.9); fecal matter (569.87); habit (536.2); of newborn (779.32-779.33); persistent (536.2); psychogenic NOS (307.54)

787.01 Nausea with vomiting
787.02 Nausea alone
787.03 Vomiting alone

789 OTHER SYMPTOMS INVOLVING ABDOMEN AND PELVIS

Excludes:
symptoms referable to genital organs: female (625.0-625.9); male (607.0-608.9); psychogenic (302.70-302.79)

789.0 Abdominal pain

789.00 unspecified site
789.01 right upper quadrant
789.02 left upper quadrant
789.03 right lower quadrant
789.04 left lower quadrant
789.05 periumbilic
789.06 epigastric
789.07 generalized
789.09 other specified site
multiple sites

NONSPECIFIC ABNORMAL FINDINGS (790-796)

793 NONSPECIFIC (ABNORMAL) FINDINGS ON RADIOLOGICAL AND OTHER EXAMINATION OF BODY STRUCTURE

Includes:
> nonspecific abnormal findings of: thermography; ultrasound examination [echogram]; x-ray examination

Excludes:
> abnormal results of function studies and radioisotope scans (794.0-794.9)

793.0 Skull and head

Excludes:
> nonspecific abnormal echoencephalogram (794.01)

793.2 Other intrathoracic organ
> Abnormal: echocardiogram; heart shadow; ultrasound cardiogram
>
> Mediastinal shift

793.7 Musculoskeletal system

793.9 Other

Excludes:
> abnormal finding by radioisotope localization of placenta (794.9)

793.91 Image test inconclusive due to excess body fat

> <u>Use additional code</u> to identify Body Mass Index (BMI), if known (V85.0-V85.54)

793.99 Other nonspecific abnormal findings on radiological and other examinations of body structure

> Abnormal: placental finding by x-ray or ultrasound method; radiological findings in skin and subcutaneous tissue

17. INJURY AND POISONING (800-999)

Use E code(s) to identify the cause and intent of the injury or poisoning (E800-E999)

Note:

1. *The principle of multiple coding of injuries should be followed wherever possible. Combination categories for multiple injuries are provided for use when there is insufficient detail as to the nature of the individual conditions, or for primary tabulation purposes when it is more convenient to record a single code; otherwise, the component injuries should be coded separately.*

   Where multiple sites of injury are specified in the titles, the word "with" indicates involvement of both sites, and the word "and" indicates involvement of either or both sites. The word "finger" includes thumb.

2. *Categories for "late effect" of injuries are to be found at 905-909.*

FRACTURE OF NECK AND TRUNK (805-809)

805 FRACTURE OF VERTEBRAL COLUMN WITHOUT MENTION OF SPINAL CORD INJURY

Includes:
> neural arch; spine; spinous process; transverse process; vertebra

NOTE: SEE ALSO CODING LATE EFFECT OF FRACTURE OF SPINE AND TRUNK WITHOUT SPINAL CORD LESION (905.1).

805.0 Cervical, closed
> Atlas; Axis

- **805.00 Cervical vertebra, unspecified level**
- **805.01 First cervical vertebra**
- **805.02 Second cervical vertebra**
- **805.03 Third cervical vertebra**
- **805.04 Fourth cervical vertebra**
- **805.05 Fifth cervical vertebra**
- **805.06 Sixth cervical vertebra**
- **805.07 Seventh cervical vertebra**
- **805.08 Multiple cervical vertebrae**

805 Fracture of vertebral column without mention of spinal cord injury

- **805.2 Dorsal [thoracic], closed**
- **805.4 Lumbar, closed**
- **805.6 Sacrum and coccyx, closed**
- **805.8 Unspecified, closed**

806 FRACTURE OF VERTEBRAL COLUMN WITH SPINAL CORD INJURY

Includes:
> any condition classifiable to 805 with: complete or incomplete transverse lesion (of cord); hematomyelia; injury to: cauda equina, nerve; paralysis; paraplegia; quadriplegia; spinal concussion

NOTE: SEE ALSO CODING LATE EFFECT OF FRACTURE OF SPINE AND TRUNK WITHOUT SPINAL CORD LESION (905.1).

- **806.0** Cervical, closed
  - **806.00** C1-C4 level with unspecified spinal cord injury
    > Cervical region NOS with spinal cord injury NOS
  - **806.01** C1-C4 level with complete lesion of cord
  - **806.02** C1-C4 level with anterior cord syndrome
  - **806.03** C1-C4 level with central cord syndrome
  - **806.04** C1-C4 level with other specified spinal cord injury
    > C_1-C_4 level with: incomplete spinal cord lesion NOS, posterior cord syndrome
  - **806.05** C5-C7 level with unspecified spinal cord injury
  - **806.06** C5-C7 level with complete lesion of cord
  - **806.07** C5-C7 level with anterior cord syndrome
  - **806.08** C5-C7 level with central cord syndrome
  - **806.09** C5-C7 level with other specified spinal cord injury
    > C_5-C_7 level with: incomplete spinal cord lesion NOS, posterior cord syndrome
- **806.2** Dorsal [thoracic], closed
  - **806.20** T1-T6 level with unspecified spinal cord injury
    > Thoracic region NOS with spinal cord injury NOS
  - **806.21** T1-T6 level with complete lesion of cord
  - **806.22** T1-T6 level with anterior cord syndrome
  - **806.23** T1-T6 level with central cord syndrome
  - **806.24** T1-T6 level with other specified spinal cord injury
    > T_1-T_6 level with: incomplete spinal cord lesion NOS, posterior cord syndrome
  - **806.25** T7-T12 level with unspecified spinal cord injury
  - **806.26** T7-T12 level with complete lesion of cord
  - **806.27** T7-T12 level with anterior cord syndrome
  - **806.28** T7-T12 level with central cord syndrome
  - **806.29** T7-T12 level with other specified spinal cord injury
    > T_7-T_{12} level with: incomplete spinal cord lesion NOS, posterior cord syndrome

806 Fracture of vertebral column with spinal cord injury

- **806.4** Lumbar, closed
- **806.6** Sacrum and coccyx, closed
  - **806.60** With unspecified spinal cord injury
  - **806.61** With complete cauda equina lesion
  - **806.62** With other cauda equina injury
  - **806.69** With other spinal cord injury

806 Fracture of vertebral column with spinal cord injury

- **806.8** Unspecified, closed

807 FRACTURE OF RIB(S), STERNUM, LARYNX, AND TRACHEA

NOTE: SEE ALSO CODING LATE EFFECT OF FRACTURE OF SPINE AND TRUNK WITHOUT SPINAL CORD LESION (905.1).

- **807.0** Rib(s), closed
  - **807.00** Rib(s), unspecified
  - **807.01** One rib
  - **807.02** Two ribs
  - **807.03** Three ribs
  - **807.04** Four ribs
  - **807.05** Five ribs
  - **807.06** Six ribs
  - **807.07** Seven ribs
  - **807.08** Eight or more ribs
  - **807.09** Multiple ribs, unspecified

809   **ILL-DEFINED FRACTURES OF BONES OF TRUNK**

Includes:

bones of trunk with other bones except those of skull and face, multiple bones of trunk

Excludes:

multiple fractures of: pelvic bones alone (808.0-808.9), ribs alone (807.0-807.1, 807.4), ribs or sternum with limb bones (819.0-819.1, 828.0-828.1), skull or face with other bones (804.0-804.9)

NOTE: SEE ALSO CODING LATE EFFECT OF FRACTURE OF SPINE AND TRUNK WITHOUT SPINAL CORD LESION (905.1).

- **809.0**   Fracture of bones of trunk, closed

FRACTURE OF UPPER LIMB (810-819)

810   **FRACTURE OF CLAVICLE**

Includes:

collar bone; interligamentous part of clavicle

NOTE: SEE ALSO CODING LATE EFFECT OF FRACTURE OF UPPER EXTREMITIES (905.2).

810.0   Closed
- **810.00**   Unspecified part
  - Clavicle NOS
- **810.01**   Sternal end of clavicle
- **810.02**   Shaft end of clavicle
- **810.03**   Acromial end of clavicle

811   **FRACTURE OF SCAPULA**

Includes:

shoulder blade

NOTE: SEE ALSO CODING LATE EFFECT OF FRACTURE OF UPPER EXTREMITIES (905.2).

811.0   Closed
- **811.00**   Unspecified part
- **811.01**   Acromial process
  - Acrominion (process)
- **811.09**   Other
  - Scapula body

812   **FRACTURE OF HUMERUS**

NOTE: SEE ALSO CODING LATE EFFECT OF FRACTURE OF UPPER EXTREMITIES (905.2).

812.0   Upper end, closed
- **812.00**   Upper end, unspecified part
  - Proximal end; Shoulder
- **812.01**   Surgical neck
  - Neck of humerus NOS
- **812.02**   Anatomical neck
- **812.03**   Greater tuberosity
- **812.09**   Other
  - Head; Upper epiphysis

812.2   Shaft or unspecified part, closed
- **812.20**   Unspecified part of humerus
  - Humerus NOS; Upper arm NOS
- **812.21**   Shaft of humerus

812.4   Lower end, closed
- Distal end of humerus; Elbow
- **812.40**   Lower end, unspecified part
- **812.41**   Supracondylar fracture of humerus

813   **FRACTURE OF RADIUS AND ULNA**

NOTE: SEE ALSO CODING LATE EFFECT OF FRACTURE OF UPPER EXTREMITIES (905.2).

813.0   Upper end, closed
- Proximal end
- **813.04**   Other and unspecified fractures of proximal end of ulna (alone)
  - Multiple fractures of ulna, upper end
- **813.05**   Head of radius
- **813.06**   Neck of radius
- **813.07**   Other and unspecified fractures of proximal end of radius (alone)
  - Multiple fractures of radious, upper end
- **813.08**   Radius with ulna, upper end [any part]

813.2   Shaft, closed
- **813.20**   Shaft, unspecified
- **813.21**   Radius (alone)
- **813.22**   Ulna (alone)
- **813.23**   Radius with ulna

813.4   Lower end, closed
- **813.41**   Colles' fracture
  - Smith's fracture
- **813.45**   Torus fracture of radius (alone)
  - *Excludes:*
    - *Torus fracture of radius and ulna (813.47)*
- **813.46**   Torus fracture of ulna (alone)
  - *Excludes:*
    - *Torus fracture of radius and ulna (813.47)*
- **813.47**   Torus fracture of radius and ulna

815	FRACTURE OF METACARPAL BONE(S)

Includes:
   hand [except finger]; metacarpus

NOTE: SEE ALSO CODING LATE EFFECT OF FRACTURE OF UPPER EXTREMITIES (905.2).

- **815.0** Closed
  - **815.00** Metacarpal bone(s), site unspecified
  - **815.01** Base of thumb [first] metacarpal
      Bennett's fracture
  - **815.02** Base of other metacarpal bone(s)
  - **815.03** Shaft of metacarpal bone(s)
  - **815.04** Neck of metacarpal bone(s)
  - **815.09** Multiple sites of metacarpus

- **816** FRACTURE OF ONE OR MORE PHALANGES OF HAND

  Includes:
     finger(s); thumb

  NOTE: SEE ALSO CODING LATE EFFECT OF FRACTURE OF UPPER EXTREMITIES (905.2).

  - **816.0** Closed
    - **816.00** Phalanx or phalanges, unspecified
    - **816.01** Middle or proximal phalanx or phalanges
    - **816.02** Distal phalanx or phalanges
    - **816.03** Multiple sites

FRACTURE OF LOWER LIMB (820-829)

- **821** FRACTURE OF OTHER AND UNSPECIFIED PARTS OF FEMUR

  NOTE: SEE ALSO CODING LATE EFFECT OF FRACTURE OF LOWER EXTREMITIES (905.4).

  - **821.0** Shaft or unspecified part, closed
    - **821.01** Shaft
  - **821.2** Lower end, closed
      Distal end
    - **821.20** Lower end, unspecified part
    - **821.21** Condyle, femoral
    - **821.22** Epiphysis, lower (separation)
    - **821.23** Supracondylar fracture of femur
    - **821.29** Other
        Multiple fractures of lower end

- **822** FRACTURE OF PATELLA

  NOTE: SEE ALSO CODING LATE EFFECT OF FRACTURE OF LOWER EXTREMITIES (905.4).

  - **822.0** Closed

- **823** FRACTURE OF TIBIA AND FIBULA

  Excludes:
     Dupuytren's fracture (824.4-824.5):
     ankle (824.4-824.5); radius (813.42, 813.52)
     Pott's fracture (824.4-824.5); that involving ankle (824.0-824.9)

  - **823.0** Upper end, closed
    - **823.00** tibia alone
    - **823.01** fibula alone
    - **823.02** fibula with tibia
  - **823.2** Shaft, closed
    - **823.20** tibia alone
    - **823.21** fibula alone
    - **823.22** fibula with tibia
  - **823.4** Torus fracture
    - **823.40** tibia alone
    - **823.41** fibula alone
    - **823.42** fibula with tibia
  - **823.8** Unspecified part, closed
      Lower leg NOS
    - **823.80** tibia alone
    - **823.81** fibula alone
    - **823.82** fibula with tibia

- **824** FRACTURE OF ANKLE

  NOTE: SEE ALSO CODING LATE EFFECT OF FRACTURE OF LOWER EXTREMITIES (905.4).

  - **824.0** **Medial malleolus, closed**
        Tibia involving: ankle; malleolus
  - **824.2** **Lateral malleolus, closed**
        Fibula involving: ankle; malleolus
  - **824.4** **Bimalleolar, closed**
        Dupuytren's fracture, fibula; Pott's fracture
  - **824.6** **Trimalleolar, closed**
        Lateral and medial malleolus with anterior or posterior lip of tibia
  - **824.8** **Unspecified, closed**
        Ankle NOS

- **825** FRACTURE OF ONE OR MORE TARSAL AND METATARSAL BONES

  NOTE: SEE ALSO CODING LATE EFFECT OF FRACTURE OF LOWER EXTREMITIES (905.4).

  - **825.0** **Fracture of calcaneus, closed**
        Heel bone; Os calcis

826	FRACTURE OF ONE OR MORE PHALANGES OF FOOT

NOTE: SEE ALSO CODING LATE EFFECT OF FRACTURE OF LOWER EXTREMITIES (905.4).

Includes:
> toe(s)

826.0 Closed

829	FRACTURE OF UNSPECIFIED BONES

NOTE: SEE ALSO CODING LATE EFFECT OF FRACTURE OF MULITPLE AND UNSPECIFIED BONES (905.5).

829.0 Unspecified bone, closed

DISLOCATION (830-839)

Includes:
> displacement; subluxation

Excludes:
> congenital dislocation (754.0-755.8); pathological dislocation (718.2); recurrent dislocation (718.3)

The descriptions "closed" and "open," used in the fourth-digit subdivisions, include the following terms:
> closed: complete; dislocation NOS; partial; simple; uncomplicated
> open: compound; infected; with foreign body

A dislocation not indicated as closed or open should be classified as closed.

830	DISLOCATION OF JAW

Includes:
> jaw (cartilage) (meniscus); mandible; maxilla (inferior); temporomandibular (joint)

NOTE: SEE ALSO CODING LATE EFFECT OF DISLOCATION (905.6).

830.0 Closed dislocation

831	DISLOCATION OF SHOULDER

Excludes:
> sternoclavicular joint (839.61, 839.71); sternum (839.61, 839.71)

NOTE: SEE ALSO CODING LATE EFFECT OF DISLOCATION (905.6).

831.0 Closed dislocation

- **831.00 Shoulder, unspecified**
  Humerus NOS
- **831.01 Anterior dislocation of humerus**
- **831.02 Posterior dislocation of humerus**
- **831.03 Inferior dislocation of humerus**
- **831.04 Acromioclavicular (joint)**
  Clavicle
- **831.09 Other**
  Scapula

832	DISLOCATION OF ELBOW

NOTE: SEE ALSO CODING LATE EFFECT OF DISLOCATION (905.6).

832.0 Closed dislocation

- **832.00 Elbow unspecified**
- **832.01 Anterior dislocation of elbow**
- **832.02 Posterior dislocation of elbow**
- **832.03 Medial dislocation of elbow**
- **832.04 Lateral dislocation of elbow**
- **832.09 Other**

832	Dislocation of elbow

- **832.2 Nursemaid's elbow**
  Subluxation of radial head

833	DISLOCATION OF WRIST

NOTE: SEE ALSO CODING LATE EFFECT OF DISLOCATION (905.6).

833.0 Closed dislocation

- **833.00 Wrist, unspecified part**
  Carpal (bone); Radius, distal end
- **833.01 radioulnar (joint), distal**
- **833.02 radiocarpal (joint)**
- **833.03 midcarpal (joint)**
- **833.04 carpometacarpal (joint)**
- **833.05 metacarpal (bone), proximal end**
- **833.09 other**
  Ulna, distal end

834	DISLOCATION OF FINGER

NOTE: SEE ALSO CODING LATE EFFECT OF DISLOCATION (905.6).

834.0 Closed dislocation

- **834.00 Finger, unspecified part**

835	DISLOCATION OF HIP

NOTE: SEE ALSO CODING LATE EFFECT OF DISLOCATION (905.6).

835.0 Closed dislocation

- **835.00 dislocation of hip, unspecified**
- **835.01 posterior dislocation**
- **835.02 obturator dislocation**
- **835.03 other anterior dislocation**

836	DISLOCATION OF KNEE

Excludes:

dislocation of knee: old or pathological (718.2); recurrent (718.3); internal derangement of knee joint (717.0-717.5, 717.8-717.9); old tear of cartilage or meniscus of knee (717.0-717.5, 717.8-717.9)

NOTE: SEE ALSO CODING LATE EFFECT OF DISLOCATION (905.6).

- **836.0 Tear of medial cartilage or meniscus of knee, current**
  - Bucket handle tear: NOS current injury; medial meniscus current injury
- **836.1 Tear of lateral cartilage or meniscus of knee, current**
- **836.2 Other tear of cartilage or meniscus of knee, current**
  - Tear of: cartilage (semilunar) current injury, not specified as medial or lateral; meniscus current injury, not specified as medial or lateral
- **836.3 Dislocation of patella, closed**
- 836.5 Other dislocation of knee, closed
  - **836.50 Dislocation of knee, unspecified**
  - **836.51 Anterior dislocation of tibia, proximal end**
    - Posterior dislocation of femur, distal end, closed
  - **836.52 Posterior dislocation of tibia, proximal end**
    - Posterior dislocation of femur, distal end, closed
  - **836.53 Medial dislocation of tibia, proximal end**
  - **836.54 Lateral dislocation of tibia, proximal end**
  - **836.59 Other**

837	DISLOCATION OF ANKLE

Includes:

astragalus; fibula, distal end; navicular, foot; scaphoid, foot; tibia, distal end

NOTE: SEE ALSO CODING LATE EFFECT OF DISLOCATION (905.6).

- **837.0 Closed dislocation**

838	DISLOCATION OF FOOT

NOTE: SEE ALSO CODING LATE EFFECT OF DISLOCATION (905.6).

- 838.0 Closed dislocation
  - **838.00 foot, unspecified**
  - **838.01 tarsal (bone), joint unspecified**
  - **838.02 midtarsal (joint)**
  - **838.03 tarsometatarsal (joint)**
  - **838.04 metatarsal (bone), joint unspecified**
  - **838.05 metatarsophalangeal (joint)**
  - **838.06 interphalangeal (joint)**
  - **838.09 other**
    - Phalanx of foot; Toe(s)

839	OTHER, MULTIPLE, AND ILL-DEFINED DISLOCATIONS

NOTE: IF NOT DUE TO INJURY USE THE 739 CODES SERIES.

SEE ALSO CODING LATE EFFECT OF DISLOCATION (905.6).

- 839.0 Cervical vertebra, closed
  - Cervical spine; Neck
  - **839.00 Cervical vertebra, unspecified**
  - **839.01 First cervical vertebra**

Medicare and the 739/839 Codes

Medicare only pays for spinal Chiropractic Manipulative Treatment to correct subluxations. All Medicare carriers and MACs except for First Coast Service Options, which services Florida, Puerto Rico and the U.S. Virgin Islands, require that you use code 739.x as the primary diagnosis. A secondary diagnosis from the list provided in the carriers or MACs Local Coverage Determination must be used with each primary diagnosis.

Medicare considers "Acute arthropathies characterized by acute inflammation and ligamentous laxity and anatomic subluxation or dislocation, including acute rheumatoid arthritis and ankylosing spondylitis" to be an absolute contraindication to dynamic thrust. The use of the 839.x diagnosis indicates an anatomic (or medical) subluxation and should not be used with a Medicare patient.

The use of the 839.x diagnosis with a non-Medicare patient should be limited to those injury cases where you have loss of motion segment integrity as visualized on flexion and extension x-rays.

↑ Highest Specificity Column   ↑ Highest Specificity Column

NOTES IN SMALL CAPS are added by ChiroCode Institute

	839.02	Second cervical vertebra	840	**SPRAINS AND STRAINS OF SHOULDER AND UPPER ARM**
	839.03	Third cervical vertebra		
	839.04	Fourth cervical vertebra		

839.02 Second cervical vertebra
839.03 Third cervical vertebra
839.04 Fourth cervical vertebra
839.05 Fifth cervical vertebra
839.06 Sixth cervical vertebra
839.07 Seventh cervical vertebra
839.08 Multiple cervical vertebrae

839.2 Thoracic and lumbar vertebra, closed
  839.20 Lumbar vertebra
  839.21 Thoracic vertebra
    Dorsal [thoracic] vertebra

839.4 Other vertebra, closed
  839.40 Vertebra, unspecified site
    Spine NOS
  839.41 Coccyx
  839.42 Sacrum
    Sacroiliac (joint)
  839.49 Other

839.6 Other location, closed
  839.61 Sternum
    Sternoclavicular joint
  839.69 Other
    Pelvis

839 Other, multiple, and ill-defined dislocations
  839.8 Multiple and ill-defined, closed
    Arm; Back; Hand; Multiple locations, except fingers or toes alone; Other ill-defined locations; Unspecified location

SPRAINS AND STRAINS OF JOINTS AND ADJACENT MUSCLES (840-848)

Includes:
  avulsion of: joint capsule, ligament, muscle, tendon;
  hemarthrosis of: joint capsule, ligament, muscle, tendon
  laceration of: joint capsule, ligament, muscle, tendon
  rupture of: joint capsule, ligament, muscle, tendon; sprain
  sprain of: joint capsule, , ligament, muscle, tendon
  strain of: joint capsule, ligament, muscle, tendon
  tear of: joint capsule, ligament, muscle, tendon

Excludes:
  aceration of tendon in open wounds (880-884 and 890-894 with .2)

---

840 **SPRAINS AND STRAINS OF SHOULDER AND UPPER ARM**

NOTE: SEE ALSO CODING LATE EFFECT OF SPRAIN AND STRAIN WITHOUT TENDON INJURY (905.7). SEE ALSO CODING LATE EFFECT OF TENDON INJURY (905.8).

840.0 Acromioclavicular (joint) (ligament)
840.1 Coracoclavicular (ligament)
840.2 Coracohumeral (ligament)
840.3 Infraspinatus (muscle) (tendon)
840.4 Rotator cuff (capsule)
  Excludes:
    complete rupture of rotator cuff, nontraumatic (727.61)
840.5 Subscapularis (muscle)
840.6 Supraspinatus (muscle) (tendon)
840.8 Other specified sites of shoulder and upper arm
840.9 Unspecified site of shoulder and upper arm
  Arm NOS; Shoulder NOS

841 **SPRAINS AND STRAINS OF ELBOW AND FOREARM**

NOTE: SEE ALSO CODING LATE EFFECT OF SPRAIN AND STRAIN WITHOUT TENDON INJURY (905.7). SEE ALSO CODING LATE EFFECT OF TENDON INJURY (905.8).

841.0 Radial collateral ligament
841.1 Ulnar collateral ligament
841.2 Radiohumeral (joint)
841.3 Ulnohumeral (joint)
841.8 Other specified sites of elbow and forearm
841.9 Unspecified site of elbow and forearm
  Elbow NOS

842 **SPRAINS AND STRAINS OF WRIST AND HAND**

NOTE: SEE ALSO CODING LATE EFFECT OF SPRAIN AND STRAIN WITHOUT TENDON INJURY (905.7). SEE ALSO CODING LATE EFFECT OF TENDON INJURY (905.8).

842.0 Wrist
  842.00 Unspecified site
  842.01 Carpal (joint)
  842.02 Radiocarpal (joint) (ligament)
  842.09 Other
    Radioulnar joint, distal
842.1 Hand
  842.10 Unspecified site

	842.11	Carpometacarpal (joint)	845.11	Tarsometatarsal (joint) (ligament)
	842.12	Metacarpophalangeal (joint)	845.12	Metatarsophalangeal (joint)
	842.13	Interphalangeal (joint)	845.13	Interphalangeal (joint), toe
	842.19	Other	845.19	Other

842.19 Other
Midcarpal (joint)

843 SPRAINS AND STRAINS OF HIP AND THIGH

NOTE: SEE ALSO CODING LATE EFFECT OF SPRAIN AND STRAIN WITHOUT TENDON INJURY (905.7). SEE ALSO CODING LATE EFFECT OF TENDON INJURY (905.8).

- **843.0** Iliofemoral (ligament)
- **843.8** Other specified sites of hip and thigh
- **843.9** Unspecified site of hip and thigh
   Hip NOS; Thigh NOS

844 SPRAINS AND STRAINS OF KNEE AND LEG

NOTE: SEE ALSO CODING LATE EFFECT OF SPRAIN AND STRAIN WITHOUT TENDON INJURY (905.7). SEE ALSO CODING LATE EFFECT OF TENDON INJURY (905.8).

- **844.0** Lateral collateral ligament of knee
- **844.1** Medial collateral ligament of knee
- **844.2** Cruciate ligament of knee
- **844.3** Tibiofibular (joint) (ligament), superior
- **844.8** Other specified sites of knee and leg
- **844.9** Unspecified site of knee and leg
   Knee NOS; Leg NOS

845 SPRAINS AND STRAINS OF ANKLE AND FOOT

NOTE: SEE ALSO CODING LATE EFFECT OF SPRAIN AND STRAIN WITHOUT TENDON INJURY (905.7). SEE ALSO CODING LATE EFFECT OF TENDON INJURY (905.8).

845.0 Ankle
- **845.00** Unspecified site
- **845.01** Deltoid (ligament), ankle
   Internal collateral (ligament), ankle
- **845.02** Calcaneofibular (ligament)
- **845.03** Tibiofibular (ligament), distal
- **845.09** Other
   Achilles tendon

845.1 Foot
- **845.10** Unspecified site

846 SPRAINS AND STRAINS OF SACROILIAC REGION

NOTE: SEE ALSO CODING LATE EFFECT OF SPRAIN AND STRAIN WITHOUT TENDON INJURY (905.7). SEE ALSO CODING LATE EFFECT OF TENDON INJURY (905.8).

- **846.0** Lumbosacral (joint) (ligament)
- **846.1** Sacroiliac ligament
- **846.2** Sacrospinatus (ligament)
- **846.3** Sacrotuberous (ligament)
- **846.8** Other specified sites of sacroiliac region
- **846.9** Unspecified site of sacroiliac region

847 SPRAINS AND STRAINS OF OTHER AND UNSPECIFIED PARTS OF BACK

NOTE: SEE ALSO CODING LATE EFFECT OF SPRAIN AND STRAIN WITHOUT TENDON INJURY (905.7). SEE ALSO CODING LATE EFFECT OF TENDON INJURY (905.8).

Excludes:
   lumbosacral (846.0)

- **847.0** Neck
   Anterior longitudinal (ligament), cervical;
   Atlanto-axial (joints);
   Atlanto-occipital (joints);
   Whiplash injury

   Excludes:
      neck injury NOS (959.0);
      thyroid region (848.2)

- **847.1** Thoracic
- **847.2** Lumbar
- **847.3** Sacrum
   Sacrococcygeal (ligament)
- **847.4** Coccyx
- **847.9** Unspecified site of back
   Back NOS

848 OTHER AND ILL-DEFINED SPRAINS AND STRAINS

NOTE: SEE ALSO CODING LATE EFFECT OF SPRAIN AND STRAIN WITHOUT TENDON INJURY (905.7). SEE ALSO CODING LATE EFFECT OF TENDON INJURY (905.8).

- **848.1** Jaw
   Temporomandibular (joint) (ligament)

↑ Highest Specificity Column
NOTES IN SMALL CAPS are added by ChiroCode Institute

↑ Highest Specificity Column

848.2 Thyroid region
Cricoarytenoid (joint) (ligament); Cricothyroid (joint) (ligament); Thyroid cartilage

848.3 Ribs
Chondrocostal (joint) without mention of injury to sternum; Costal cartilage without mention of injury to sternum

848.4 Sternum
- **848.40** Unspecified site
- **848.41** Sternoclavicular (joint) (ligament)
- **848.42** Chondrosternal (joint)
- **848.49** Other
  Xiphoid cartilage

848 Other and ill-defined sprains and strains
- **848.5 Pelvis**
  Symphysis pubis
  Excludes:
  that in childbirth (665.6)
- **848.8 Other specified sites of sprains and strains**
- **848.9 Unspecified site of sprain and strain**

INTRACRANIAL INJURY, EXCLUDING THOSE WITH SKULL FRACTURE (850-854)

Excludes:
intracranial injury with skull fracture (800-801 and 803-804, except .0 and .5); open wound of head without intracranial injury (870.0-873.9); skull fracture alone (800-801 and 803-804 with .0, .5)

The description "with open intracranial wound," used in the fourth-digit subdivisions, includes those specified as open or with mention of infection or foreign body.

NOTE: SEE ALSO LATE EFFECT OF INTRACRANIAL INJURY WITHOUT SKULL FRACTURE (907.0).

850 CONCUSSION
Includes:
commotio cerebri
Excludes:
concussion with: cerebral laceration or contusion (851.0-851.9); cerebral hemorrhage (852-853)
head injury NOS (959.01)

NOTE: SEE ALSO PERSONAL HISTORY OF TRAUMATIC BRAIN INJURY (V15.52).

850.0 With no loss of consciousness
Concussion with mental confusion or disorientation, without loss of consciousness

850.1 With brief loss of consciousness
Loss of consciousness for less than one hour
- **850.11 With loss of consciousness of 30 minutes or less**
- **850.12 With loss of consciousness from 31 to 59 minutes**

850 Concussion
- **850.5 With loss of consciousness of unspecified duration**
- **850.9 Concussion, unspecified**

LATE EFFECTS OF INJURIES, POISONINGS, TOXIC EFFECTS, AND OTHER EXTERNAL CAUSES (905-909)

Note:
These categories are to be used to indicate conditions classifiable to 800-999 as the cause of late effects, which are themselves classified elsewhere. The "late effects" include those specified as such, or as sequelae, which may occur at any time after the acute injury.

905 LATE EFFECTS OF MUSCULOSKELETAL AND CONNECTIVE TISSUE INJURIES

- **905.0 Late effect of fracture of skull and face bones**
  Late effect of injury classifiable to 800-804
- **905.1 Late effect of fracture of spine and trunk without mention of spinal cord lesion**
  Late effect of injury classifiable to 805, 807-809
- **905.2 Late effect of fracture of upper extremities**
  Late effect of injury classifiable to 810-819
- **905.3 Late effect of fracture of neck of femur**
  Late effect of injury classifiable to 820
- **905.4 Late effect of fracture of lower extremities**
  Late effect of injury classifiable to 821-827

905.6 Late effect of dislocation
Late effect of injury classifiable to 830-839

905.7 Late effect of sprain and strain without mention of tendon injury
Late effect of injury classifiable to 840-848, except tendon injury

905.8 Late effect of tendon injury
Late effect of tendon injury due to: open wound [injury classifiable to 880-884 with .2, 890-894 with .2]; sprain and strain [injury classifiable to 840-848]

907 LATE EFFECTS OF INJURIES TO THE NERVOUS SYSTEM

907.2 Late effect of spinal cord injury
Late effect of injury classifiable to 806, 952

907.3 Late effect of injury to nerve root(s), spinal plexus(es), and other nerves of trunk
Late effect of injury classifiable to 953-954

907.4 Late effect of injury to peripheral nerve of shoulder girdle and upper limb
Late effect of injury classifiable to 955

907.5 Late effect of injury to peripheral nerve of pelvic girdle and lower limb
Late effect of injury classifiable to 956

907.9 Late effect of injury to other and unspecified nerve
Late effect of injury classifiable to 957

SUPERFICIAL INJURY (910-919)

910 SUPERFICIAL INJURY OF FACE, NECK, AND SCALP EXCEPT EYE

910.0 Abrasion or friction burn without mention of infection

911 SUPERFICIAL INJURY OF TRUNK

911.0 Abrasion or friction burn, without mention of infection

912 SUPERFICIAL INJURY OF SHOULDER AND UPPER ARM

912.0 Abrasion or friction burn without mention of infection

913 SUPERFICIAL INJURY OF ELBOW, FOREARM, AND WRIST

913.0 Abrasion or friction burn, without mention of infection

916 SUPERFICIAL INJURY OF HIP, THIGH, LEG, AND ANKLE;

916.0 Abrasion or friction burn without mention of infection

CONTUSION WITH INTACT SKIN SURFACE (920-924)

Includes:
bruise without fracture or open wound; hematoma without fracture or open wound

Excludes:
concussion (850.0-850.9); hemarthrosis (840.0-848.9); internal organs (860.0-869.1); that incidental to: crushing injury (925-929.9); dislocation (830.0-839.9); fracture (800.0-829.1); internal injury (860.0-869.1); intracranial injury (850.0-854.1); nerve injury (950.0-957.9); open wound (870.0-897.7)

920 CONTUSION OF FACE, SCALP, AND NECK EXCEPT EYE(S)

920 Contusion of face, scalp, and neck except eye(s)
Cheek; Ear (auricle); Gum; Lip; Mandibular joint area; Nose; Throat

NOTE: SEE ALSO LATE EFFECT OF CONTUSION (906.3).

922 CONTUSION OF TRUNK

NOTE: SEE ALSO LATE EFFECT OF CONTUSION (906.3).

922.0 Breast
922.1 Chest wall
922.3 Back
Excludes:
scapular region (923.01)
922.31 Back
Excludes:
interscapular region (922.33)
922.32 Buttock
922.33 Interscapular region

923 CONTUSION OF UPPER LIMB

NOTE: SEE ALSO LATE EFFECT OF CONTUSION (906.3).

923.0 Shoulder and upper arm
923.00 Shoulder region
923.01 Scapular region
923.02 Axillary region
923.03 Upper arm

	923.09	Multiple sites
923.1		Elbow and forearm
	923.10	Forearm
	923.11	Elbow
923.2		Wrist and hand(s), except finger(s) alone
	923.20	Hand(s)
	923.21	Wrist
923		Contusion of upper limb
	923.3	Finger
		Fingernail; Thumb (nail)
	923.8	Multiple sites of upper limb
	923.9	Unspecified part of upper limb
		Arm NOS
924		CONTUSION OF LOWER LIMB AND OF OTHER AND UNSPECIFIED SITES

NOTE: SEE ALSO LATE EFFECT OF CONTUSION (906.3).

924.0		Hip and thigh
	924.00	Thigh
	924.01	Hip
924.1		Knee and lower leg
	924.10	Lower leg
	924.11	Knee
924.2		Ankle and foot, excluding toe(s)
	924.20	Foot
		Heel
	924.21	Ankle
924		Contusion of lower limb and of other and unspecified sites
	924.3	Toe
		Toenail
	924.4	Multiple sites of lower limb
	924.5	Unspecified part of lower limb
		Leg NOS
	924.8	Multiple sites, not elsewhere classified
	924.9	Unspecified site

INJURY TO NERVES AND SPINAL CORD (950-957)

Includes:

division of nerve (with open wound); lesion in continuity (with open wound); traumatic neuroma (with open wound); traumatic transient paralysis (with open wound)

Excludes:

accidental puncture or laceration during medical procedure (998.2)

951		INJURY TO OTHER CRANIAL NERVE(S)

NOTE: SEE ALSO LATE EFFECT OF INJURY TO CRANIAL NERVE (907.1). SEE ALSO LATE EFFECTS OF INJURIES TO THE NERVOUS SYSTEM (907).

	951.9	Injury to unspecified cranial nerve
953		INJURY TO NERVE ROOTS AND SPINAL PLEXUS

NOTE: SEE ALSO LATE EFFECT OF INJURY TO NERVE ROOTS(S) SPINAL PLEXUS(ES) AND OTHER NERVES OF TRUNK (907.3). SEE ALSO LATE EFFECTS OF INJURIES TO THE NERVOUS SYSTEM (907).

	953.0	Cervical root
	953.1	Dorsal root
	953.2	Lumbar root
	953.3	Sacral root
	953.4	Brachial plexus
	953.5	Lumbosacral plexus
	953.8	Multiple sites
	953.9	Unspecified site
954		INJURY TO OTHER NERVE(S) OF TRUNK, EXCLUDING SHOULDER AND PELVIC GIRDLES

NOTE: SEE ALSO LATE EFFECTS OF INJURIES TO THE NERVOUS SYSTEM (907).

	954.0	Cervical sympathetic
	954.1	Other sympathetic
		Celiac ganglion or plexus; Inferior mesenteric plexus; Splanchnic nerve(s); Stellate ganglion
	954.8	Other specified nerve(s) of trunk
	954.9	Unspecified nerve of trunk
956		INJURY TO PERIPHERAL NERVE(S) OF PELVIC GIRDLE AND LOWER LIMB

NOTE: SEE ALSO LATE EFFECT OF INJURY TO PERIPHERAL NERVE OF PELVIC GIRDLE AND LOWER LIMB (907.5). SEE ALSO CODING LATE EFFECTS OF INJURIES TO THE NERVOUS SYSTEM (907).

	956.0	Sciatic nerve
	956.1	Femoral nerve
	956.2	Posterior tibial nerve
	956.3	Peroneal nerve
	956.4	Cutaneous sensory nerve, lower limb
	956.5	Other specified nerve(s) of pelvic girdle and lower limb
	956.8	Multiple nerves of pelvic girdle and lower limb
	956.9	Unspecified nerve of pelvic girdle and lower limb

CERTAIN TRAUMATIC COMPLICATIONS AND UNSPECIFIED INJURIES (958-959)

958   CERTAIN EARLY COMPLICATIONS OF TRAUMA

Excludes:

    adult respiratory distress syndrome (518.5); flail chest (807.4); post-traumatic seroma (729.91); shock lung (518.5); that occurring during or following medical procedures (996.0-999.9)

NOTE: SEE ALSO LATE EFFECT OF CERTAIN COMPLICATIONS OF TRAUMA (908.6). SEE ALSO LATE EFFECTS OF OTHER AND UNSPECIFIED INJURIES (908).

958.6   **Volkmann's ischemic contracture**

    Posttraumatic muscle contracture

958.9   Traumatic compartment syndrome

Excludes:

    nontraumatic compartment syndrome (729.71-729.79)

958.90   **Compartment syndrome, unspecified**

958.91   **Traumatic compartment syndrome of upper extremity**

    Traumatic compartment syndrome of shoulder, arm, forearm, wrist, hand, and fingers

958.92   **Traumatic compartment syndrome of lower extremity**

    Traumatic compartment syndrome of hip, buttock, thigh, leg, foot, and toes

958.93   **Traumatic compartment syndrome of abdomen**

958.99   **Traumatic compartment syndrome of other sites**

959   INJURY, OTHER AND UNSPECIFIED

Includes:

    injury NOS

Excludes:

    injury NOS of: blood vessels (900.0-904.9); eye (921.0-921.9); internal organs (860.0-869.1); intracranial sites (854.0-854.1); nerves (950.0-951.9, 953.0-957.9); spinal cord (952.0-952.9)

NOTE: SEE ALSO LATE EFFECT OF UNSPECIFIED INJURY (908.9). SEE ALSO LATE EFFECTS OF OTHER AND UNSPECIFIED INJURIES (908).

959.2   **Shoulder and upper arm**

    Axilla; Scapular region

959.3   **Elbow, forearm, and wrist**

959.4   **Hand, except finger**

959.5   **Finger**

    Fingernail; Thumb (nail)

959.6   **Hip and thigh**

    Upper leg

959.7   **Knee, leg, ankle, and foot**

959.8   **Other specified sites, including multiple**

Excludes:

    multiple sites classifiable to the same four-digit category (959.0-959.7)

959.9   **Unspecified site**

4. Numeric ICD-9-CM List
V Codes

This classification is provided to deal with occasions when circumstances other than a disease or injury classifiable to categories 001-999 (the main part of ICD) are recorded as "diagnoses" or "problems." This can arise mainly in three ways:

a. When a person who is **not currently sick or injured** encounters the health services for some specific purpose, such as to act as a donor of an organ or tissue, to receive prophylactic vaccination, or to discuss a problem which in itself is not a disease or injury but is supplemental information which could affect the patient in the future.

b. When a person with a known disease or injury, whether current or resolving, encounters the health care system for a **specific treatment** of that disease or injury (e.g., dialysis for renal disease; chemotherapy for malignancy; cast change).

c. When some circumstance or problem is present which influences the person's health status but is not in itself a current illness or injury (e.g., smoking). Such factors may be elicited during population surveys, when the person may or may not be currently sick, or be recorded as an additional factor to be borne in mind when the person is receiving care for some current illness or injury classifiable to categories 001-999.

In the latter circumstances the V code should be used only as a supplementary code and should not be the one selected for use in primary, single cause tabulations.

Principal/First-Listed Diagnoses

In the official ICD-9 guidelines by HHS, a list is provided of V codes/categories that may only be reported as the principal/first-listed diagnosis. In this V-code section this note is shown after those codes: *Principal/1st Dx Only*

See Resource 356 for the complete ICD-9-CM coding guidelines.

Supplementary Classification of Factors Influencing Health Status and Contact with Health Services (V01 - V91)

RELATED TO PERSONAL AND FAMILY HISTORY (V10-V19)

Excludes:
   obstetric patients where the possibility that the fetus might be affected is the reason for observation or management during pregnancy (655.0-655.9)

- **V13** PERSONAL HISTORY OF OTHER DISEASES
- **V13.5** Other musculoskeletal disorders
   - **V13.51** **Pathologic fracture**
      Healed pathologic fracture
      Excludes:
         personal history of traumatic fracture (V15.51)
   - **V13.52** **Stress fracture**
      Healed stress fracture
      Excludes:
         personal history of traumatic fracture (V15.51)
   - **V13.59** **Other musculoskeletal disorders**
- **V13.6** Congenital (corrected) malformations
   - **V13.68** **Personal history of (corrected) congenital malformations of integument, limbs, and musculoskeletal systems**
- **V15** OTHER PERSONAL HISTORY PRESENTING HAZARDS TO HEALTH
   Excludes:
      personal history of drug therapy (V87.41-V87.49)
- **V15.5** Injury
   - **V15.51** **Traumatic fracture**
      Healed traumatic fracture
      Excludes:
         personal history of pathologic and stress fracture (V13.51, V13.52)
   - **V15.59** **Other injury**
- **V15.8** Other specified personal history presenting hazards to health
   Excludes:
      contact with and (suspected) exposure to: aromatic compounds and dyes (V87.11-V87.19); arsenic and other metals (V87.01-V87.09); molds (V87.31)
   - **V15.88** **History of fall**
      At risk for falling
   - **V15.89** **Other**
      Excludes:
         contact with and (suspected) exposure to other potentially hazardous chemicals (V87.2); contact with and (suspected) exposure to other potentially hazardous substances (V87.39)
- **V15** Other personal history presenting hazards to health
   - **V15.9** **Unspecified personal history presenting hazards to health**
- **V17** FAMILY HISTORY OF CERTAIN CRONIC DISABLING DISEASES
- **V17.8** Other musculoskeletal diseases
   - **V17.81** **Osteoporosis**
   - **V17.89** **Other musculoskeletal diseases**
- **V18** FAMILY HISTORY OF CERTAIN OTHER SPECIFIC CONDITIONS
   - **V18.0** **Diabetes mellitus**

PERSONS WITH A CONDITION INFLUENCING THEIR HEALTH STATUS (V40-V49)

- **V48** PROBLEMS WITH HEAD, NECK, AND TRUNK
   - **V48.0** **Deficiencies of head**
      Excludes:
         deficiencies of ears, eyelids, and nose (V48.8)
   - **V48.1** **Deficiencies of neck and trunk**
   - **V48.2** **Mechanical and motor problems with head**
   - **V48.3** **Mechanical and motor problems with neck and trunk**
   - **V48.4** **Sensory problem with head**
   - **V48.5** **Sensory problem with neck and trunk**
   - **V48.6** **Disfigurements of head**

V48.7	Disfigurements of neck and trunk		V54.14	Aftercare for healing traumatic fracture of leg, unspecified
V48.8	Other problems with head, neck, and trunk		V54.15	Aftercare for healing traumatic fracture of upper leg
V48.9	Unspecified problem with head, neck, or trunk			

V49 OTHER CONDITIONS INFLUENCING HEALTH STATUS

- V49.0 Deficiencies of limbs
- V49.1 Mechanical problems with limbs
- V49.2 Motor problems with limbs
- V49.3 Sensory problems with limbs
- V49.4 Disfigurements of limbs
- V49.5 Other problems of limbs

PERSONS ENCOUNTERING HEALTH SERVICES FOR SPECIFIC PROCEDURES AND AFTERCARE (V50-V59)

Note:
Categories V51-V58 are intended for use to indicate a reason for care in patients who may have already been treated for some disease or injury not now present, but who are receiving care to consolidate the treatment, to deal with residual states, or to prevent recurrence.

Excludes:
follow-up examination for medical surveillance following treatment (V67.0-V67.9)

V54 OTHER ORTHOPEDIC AFTERCARE

Excludes:
fitting and adjustment of orthopedic devices (V53.7); malfunction of internal orthopedic device (996.40-996.49); other complication of nonmechanical nature (996.60-996.79)

- V54.1 Aftercare for healing traumatic fracture
  Excludes:
  aftercare following joint replacement (V54.81); aftercare for amputation stump (V54.89)
  - V54.10 Aftercare for healing traumatic fracture of arm, unspecified
  - V54.11 Aftercare for healing traumatic fracture of upper arm
  - V54.12 Aftercare for healing traumatic fracture of lower arm
  - V54.13 Aftercare for healing traumatic fracture of hip

- V54.14 Aftercare for healing traumatic fracture of leg, unspecified
- V54.15 Aftercare for healing traumatic fracture of upper leg
  Excludes:
  aftercare for healing traumatic fracture of hip (V54.13)
- V54.16 Aftercare for healing traumatic fracture of lower leg
- V54.17 Aftercare for healing traumatic fracture of vertebrae
- V54.19 Aftercare for healing traumatic fracture of other bone

V54.2 Aftercare for healing pathologic fracture
Excludes:
aftercare following joint replacement (V54.81)
- V54.20 Aftercare for healing pathologic fracture of arm, unspecified
- V54.21 Aftercare for healing pathologic fracture of upper arm
- V54.22 Aftercare for healing pathologic fracture of lower arm
- V54.23 Aftercare for healing pathologic fracture of hip
- V54.24 Aftercare for healing pathologic fracture of leg, unspecified
- V54.25 Aftercare for healing pathologic fracture of upper leg
  Excludes:
  aftercare for healing pathologic fracture of hip (V54.23)
- V54.26 Aftercare for healing pathologic fracture of lower leg
- V54.27 Aftercare for healing pathologic fracture of vertebrae
- V54.29 Aftercare for healing pathologic fracture of other bone

- **V54.8** Other orthopedic aftercare
  - **V54.81 Aftercare following joint replacement**
    - *Use additional code* to identify joint replacement site (V43.60-V43.69)
  - **V54.89 Other orthopedic aftercare**
    - Aftercare for healing fracture NOS
- **V54** Other orthopedic aftercare
  - **V54.82 Aftercare following explantation of joint prosthesis**
    - Aftercare following explantation of joint prosthesis, staged procedure
    - Encounter for joint prosthesis insertion following prior explantation of joint prosthesis
  - **V54.9 Unspecific orthopedic aftercare**
- **V57** CARE INVOLVING USE OF REHABILITATION PROCEDURES
  - *Use additional code* to identify underlying condition
  - **V57.1 Other physical therapy**
    - *Principal/1st Dx Only*
    - Therapeutic and remedial exercises, except breathing
- **V57.2** Occupational therapy and vocational rehabilitation
  - **V57.21 Encounter for occupational therapy**
    - *Principal/1st Dx Only*
  - **V57.22 Encounter for vocational therapy**
    - *Principal/1st Dx Only*
- **V57** Care involving use of rehabilitation procedures
  - **V57.4 Orthoptic training**
    - *Principal/1st Dx Only*
- **V57.8** Other specified rehabilitation procedure
  - **V57.81 Orthotic training**
    - *Principal/1st Dx Only*
    - Gait training in the use of artificial limbs
  - **V57.89 Other**
    - *Principal/1st Dx Only*
    - Multiple training or therapy
- **V57** Care involving use of rehabilitation procedures

- **V57.9 Unspecified rehabilitation procedure**
  - *Principal/1st Dx Only*
- **V58** ENCOUNTER FOR OTHER AND UNSPECIFIED PROCEDURES AND AFTERCARE
  - *Excludes:*
    - convalescence and palliative care (V66)
- **V58.7** Aftercare following surgery to specified body systems, not elsewhere classified
  - *Note:*
    - Codes from this subcategory should be used in conjunction with other aftercare codes to fully identify the reason for the aftercare encounter
  - *Excludes:*
    - aftercare following organ transplant (V58.44), aftercare following surgery for neoplasm (V58.42)
  - **V58.78 Aftercare following surgery of the musculoskeletal system, NEC**
    - Conditions classifiable to 710-739
    - *Excludes:*
      - orthopedic aftercare (V54.01-V54.9)

PERSONS ENCOUNTERING HEALTH SERVICES IN OTHER CIRCUMSTANCES (V60-V69)

- **V64** PERSONS ENCOUNTERING HEALTH SERVICES FOR SPECIFIC PROCEDURES, NOT CARRIED OUT
  - **V64.1 Surgical or other procedure not carried out because of contraindication**
  - **V64.2 Surgical or other procedure not carried out because of patient's decision**
- **V65** OTHER PERSONS SEEKING CONSULTATION
- **V65.1** Person consulting on behalf of another person
  - Advice or treatment for nonattending third party
  - *Excludes:*
    - concern (normal) about sick person in family (V61.41-V61.49)
  - **V65.19 Other person consulting on behalf of another person**

V65.4 Other counseling, not elsewhere classified

Health: advice; education; instruction

Excludes:

counseling (for): contraception (V25.40-V25.49); genetic (V26.31-V26.39); on behalf of third party (V65.11, V65.19); procreative management (V26.41-V26.49)

- **V65.40 Counseling NOS**
- **V65.41 Exercise counseling**
- **V65.43 Counseling on injury prevention**
- **V65.49 Other specified counseling**

V68 ENCOUNTERS FOR ADMINISTRATIVE PURPOSES

V68.0 Issue of medical certificates

Excludes:

encounter for general medical examination (v70.0-V70.9)

- **V68.01 Disability examination**
  Principal/1st Dx Only

  Use additional code(s) to identify: specific examination(s), screening and testing performed (V72.0-V82.9)

- **V68.09 Other issue of medical certificates**
  Principal/1st Dx Only

V69 PROBLEMS RELATED TO LIFESTYLE

- **V69.0 Lack of physical exercise**
- **V69.1 Inappropriate diet and eating habits**

  Excludes:

  anorexia nervosa (307.1); bulimia (783.6); malnutrition and other nutritional deficiencies (260-269.9); other and unspecified eating disorders (307.50-307.59)

- **V69.4 Lack of adequate sleep**

  Sleep deprivation

  Excludes:

  insomnia (780.52)

- **V69.8 Other problems related to lifestyle**

  Self-damaging behavior

- **V69.9 Problem related to lifestyle, unspecified**

PERSONS WITHOUT REPORTED DIAGNOSIS ENCOUNTERED DURING EXAMINATION AND INVESTIGATION OF INDIVIDUALS AND POPULATIONS (V70-V82)

Note:

Nonspecific abnormal findings disclosed at the time of these examinations are classifiable to categories 790-796.

V70 GENERAL MEDICAL EXAMINATION

Use additional code(s) to identify any special screening examination(s) performed (V73.0-V82.9)

- **V70.0 Routine general medical examination at a health care facility**
  Principal/1st Dx Only

  Health checkup

  Excludes:

  health checkup of infant or child over 28 days old (V20.2); health supervision of newborn 8 to 28 days old (V20.32); health supervision of newborn under 8 days old (V20.31); pre-procedural general physical examination (V72.83)

- **V70.3 Other medical examination for administrative purposes**
  Principal/1st Dx Only

  General medical examination for: admission to old age home; adoption; camp; driving license; immigration and naturalization; insurance certification; marriage; prison; school admission; sports competition

  Excludes:

  attendance for issue of medical certificates (V68.0); pre-employment screening (V70.5)

V70.4 Examination for medicolegal reasons
Principal/1st Dx Only
> Blood-alcohol tests; Blood-drug tests; Paternity testing

Excludes:
> examination and observation following: accidents (V71.3, V71.4); assault (V71.6); rape (V71.5)

V70.5 Health examination of defined subpopulations
Principal/1st Dx Only
> Armed forces personnel; Inhabitants of institutions; Occupational health examinations; Pre-employment screening; Preschool children; Prisoners; Prostitutes; Refugees; School children; Students

V70.7 Examination of participant in clinical trial
> Examination of participant or control in clinical research

V71 OBSERVATION AND EVALUATION FOR SUSPECTED CONDITIONS NOT FOUND

Note:
> This category is to be used when persons without a diagnosis are suspected of having an abnormal condition, without signs or symptoms, which requires study, but after examination and observation, is found not to exist. This category is also for use for administrative and legal observation status.

Excludes:
> suspected maternal and fetal conditions not found (V89.01-V89.09)

V71.3 Observation following accident at work
Principal/1st Dx Only

V71.4 Observation following other accident
Principal/1st Dx Only
> Examination of individual involved in motor vehicle traffic accident

V72 SPECIAL INVESTIGATIONS AND EXAMINATIONS

Includes:
> routine examination of specific system

Excludes:
> general medical examination (V70.0-V70.4); general screening examination of defined population groups (V70.5, V70.6, V70.7); health supervision of newborn 8 to 28 days old (V20.32); health supervision of newborn under 8 days old (V20.31); routine examination of infant or child (V20.2)

Use additional code(s) to identify any special screening examination(s) performed (V73.0-V82.9)

V72.5 Radiological examination, not elsewhere classified
> Routine chest x-ray

Excludes:
> radiologic examinations as part of pre-procedural testing (V72.81-V72.84)

V72.8 Other specified examinations
Excludes:
> pre-procedural laboratory examinations (V72.63)

V72.85 Other specified examinations

V72 Special investigations and examinations
V72.9 Unspecified examination

V77 SPECIAL SCREENING FOR ENDOCRINE, NUTRITIONAL, METABOLIC, AND IMMUNITY DISORDERS

V77.8 Obesity

V82 SPECIAL SCREENING FOR OTHER CONDITIONS

V82.3 Congenital dislocation of hip
V82.6 Multiphasic screening
V82.8 Other specified conditions
V82.81 Osteoporosis
> *Use additional code to identify:* hormone replacement therapy (postmenopausal) status (V07.4); postmenopausal (natural) status (V49.81)

V82.89 Other specified conditions

↑ Highest Specificity Column
↑ Highest Specificity Column
NOTES IN SMALL CAPS are added by ChiroCode Institute

BODY MASS INDEX (V85)

V85 BODY MASS INDEX [BMI]
Kilograms per meters squared

Note:
BMI adult codes are for use for persons over 20 years old

- **V85.0** Body Mass Index less than 19, adult
- **V85.1** Body Mass Index between 19-24, adult

V85.2 Body Mass Index between 25-29, adult
- **V85.21** Body Mass Index 25.0-25.9, adult
- **V85.22** Body Mass Index 26.0-26.9, adult
- **V85.23** Body Mass Index 27.0-27.9, adult
- **V85.23** Body Mass Index 28.0-28.9, adult
- **V85.24** Body Mass Index 29.0-29.9, adult
- **V85.25** Body Mass Index between 30-39, adult

V85.3 Body Mass Index 30.0-30.9, adult
- **V85.30** Body Mass Index 30.0-30.9, adult
- **V85.31** Body Mass Index 31.0-31.9, adult
- **V85.32** Body Mass Index 32.0-32.9, adult
- **V85.33** Body Mass Index 33.0-33.9, adult
- **V85.34** Body Mass Index 34.0-34.9, adult
- **V85.35** Body Mass Index 35.0-35.9, adult
- **V85.36** Body Mass Index 36.0-36.9, adult
- **V85.37** Body Mass Index 37.0-37.9, adult
- **V85.38** Body Mass Index 38.0-38.9, adult
- **V85.39** Body Mass Index 39.0-39.9, adult

V85.4 Body Mass Index 40 and over, adult
- **V85.41** Body Mass Index 40.0-44.9, adult
- **V85.42** Body Mass Index 45.0-49.9, adult
- **V85.43** Body Mass Index 50.0-59.9, adult
- **V85.44** Body Mass Index 60.0-69.9, adult
- **V85.45** Body Mass Index 70 and over, adult

V85.5 Body Mass Index, pediatric

Note:
BMI pediatric codes are for use for persons 2-20 years old. These percentiles are based on the growth charts published by the Centers for Disease Control and Prevention (CDC)

- **V85.51** Body Mass Index, pediatric, less than 5th percentile for age
- **V85.52** Body Mass Index, pediatric, 5th percentile to less than 85th percentile for age
- **V85.53** Body Mass Index, pediatric, 85th percentile to less than 95th percentile for age
- **V85.54** Body Mass Index, pediatric, greater than or equal to 95th percentile for age

---

ICD-9 codes for Maintenance/Wellness care (S8990)

Typically, insurance payers do not cover maintenance, wellness or preventive care, unless required by state or federal law such as the Affordable Care Act. Here are two possible ICD-9 coding options to express such encounters: V70.0 for a "Health Checkup," or V82.89 for "Other Specified Conditions." When using such codes document them in the chart as a "maintenance" or "wellness" encounter.

If you bill Medicare for maintenance or wellness care, be sure to append the GA modifier to the CMT procedure code. Use of this modifier is a declaration that you have an ABN on file that has been signed by the patient (or their responsible party).

4. Numeric ICD-9-CM List
E Codes

The "E" Codes explain **external** causes. Historically, they have not generally been used on insurance claims by all payers, as they typically supplement the primary diagnosis.

Some "E" codes were mandated for national use during 1993. A federal mandate required reporting **drugs and substances** that cause **adverse effects in therapeutic use.**

There is a growing trend by states to require supplemental "E" codes when applicable.

It will be helpful to remember that "E" codes are not usually relevant to the third party payer because most of them explain where and how an accident occurred rather than why a claim should be paid.

One of the greatest values in using "E" codes is for clinical record keeping and chiropractic research and analysis. If cases are identified with an "E" code, it would provide for an easy retrieval of data.

Instructional notes (includes, excludes, etc.) are not included in this section on "E" codes. For a complete listing of these codes, see an unabridged ICD-9-CM book.

E codes are not required by most payers. When the new Activity Codes and External Cause Status Codes were requested in 2010, it was anticipated that this would change. However, discussions have taken a back seat to ICD-10 implementation.

External Cause codes are included in ICD-10-CM (Activity codes will be in the Y codes category) and will likely play a more prominent role in the reimbursement process after ICD-10 is implemented on October 2015.

See Resource 356 for the official ICD-9-CM coding guidelines.

Supplemental Classification of External Causes of Injury and Poisoning (E000 to E999)

EXTERNAL CAUSE STATUS (E000)

Note:
A code from category E000 should be used in conjunction with the external cause code(s) assigned to a record to indicate the status of the person at the time the event occurred. A single code from category E000 should be assigned for an encounter.

E000 EXTERNAL CAUSE STATUS

E000.0 Civilian activity done for income or pay
Civilian activity done for financial or other compensation

Excludes:
military activity (E000.1)

E000.1 Military activity
Excludes:
activity of off duty military personnel (E000.8)

E000.2 Volunteer activity
Excludes:
activity of child or other family member assisting in compensated work of other family member (E000.8)

E000.8 Other external cause status
Activity NEC; Activity of child or other family member assisting in compensated work of other family member; Hobby not done for income; Leisure activity; Off-duty activity of military personnel; Recreation or sport not for income or while a student; Student activity

E000.9 Unspecified external cause status

ACTIVITY (E001-E030)

Note:
Categories E001 to E030 are provided for use to indicate the activity of the person seeking healthcare for an injury or health condition, such as a heart attack while shoveling snow, which resulted from, or was contributed to, by the activity. These codes are appropriate for use for both acute injuries, such as those from chapter 17, and conditions that are due to the long-term, cumulative effects of an activity, such as those from chapter 13. They are also appropriate for use with external cause codes for cause and intent if identifying the activity provides additional information on the event.

These codes should be used in conjunction with other external cause codes for external cause status (E000) and place of occurrence (E849).

This section contains the following broad activity categories:

E001 Activities involving walking and running
E002 Activities involving water and water craft
E003 Activities involving ice and snow
E004 Activities involving climbing, rappelling, and jumping off
E005 Activities involving dancing and other rhythmic movement
E006 Activities involving other sports and athletics played individually
E007 Activities involving other sports and athletics played as a team or group
E008 Activities involving other specified sports and athletics
E009 Activity involving other cardiorespiratory exercise
E010 Activity involving other muscle strengthening exercises
E011 Activities involving computer technology and electronic devices
E012 Activities involving arts and handcrafts
E013 Activities involving personal hygiene and household maintenance
E014 Activities involving person providing caregiving
E015 Activities involving food preparation, cooking and grilling
E016 Activities involving property and land maintenance, building and construction
E017 Activities involving roller coasters and other types of external motion

E018 *Activities involving playing musical instrument*
E019 *Activities involving animal care*
E029 *Other activity*
E030 *Unspecified activity*

E001 **ACTIVITIES INVOLVING WALKING AND RUNNING**

Excludes:
walking an animal (E019.0); walking or running on a treadmill (E009.0)

E001.0 Walking, marching and hiking

Walking, marching and hiking on level or elevated terrain

Excludes:
mountain climbing (E004.0)

E001.1 Running

E002 **ACTIVITIES INVOLVING WATER AND WATER CRAFT**

Excludes:
activities involving ice (E003.0-E003.9); boating and other watercraft transport accidents (E830-E838)

E002.0 Swimming

E002.1 Springboard and platform diving

E002.2 Water polo

E002.3 Water aerobics and water exercise

E002.4 Underwater diving and snorkeling

SCUBA diving

E002.5 Rowing, canoeing, kayaking, rafting and tubing

Canoeing, kayaking, rafting and tubing in calm and turbulent water

E002.6 Water skiing and wake boarding

E002.7 Surfing, windsurfing and boogie boarding

E002.8 Water sliding

E002.9 Other activity involving water and watercraft

Activity involving water NOS; Parasailing; Water survival training and testing

E003 **ACTIVITIES INVOLVING ICE AND SNOW**

Excludes:
shoveling ice and snow (E016.0)

E003.0 Ice skating

Figure skating (singles) (pairs); Ice dancing

Excludes:
ice hockey (E003.1)

E003.1 Ice hockey

E003.2 Snow (alpine) (downhill) skiing, snow boarding, sledding, tobogganing and snow tubing

Excludes:
cross country skiing (E003.3)

E003.3 Cross country skiing

Nordic skiing

E003.9 Other activity involving ice and snow

Activity involving ice and snow NOS

E004 **ACTIVITIES INVOLVING CLIMBING, RAPPELLING AND JUMPING OFF**

Excludes:
hiking on level or elevated terrain (E001.0); jumping rope (E006.5); sky diving (E840-E844); trampoline jumping (E005.3)

E004.0 Mountain climbing, rock climbing and wall climbing

E004.1 Rappelling

E004.2 BASE jumping

Building, Antenna, Span, Earth jumping

E004.3 Bungee jumping

E004.4 Hang gliding

E004.9 Other activity involving climbing, rappelling and jumping off

E005 **ACTIVITIES INVOLVING DANCING AND OTHER RHYTHMIC MOVEMENT**

Excludes:
martial arts (E008.4)

E005.0 Dancing

E005.1 Yoga

E005.2 Gymnastics

Rhythmic gymnastics

Excludes:
trampoline (E005.3)

	E005.3	Trampoline
	E005.4	Cheerleading
	E005.9	Other activity involving dancing and other rhythmic movements
E006		ACTIVITIES INVOLVING OTHER SPORTS AND ATHLETICS PLAYED INDIVIDUALLY

Excludes:
> dancing (E005.0); gymnastic (E005.2); trampoline (E005.3); yoga (E005.1)

	E006.0	Roller skating (inline) and skateboarding
	E006.1	Horseback riding
	E006.2	Golf
	E006.3	Bowling
	E006.4	Bike riding

Excludes:
> transport accident involving bike riding (E800-E829)

	E006.5	Jumping rope
	E006.6	Non-running track and field events

Excludes:
> running (any form) (E001.1)

	E006.9	Other activity involving other sports and athletics played individually

Excludes:
> activities involving climbing, rappelling, and jumping (E004.0-E004.9); activities involving ice and snow (E003.0-E003.9); activities involving walking and running (E001.0-E001.9); activities involving water and watercraft (E002.0-E002.9)

E007		ACTIVITIES INVOLVING OTHER SPORTS AND ATHLETICS PLAYED AS A TEAM OR GROUP

Excludes:
> ice hockey (E003.1); water polo (E002.2)

	E007.0	American tackle football
		Football NOS
	E007.1	American flag or touch football
	E007.2	Rugby
	E007.3	Baseball
		Softball
	E007.4	Lacrosse and field hockey
	E007.5	Soccer
	E007.6	Basketball
	E007.7	Volleyball (beach) (court)
	E007.8	Physical games generally associated with school recess, summer camp and children
		Capture the flag; Dodge ball; Four square; Kickball
	E007.9	Other activity involving other sports and athletics played as a team or group
		Cricket
E008		ACTIVITIES INVOLVING OTHER SPECIFIED SPORTS AND ATHLETICS
	E008.0	Boxing
	E008.1	Wrestling
	E008.2	Racquet and hand sports
		Handball; Racquetball; Squash; Tennis
	E008.3	Frisbee
		Ultimate frisbee
	E008.4	Martial arts
		Combatives
	E008.9	Other specified sports and athletics activity

Excludes:
> sports and athletics activities specified in categories E001-E007

E009		ACTIVITY INVOLVING OTHER CARDIORESPIRATORY EXERCISE
		Activity involving physical training
	E009.0	Exercise machines primarily for cardiorespiratory conditioning
		Elliptical and stepper machines; Stationary bike; Treadmill
	E009.1	Calisthenics
		Jumping jacks; Warm up and cool down
	E009.2	Aerobic and step exercise
	E009.3	Circuit training
	E009.4	Obstacle course
		Challenge course; Confidence course
	E009.5	Grass drills
		Guerilla drills

E009.9 Other activity involving other cardiorespiratory exercise
Excludes:
activities involving cardiorespiratory exercise specified in categories E001-E008

E010 ACTIVITY INVOLVING OTHER MUSCLE STRENGTHENING EXERCISES

E010.0 Exercise machines primarily for muscle strengthening

E010.1 Push-ups, pull-ups, sit-ups

E010.2 Free weights
Barbells; Dumbbells

E010.3 Pilates

E010.9 Other activity involving other muscle strengthening exercises
Excludes:
activities involving muscle strengthening specified in categories E001-E009

E011 ACTIVITIES INVOLVING COMPUTER TECHNOLOGY AND ELECTRONIC DEVICES
Excludes:
electronic musical keyboard or instruments (E018.0)

E011.0 Computer keyboarding
Electronic game playing using keyboard or other stationary device

E011.1 Hand held interactive electronic device
Cellular telephone and communication device; Electronic game playing using interactive device
Excludes:
electronic game playing using keyboard or other stationary device (E011.0)

E011.9 Other activity involving computer technology and electronic devices

E012 ACTIVITIES INVOLVING ARTS AND HANDCRAFTS
Excludes:
activities involving playing musical instrument (E018.0-E018.3)

E012.0 Knitting and crocheting

E012.1 Sewing

E012.2 Furniture building and finishing
Furniture repair

E012.9 Activity involving other arts and handcrafts

E013 ACTIVITIES INVOLVING PERSONAL HYGIENE AND HOUSEHOLD MAINTENANCE
Excludes:
activities involving cooking and grilling (E015.0-E015.9); activities involving property and land maintenance, building and construction (E016.0-E016.9); activity involving persons providing caregiving (E014.0-E014.9); dishwashing (E015.0); food preparation (E015.0); gardening (E016.1)

E013.0 Personal bathing and showering

E013.1 Laundry

E013.2 Vacuuming

E013.3 Ironing

E013.4 Floor mopping and cleaning

E013.5 Residential relocation
Packing up and unpacking involved in moving to a new residence

E013.8 Other personal hygiene activity

E013.9 Other household maintenance

E014 ACTIVITIES INVOLVING PERSON PROVIDING CAREGIVING

E014.0 Caregiving involving bathing

E014.1 Caregiving involving lifting

E014.9 Other activity involving person providing caregiving

E015 ACTIVITIES INVOLVING FOOD PREPARATION, COOKING AND GRILLING

E015.0 Food preparation and clean up
Dishwashing

E015.1 Grilling and smoking food

E015.2 Cooking and baking
Use of stove, oven and microwave oven

E015.9 Other activity involving cooking and grilling

E016	ACTIVITIES INVOLVING PROPERTY AND LAND MAINTENANCE, BUILDING AND CONSTRUCTION
E016.0	**Digging, shoveling and raking**
	Dirt digging
	Raking leaves
	Snow shoveling
E016.1	**Gardening and landscaping**
	Pruning, trimming shrubs, weeding
E016.2	**Building and construction**
E016.9	**Other activity involving property and land maintenance, building and construction**

E017	ACTIVITIES INVOLVING ROLLER COASTERS AND OTHER TYPES OF EXTERNAL MOTION
E017.0	**Roller coaster riding**
E017.9	**Other activity involving external motion**

E018	ACTIVITIES INVOLVING PLAYING MUSICAL INSTRUMENT
	Activity involving playing electric musical instrument
E018.0	**Piano playing**
	Musical keyboard (electronic) playing
E018.1	**Drum and other percussion instrument playing**
E018.2	**String instrument playing**
E018.3	**Wind and brass instrument playing**

E019	ACTIVITIES INVOLVING ANIMAL CARE
	Excludes:
	horseback riding (E006.1)
E019.0	**Walking an animal**
E019.1	**Milking an animal**
E019.2	**Grooming and shearing an animal**
E019.9	**Other activity involving animal care**

E029	OTHER ACTIVITY
E029.0	**Refereeing a sports activity**
E029.1	**Spectator at an event**
E029.2	**Rough housing and horseplay**
E029.9	**Other activity**

E030	UNSPECIFIED ACTIVITY
E030	**Unspecified activity**

RAILWAY ACCIDENTS (E800-E807)

Note:
For definitions of railway accident and related terms, see complete ICD-9-CM.

Excludes:
accidents involving railway train and: aircraft (E840.0-E845.9); motor vehicle (E810.0-E825.9); watercraft (E830.0-E838.9)

The following definitions are for use with categories E800-E807:

Railway employee (.0)

Any person who by virtue of his employment in connection with a railway, whether by the railway company or not, is at increased risk of involvement in a railway accident, such as: catering staff of train; driver; guard; porter; postal staff on train; railway fireman; shunter; sleeping car attendant

Passenger on railway (.1)

Any authorized person traveling on a train, except a railway employee.

Excludes:
intending passenger waiting at station (.8); unauthorized rider on railway vehicle (.8)

Pedestrian (.2)

Any person involved in an accident who was not at the time of the accident riding in or on a motor vehicle, railroad train, streetcar, animal-drawn or other vehicle, or on a bicycle or animal.

Includes:
Person: changing tire of vehicle; in or operating a pedestrian conveyance; making adjustment to motor of vehicle; on foot

Pedal cyclist (.3)

Any person riding on a pedal cycle or in a sidecar attached to such a vehicle

Other specified person (.8)

Intending passenger or bystander waiting at station; Unauthorized rider on railway vehicle

Unspecified person (.9)

E800	RAILWAY ACCIDENT INVOLVING COLLISION WITH ROLLING STOCK
	Includes:
	collision between railway trains or railway vehicles, any kind; collision NOS on railway; derailment with antecedent collision with rolling stock or NOS
E800.0	**Railway employee**
E800.1	**Passenger on railway**
E800.2	**Pedestrian**

E800.8 Other specified person
E800.9 Unspecified person

E801 **RAILWAY ACCIDENT INVOLVING COLLISION WITH OTHER OBJECT**

Includes:

collision of railway train with: buffers; fallen tree on railway; gates; platform; rock on railway; streetcar; other nonmotor vehicle; other object

Excludes:

collision with aircraft (E840.0-E842.9); motor vehicle (E810.0-E810.9, E820.0-E822.9)

E801.0 Railway employee
E801.1 Passenger on railway
E801.2 Pedestrian
E801.3 Pedal cyclist
E801.8 Other specified person
E801.9 Unspecified person

E802 **RAILWAY ACCIDENT INVOLVING DERAILMENT WITHOUT ANTECEDENT COLLISION**

E802.0 Railway employee
E802.1 Passenger on railway
E802.2 Pedestrian
E802.8 Other specified person
E802.9 Unspecified person

E804 **FALL IN, ON, OR FROM RAILWAY TRAIN**

Excludes:

fall related to collision, derailment or explosion of railway train (E800.0-E803.9)

E804.0 Railway employee
E804.1 Passenger on railway
E804.2 Pedestrian
E804.8 Other specified person
E804.9 Unspecified person

E805 **HIT BY ROLLING STOCK**

Includes:

crushed by railway train or part; injured by railway train or part; killed by railway train or part; knocked down by railway train or part; run over by railway train or part

Excludes:

pedestrian hit by object set in motion by railway train (E806.0-E806.9)

E805.0 Railway employee
E805.1 Passenger on railway
E805.2 Pedestrian
E805.8 Other specified person
E805.9 Unspecified person

E806 **OTHER SPECIFIED RAILWAY ACCIDENT**

Includes:

hit by object falling in railway train; injured by door or window on railway train; nonmotor road vehicle or pedestrian hit by object set in motion by railway train

railway train hit by falling: earth NOS; rock; tree; other object

Excludes:

railway accident due to cataclysm (E908-E909)

E806.0 Railway employee
E806.1 Passenger on railway
E806.2 Pedestrian
E806.8 Other specified person
E806.9 Unspecified person

MOTOR VEHICLE TRAFFIC ACCIDENTS (E810-E819)

Note:

For definitions of motor vehicle traffic accident, and related terms, see complete ICD-9-CM.

Excludes:

accidents involving motor vehicle and aircraft (E840.0-E845.9)

[SEE ALSO LATE EFFECTS OF MOTOR VEHICLE ACCIDENT (E929.0).]

The following is for use with categories E810-E819:

Driver of motor vehicle other than motorcycle (.0)

A driver of a motor vehicle is the occupant of the motor vehicle operating it or intending to operate it

Passenger in motor vehicle other than motorcycle (.1)

Other authorized occupants of a motor vehicle

Motorcyclist (.2)

The driver of a motorcycle

Passenger on motorcycle (.3)

Other authorized occupants of a motorcycle

Pedal cyclist (.6)

Any person riding a pedal cycle or in a sidecar attached to such a vehicle

Pedestrian (.7)
　Any person involved in an accident who was not at the time of the accident riding in or on a motor vehicle, railroad train, streetcar, animal-drawn or other vehicle, or on a bicycle or animal.

　Includes:
　　person: changing tire of vehicle; in or operating a pedestrian conveyance; making adjustment to motor of vehicle; on foot

Other specified person (.8)
　Occupant of vehicle other than above; Person in railway rain or involved in accident; Unauthorized rider of motor vehicle

Unspecified person (.9)

E810　INVOLVING COLLISION WITH TRAIN

　Excludes:
　　motor vehicle collision with object set in motion by railway train (E815.0-E815.9); railway train hit by object set in motion by motor vehicle (E818.0-E818.9)

E810.0	Driver of motor vehicle other than motorcycle
E810.1	Passenger in motor vehicle other than motorcycle
E810.2	Motorcyclist
E810.3	Passenger on motorcycle
E810.6	Pedal cyclist
E810.7	Pedestrian
E810.8	Other specified person
E810.9	Unspecified person

E811　INVOLVING RE-ENTRANT COLLISION WITH ANOTHER MOTOR VEHICLE

　Includes:
　　collision between motor vehicle which accidentally leaves the roadway then re-enters the same roadway, or the opposite roadway on a divided highway, and another motor vehicle.

　Excludes:
　　collision on the same roadway when none of the motor vehicles involved have left and re-entered the roadway (E812.0-E812.9)

E811.0	Driver of motor vehicle other than motorcycle
E811.1	Passenger in motor vehicle other than motorcycle
E811.2	Motorcyclist
E811.3	Passenger on motorcycle
E811.6	Pedal cyclist
E811.7	Pedestrian
E811.8	Other specified person
E811.9	Unspecified person

E812　INVOLVING COLLISION WITH MOTOR VEHICLE

　Includes:
　　collision with another motor vehicle parked, stopped, stalled, disabled, or abandoned on the highway; motor vehicle collision NOS

E812.0	Driver of motor vehicle other than motorcycle
E812.1	Passenger in motor vehicle other than motorcycle
E812.2	Motorcyclist
E812.3	Passenger on motorcycle
E812.6	Pedal cyclist
E812.7	Pedestrian
E812.8	Other specified person
E812.9	Unspecified person

E813　INVOLVING COLLISION WITH OTHER VEHICLE

　Includes:
　　collision between motor vehicle, any kind, and: other road (nonmotor transport) vehicle, such as: animal carrying a person; animal-drawn vehicle; pedal cycle; streetcar

　Excludes:
　　collision with: object set in motion by nonmotor road vehicle (E815.0-815.9); pedestrian)(E814.0-814.9)

　　Nonmotor road vehicle hit by object set in motion by motor vehicle (E818.0-818.9)

E813.0	Driver of motor vehicle other than motorcycle
E813.1	Passenger in motor vehicle other than motorcycle
E813.2	Motorcyclist
E813.3	Passenger on motorcycle
E813.6	Pedal cyclist
E813.7	Pedestrian
E813.8	Other specified person
E813.9	Unspecified person

E814　INVOLVING COLLISION WITH PEDESTRIAN

　Includes
　　collision between motor vehicle, any kind and pedestrian; pedestrian dragged, hit, or run over by motor vehicle, any kind

Excludes:
   pedestrian hit by object set in motion by motor vehicle (E818.0-E818.9)

E814.0   **Driver of motor vehicle other than motorcycle**

E814.1   **Passenger in motor vehicle other than motorcycle**

E814.2   **Motorcyclist**

E814.3   **Passenger on motorcycle**

E814.6   **Pedal cyclist**

E814.7   **Pedestrian**

E814.8   **Other specified person**

E814.9   **Unspecified person**

E815   **INVOLVING COLLISION ON THE HIGHWAY**

Includes:
   collision (due to loss of control) (on highway) between motor vehicle, any kind, and: abutment; (bridge) (overpass); animal (herded) (unattended); fallen stone, traffic sign, tree, utility pole; guard rail or boundary fence; interhighway divider; landslide (not moving); object set in motion by railway train or road vehicle (motor) (nonmotor); object thrown in front of motor vehicle; safety island; temporary traffic sign or marker; wall of cut made for road; other object, fixed, movable, or moving

Excludes:
   collision with: any object off the highway (resulting from loss of control) (E816.0-E816.9); any object which normally would have been off the highway and is not stated to have been on it (E816.0-E816.9); motor vehicle parked, stopped, stalled, disabled, or abandoned on highway (E812.0-E812.9); moving landslide (E909)

   motor vehicle hit by object: set in motion by railway train or road vehicle (motor) (nonmotor) (E818.0-E818.9); thrown into or on vehicle (E818.0-E818.9)

E815.0   **Driver of motor vehicle other than motorcycle**

E815.1   **Passenger in motor vehicle other than motorcycle**

E815.2   **Motorcyclist**

E815.3   **Passenger on motorcycle**

E815.6   **Pedal cyclist**

E815.7   **Pedestrian**

E815.8   **Other specified person**

E815.9   **Unspecified person**

E816   **DUE TO LOSS OF CONTROL, WITHOUT COLLISION ON THE HIGHWAY**

Includes:
   motor vehicle:

     failing to make curve and: colliding with object off the highway; overturning; stopping abruptly off the highway

     going out of control (due to) blowout and: colliding with object off the highway; overturning; stopping abruptly off the highway

     burst tire and: colliding with object off the highway; overturning; stopping abruptly off the highway

     driver falling asleep and: colliding with object off the highway; overturning; stopping abruptly off the highway

     driver inattention and: colliding with object off the highway; overturning; stopping abruptly off the highway

     excessive speed and: colliding with object off the highway; overturning; stopping abruptly off the highway

     failure of mechanical part and: colliding with object off the highway; overturning; stopping abruptly off the highway

Excludes:
   collision on highway following loss of control (E810.0-E815.9); loss of control of motor vehicle following collision on the highway (E810.0-E815.9)

E816.0   **Driver of motor vehicle other than motorcycle**

E816.1   **Passenger in motor vehicle other than motorcycle**

E816.2   **Motorcyclist**

E816.3   **Passenger on motorcycle**

E816.6   **Pedal cyclist**

E816.7   **Pedestrian**

E816.8   **Other specified person**

E816.9   **Unspecified person**

E817 NONCOLLISION ACCIDENT WHILE BOARDING OR ALIGHTING

Includes:
> fall down stairs of motor bus while boarding or alighting; fall from car in street while boarding or alighting; injured by moving part of the vehicle while boarding or alighting; trapped by door of motor bus while boarding or alighting

- **E817.0** Driver of motor vehicle other than motorcycle
- **E817.1** Passenger in motor vehicle other than motorcycle
- **E817.2** Motorcyclist
- **E817.3** Passenger on motorcycle
- **E817.6** Pedal cyclist
- **E817.7** Pedestrian
- **E817.8** Other specified person
- **E817.9** Unspecified person

E818 OTHER NONCOLLISION MOTOR VEHICLE TRAFFIC ACCIDENT

Includes:
> accidental poisoning from exhaust gas generated by motor vehicle while in motion; breakage of any part of motor vehicle while in motion; explosion of any part of motor vehicle while in motion; fall, jump, or being accidentally pushed from motor vehicle while in motion; fire starting in motor vehicle while in motion; hit by object thrown into or on motor vehicle while in motion; injured by being thrown against some part of, or object in motor vehicle while in motion; injury from moving part of motor vehicle while in motion; object falling in or on motor vehicle while in motion; object thrown on motor vehicle while in motion; collision of railway train or road vehicle except motor vehicle, with object set in motion by motor vehicle; motor vehicle hit by object set in motion by railway train or road vehicle (motor) (nonmotor); pedestrian, railway train, or road vehicle (motor) (nonmotor) hit by object set in motion by motor vehicle

Excludes:
> collision between motor vehicle and: object set in motion by railway train or road vehicle (motor) (nonmotor) (E815.0-E815.9); object thrown towards the motor vehicle (E815.0-E815.9); person overcome by carbon monoxide generated by stationary motor vehicle off the roadway with motor running (E868.2)

- **E818.0** Driver of motor vehicle other than motorcycle
- **E818.1** Passenger in motor vehicle other than motorcycle
- **E818.2** Motorcyclist
- **E818.3** Passenger on motorcycle
- **E818.6** Pedal cyclist
- **E818.7** Pedestrian
- **E818.8** Other specified person
- **E818.9** Unspecified person

E819 MOTOR VEHICLE TRAFFIC ACCIDENT OF UNSPECIFIED NATURE

Includes:
> motor vehicle traffic accident NOS; traffic accident NOS

- **E819.0** Driver of motor vehicle other than motorcycle
- **E819.1** Passenger in motor vehicle other than motorcycle
- **E819.2** Motorcyclist
- **E819.3** Passenger on motorcycle
- **E819.6** Pedal cyclist
- **E819.7** Pedestrian
- **E819.8** Other specified person
- **E819.9** Unspecified person

MOTOR VEHICLE NONTRAFFIC ACCIDENTS (E820-E825)

Note:
> For definitions of motor vehicle nontraffic accident and related terms see complete ICD-9-CM.

Includes:
> accidents involving motor vehicles being used in recreational or sporting activities off the highway; collision and noncollision motor vehicle accidents occurring entirely off the highway

Excludes:

accidents involving motor vehicle and: aircraft (E840.0-E845.9); watercraft (E830.0-E838.9); accidents, not on the public highway, involving agricultural and construction machinery but not involving another motor vehicle (E919.0, E919.2, E919.7)

[SEE ALSO LATE EFFECTS OF MOTOR VEHICLE ACCIDENT (E929.0). SEE ALSO LATE EFFECTS OF OTHER TRANSPORT ACCIDENT (E929.1).]

The following is for use with categories E820-E825

Driver (.0)

The occupant of the motor vehicle operating it or intending to operate it.

Motorcyclist (.2)

The driver of a motorcycle.

Passenger (.1 and .3)

Other authorized occupants of a motor vehicle

Pedal Cyclist (.6)

Any person riding a pedal cycle or in a sidecar attached to such a vehicle

Pedestrian (.7)

Any person involved in an accident who was not at the time of the accident riding in or on a motor vehicle, railroad train, streetcar, animal-drawn or other vehicle, or on a bicycle or animal.

Includes:

person: changing tire of vehicle; in or operating a pedestrian conveyance; making adjustment to motor of vehicle; on foot

Other specified person (.8)

Occupant of vehicle other than above; Person on railway train involved in accident; Unauthorized rider of motor vehicle

E820 INVOLVING MOTOR-DRIVEN SNOW VEHICLE

Includes:

breakage of part of motor-driven snow vehicle (not on public highway); fall from motor-driven snow vehicle (not on public highway); hit by motor-driven snow vehicle (not on public highway); overturning of motor-driven snow vehicle (not on public highway); run over or dragged by motor-driven snow vehicle (not on public highway)

collision of motor-driven snow vehicle with: animal (being ridden) (-drawn vehicle); another off-road motor vehicle; other motor vehicle, not on public highway; railway train; other object, fixed or movable

injury caused by rough landing of motor-driven snow vehicle (after leaving ground on rough terrain)

Excludes:

accident on the public highway involving motor driven snow vehicle (E810.0-E819.9)

E820.0 Driver of motor vehicle other than motorcycle
E820.1 Passenger in motor vehicle other than motorcycle
E820.2 Motorcyclist
E820.3 Passenger on motorcycle
E820.6 Pedal cyclist
E820.7 Pedestrian
E820.8 Other specified person
E820.9 Unspecified person

E821 INVOLVING OTHER OFF-ROAD MOTOR VEHICLE

Includes:

breakage of part of off-road motor vehicle, except snow vehicle (not on public highway); fall from off-road motor vehicle, except snow vehicle (not on public highway); hit by off-road motor vehicle, except snow vehicle (not on public highway); overturning of off-road motor vehicle, except snow vehicle (not on public highway); run over or dragged by off-road motor vehicle, except snow vehicle (not on public highway); thrown against some part of or object in off-road motor vehicle, except snow vehicle (not on public highway)

collision with: animal (being ridden) (-drawn vehicle); another off-road motor vehicle, except snow vehicle; other motor vehicle, not on public highway; other object, fixed or movable

Excludes:
> accident on public highway involving off-road motor vehicle (E810.0-E819.9); collision between motor driven snow vehicle and other off-road motor vehicle (E820.0-E820.9); hovercraft accident on water (E830.0-E838.9)

	E821.0	Driver of motor vehicle other than motorcycle
	E821.1	Passenger in motor vehicle other than motorcycle
	E821.2	Motorcyclist
	E821.3	Passenger on motorcycle
	E821.6	Pedal cyclist
	E821.7	Pedestrian
	E821.8	Other specified person
	E821.9	Unspecified person
E822		INVOLVING OTHER COLLISION WITH MOVING OBJECT

Includes:
> collision, not on public highway, between motor vehicle, except off-road motor vehicle and: animal; nonmotor vehicle; other motor vehicle, except off-road motor vehicle; pedestrian; railway train; other moving object

Excludes:
> collision with:; motor-driven snow vehicle (E820.0-E820.9); other off-road motor vehicle (E821.0-E821.9)

	E822.0	Driver of motor vehicle other than motorcycle
	E822.1	Passenger in motor vehicle other than motorcycle
	E822.2	Motorcyclist
	E822.3	Passenger on motorcycle
	E822.6	Pedal cyclist
	E822.7	Pedestrian
	E822.8	Other specified person
	E822.9	Unspecified person
E823		INVOLVING OTHER COLLISION WITH STATIONARY OBJECT

Includes:
> collision, not on public highway, between motor vehicle, except off-road motor vehicle, and any object, fixed or movable, but not in motion

	E823.0	Driver of motor vehicle other than motorcycle
	E823.1	Passenger in motor vehicle other than motorcycle
	E823.2	Motorcyclist
	E823.3	Passenger on motorcycle
	E823.6	Pedal cyclist
	E823.7	Pedestrian
	E823.8	Other specified person
	E823.9	Unspecified person
E824		OTHER ACCIDENT WHILE BOARDING OR ALIGHTING

Includes:
> fall while boarding or alighting from motor vehicle except off-road motor vehicle, not on public highway; injury from moving part of motor vehicle while boarding or alighting from motor vehicle except off-road motor vehicle, not on public highway; trapped by door of motor vehicle while boarding or alighting from motor vehicle except off-road motor vehicle, not on public highway

	E824.0	Driver of motor vehicle other than motorcycle
	E824.1	Passenger in motor vehicle other than motorcycle
	E824.2	Motorcyclist
	E824.3	Passenger on motorcycle
	E824.6	Pedal cyclist
	E824.7	Pedestrian
	E824.8	Other specified person
	E824.9	Unspecified person
E825		OTHER MOTOR VEHICLE NONTRAFFIC ACCIDENT OF OTHER AND UNSPECIFIED NATURE

Includes:
> accidental poisoning from carbon monoxide generated by motor vehicle while in motion, not on public highway; breakage of any part of motor vehicle while in motion, not on public highway; explosion of any part of motor vehicle while in motion, not on public highway; fall, jump, or being accidentally pushed from motor vehicle while in motion, not on public highway; fire starting in motor vehicle while in motion, not on public highway; hit by object thrown into, towards, or on motor vehicle while in motion, not on public highway; injured by being thrown against some part of, or object in motor vehicle while in motion,

not on public highway; injury from moving part of motor vehicle while in motion, not on public highway; object falling in or on motor vehicle while in motion, not on public highway; motor vehicle nontraffic accident NOS

Excludes:
fall from or in stationary motor vehicle (E884.9, E885); overcome by carbon monoxide or exhaust gas generated by stationary motor vehicle off the roadway with motor running (E868.2); struck by falling object from or in stationary motor vehicle (E916)

- **E825.0** Driver of motor vehicle other than motorcycle
- **E825.1** Passenger in motor vehicle other than motorcycle
- **E825.2** Motorcyclist
- **E825.3** Passenger on motorcycle
- **E825.6** Pedal cyclist
- **E825.7** Pedestrian
- **E825.8** Other specified person
- **E825.9** Unspecified person

OTHER ROAD VEHICLE ACCIDENTS (E826-E829)

Note:
Other road vehicle accidents are transport accidents involving road vehicles other than motor vehicles. For definitions of other road vehicle and related terms, see complete ICD-9-CM.

Includes:
accidents involving other road vehicles being used in recreational or sporting activities

Excludes:
collision of other road vehicle [any] with: aircraft (E840.0-E845.9); motor vehicle (E813.0-E813.9, E820.0-E822.9); railway train (E801.0-E801.9)

The following is for use with categories E826-E829

Pedestrian (.0)
Any person involved in an accident who was not at the time of the accident riding in or on a motor vehicle, railroad train, streetcar, animal-drawn or other vehicle, or on a bicycle or animal.

Includes:
person: changing tire of vehicle; in or operating a pedestrian conveyance; making adjustment to motor of vehicle; on foot

Pedal Cyclist (.1)
Any person riding a pedal cycle or in a sidecar attached to such a vehicle

E826 PEDAL CYCLE ACCIDENT

Includes:
breakage of any part of pedal cycle

collision between pedal cycle and: animal (being ridden) (herded) (unattended); another pedal cycle; nonmotor road vehicle, any; pedestrian; other object, fixed, movable, or moving, not set in motion by motor vehicle, railway train, or aircraft

entanglement in wheel of pedal cycle; fall from pedal cycle; hit by object falling or thrown on the pedal cycle; pedal cycle accident NOS; pedal cycle overturned

- **E826.0** Pedestrian
- **E826.1** Pedal cyclist
- **E826.8** Other specified person
- **E826.9** Unspecified person

E828 ACCIDENT INVOLVING ANIMAL INVOLVING BEING RIDDEN

Includes:
collision between animal being ridden and: another animal; nonmotor road vehicle, except pedal cycle, and animal-drawn vehicle; pedestrian, pedestrian conveyance, or pedestrian vehicle;other object, fixed, movable, or moving, not set in motion by motor vehicle, railway train, or aircraft

fall from animal being ridden; knocked down by animal being ridden; thrown from animal being ridden; trampled by animal being ridden; ridden animal stumbled and fell

Excludes:
collision of animal being ridden with: animal-drawn vehicle (E827.0-E827.9); pedal cycle (E826.0-E826.9)

- **E828.0** Pedestrian
- **E828.2** Rider of Animal
- **E828.8** Other specified person
- **E828.9** Unspecified person

E829   OTHER ROAD VEHICLE ACCIDENTS

Includes:
> accident while boarding or alighting from: streetcar; nonmotor road vehicle not classifiable to E826-E828
>
> blow from object in: streetcar; nonmotor road vehicle not classifiable to E826-E828
>
> breakage of any part of: streetcar; nonmotor road vehicle not classifiable to E826-E828
>
> caught in door of: streetcar; nonmotor road vehicle not classifiable to E826-E828
>
> derailment of: streetcar; nonmotor road vehicle not classifiable to E826-E828
>
> fall in, on, or from: streetcar; nonmotor road vehicle not classifiable to E826-E828
>
> fire in: streetcar; nonmotor road vehicle not classifiable to E826-E828
>
> collision between streetcar or nonmotor road vehicle, except as in E826-E828, and: animal (not being ridden); another nonmotor road vehicle not classifiable to E826-E828; pedestrian; other object, fixed, movable, or moving, not set in motion by motor vehicle, railway train, or aircraft
>
> nonmotor road vehicle accident NOS; streetcar accident NOS

Excludes:
> collision with: animal being ridden (E828.0-E828.9); animal-drawn vehicle (E827.0-E827.9); pedal cycle (E826.0-E826.9)

E829.0   Pedestrian
E829.8   Other specified person
E829.9   Unspecified person

WATER TRANSPORT ACCIDENTS (E830-E838)

Note:
> For definitions of water transport accident and related terms, see complete ICD-9-CM.

Includes:
> watercraft accidents in the course of recreational activities

Excludes:
> accidents involving both aircraft, including objects set in motion by aircraft, and watercraft (E840-E845.9)

The following is for use with categories E830-E838:

Occupant of small boat (.0 and .1)
> Any watercraft propelled by paddle, oars, or small motor, with a passenger capacity of less than ten.

Includes:
> boat NOS; canoe; coble; dinghy; punt; raft; rowboat; rowing shell; scull; skiff; small motorboat

Excludes:
> barge; lifeboat (used after abandoning ship); raft (anchored) being used as diving platform; yacht

Occupant of small boat, powered (.1)
> Excludes: water skier (.4)

Other specified person (.8)
> Immigration and custom officials on board ship
>
> Person: accompanying passenger or member of crew; visiting boat
>
> Pilot (guiding ship into port)

E833   FALL ON STAIRS OR LADDERS IN WATER TRANSPORT

Excludes:
> fall due to accident to watercraft (E831.0-E831.9)

E833.0   Occupant of small boat, unpowered
E833.1   Occupant of small boat, powered
E833.8   Other specified person
E833.9   Unspecified person

E834   OTHER FALL FROM ONE LEVEL TO ANOTHER IN WATER TRANSPORT

Excludes:
> fall due to accident to watercraft (E831.0-E831.9)

E834.0   Occupant of small boat, unpowered
E834.1   Occupant of small boat, powered
E834.8   Other specified person
E834.9   Unspecified person

E835   OTHER AND UNSPECIFIED FALL IN WATER TRANSPORT

Excludes:
> fall due to accident to watercraft (E831.0-E831.9)

E835.0   Occupant of small boat, unpowered

Code	Description
E835.1	Occupant of small boat, powered
E835.8	Other specified person
E835.9	Unspecified person

PLACE OF OCCURRENCE (E849)

The following category is for use to denote the place where the injury or poisoning occurred.

E849 PLACE OF OCCURRENCE

E849.0 Home

Apartment; Boarding house; Farm house; Home premises; House (residential); Noninstitutional place of residence

Private: driveway; garage; garden; home; walk; Swimming pool in private house or garden; Yard of home

Excludes:

home under construction but not yet occupied (E849.3); institutional place of residence (E849.7)

E849.1 Farm

Farm: buildings; land under cultivation

Excludes:

farm house and home premises of farm (E849.0)

E849.2 Mine or quarry

Gravel pit; Sand pit; Tunnel under construction

E849.3 Industrial place and premises

Building under construction; Dockyard; Dry dock

Factory building; premises

Garage (place of work); Industrial yard; Loading platform (factory) (store); Plant, industrial; Railway yard; Shop (place of work); Warehouse; Workhouse

E849.4 Place for recreation and sport

Amusement park; Baseball field; Basketball court; Beach resort; Cricket ground; Fives court; Football field; Golf course; Gymnasium; Hockey field; Holiday camp; Ice palace; Lake resort; Mountain resort; Playground, including school playground; Public park; Racecourse; Resort NOS; Riding school; Rifle range; Seashore resort; Skating rink; Sports palace; Stadium; Swimming pool, public; Tennis court; Vacation resort

Excludes:

that in private house or garden (E849.0)

E849.5 Street and highway

E849.6 Public building

Building (including adjacent grounds) used by the general public or by a particular group of the public, such as: airport; bank; café; casino; church; cinema; clubhouse; courthouse; dance hall; garage building (for car storage); hotel; market (grocery or other commodity); movie house; music hall; nightclub; office; office building; opera house; post office; public hall; radio broadcasting station; restaurant; school (state) (public) (private); shop, commercial; station (bus) (railway); store; theater

Excludes:

home garage (E849.0); industrial building or workplace (E849.3)

E849.7 Residential institution

Children's home; Dormitory; Hospital; Jail; Old people's home; Orphanage; Prison; Reform School

E849.8 Other specified places (see unabridged ICD)

Beach NOS; Canal; Caravan site NOS; Derelict house; Desert; Dock; Forest; Harbor; Hill; Lake NOS; Mountain; Parking lot; Parking place; Pond or pool (natural); Prairie; Public place NOS; Railway line; Reservoir; River; Sea;

Seashore NOS; Stream; Swamp; Trailer court; Woods

E849.9   **Unspecified place**

ACCIDENTAL FALLS (E880-E888)

Excludes:

falls (in or from): burning building (E890.8, E891.8); into fire (E890.0-E899); into water (with submersion or drowning) (E919.0-E919.9); machinery (in operation) (E919.0-E919.9); on edged, pointed, or sharp object (E920.0-E920.9); transport vehicle (E800.0-E845.9); vehicle not elsewhere classifiable (E846-E848)

[SEE ALSO LATE EFFECTS OF ACCIDENTAL FALL (E929.3). SEE ALSO PERSONAL HISTORY OF FALL (V15.88).]

E880   **FALL ON OR FROM STAIRS OR STEPS**

     E880.0   **Escalator**

     E880.1   **Fall on or from sidewalk curb**

         Excludes:

            fall from moving sidewalk (E885.9)

     E880.9   **Other stairs or steps**

E881   **FALL ON OR FROM LADDERS OR SCAFFOLDING**

     E881.0   **Fall from ladder**

     E881.1   **Fall from scaffolding**

E882   **FALL FROM OR OUT OF BUILDING OR OTHER STRUCTURE**

         Fall from: balcony; bridge; building; flagpole; tower; turret; viaduct; wall; window

         Fall through roof

     Excludes:

         collapese of a building or sturcture (E916); fall or jump from burning building (E890.8, E891.8)

     E882   **Fall from or out of building or other structure**

E883   **FALL INTO HOLE OR OTHER OPENING IN SURFACE**

     Includes:

         fall into: cavity, dock; hole; pit; quarry; shaft; swimming pool; tank; well

     Excludes:

         fall into water NOS (E910.0-E910.9)

     E883.0   **Accident from diving or jumping into water [swimming pool]**

         Strike or hit: against bottom when jumping or diving into water; wall or board of swimming pool; water surface

         Excludes:

            diving with insufficient air supply (E913.2); effects of air pressure from diving (E902.2)

     E883.1   **Accidental fall into well**

     E883.2   **Accidental fall into storm drain or manhole**

     E883.9   **Fall into other hole or other opening in surface**

E884   **OTHER FALL FROM ONE LEVEL TO ANOTHER**

     E884.1   **Fall from cliff**

     E884.2   **Fall from chair**

     E884.3   **Fall from wheelchair**

         Fall from motorized mobility scooter; Fall from motorized wheelchair

     E884.4   **Fall from bed**

     E884.5   **Fall from other furniture**

     E884.6   **Fall from commode**

         Toilet

     E884.9   **Other fall from one level to another**

         Fall from: embankment; haystack; stationary vehicle; tree

E885   **FALL ON SAME LEVEL FROM SLIPPING, TRIPPING OR STUMBLING**

     E885.0   **Fall from (nonmotorized) scooter**

         Excludes:

            fall from motorized mobility scooter (E884.3)

     E885.1   **Fall from roller skates**

         Heelies; In-line skates; Wheelies

     E885.2   **Fall from skateboard**

     E885.3   **Fall from skis**

     E885.4   **Fall from snowboard**

     E885.9   **Fall from other slipping, tripping or stumbling**

         Fall on moving sidewalk

E886   **FALL ON SAME LEVEL FROM COLLISION, PUSHING, OR SHOVING, BY OR WITH OTHER PERSON**

     Excludes:

         crushed or pushed by a crowd or human stampede (E917.1, E9117.6)

     E886.0   **In sports**

Tackles in sports

E886.9 Other and unspecified

Fall from collision of pedestrian (conveyance) with another pedestrian (conveyance)

E887 FRACTURE, CAUSE UNSPECIFIED

E887 Fracture, cause unspecified

E888 OTHER AND UNSPECIFIED FALL

Accidental fall NOS; Fall on same level NOS

E888.0 Fall resulting in striking against sharp object

Use additional external cause code to identify object (E920)

E888.1 Fall resulting in striking against other object

E888.8 Other fall

E888.9 Unspecified fall

Fall NOS

OTHER ACCIDENTS (E916-E928)

E916 STRUCK ACCIDENTALLY BY FALLING OBJECT

Collapse of building, except on fire; Falling: rock; snowslide NOS; stone; tree

Object falling from: machine, not in operation; stationary vehicle

Code first:

collapse of building on fire (E890.0-E891.9)

falling object in: cataclysm (E908-E909), machinery accidents (E919.0-E919.9), transport accidents (E800.0-E845.9), vehicle accidents not elsewhere classifiable (E846-E848)

object set in motion by: explosion (E921.0-E921.9, E923.0-E923.9), firearm (E922.0-E922.9), projected object (E917.0-E917.9)

[SEE ALSO CODING LATE EFFECTS OF OTHER ACCIDENTS (E929.8).]

E916 Struck accidentally by falling object

E917 STRIKING AGAINST OR STRUCK ACCIDENTALLY BY OBJECTS OR PERSONS

Includes:

bumping into or against: object (moving) (projected) (stationary); pedestrian conveyance; person

colliding with: object (moving) (projected) (stationary); pedestrian conveyance; person

kicking against: object (moving) (projected) (stationary); pedestrian conveyance; person

stepping on: object (moving) (projected) (stationary); pedestrian conveyance; person

struck by: object (moving) (projected) (stationary); pedestrian conveyance; person

Excludes:

fall from: bumping into or against object (E888); collision with another person, except when caused by a crowd (E886.0-E886.9); stumbling over object (E885)

injury caused by: assault (E960.0-E960.1, E967.0-E967.9); cutting or piercing instrument (E920.0-E920.9); explosion (E921.0-E921.9, E923.0-E923.9); firearm (E922.0-E922.9); machinery (E919.0-E919.9); transport vehicle (E800.0-E845.9); vehicle not elsewhere classifiable (E846-E848)

E917.0 In sports without subsequent fall

Kicked or stepped on during game (football) (rugby); Knocked down while boxing; Struck by hit or thrown ball; Struck by hockey stick or puck

E917.1 Caused by crowd, by collective fear or panic without subsequent fall

Crushed by crowd or human stampede; Pushed by crowd or human stampede; Stepped on by crowd or human stampede

E917.2 In running water without subsequent fall

Excludes:

drowning or submersion (E910.0-E910.9) that in sports (E917.0, E917.5)

E917.3 Furniture without subsequent fall

Excludes:

fall from furniture (E884.2, E884.4-E884.5)

E917.4 Other stationary object without subsequent fall

Bath tub; Fence; Lamp-post

E917.5 Object in sports with subsequent fall

Knocked down while boxing

E917.6 Caused by a crowd, by collective fear or panic with subsequent fall

E917.7 Furniture with subsequent fall

Excludes:

fall from furniture (E884.2, E884.4-E884.5)

E917.8 Other stationary object with subsequent fall

Bath tub; Fence; Lamp-post

E917.9 Other striking against with or without subsequent fall

E918 CAUGHT ACCIDENTALLY IN OR BETWEEN OBJECTS

Caught, crushed, jammed, or pinched in or between moving or stationary objects, such as: escalator; folding object; hand tools, appliances, or implements; sliding door and door frame; under packing crate; washing machine wringer

Excludes:

injury caused by: cutting or piercing instrument (E920.0-E920.9); machinery (E919.0-E919.9); mechanism or component of firearm and air gun (E928.7); transport vehicle (E800.0-E845.9); vehicle not elsewhere classifiable (E846-E848)

struck accidentally by: falling object (E916); object (moving) (projected) (E917.0-E917.9)

E918 Caught accidentally in or between objects

E919 ACCIDENTS CAUSED BY MACHINERY

Includes:

burned by machinery (accident); caught in (moving parts of) machinery (accident); collapse of machinery (accident); crushed by machinery (accident); cut or pierced by machinery (accident); drowning or submersion caused by machinery (accident); explosion of, on, in machinery (accident); fall from or into moving part of machinery (accident); fire starting in or on machinery (accident);

mechanical suffocation caused by machinery (accident); mechanism or component of firearm and air gun (E928.7); object falling from, on, in motion by machinery (accident); overturning of machinery (accident); pinned under machinery (accident); run over by machinery (accident); struck by machinery (accident); thrown from machinery (accident); caught between machinery and other object; machinery accident NOS

Excludes:

accidents involving machinery, not in operation (E884.9, E916-E918)

injury caused by: electric current in connection with machinery (E925.0-E925.9); escalator (E880.0, E918); explosion of pressure vessel in connection with machinery (E921.0-E921.9); moving sidewalk (E885.9); powered hand tools, appliances, and implements (E916-E918, E920.0-E921.9, E923.0-E926.9); transport vehicle accidents involving machinery (E800.0-E848.9)

poisoning by carbon monoxide generated by machine (E868.8)

E919.0 Agriculture machines

Animal-powered agricultural machine; Combine; Derrick, hay; Farm machinery NOS; Farm tractor; Harvester; Hay mower or rake; Reaper; Thresher

Excludes:

that in transport under own power on the highway (E810.0-E819.9); that being towed by another vehicle on the highway (E810.0-E819.9, E827.0-E827.9, E829.0-E829.9); that involved in accident classifiable to E820-E829 (E820.0-E829.9)

E919.1 Mining and earth-drilling machinery

Bore or drill (land) (seabed); Shaft hoist; Shaft lift; Under-cutter

Excludes:

coal car, tram, truck, and tub in mine (E846)

E919.2 Lifting machines and appliances

Chain hoist except in agricultural or mining operations; Crane except in agricultural or mining operations; Derrick except in agricultural or mining operations; Elevator (building) (grain) except in agricultural or mining operations; Forklift truck except in agricultural or mining operations; Lift except in agricultural or mining operations; Pulley block except in agricultural or mining operations; Winch except in agricultural or mining operations

Excludes:

that being towed by another vehicle on the highway (E810.0-E819.9, E827.0-E827.9, E829.0-E829.9); that in transport under own power on the highway (E810.0-E819.9); that involved in accident classifiable to E820-E829 (E820.0-E829.9)

E919.3 Metalworking machines

Abrasive wheel; Forging machine; Lathe; Mechanical shears

Metal: drilling machine; milling machine; power press; rolling-mill; sawing machine

E919.4 Woodworking and forming machines

Band saw; Bench saw; Circular saw; Molding machine; Overhead plane; Powered saw; Radial saw; Sander

Excludes:

hand saw (E920.1)

E919.5 Prime movers, except electrical motors

Gas turbine; Internal combustion engine; Steam engine; Water driven turbine

Excludes:

that being towed by other vehicle on the highway (E810.0-E819.9, E827.0-E827.9, E829.0-E829.9); that in transport under own power on the highway (E810.0-E819.9)

E919.6 Transmission machinery

Transmission: belt; cable; chain; gear; pinion; pulley; shaft

E919.7 Earth moving, scraping, and other excavating machines

Bulldozer; Road scraper; Steam shovel

Excludes:

that being towed by other vehicle on the highway (E810.0-E819.9, E827.0-E827.9, E829.0-E829.9); that in transport under own power on the highway (E810.0-E819.9)

E919.8 Other specified machinery

Machines for manufacture of: clothing; foodstuffs and beverages; paper; Printing machine; Recreational machinery; Spinning, weaving, and textile machines

E919.9 Unspecified machinery

E927 OVEREXERTION AND STRENUOUS AND REPETITIVE MOVEMENTS OR LOADS

Use additional code to identify activity (E001-E030)

E927.0 Overexertion from sudden strenuous movement

Sudden trauma from strenuous movement

E927.1 Overexertion from prolonged static position

Overexertion from maintaining prolonged positions, such as: holding; sitting; standing

E927.2 Excessive physical exertion from prolonged activity

E927.3 Cumulative trauma from repetitive motion

Cumulative trauma from repetitive movements

E927.4	Cumulative trauma from repetitive impact
E927.8	Other overexertion and strenuous and repetitive movements or loads
E927.9	Unspecified overexertion and strenuous and repetitive movements or loads

LATE EFFECTS OF ACCIDENTAL INJURY (E929)

Note:

This category is to be used to indicate accidental injury as the cause of death or disability from late effects, which are themselves classifiable elsewhere. The "late effects" include conditions reported as such or as sequelae which may occur at any time after the acute injury.

E929　LATE EFFECTS OF ACCIDENTAL INJURY

Excludes:
late effects of: surgical and medical procedures (E870.0-E879.9); therapeutic use of drugs and medicines (E930.0-E949.9)

E929.0　Motor vehicle accident
Late effects of accidents classifiable to E810-E825

E929.1　Other transport accident
Late effects of accidents classifiable to E800-E807, E826-E838, E840-E848

E929.3　Accidental fall
Late effects of accidents classifiable to E880-E888

E929.8　Other accidents
Late effects of accidents classifiable to E910-E928.8

E929.9　Unspecified accident
Late effects of accidents classifiable to E910-E928.8

INJURY UNDETERMINED WHETHER ACCIDENTAL OR PURPOSELY INFLICTED (E980-E989)

Note:

Categories E980-E989 are for use when it is unspecified or it cannot be determined whether the injuries are accidental (unintentional), suicide (attempted), or assault.

[SEE ALSO CODING LATE EFFECTS OF INJURY UNDETERMINED WHETHER ACCIDENTALLY OR PURPOSELY INFLICTED (E989).]

E987　FALLING FROM HIGH PLACE, UNDETERMINED WHETHER ACCIDENTALLY OR PURPOSELY INFLICTED

E987.0	Residential premises
E987.1	Other man-made structures
E987.2	Natural Sites
E987.9	Unspecified sites

5. Alphabetic List (ICD-9-CM)

Do not code from this alphabetic list. It is for reference only. Verify your code in the *Numeric* (Tabular) List. Read all "includes," "excludes" and other notes. Codes are sometimes duplicated here because of more than one description for that code. Parentheses indicate a reference to another word or code. The "x" indicates that another digit(s) is needed.

A

Abdomen and other subluxation	739.9
Abdominal pain	789.0x
Abnormal	
head movements	781
involuntary movements	781
Abnormality of gait	781.2
Accidental	
falls	E880-E888
injury, late effects of	E929
Accidents	
motor vehicle nontraffic	E820-E825
motor vehicle traffic	E810-E819
other	E916-E928
railway	E800-E807
road vehicle, other	E826-E829
water transport	E830-E838
Achondroplasia	756.4
Acquired equinovarus deformity	736.71
Acquired musculoskeletal deformities, ostepathies, chondropathies	730-739
Acromial process	811.01
Acromioclavicular region subluxation	739.7
Activity	
animal care	E019.x
arts and handcrafts	E012.x
building and construction	E016.x
cardiorespiratory exercise, other	E009.x
caregiving	E014.x
climbing, rappelling and jumping off	E004.x
computer technology and electronic devices	E011.x
dancing and other rhythmic movement	E005.x
food preparation, cooking and grilling	E015.x
household maintenance	E013.x
hygiene, personal	E013.x
ice and snow	E003.x
muscle strengthening exercises	E010.x
other	E029.x
property and land maintenance	E016.x
roller coasters and other types of external motion	E017.x
sports and athletics played as a team or group	E007.x
sports and athletics played individually	E006.x
sports and athletics, other	E008.x
water and water craft	E002.x
Aftercare	V54-V59
Anasarca	782.3
Anatomical neck	812.02
Ankle and tarsus enthesopathy	726.7x
Ankle, sprains and strains of	845.x
Ankylosing spondylitis	720.0
Ankylosis of joint	718.5x
Anorexia	783.0
Anorexia nervosa	307.1
Aquired deformity, other	738.x
Arm, upper, sprains and strains of	840.x
Arthritis, rheumatoid, with visceral or systemic involvement	714.2
Arthoropathies and related disorders	710-719
Arthralgia, pain in joint	719.4x
Arthritis, rheumatoid	714.x
Arthropathies associated w/ infections	711.x
Ataxia NOS	781.3

Atlas, fracture of 805.0x
Autonomic nervous system, disorders of 337.x

B

Baastrup's syndrome 721.5
Back
    other and unspecified disorders of 724.x
    sprains and strains, other 847.x
Backache, unspecified 724.5
Barré-Liéou syndrome 723.2
Bells palsy 351.0
Body mass index V85.x
Bone and cartilage, other disorders of 733.x
    Tietze's disease 733.6
Brachia neuritis or radiculitis NOS 723.4
Brachial plexus lesions 353.0
Brain damage, mental disorders due to 310x
Bunion disorder 727.1
Burning or prickling sensation 782.0
Bursa, other disorders of 727.x
Bursitis
    of elbow 726.33
    of hand or wrist 726.4

C

Calcification of joint 719.8x
Carotid sinus syndrome 337.01
Carpal tunnel syndrome 354.0
Cauda equina syndrome 344.6x
Central nervous system disorders 340-349
Certificates, issue of medical V68.x
Cervical region
    disorders X723.x
    subluxation 739.1
Cervical rib X756.2
Cervical rib syndrome 353.0
Cervical vertebra subluxation
    fifth 839.05
    first 839.01
    fourth 839.04
    second 839.02
    seventh 839.07
    sixth 839.06
    third 839.03
    unspecified 839.00
Cervicalgia 723.1
Cervicocranial syndrome 723.2
Cervicothoracic region subluxation 739.1
Chest pain 786.5x
Childhood, lack of expected normal
    physiological development 784.x
Chondromalacia of patella 717.7
Chronic pain syndrome 338.4
Cluster headaches 339.0x

Coccyx
    disorders of 724.7x
    sprain and strain 847.4
    subluxation 839.41
Colic: NOS; infantile 789.0x
Concussion 850.x
Conditions influencing health status ... V40-V49
Congenital
    dislocation of hip 754.3x
    genu recurvatum, bowing of bone 754.4x
    musculoskeletal anomalies, other 756.x
    musculoskeletal deformities 754.x
Consulting on behalf of another person .. V65.19
Contracture of joint 718.4x
Contusion
    of trunk 922.x
    of upper limb 923.x
    of face, scalp, and neck except eye(s) 920
    of lower limb and other and
        unspecified sites 924.x
    w/ intact skin on surface 920-924
Costochondral region subluxation 739.8
Costoclavicular syndrome 353.0
Costovertebral region subluxation 739.8
Coxae malum senilis 715.2x
Cramps, abdominal 789.0x
Cranial nerves disorders 352.x
Crystal arthropathies 712.x
Cubitus valgus (acquired) 736.01
Cubitus varus (acquired) 736.02
Curvature of spine 737.x
Cyst of bone 733.2x
    solitary bone cyst 733.21
    other, fibrous dysplasia 733.29

D

Deformities of feet, varus 754.5x
    congenital elevation of scapula 754.52
    radioulnar synostosis 754.53
    madelung's deformity 755.54
Derangement of
    anterior horn of lateral meniscus 717.42
    joint, other 718.x
Diabetes 250.x
Difficulty in walking 719.7
Digestive system, symptoms involving 787.x
Disability examination V68.01

DISH

No ICD-9 code exists for DISH (Diffused Idiopathic Skeletal Hyperostosis). Common coding variations are:

- 721.6 Ankylosing vertebral hyperostosis
- 721.8 Other allied disorders of spine
- 724.1 Pain in thoracic spine
- 724.8 Other symptoms referable to back

Dislocation	830-839
of ankle	837.x
of elbow	832.x
of finger	834.x
of foot	838.x
of hip	835.x
of jaw	830.x
of joint, recurrent	718.3x
of knee	836.x
of knee, closed, other	836.5x
of shoulder	831.x
of wrist	833.x
Dislocations and subluxations	839.x
Disuse atrophy of bone	733.7
Dizziness and giddiness	780.4
Dorsopathies	720-724
Dropsy	782.3
Dupuytren's contracture	728.6
Dysthymic disorder	300.4

E

Edema	782.3
Effusion of joint	719.x
Enthesopathies and allied syndromes, peripheral	726.x
Enthesopathies, peripheral, and allied syndromes	726.x
Enthesopathy	
of elbow region	726.3x
of knee	726.6x
Epicondylitis	
lateral	726.32
medial	726.31
Equinus deformity of foot, acquired	736.72
Essential Hypertension	401.x
benign	401.1
malignant	401.0
unspecified	401.9
Examination	
general medical	V70.x
of participant in clinical trial	V70.7
routine	V70.0
External cause status	E000.x

F

Facial	
pain	784.0
weakness	781.94
Family history	V18.x
Family history of certain chronic disabling diseases	V17.x
Fascia, disorders of	728.x
Fasciculation	781
Fasciitis, unspecified	729.4
Fatigue	780.7x
Feet	
other deformitites	754.7x
valgas deformitites	754.6x
Female genital tract disorders, other	617-629
Fibromatoses, other	728.7x
Fibromatosis, plantar fascial	728.71
Garrod's or knuckle pads	728.79
Fibromyalgia	729.1
Flat foot	734
Foot, sprains and strains of	845.1x
Fracture	
of clavicle	810.x
of humerus	812.x
of lower limb	820-829
of metacarpal bone(s)	815.x
of neck and trunk	805-809
of radius and ulna	813.x
of rib(s), sternum, larynx, and trachea	807.x
of scapula	811.x
of Upper limb	810-819
of vertebral column	805.x
of vertebral column w/out mentiion of spinal cord injury	805.x
of vertebral column, w/ spinal cord injury	806.x
Fracture	
pathologic	V13.51
stress	V13.52
traumatic	V15.51
Fusion of spine [vertebra], congenital	756.15

G

Gait,	
abnormality	781.2
ataxic; paralytic; spastic; staggering	781.2
Golfers' elbow	726.32
Gout and gouty	274.x

H

Hamstring	728.8x
Head region subluxation	739
Head, neck, and trunk problems	V48.x

Head, neck, and trunk problems
    influencing health V48.x
Headache 784.0
Headache syndromes, other 339.x
Headache
    post-traumatic X339.2x
    tension 307.81
    tension type 339.1x
Health
    checkup V70.0
    examination of defined
        subpopulations V70.5
Height, loss of 781.91
Hemarthrosis 719.1x
Hemiplegic migraine 346.3
Herpes zoster 053.x
Hip region subluxation 739.5
History
    family
        of chronic disabling diseases V17.x
    other personal, presenting hazards to
        health V15.x
    personal, of other diseases V13.x
Hyperesthesia 782.0
Hyperhidrosis, generalized 780.8
Hypermobility syndrome 728.5
Hypoesthesia 782.0

I

Injury
    to nerve roots and spinal plexus 953.x
    to nerves and spinal cord 950-957
    to other cranial nerve(s) 951.x
Intervertebral disc disorders 722.x
Intracranial injury 850-854
Investigations and examinations, special V72.x

J

Jaw, diseases of 526.x
Joint crepitus 719.6x
Joint mice 718.1x
Joint
    other and unspecified disorders of 719.x
    other symptoms referable 719.6

K

Kissing spine 721.5
Klippel's disease 723.8
Klippel-Feil syndrome 756.16
Knee enthesopathy 726.6x
Knee
    internal, derangement of 717.x
    sprains and strains of 844.x
Kümmell's disease or spondylitis 721.7

Kyphoscoliosis and scoliosis 737.3x
Kyphosis (aquired) 737.1x

L

Labyrinthitis, unspecified 386.3
Lack of coordination 781.3
Late effects of injuries 905-909
Late effects
    of injuries to the nervous system 907.x
    of musuloskeletal and connective tissue
        injuries 905.x
Leg, sprains and strains of 844.x
Lesion, nerve 354.x
Lesions,
    femoral nerve 355.2
    nonallopathic, not elsewhere classified ... 739.x
    popliteal nerve 355.3
Lethargy 780.79
Lifestyle, problems related to V69.x
Ligament, disorders of 728.x
Light-headedness 780.4
Limbs, other congenital anomalies X755.x
Loose body in joint 718.1x
Lordosis (aquired) 737.2x
Lower extremities subluxation 739.6
Lumbago 724.2
Lumbar
    region subluxation 739.3
    spondylosis w/myelopathy 721.4x
    sprain and strain X847.2
    vertebra subluxation 839.20
Lumbosacral region subluxation 739.3
Lupus 710.0

M

Malaise 780.7x
Ménière's disease 386.0x
Meniscus 718.x
Menopausal and postmenopausal
    disorders 627.x
Menstrual headache 346.4x
Mental disorders
    due to brain damage 310x
    nonpsychotic 300-316
Migraine 346.x
    with aura 346.0x
    common 346.1x
    variants 346.2x
Mononeuritis
    of lower limb 355.x
    of upper limb 354.x
Multiple
    cervical vertebrae subluxation 839.08
Muscle, disorders of 728.x
Muscular atrophy, spinal 335.1

Muscular calcification and ossification	728.1x
Muscular incoordination	781.3
Musculoskeletal system, abnormal x-ray	793.7
Myelitis, herpes zoster	053.14
Mylagia and myositis, unspecified	729.1

N

Nausea and vomiting	787.0x
Neck, contracture of	723.5
Nerve root and plexus	353.x
Nervous and musculoskeletal systems, symptoms involving	781.x
Nervous system peripheral disorders	350-359
Neuralgia	
occipital	723.8
postherpetic trigeminal	053.12
Neuritis, thoracic or lumbosacral, unspecified	724.4
Neurologic neglect syndrome	781.8
Neuropathy	
hereditary and idiopathic peripheral	356.x
idiopathic peripheral autonomic	337
Neurotic disorders	300-316
Numbness	782.0

O

Obesity	278.0x
Obesity, screening	V77.8
Observation and eval, suspected conditions not found	V71.x
Occipitocervical region subluxation	739
Occupational therapy	V57.21
Ocular torticollis	781.93
Osteitis deformans and osteopathies	731.x
Osteoarthropathy, hypertrophic pulmonary	731.2
Osteoarthrosis and allied disorders	715.x
Osteochondropathies	732.x
Osteomyelitis, chronic	730.1x
Osteoporosis	733.0x
screening	V82.81
Other vertabra subluxation	839.4x
Otto's pelvis	715.3x
Overexertion	E927.x
Overweight	278.02

P

Paget's disease of bone	731.0
Pain	338.x
Pain in head NOS	784
Pain	
acute	338.1x
chronic	338.2x
Palmar fascia, contracture of	728.6
Palsy, bell's	351.0
Panniculitis, unspecified	729.3x
Paresthesia	782.0
Pathologic fracture	733.1x
Pelvic region subluxation	739.5
Pelvis subluxation	839.69
Periarthritis of shoulder	726.2
Peripheral enthesopathies and allied syndromes	726.x
Personal and family history, health hazards related	V10-V19
Personality disorders	300-316
Pes planus (acquired)	734
Physical therapy, other	V57.1
Place of occurrence	E849.x
Plexus disorders	353.x
Polyneuropathy, postherpetic	053.13
Postconcussion syndrome	310.2
Postlaminectomy syndrome	722.8x
Posture, abnormal	781.92
Premenstrual	
headache	346.4x
syndrome	625.4
Psychogenic paralysis	306.0
Pubic region subluxation	739.5

R

Radiculitis, thoracic or lumbosacral, unspecified	724.4
Radiological abnormal findings	793.x
Reflex sympathetic dystrophy	337.2x
Rehabilitation care	V57.x
Rheumatism, Excluding the back	725-729
Rib cage subluxation	739.8
Root lesions	353.x
Rotator cuff	840.4
Rotator cuff syndrome of shoulder and allied disorders	726.1x

S

Sacral region subluxation	v739.4
Sacrococcygeal (ligament) sprain and strain	v847.3
Sacrococcygeal region subluxation	v739.4
Sacroiliac (joint) subluxation	839.42
Sacroiliac region, sprains and strains of	846.x
Sacroiliac region subluxation	739.4
Sacrum	
disorders of	724.6
sprain and strain	847.3
subluxation	839.42
Scalenus anticus syndrome	353.0
Schmorl's nodes	722.3x
Sciatia	724.3
Scleroderma	710.1

Scoliosis 737.43
Screening, nutritional, metabolic,
    immunity, etc V77.x
Shoulder, sprains and strains of 840.x
Skin and other integumentary tissue, symptoms
    involving 782.x
Skin sensation, disturbance of 782.0
Skull and head, abnormal x-ray 793
Sleep deprivation, lack of adequate V69.4
Sleep disturbances 780.5x
Snapping hip 719.6x
Soft tissues, other disorders of 729.x
Spasm
    of muscle 728.85
    NOS 781
Spina bifida occulta 756.17
Spondylitis, ankylosing 720.0
Spondylolisthesis, acquired 738.4
Spondylolysis 756.12
    lumbosacral region 756.11
Spondylosis and allied disorders 721.x
Sprains and strains
    of ankle and foot 845.x
    of elbow and forearm 841.x
    of hip and thigh 843.x
    of joints and adjacent muscles 840-848
    of knee and leg 844.x
    of other 847.x
    of sacroiliac region 846.x
    of wrist and hand 842.x
Sprains and strains, other and ill-defined 848.x
Spur, calcaneal 726.73
Stenosis, spinal, other than cervical 724.0x
Sternoclavicular joint subluxation 839.61
Sternoclavicular region subluxation 739.7
Sternum subluxation 839.61
Stiffness of joint, not elsewhere classified . 719.5x
Stress fracture of shaft of femur 733.97
Students, health exam V70.5
Subluxation other than accident 739.x
Subluxations and dislocations 839.x
Subluxations multiple and ill-defined 839.8
Superficial injury 91x.0
Supracondylar fracture of humerus 812.41
Supraspinatus 840.6
Swan-neck deformity 736.22
Symptoms involving head and neck 784.x
Symptoms, general 780.x
Synovium, other disorders of 727.x

T

Talipes planus (acquired) v734
Temporomandibular joint disorders 524.6x

Tendinitis
    calcifying, of shoulder v726.11
    patellar 726.64
Tendon, other disorders of v727.x
Tennis elbow 726.32
Tenosynovitis, bicipital v726.12
Thoracic and lumbar subluxation 839.2x
Thoracic or lumbar intervertebral disc
    degeneration 722.5x
Thoracic
    outlet syndrome 353.0
    region subluxation 739.2
    spondylosis w/ myelopathy 721.4x
    sprain and strain 847.1
    vertebra subluxation 839.21
Thoracolumbar region subluxation 739.2
Tingling 782.0
Tinnitus 388.3x
Tiredness 780.79
Toe, acquired deformities 735.x
Torticollis, unspecified 723.5
Tuberosity, greater 812.03
Traumatic complications and unspecified
    injuries 958-959
Traumatic fracture V15.51
Trigeminal neuralgia 350.1

U

Upper extremities subluxation 739.7

V

Valgus deformity, wrist 736.03
Varus deformity, wrist 736.04
Vertigo NOS 780.4
Vertigo of central origin 386.2
Vertigo, other and unspecified peripheral 386.1x
Vestibular system, disorders of 386.x
Vocational rehabilitation V57.22

W

Wrist, sprains and strains of 842.x

X

X-ray examination V72.50

H PROCEDURE CODES

1. Procedure Coding
Page H-3

2. Commonly Used Codes
Page H-11

3. Evaluation and Management
Page H-21

4. CPT Procedure Codes
Page H-35

5. HCPCS Procedure Codes
Page H-92

6. Procedure Modifiers
Page H-97

7. Clinical Examples
Page H-112

8. Alphabetic List
Page H-128

PROCEDURE CODES

OBJECTIVES

This section includes the HIPAA approved procedure code sets for claims submission. But it is much more than a listing of codes, it also includes the National Correct Coding Initiative (NCCI) edits, Relative Value Units (RVUs) and guidance on the proper use of these codes. This section contains just the excerpts which are of primary concern for chiropractic offices.

OUTLINE

1. Procedure Coding *H-3*
    - Introduction to Procedure Coding *H-3*
    - Coding Conventions *H-5*
    - Getting Started with CPT *H-5*
    - NCCI Coding Edits *H-7*
    - Review *H-10*
2. Commonly Used Procedure Codes *H-11*
    - Commonly Used Procedure Codes *H-11*
    - Commonly Used Procedure Modifiers *H-20*
3. Evaluation and Management *H-21*
    - Introduction to E/M Documentation *H-21*
    - Levels of Care *H-22*
    - Code Selection by Counseling Time *H-32*
    - Review *H-34*
4. CPT Procedure Codes *H-35*
    - Evaluation and Management Codes *H-35*
    - Surgery Codes *H-48*
    - Diagnostic Imaging *H-52*
    - Laboratory Codes *H-62*
    - Medicine Codes (Chiropractic and Therapies) *H-63*
    - Category III (Temporary) *H-90*
5. HCPCS Procedure Codes *H-92*
6. Procedure Modifiers *H-97*
    - Commonly Used Level I CPT Modifiers *H-97*
    - Commonly Used Level II HCPCS Modifiers *H-97*
    - Understanding Modifiers *H-98*
    - Level I CPT Modifiers *H-99*
    - Level II HCPCS Procedure Modifiers *H-108*
7. Clinical Examples *H-112*
    - Clinical Examples for CMT Code *H-114*
    - Clinical Examples for E/M *H-116*
    - Clinical Examples for Other Chiropractic Related Services *H-118*
    - Clinical Examples for Telephone Services *H-122*
    - Clinical Examples for Online Medical Evaluations *H-122*
    - Clinical Examples for Preventive Medicine Service Codes *H-123*
    - Established Patient *H-124*
    - Clinical Examples for Preventive Medicine Counseling (PMC) and/or Risk Factor Reduction for Interventions *H-126*
8. Alphabetic List *H-128*

1. Procedure Coding

INTRODUCTION TO PROCEDURE CODING

There are three recognized procedural coding sets. Two may be used for HIPAA transactions: CPT and HCPCS. Each of these code sets cover different procedural scenarios. These code sets are the following:

- Current Procedural Terminology (CPT®)
- Healthcare Common Procedure Coding System (HCPCS)
- Advanced Billing Concepts (ABC)

Only HIPAA-approved codes pertaining to chiropractic are included in this specialized book. See Resource 346 for information on ABC codes, which may be valuable for internal record keeping.

CPT

CPT® is published by the American Medical Association (AMA). Medicare also refers to these codes as the Healthcare Common Procedure Coding System (HCPCS) Level I code set. *Current Procedural Terminology (CPT®), Fourth Edition*, is a set of codes, descriptions, and guidelines intended to describe procedures and services performed by physicians and other health care providers. Each procedure or service is identified with a five-digit code. The use of CPT codes simplifies the reporting of services.

> "Inclusion of a descriptor and its associated five-digit code number in the CPT codebook is based on whether the procedure is consistent with contemporary medical practice and is performed by many practitioners in clinical practice in multiple locations. Inclusion in the CPT codebook does not represent endorsement by the American Medical Association (AMA) of any particular diagnostic or therapeutic procedure. Inclusion or exclusion of a procedure does not imply any health insurance coverage or reimbursement policy." –CPT 2015, by the AMA

The CPT codes in this *ChiroCode DeskBook* are selected because of their relevance to the chiropractic office.

See Resource 344 for additional information, articles and webinars about procedure coding.

- See Resource 335 for the complete CPT codes.
- See FindACode.com (Resource 336) for electronic searching for CPT codes, descriptions and related information.

HCPCS Codes

HCPCS codes are properly known as HCPCS Level II codes. They are created and maintained by the Centers for Medicare and Medicaid Services (CMS). HCPCS (pronounced "hick-picks") is a five-digit alphanumeric code set that describes physician and non-physician services and supplies. This code set also includes some Quality Data Codes such as those used to report on the Physician Quality Reporting System (PQRS). HCPCS codes pertaining to procedures are included in this section.

One benefit of this code set is the increased specificity for services and supplies that are either unavailable or ill-defined within the CPT code set. Providers should be aware of individual payer preferences regarding the use of HCPCS to avoid claims processing errors.

- See *Section I–Supplies* for HCPCS supply codes.
- See *Section C–Medicare* for information about PQRS.

ABC Codes

ABC codes are created and maintained by Alternative Link to fill the gaps or replace general (unspecific) codes in the CPT and HCPCS code sets. The ABC codes use a five-digit alphabetic system with a two digit identifier based on provider type. This code set does not use modifiers. ABC codes permit documentation of services at a higher level of specificity for practitioners, patients, payers, and researchers. *Currently, these codes may **only** be used for documentation and not HIPAA regulated transactions.*

- See FindACode.com (Resource 346) to search for and learn more about ABC codes.
- See *Section D–Documentation* for more about proper documentation.

Instructions for Procedural Coding

It is significant to note that the instructions from CPT state "Select the name of a procedure that accurately identifies the service performed. Do not select a CPT code that merely approximates the service provided." Therefore, when no "accurate" code exists to describe the service, you will need to do one of the following:

1. If a modifier clarifies and makes the CPT code accurate, append the modifier.
2. If still not accurate, use a HCPCS procedural code if a current one exists.
3. If there is no accurate CPT or HCPCS code, use an unlisted CPT code.
4. When using an unlisted/unspecified code, enter supporting supplemental information in the shaded area within Item #24 on a 1500 claim form or attach a report.

- See Resource 178 for detailed CMS and NUCC claim instructions.

Specific guidelines for each section are available from the original source documents, as published by the AMA and the government. General coding guidance to assist you in understanding and using each of these code sets is included in the *ChiroCode DeskBook*.

Coding Conventions

The following coding conventions are used in this procedure section:

Type Styles

Excerpts from the AMA's CPT codebook are in a type style like this.

Explanations added by the ChiroCode Institute are in a type style like this.

Code Symbols

- ● Identifies a new procedure code added for 2015.
- ▲ Identifies a revised procedure descriptor for 2015.
- # Identifies a re-sequenced code.
- ✚ Identifies CPT add-on codes. Describes additional intra-service work associated with the primary procedure.
- ⊘ Identifies codes that are exempt from the use of modifier 51 but have not been designated as CPT add-on procedures or services.
- ►◄ Identifies new or revised text for this year other than the procedure descriptors.
- ncci Identifies codes to which NCCI edits apply (see page H-9).

Getting Started with CPT

In general, CPT codes are not restricted to any specialty or group, and may be used by any qualified healthcare practitioner. However, certain CPT codes may only be used by a "physician," and the definition of which practitioners are "physicians" varies by state, as specified by statutes.

Format of the Terminology

In order to save space and improve readability, codes have been formatted with the main information on the first line; code differentiation is included below and is indented. The primary component of the text is placed before the semicolon, and is part of the code.

For example:

	Work hardening/conditioning;
97545	initial 2 hours
97546	each additional hour

Therefore, the full description for code 97545 would be "Work hardening/conditioning; initial 2 hours."

CPT Modifiers

Modifiers should be used to properly and accurately identify an encounter that has been altered due to a specific circumstance. The CPT code book states that "the judicious application of modifiers obviates the necessity for separate procedure listings…".

Append an appropriate modifier to more fully describe a service that has been altered. For instance, if a service has been reduced, use a CPT code appended with modifier 52. If the service is substantially greater than normally required, append modifier 22. Append modifier 53 if a course of treatment must be discontinued.

See Chapter 6–Procedure Modifiers in this *Procedures* section for a table of commonly appended modifiers and instructions.

Add-on Codes

Add-on codes mean exactly what the name implies. They never stand alone and are always placed on the second line after the primary code associated with it. In this book, add-on codes are represented with a plus symbol (✢).

For example:

Prolonged physician service in the office or other outpatient setting requiring direct (face-to-face) patient contact beyond the usual service (e.g., prolonged care and treatment on an acute asthmatic patient in an outpatient setting);

✢ 99354   first hour (List separately in addition to code for office or other outpatient Evaluation and Management service)

Code 99354 for prolonged treatment for an unusual circumstance is shown with a "plus" symbol (✢). Use this code **in addition to** the standard office or outpatient evaluation and management codes, when services exceed the usual and customary services.

See the current CPT codebook for detailed guidelines.

Unlisted Codes

An unlisted code could be used in situations in which no **accurate** CPT or HCPCS code is available. Typically, an unlisted procedure code is provided at the end of each CPT category of service to allow for these situations. When using unlisted codes, it is important to include a report describing the encounter. These reports for unlisted codes should not be confused with "special reports," covered in the next paragraph.

When an unlisted code is used, some payers may require you to either briefly define/explain the service rendered (in the supplemental shaded area above the code for Item 24 on the 1500 claim form) and/or attach supporting documentation.

Special Reports

A special report is used to code services that are new, variable, unusual, or rarely provided. These special reports are used to determine medical necessity or medical appropriateness of the service, and are used to justify payment.

Special reports should document the need and extent of the service, including duration of treatment and equipment needed. Special reports can also include treatment plans, therapeutic findings, and exacerbating or other conditions that arise during treatment.

The CPT lists the following as reasons to create a special report: "complexity of symptoms, final diagnosis, diagnostic and therapeutic procedures, concurrent problems, and follow-up care."

Examples:

99080   Special reports such as insurance forms, more than the information conveyed in the usual medical communications or standard reporting form

97799   Unlisted physical medicine/rehabilitation service or procedure

Results/Testing/Reports

In 2007, the CPT Editorial Panel issued a statement that helps to clarify the difference between results, testing, and reports. "Results are the technical component of a service. Testing leads to results; results lead to interpretation. Reports are the work product of the interpretation of numerous test results."

NCCI Coding Edits

National Correct Coding Initiative (NCCI) edits are tools used to determine the appropriate billing of CPT and HCPCS procedural codes. The Centers for Medicare & Medicaid Services (CMS) developed these edits to control improper coding that could lead to inappropriate increased payment of Medicare Part B claims. In an effort to promote correct coding nationwide and assist physicians in correctly coding their services for payment, the policies developed are based on:

- Coding conventions in the American Medical Association's CPT-4 manual
- National and local policies and edits
- Coding guidelines developed by national societies
- Analysis of medical and surgical practices and current coding practices

NCCI edits are dynamic. Codes and policies are updated quarterly. The edits in this annual edition of the *ChiroCode DeskBook* are from NCCI version 20.3 (October-December 2014).

While NCCI edits were not intended for use by commercial/private payers, the impact of these CMS standards goes far beyond Medicare, and affects every doctor and health provider as other payers adopt and adapt them.

There are two types of edits that providers need to pay particular attention to when it comes to reimbursement. Both are components of the National Correct Coding Initiative (NCCI) Edits. They are the Medically Unlikely Edits, and the NCCI code pair edits.

Medically Unlikely Edits

Medically Unlikely Edits (MUE) are the maximum number of units that may be billed on a single session. For example, it is "unlikely" (impossible in this particular situation) to perform more than one unit of 98940 in one patient encounter; therefore, its MUE is 1. If you bill 2 units for a single session, the claim is likely to be rejected.

Some codes do not have any MUE edits assigned. The "Edit Example" on page H-10, shows [MUE=1] which means that this code is typically billed with one unit. None of the commonly used codes for chiropractic have an MUE of more than one for outpatient services.

NCCI Code Pair (Bundling) Edits

NCCI code pair edits are automated coding edits that prevent improper payment when certain codes are submitted together for Part B-covered services.

Understanding NCCI edits can help healthcare providers and coders make appropriate coding decisions.

> **Alert:** NCCI edits are only a guide. CMS states that "it is important to understand, however, that the NCCI does not include all possible combinations of correct coding edits or types of unbundling that exist. Providers are obligated to code correctly even if edits do not exist to prevent use of an inappropriate code combination."

Unbundling

There are two types of unbundling: the first is unintentional which results from a misunderstanding of coding, and the second is intentional, when providers deviate from ethical coding to increase payments. Unbundling is essentially the billing of multiple procedures codes for a group of procedures that are covered by a single comprehensive code.

Correct coding means bundling a group of procedures with an appropriate single code. Examples of unbundling and improper coding are:

- Fragmenting one service into component parts and coding each component part as if it were a separate service.
- Reporting separate codes for related services when one comprehensive code includes all related services.
- Downcoding a service in order to use an additional code when one higher level and more comprehensive code is appropriate. An example is in laboratory coding with various panels and chemistry test options.

Edit Format

Code pair edits apply to code combinations where one of the codes is either a component of a more comprehensive code or is mutually exclusive.

Mutually Exclusive codes are those codes that cannot reasonably be performed in the same session. An example of a mutually exclusive situation for chiropractic is the use of both the Osteopathic Manipulative Treatment (OMT) and the Chiropractic Manipulative Treatment (CMT). Obviously, they both would not happen at the same encounter. A second example is the reporting of an "initial" service and a "subsequent" service. It is contradictory for a service to be classified as an initial and subsequent service at the same time. CPT codes that are mutually exclusive of one another are based either on the CPT definition or the medical impossibility/improbability that the procedure(s) could be performed at the same session.

Superscript Indicators

Column 2 codes are not payable with the column 1 codes unless the edit permits it by using an indicator of "1."

- A superscript indicator of "0" (such as 98926^0) indicates that no modifiers associated with the NCCI are allowed to be used with this code pair. There are no circumstances in which both procedures of the code pair should be paid on the same day by the same provider.
- A superscript indicator of "1" (such as 97140^1) indicates that the modifiers associated with the NCCI are allowed with this code pair when appropriate (e.g., 97140 with a CMT service).

NCCI Edit Challenges

On January 1st, 1999 five physical medicine codes (97122-manual traction, 97250-myofascial release, 97260-manipulation one area, 97261-manipulation additional areas, 97265-joint mobilization) were merged into one new code. This single code is known as 97140-manual therapy techniques. The previous five codes had different coding standards and coding practices. However, the initial edits in 1999 for this new 97140 code resulted in a conflict with CMS's own policy to follow the AMA's CPT coding standards, and the standards and acceptable coding practices of the chiropractic profession.

This edit placed 97140-manual therapy techniques as "mutually exclusive" to 98940 (CMT). Mutually exclusive means the codes are interchangeable and are for the same service.

In 2000, this 97140 edit was changed by CMS. However, they made 97140 a component of the CMT codes (98940-98942), which was still not entirely accurate. By law, "other manual therapy techniques" by a chiropractor are not covered by Medicare. Furthermore, 97140 is a time based code, while CMT codes are not. Accordingly, 97140 can never be a component of a CMT code. The current 97140 NCCI edit has a superscript of '1' which indicates that there can be exceptions, such as when it is performed in a different body region. The NCCI edits are currently consistent with the AMA's protocol regarding CMT and 97140. However, it is an edit put in place by CMS that continues to be a problem for providers and payers.

In 2005, the ACA won a landmark case against CMS for allowing non-DCs to perform chiropractic manipulations. Hopefully, in time this will lead to a revised edit for procedure codes 97140, 97112 and 97124.

While efforts are made by the CMS staff and its agents at AdminiStar Federal (a BC/BS entity) to ensure the accuracy of NCCI edits, their official disclaimer states "absolute accuracy cannot be guaranteed." If inaccuracies occur in the future, providers can help resolve the problem by working with associations and payers. It is helpful to remember that NCCI edits are designed for Medicare use only. Other government agencies and payers need to modify the edits for non-Medicare payment policies.

See Resource 337 for official information on NCCI edits by CMS.

NCCI Edits for Codes

The example and excerpt included here list the NCCI edits, version 20.3, effective from October 1 to December 31, 2014. These excerpts are to help you get started in finding and understanding the NCCI edits for commonly used codes. The NCCI edit information is dynamic and changes throughout the year.

See Resource 364 for a list of commonly used NCCI edits for chiropractic.

Example

98940   Chiropractic manipulative treatment (CMT) spinal, 1-2 regions;   **ncci**

The "**ncci**" symbol on the right side of the code indicates that NCCI edits apply. Upon checking the edits for 98940 below, you will note four codes that are Mutually Exclusive (ME) to 98940. These procedure codes are 98926^0, 98927^0, 98928^0 and 98929^0, the Osteopathic Manipulative Treatment (OMT) codes. These can never be performed on the same day as the CMT service, and as such they have a superscript of "0" after the code. Note the Column 1/Column 2 (CC) edit after 98940 of 97140^1. The superscript of "1" indicates that 97140 could be used with a modifier at the same encounter as a 98940 service. Typically, that would be modifier 59 for a "distinct procedural service."

See FindACode.com (Resource 336) for the complete NCCI edits.

Edit Example

Chiropractic Manipulative Treatment - CMT/Chiropractic Adjustment

98940	Spinal, one to two regions [MUE = 1]							
	G0380[1]	G0381[1]	G0382[1]	G0383[1]	G0384[1]	G0406[1]	G0407[1]	G0408[1]	G0425[1]
	G0426[1]	G0427[1]	00640[0]	97112[1]	97124[1]	97140[1]	98926[0]	98927[0]	98928[0]
	98929[0]	99201[1]	99202[1]	99203[1]	99204[1]	99205[1]	99211[1]	99212[1]	99213[1]
	99214[1]	99215[1]	99217[1]	99218[1]	99219[1]	99220[1]	99221[1]	99222[1]	99223[1]
	99224[1]	99225[1]	99226[1]	99231[1]	99232[1]	99233[1]	99234[1]	99235[1]	99236[1]
	99238[1]	99239[1]	99241[1]	99242[1]	99243[1]	99244[1]	99245[1]	99251[1]	99252[1]
	99253[1]	99254[1]	99255[1]	99281[1]	99282[1]	99283[1]	99284[1]	99285[1]	99291[1]
	99292[1]	99304[1]	99305[1]	99306[1]	99307[1]	99308[1]	99309[1]	99310[1]	99315[1]
	99316[1]	99318[1]	99324[1]	99325[1]	99326[1]	99327[1]	99328[1]	99334[1]	99335[1]
	99336[1]	99337[1]	99341[1]	99342[1]	99343[1]	99344[1]	99345[1]	99347[1]	99348[1]
	99349[1]	99350[1]	99374[1]	99375[1]	99377[1]	99378[1]	99455[1]	99456[1]	99460[1]
	99461[1]	99462[1]	99463[1]	99465[1]	99466[1]	99468[1]	99469[1]	99471[1]	99472[1]
	99475[1]	99476[1]	99477[1]	99478[1]	99479[1]	99480[1]	99485[1]		

Review: Procedure Coding

- Which procedure should you code when no "accurate" code exists to describe the service? *H-4*
- What does a "▲" mean at the beginning of a code? *H-5*
- What is the purpose of the CPT modifiers? *H-5*
- When should an "add-on" code be used? *H-6*
- What is a special report, and when is it used? *H-6*
- NCCI edits are dynamic. How often are codes and policies updated? *H-7*
- If you don't understand coding, is it possible for you to unbundle codes? *H-7*
- What is a superscript indicator? *H-8*

2. Commonly Used Codes

This Commonly Used Codes Chapter is designed to be a quick reference to assist in the code selection and billing process. Detailed information on these codes are included in other sections of this book and should be referred to for a more thorough explanation. For example, because CMT is a complex coding subject, readers should refer to Chapter 4 where there is more information.

Important notes regarding the usage of this chapter:

- The Commonly Associated ICD-9/ICD-10 Codes segment is informational. Providers should use clinical judgment when determining the appropriate diagnosis for a case. Do not use the "Commonly Associated ICD-9/ICD-10 Codes" listing as a substitute for proper diagnosis code selection.

- The Modifiers segment is general information regarding commonly used modifiers when billing codes together. It is not all inclusive for all payers. Be aware of individual payer policies and guidelines regarding the use of code pairs and modifers.

Alert: CMS has established four new HCPCS modifiers to define subsets of modifier 59. See page H-104 for additional information.

CHIROPRACTIC MANIPULATIVE TREATMENT (CMT)

98940 (1-2 REGIONS), 98941 (3-4 REGIONS), 98942 (5 REGIONS); SPINAL

Explanation

As explained by CPT Guidelines, "Chiropractic manipulative treatment (CMT) is a form of manual treatment to influence joint and neurophysiological function. This treatment may be accomplished using a variety of techniques."

Coding Tips

- The work value of CMT codes (98940-98942) includes pre-service, intraservice, and post-service work. E/M codes may be reported separately with modifier 25 if the patient's condition requires significant, separately identifiable E/M work above and beyond the usual pre and post service work associated with the CMT.

- Different diagnoses for the CMT and the E/M are not required.

- For Medicare claims, modifier AT must be appended to indicate that the treatment is medically necessary. Without the modifier, it is considered maintenance care, which is not reimbursable by Medicare.

- According to Medicare, manual devices (i.e., hand-held devices where the force of the thrust is controlled manually) may be used by doctors of chiropractic in performing manual manipulation of the spine. However, no additional payment is available for the use of the device, nor does Medicare recognize an extra charge for the device itself.

- Do not substitute 97140 for CMT.

- To appeal denials for 97110, 97112, and 97124 when performed with CMT, see Resource 206.

See page H-82 for more information.

See the legend for using resource icons on page xvi.

★ Always code the most appropriate diagnosis code for the patient condition(s).

Terminology to Understand

Spinal regions (by CPT) are:

- Cervical (includes atlanto-occipital joint)
- Thoracic (includes costovertebral and costotransverse joints)
- Lumbar
- Sacral
- Pelvic (sacro-iliac joint).

Commonly Associated ICD Codes*

ICD-9 code(s):

722, 723, 724, 739, 839, 847 (note that 739.4 should be used for the sacro-iliac region, not 739.5)

ICD-10 code categories:

M48, M51, M53, M54, M99, S13, S16, S23, S29, S33, S36, S39

Modifiers

When billed on the same visit as a CMT service, it may be necessary to add modifier 59 to:

97112   97124   97140 (always)

When billed on the same visit as a CMT service, it is always necessary to add modifier 25 to:

99201   99202   99203   99204
99205   99211   99212   99213
99214   99215

Note: No modifier will allow the use of multiple CMT codes for the same patient encounter. Many carriers do not allow more than one CMT per date of service.

98943 CMT; Extra-spinal, 1 or more regions

Coding Tips

- This code may only be used once per encounter, per patient, regardless of how many extraspinal areas are addressed.
- This code would be appropriate for adjusting joints in the head region, excluding the altanto-occipital joint.
- This code would also be appropriate for adjusting the anterior rib cage, including the costosternal junction, excluding the costotransverse and costovertebral joints.
- Submitted claims should only point to extraspinal diagnosis codes for this procedure code. Pay close attention to Item 24E on the 1500 claim form because some computer programs may default to pointing to ALL listed diagnosis codes for every listed procedure code.
- Each extraspinal region should have a subjective complaint, objective findings, and be included in the care plan, with measurable outcomes (such as an outcome assessment tool for the extraspinal joint).

See page H-82 for more information.

Terminology to Understand

Extraspinal (nonspinal) regions (by CPT) are:

- Head (including temporomandibular joint, excluding atlanto-occipital)
- Lower extremities
- Upper extremities
- Rib cage (excluding costotransverse and costovertebral joints)
- Abdomen

Commonly Associated ICD Codes*

ICD-9 code(s):

307, 339, 346, 353, 355, 356, 715, 716, 718, 719, 720, 723, 724, 726, 728, 729, 739, 784, 840-848, 905

ICD-10 code categories:

G54, M15-M21, M25-M26, M65, M67, M70, M75-M77, M79, M99, S03, S23, S43, S46, S53, S56, S63, S66, S73, S76, S83, S86, S93, S96

Modifiers

When billed on the same visit as a CMT service, it is necessary to add modifier 25 to:

99201   99202   99203   99204
99205   99211   99212   99213
99214   99215

S8990 Manipulative therapy for maintenance

Explanation

This code could be used for manipulation that is not medically necessary, or when the patient has no complaints, such as for wellness care. It is for non-Medicare payers, but note that few, if any, will reimburse for this code.

Coding Tips

- Documentation should clearly indicate that the patient encounter was for "maintenance" or "wellness care."

Commonly Associated ICD Codes*

ICD-9 code(s):

739, V70.0, V82.89

ICD-10 code categories:

M99, M99, Z00, Z13

EVALUATION & MANAGEMENT

Evaluation and Management (E/M) codes are used to report professional services rendered by a physician/qualified health care professional (usually face to face). These services have extensive special guidelines that are essential to understand. For quick reference, a few codes and tips are listed here.

See page H-21 to gain a more thorough understanding of coding E/M services.

99201-99204, 99211-99214
OFFICE VISITS

Coding Tips

- E/M codes, when performed with a primary procedure (such as CMT), requires appending modifier 25 to the E/M code to indicate that this service is significant and separately identifiable from the primary procedure performed.

- When an E/M service is performed alone on a specific date-of-service, modifier 25 would not be necessary.

- If a returning patient has not received services from any doctor of chiropractic in your practice within the past 3 years, they are considered a new patient.

- The highest levels of service (99205 & 99215) are rarely used in a chiropractic setting. See *Chapter 3–Evaluation & Management* in this Procedure Codes section for full information.

- 99211 is not commonly used in a chiropractic setting.

See page H-37 for additional information.

IMAGING

Explanation

X-ray, or radiograph, is a photographic or digital image of the internal composition of a body part.

Coding Tips

- Unless specifically appended with the appropriate modifier, all listed radiographic services contain both a "professional" (26) and a "technical" (TC) component, and are typically billed as an all-inclusive, "global" code.

- There should always be documented, clinical evidence demonstrating the need for diagnostic x-ray examinations before an x-ray is performed. *Routine* use of x-rays should be avoided.

72010 X-RAY, SPINE; ENTIRE, SURVEY STUDY, ANTEROPOSTERIOR AND LATERAL

Coding Tips

- This type of study is typically performed for a postural/biomechanical evaluation, to obtain scoliosis measurements, or to evaluate for spinal metastasis.

- The number of films may vary depending on the size of the patient. Regardless, this is interpreted as a single study.

- This is a *comprehensive* code which includes codes 72020, 72040, and 72050 as component codes, along with other x-ray codes.

See page H-55 for more information.

Commonly Associated ICD-9 Codes*

ICD-9 code(s):

720-724, 737, 738, 739, 839, 846, 847

ICD-10 code categories:

M40, M43, M45-M54, M95, M96, M99, S13, S23, S33

Modifiers

When billed on the same visit as 97012, it may be necessary to add modifier 59 to:

72020	72040	72050	72052
72069	72070	72072	72074
72080	72090	72100	72110
72114	72120		

* Always code the most appropriate diagnosis code for the patient condition(s).

72020 X-RAY, SPINE; SINGLE VIEW,

Coding Tips

To specify the level of the radiology exam, add this information to Item 19 of the 1500 claim form.

See page H-55 for more information.

Commonly Associated ICD Codes*

ICD-9 code(s):

720,-724, 737, 738, 739, 839, 846, 847

ICD-10 code categories:

M40, M43, M45-M54, M95, M96, M99, S13, S23, S33

Modifiers

You may need to append modifier 59 to 72020 when billed on the same visit as:

72010   72050   72052   72110

72040, 72050, 72052 X-RAY, SPINE; CERVICAL

Coding Tips

If the AP and lateral views are taken, then reviewed to determine the need for obliques, the additional views, taken on the same visit, should not be separately coded. Only the 72050, 4 or 5 views; or the 72052, 6 or more views should be billed.

See page H-55 for more information.

Commonly Associated ICD Codes*

ICD-9 code(s):

720-723, 737, 738, 739, 839, 847

ICD-10 code categories:

M40, M43-M50, M53, M54, M95, M96, M99, S13

Modifiers

<u>72040: 2 or 3 views</u>

You may need to add modifier 59 to 72040 when billed on the same visit as:

72010   72050   72052

<u>72050: 4 or 5 views</u>

When billed on the same visit as 72050, it may be necessary to add modifier 59 to:

72020   72040

You may need to add modifier 59 to 72050 when billed on the same visit as:

72010   72052

<u>72052: 6 or more views</u>

When billed on the same visit as 72052, it may be necessary to add modifier 59 to:

72020   72040   72050

You may need to add modifier 59 to 72052 when billed on the same visit as:

72010

72070, 72072, 72074 X-RAY, SPINE; THORACIC SPINE

Commonly Associated ICD Codes*

ICD-9 code(s):

720, 722, 724, 737, 738, 739, 839, 847

ICD-10 code categories:

M40, M43, M45-M49, M51-M54, M95, M96, M99, S23

Modifiers

<u>72070: 2 views</u>

When billed on the same visit as 72070, it may be necessary to add modifier 59 to:

72020

You may need to add modifier 59 to 72070 when billed on the same visit as:

72010   72072   72074   72080

<u>72072: 3 views</u>

When billed on the same visit as 72072, it may be necessary to add modifier 59 to:

72070   72090

You may need to add modifier 59 to 72072 when billed on the same visit as:

72010   72074   72080

<u>72074: 4 views minimum</u>

When billed on the same visit as 72074, it may be necessary to add modifier 59 to:

72069   72070   72072   72090

You may need to add modifier 59 to 72074 when billed on the same visit as:
72010   72080

72100, 72110   X-RAY, SPINE; LUMBOSACRAL

Coding Tips

- 72100 may be reported to describe any combination of two or three views taken.
- 72110 is used to report a minimum of four views. If any additional views are necessary, no additional code would be reported.

See page H-55 for more information.

Commonly Associated ICD Codes*

ICD-9 code(s):

720, 724, 737, 738, 739, 839, 846, 847

ICD-10 code categories:

M40, M43, M45-M49, M51-M54, M95, M96, M99, S33

Modifiers

72100: 2 or 3 views

When billed on the same visit as 72052, it may be necessary to add modifier 59 to:
72010   72110   72114

72110: 4 views minimum

When billed on the same visit as 72052, it may be necessary to add modifier 59 to:
72020   72100   72114

PHYSICAL MEDICINE AND REHABILITATION

The codes in this section are not limited to any particular specialty group. However, state and institutional authorities should be consulted regarding the appropriateness of these services being performed by other healthcare professionals such as assistants.

Supervised modality codes, 97010 thru 97028 should only be billed once per patient per encounter, regardless of time or number of regions. However, codes 97032 thru 97140 are billed based on 15 minute increments, regardless of the number of regions treated.

Coding Tips

Pay particular attention to codes specifying service time and bill appropriately:

- See Resource 345 for the Medicare definition of timed codes with examples.
- See ACAtoday.org/coding for information on timed codes.

97010   HOT OR COLD PACKS, ONE OR MORE AREAS

Explanation

The application of heat, through the use of hot packs, also called hydro-collator packs, is often most effective in subacute or chronic problems. Use of hot packs is considered a superficial heat application. In general terms, the application of cold (withdrawal of thermal energy), is the treatment of choice in patients with acute trauma or severe spasticity. This application can be in the form of ice packs, in some applications this is also referred to as "cryotherapy."

Coding Tips

- The work of hot/cold packs as described by CPT code 97010 is not included in the CMT codes 98940-43 and thus is appropriate to be billed separately.
- Unless clinically indicated, *routine* and/or extended use of hot packs for patient care should be avoided.
- Medicare policy excludes payment for hot packs to providers. However, when clinically appropriate in the chiropractic office, it may be paid by other insurance carriers.

Commonly Associated ICD Codes*

ICD-9 code(s):

722, 723, 724, 739, 839, 847

ICD-10 code categories:

M46, M48, M50, M51, M53, M54, M99, S13, S16, S23, S29, S33, S36, S39

---

* Always code the most appropriate diagnosis code for the patient condition(s).

97012 TRACTION, MECHANICAL, ONE OR MORE AREAS

Explanation

The force used to create a degree of tension of soft tissues and/or to allow for separation between joint surfaces. The degree of traction is controlled through the amount of force (pounds) allowed, duration (time), and angle of pull (degrees) using mechanical means. Terms often used in describing pelvic/cervical traction are intermittent or static (describing the length of time traction is applied), or auto traction (use of the body's own weight to create the force).

Coding Tips

- This code may only be billed once per patient, per encounter, regardless of time or number of areas treated.
- Roller table type traction normally meets the requirement of autotraction, the use of the body's own weight to create the force; yet payers may have specific coverage guidelines.
- Unless clinically indicated, *routine* and/or extended use of roller tables for patient care should be avoided.
- Vertebral axial decompression, per session, (code S9090) is also appropriate to report with this procedure.
- "Flexion-distraction" technique is a Chiropractic Manipulative Technique and should be reported with 9894X, CMT codes.

Commonly Associated ICD Codes*

ICD-9 code(s):

722, 723, 724, 739, 839, 847

ICD-10 code categories:

M46, M48, M50, M51, M53, M54, M99, S13, S16, S23, S29, S33, S36, S39

Modifiers

When billed on the same visit as 97012, it may be necessary to add modifier 59 to:
97018   97140

97014 ELECTRICAL STIMULATION, UNATTENDED, ONE OR MORE AREAS

Explanation

The application of electrical stimulation to specific areas. The term unattended means that the patient is positioned and the appropriate type of stimulation is applied to an area, over a specific time period. Nerve and muscle stimulation can be useful in any disorder in which the patient has lost or never had adequate voluntary control over skeletal muscle. Until such time as the patient achieves useful control, it is most helpful to use this type of stimulation along with other interventions, such as passive exercise.

See page H-75 for more information.

Coding Tips

- This code may only be billed once per patient, per encounter, regardless of time or number of areas treated.
- Medicare, along with some private payers, have replaced 97014 with G0283.
- Some payers may deny this service by stating that there is insufficient evidence to support its use. Contact the ACA for references which refute this claim.
- Unless clinically indicated, *routine* and/or extended use of electrical stimulation for patient care should be avoided.
- Two disposable electrodes are included in the RBRVS payment methodology for this code. Consider using A4556 for additional electrodes.
- For sales or rentals of a TENS unit, see E0720.
- For acupuncture with electrical stimulation, see 97813 and 97814.

Terminology to Understand

<u>TENS</u> (Transcutaneous Electrical Nerve Stimulation): Used primarily for pain control and is unattended.

<u>NMS</u> (Neuro-Muscular Stimulation): Strengthens and retrains muscles following surgery, soft tissue injury, or after weakness occurs and is unattended.

M-Stim (Muscle Stimulation), M-RE-ED (Muscle Re-education): This type of stimulation allows the muscle to be taken to the point of a contraction.

HVPC (High-Voltage Pulsed Current), also called EGS (Electro-Galvanic Stimulation): Unique waveform that has been found to be particularly effective in the treatment of open wounds, decubitus ulcers, for reducing swelling, and control of pain. This stimulation is usually unattended, very low level current.

IFC (Interferential Current / Medium Current): These units have a special carrier frequency that allows the current to go deeper into the tissues. IFC is used to control swelling and pain.

MENS (Microamperage Electric Nerve Stimulation), also called microcurrent: These units are very similar to a TENS device but stimulate at a very low level current. This stimulation is usually unattended.

Commonly Associated ICD Codes*

ICD-9 code(s):

722, 723, 724, 739, 839, 847

ICD-10 code categories:

M46, M48, M50, M51, M53, M54, M99, S13, S16, S23, S29, S33, S36, S39

97032 ELECTRICAL STIMULATION, MANUAL, ATTENDED, 15 MINUTES, ONE OR MORE AREAS

Explanation

Modality used to apply electrical current to a specific area. Attended electrical stimulation is also referred to as manual stimulation. Attended stimulation calls for the application of stimulation for shorter or more specific time frames and at varying degrees of current.

Coding Tips

- This code differs from 97014 in that it requires direct (one-on-one) contact by the physician or other qualified health care professional.
- The number of regions is irrelevant when billing units of time with this procedure code.

- Two disposable electrodes are included in the RBRVS payment methodology for this code.
- Unless clinically indicated, *routine* and/or extended use of electrical stimulation for patient care should be avoided.
- This type of electrical stimulation is usually performed by using a stylus or rod. Simply standing around with the patient when no provider is necessary would be more appropriately billed with 97014.
- Understand both state and federal guidelines defining "constant attendance" before choosing this code to ensure proper code selection.

See page H-77 for more information.

Commonly Associated ICD Codes*

ICD-9 code(s):

722, 723, 724, 739, 839, 847

ICD-10 code categories:

M46, M48, M50, M51, M53, M54, M99, S13, S16, S23, S29, S33, S36, S39

Modifiers

When billed on the same visit as 97002 or 97004, it may be necessary to add modifier 59 to: 97032

97035 ULTRASOUND, EACH 15 MIN, ONE OR MORE AREAS

Explanation

Use of sound waves to increase absorption of heat to a deeper penetration level. Much of the value of ultrasound is in providing pain relief, due to its superior depth of penetration. This modality is used in the treatment of arthritis, neuromas, adhesive scars, and where increasing the tissue temperature is the desired effect.

Coding Tips

- This code requires constant attendance ("hands-free" ultrasound which does not require direct one-on-one patient-practitioner contact, is not reported with this code.) To ensure proper code selection, understand both state and federal guidelines

See the legend for using resource icons on page xvi.

* Always code the most appropriate diagnosis code for the patient condition(s).

- defining "constant attendance" before choosing this code.
- The number of regions is irrelevant when billing units of time with this procedure code.
- Unless clinically indicated, *routine* and/or extended use of hot packs for patient care should be avoided.

See page H-77 for more information.

Commonly Associated ICD Codes*

ICD-9 code(s):

722, 723, 724, 739, 839, 847

ICD-10 code categories:

M46, M48, M50, M51, M53, M54, M99, S13, S16, S23, S29, S33, S36, S39

Modifiers

When billed on the same visit as 97002 or 97004, it may be necessary to add modifier 59 to 97035

97110 Therapeutic exercises, each 15 minutes, one or more areas

Explanation

Therapeutic exercise incorporates one parameter (strength, endurance, and range of motion or flexibility) to one or more areas of the body. Examples include, treadmill (for endurance), isokinetic exercise (for range of motion), lumbar stabilization exercise (for flexibility), and gymnastic ball (for stretching and strengthening).

Coding Tips

- This code requires direct one-on-one contact with the provider. The number of regions is irrelevant when billing units of time with this procedure code.
- To ensure proper code selection, understand both state and federal guidelines defining "one-on-one patient contact" before choosing this code.
- Documentation should explain why a skilled provider is necessary and include goals which focus on improvement of functional deficiencies.
- Per CPT guidelines, "A minimum of eight minutes of therapeutic exercises is required to report code 97110. Services of less than eight minutes would not be reported."

This means that this code can **not** be reported with modifier 52.

Commonly Associated ICD Codes*

ICD-9 code(s):

722, 723, 724, 739, 839, 847

ICD-10 code categories:

M46, M48, M50, M51, M53, M54, M99, S13, S16, S23, S29, S33, S36, S39

Modifiers

When billed on the same visit as 97110, it may be necessary to add modifier 59 to:
97002   97004

97112 Neuromuscular reeducation, each 15 min, one or more areas

Explanation

Neuromuscular re-education of movement, balance, coordination, kinesthetic sense, posture, and proprioception. Examples include proprioceptive neuromuscular facilitation (PNF), feldenkreis, bobath, bap's boards, and desensitization techniques.

Coding Tips

- This code requires direct one-on-one contact with the provider. The number of regions is irrelevant when billing units of time with this procedure code.
- To ensure proper code selection, understand both state and federal guidelines defining "one-on-one patient contact" before choosing this code.
- Goals should include an increase in functional ability in self care, mobility, or patient safety.
- Although 97112 does not describe services provided under 9894X, CMT, some payers require the use of a modifier when billed together.
- If this service is performed in a group setting, 97150 must be used instead.

See page H-78 for more information.

Commonly Associated ICD Codes*

ICD-9 code(s):

722, 723, 724, 739, 839, and 847.

ICD-10 code categories:

M46, M48, M50, M51, M53, M54, M99, S13, S16, S23, S29, S33, S36, S39

Modifiers

When billed on the same visit as 97112, it may be necessary to add modifier 59 to:
97022   97036

You may need to add modifier 59 to 97112 when billed on the same visit as:
98940   98941   98942

97124 MASSAGE, EACH 15 MINUTES, ONE OR MORE AREAS

Explanation

Effleurage, petrissage, tapotement (stroking, compression, percussion.)

Coding Tips

- This code requires direct one-on-one contact with the provider. The number of regions is irrelevant when billing units of time with this procedure code.
- To ensure proper code selection, understand both state and federal guidelines defining "one-on-one patient contact" before choosing this code.
- Many payers require this code to include modifier 59 when appearing on the same claim as a 9894X CMT code. However, there are no restrictions on treating the same areas with massage and CMT.
- Be sure to clearly document medical necessity for massage therapy provided late in a care plan.
- This code is not interchangeable with 97140, manual therapy.

See page H-78 for more information.

Commonly Associated ICD Codes*

ICD-9 code(s):

722, 723, 724, 739, 839, 847

ICD-10 code categories:

M46, M48, M50, M51, M53, M54, M99, S13, S16, S23, S29, S33, S36, S39

Modifiers

You may need to add modifier 59 to 97124 when billed on the same visit as:
98940   98941   98942

97140 MANUAL THERAPY TECHNIQUES, EACH 15 MINUTES, ONE OR MORE REGIONS

Explanation

Manual therapy techniques consist of, but are not limited to, soft tissue mobilization, joint mobilization and manipulation, manual lymphatic drainage, manual traction, craniosacral therapy, myofascial release, and neural gliding techniques.

Coding Tips

- This code requires direct one-on-one contact with the provider. The number of regions is irrelevant when billing units of time with this procedure code.
- To ensure proper code selection, understand both state and federal guidelines defining "one-on-one patient contact" before choosing this code.
- This code should not be used interchangeably with CMT codes for joint manipulation.
- Code 97140 describes 'hands-on' therapy techniques, rather than the use of 'devices'.
- According to CPT guidelines, under certain circumstances, it may be appropriate to report CMT codes in addition to code 97140. See Clinical Example #8 on page H-119.
- This code is not interchangeable with 97124, massage.

See page H-78 for more information.

Commonly Associated ICD Codes*

ICD-9 code(s):

722, 723, 724, 739, 839, 847

ICD-10 code categories:

M46, M48, M50, M51, M53, M54, M99, S13, S16, S23, S29, S33, S36, S39

See the legend for using resource icons on page xvi.

* Always code the most appropriate diagnosis code for the patient condition(s).

Modifiers

When billed on the same visit as 97140, it may be necessary to add modifier 59 to:

95851   95852   97018   97530
97750

You **must** add modifier 59 to 97140 when billed on the same visit as:

98940   98941   98942

Note: no modifier allows 97124 and 97140 on the same visit.

S8948 Laser, low level, 15 min

Explanation

Low-level laser therapy (LLLT) utilizes red-beam or near-infrared lasers at a much lower intensity than lasers used for surgery. These lasers produce no sensation and do not burn the skin. This type of therapy is considered by some to penetrate deeply into the tissues for a photobiostimulative effect.

Coding Tips

- Many payers state that there is inadequate evidence to support coverage of LLLT.

  Because coverage may vary by individual policy, verify benefits and limitations with the payer.

- Consider using 97139 (unlisted modality) instead of S8948. Verify coverage with individual payers.

- This is not infrared and not interchangeable with the infrared code (97026). This code is also not for "hot" lasers (such as class 4).

See page H-96 for more information.

Commonly Associated ICD Codes*

ICD-9 code(s):

May be used with codes in categories 722, 723, 724, 739, 839, 847

ICD-10 code categories:

M46, M48, M50, M51, M53, M54, M99, S13, S16, S23, S29, S33, S36, S39

Commonly Used Procedure Modifiers

Level I CPT

22	Increased Procedural Services
25	Significant, Separately Identifiable Evaluation and Management Service by the Same Physician on the Same Day of a Procedure or Other Service
26	Professional Component [EG, INTERPRETATION AND REPORT OF X-RAYS]
32	Mandated Services
51	Multiple Procedures [USE WITH CAUTION]
52	Reduced Services
53	Discontinued Procedure
59 ▲	Distinct Procedural Service
76	Repeat Procedure by Same Physician
77	Repeat Procedure by Another Physician

Level II HCPCS

AT	Acute Treatment
GA	Waiver of Liability On File (ABN Form)
GP	Services Delivered under an Outpatient Physical Therapy Plan of Care
GX	Notice of Liability Issued, Voluntary Under Payer Policy
GY	Item or Service Statutorily Excluded or Does Not Meet the Definition of any Medicare Benefit
GZ	Item or Service Expected to Be Denied as Not Reasonable and Necessary
LT	Left Side (Used to Identify Procedures Performed on the Left Side of the Body)
RT	Right Side (Used to Identify Procedures Performed on the Right Side of the Body)
TC	Technical Component

See Chapter 6–Procedure Modifiers in this *Procedure Codes* section for more codes and full information.

3. Evaluation and Management

Introduction to E/M Code Selection And Documentation

Evaluation and Management (E/M) codes are used by physicians and other qualified healthcare providers to describe specific types of patient encounters such as office visits or consultations. Specific documentation guidelines must be used to report these types of services. Providers have the option to use either the 1995 or 1997 E/M documentation guidelines to facilitate their understanding of the necessary pieces of complete E/M documentation.

E/M coding is often one of the most difficult elements to understand, as it relates to reimbursement. This introduction serves to clarify the concepts necessary to correctly code and document E/M services.

The proper use of Evaluation and Management (E/M) codes for chiropractic is an essential part of proper insurance reimbursement. These are the codes typically used for the initial exam, re-exam, and a handful of other encounters. See the "E/M for Chiropractic" segment later in this chapter for more information.

> An excellent resource for understanding Evaluation and Management is *Practical E/M – Documentation and Coding Solutions for Quality Patient Care*, by Dr. Stephen R. Levinson. See Resource 334.

> See Resource 344 for additional information and resources on Evaluation and Management coding.

Categories

E/M codes are divided into twenty-one categories based on locations or types of service in the AMA's Current Procedural Terminology (CPT) manual. Often, they are further divided into subcategories based on patient status (i.e. new or established). Most of the time, doctors of chiropractic will use E/M codes for Office or Other Outpatient Services. This introduction focuses on these E/M codes which are divided into two subcategories of patient types:

- New Patient: One who *has **not** received* services from any physician in the same group practice in the same specialty within the last three years (36 months).
- Established Patient: One who *has received* services from any physician in the same group practice, in the same specialty, within the last three years (36 months).

In the instance where a physician is covering for another physician, the patient's encounter will be classified as it would have been by the physician who is not available.

Levels of Care

There are five levels of codes in each subcategory which increase in difficulty as well as value. These five levels are defined by seven components (as shown in Figure 8.1), the first three are considered **key components** in selecting the level of E/M service. The next three components are considered contributory factors. Contributory components are not critical to most E/M code selections in a chiropractic setting. The last component, time, is discussed at the end of this chapter.

FIGURE 8.1
Components for E/M Code Selection

Key Components	1. History (Hx)
	2. Examination
	3. Medical Decision Making (MDM)
Contributory Components	4. Counseling
	5. Coordination of Care
	6. Nature of Presenting Problem
Other Component	7. Time

Key Components

The key components (history, exam and medical decision making) can be broken down into additional subcomponents. Use Figure 8.2 as a helpful reference when navigating the complexity of Evaluation and Management coding throughout this chapter.

FIGURE 8.2
Three Key Components

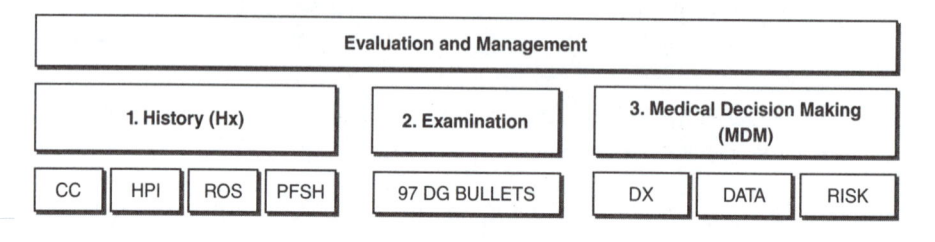

```
                    Evaluation and Management
   ┌──────────────────┬──────────────────┬─────────────────────────┐
   │  1. History (Hx) │  2. Examination  │ 3. Medical Decision     │
   │                  │                  │    Making (MDM)         │
   ├──┬───┬───┬───────┼──────────────────┼──────┬──────┬───────────┤
   │CC│HPI│ROS│ PFSH  │  97 DG BULLETS   │  DX  │ DATA │   RISK    │
   └──┴───┴───┴───────┴──────────────────┴──────┴──────┴───────────┘
```

1. **History (Hx)** is comprised of the following four subcomponents. These subcomponents must be considered as a group to determine the level of History:

    a) CC: Chief complaint

    b) HPI: History of Present Illness

    c) ROS: Review of Systems

    d) PFSH: Personal, Family and Social History

2. **Examination** is established by using either the 1995 or 1997 documentation guidelines. In this chapter, we will use the bullets (see Figure 8.5) from the 1997 E/M Documentation Guidelines (97 DGs) using the Musculoskeletal Specialty Examination.

3. **Medical Decision Making** (MDM) has three subcomponents which must be considered as a group:

a) Dx: Number of diagnoses and/or management options
b) Data: Amount and/or complexity of data to be reviewed
c) Risk: Possibility of complications and/or morbidity or mortality.

Matrix Selection

Figure 8.3 shows ChiroCode's useful E/M Office, New Patient Matrix which guides the decision making process. It acts as an audit tool to quickly evaluate whether or not you have selected the right E/M code for the patient encounter.

FIGURE 8.3
E/M Office, New Patient Matrix (3 of 3)

| | CC | **History** (3 of 3) | | | **Exam** | **MDM** (2 of 3) |
		HPI	ROS	PFSH		
99201	1+	1-3	n/a	n/a	1-5	straightforward
99202	1+	1-3	1	n/a	6-11	straightforward
99203	1+	4+	2-9	1	12+	low
99204	1+	4+	10+	2+	all	moderate
99205	1+	4+	10+	2+	all	high

The following clinical example will be referenced as we discuss the New Patient Matrix:

Clinical Example

Chief Complaint: Low back pain that radiates into the right leg with right foot numbness.

Subjective: This new patient is a 24-year-old female, mother of two, who bent over to pick up her baby from the car seat six weeks ago with immediate onset of moderate right-sided lower back pain that has greatly increased. Patient complains of pain that radiates into the right leg with numbness in the right foot. She has been taking ibuprofen 400 mg twice daily with minimal relief and reports a failed course of physical therapy.

She has a history of low back pain, but no surgeries. Lumbar x-ray in the past showed a grade #1 spondylolisthesis. Her review of systems is positive for numbness in right leg and foot, and negative for bowel or bladder impairment and peripheral vascular disease.

Objective: Patient appears to be a healthy, well nourished and groomed female. She is currently unemployed. She is alert, and oriented in time and place, BP 118/72, pulse 60, weight 125. There are no signs of varicosities, rashes, or skin lesions in either of the lower extremities. Patient rises from seated position with difficulty, bracing hands on thighs with slow deliberate movement patterns. Standing posture is antalgic forward at 10 degrees and left laterally flexed to approximate 5 degrees. Romberg's test is negative for proprioceptive disturbance. There is midline tenderness at L/4, L/5 and SI posterior elements. Right straight leg raise is positive for pain extending to calf at 60 degrees with a positive Braggard's intensifying pain with extension to ankle laterally. Kemps cannot be performed given limited lumbar mobility as ROM is restricted, secondary to pain and muscle guarding. Lumbar range of motion is restricted as follows: flexion painful to 40 degrees with difficulty to achieve upright posture, no extension from forward flexed position, left lateral flexion 2 degrees, right lateral flexion 25 degrees, rotation 30 degrees bilaterally. Abdominal palpation, percussion and auscultation unremarkable. Grade 2+ spasm is present in the paraspinals bilaterally. Diminished sensation to pin prick is evident in the right lateral leg and dorsum of the foot. Deep tendon patellar reflex is 2+ bilaterally, left Achilles +2 right Achilles absent. Bilateral lower extremity

> motor strength normal at quads and hamstrings. However foot inversion on the right is 4/5 and 5/5 on the left.
>
> **Assessment:** Spondylolisthesis with new onset radiculopathy in the right lower extremity. Refer for MRI to differentially diagnose nerve root entrapment secondary to herniated nucleus pulposus, possibly complicated by spondylolisthesis, consistent with neurological findings of right SI radiculopathy.
>
> **Plan:** Patient referred for lumbar spine MRI to assess status of radiculopathy and differentiate a herniated nucleus populus from other complications by way of spondylolisthesis. Follow-up noon tomorrow to review results and create treatment plan.

1. History

Chief Complaint (CC)

The first key component to evaluate is the history. History must always include a chief complaint, which is clearly labeled in this clinical example and is a requirement for every level of office E/M code.

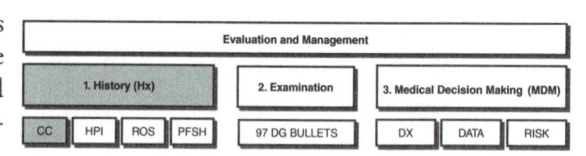

History of Present Illness (HPI)

Next, use the Matrix (Figure 8.3) to determine how many "History of Present Illness" (HPI) elements are present in the clinical example. The elements of HPI, as outlined by the CPT manual are listed below. Next to the bullet points, in italics, are relevant elements from the clinical example:

- Location: *right lower back*
- Quality: *none*
- Severity: *moderate*
- Duration: *six weeks*
- Timing: *none*
- Context: *bent over*
- Modifying factors: *improves with ibuprofen*
- Associated signs and symptoms: *numbness in right foot*

The clinical example contained six elements of HPI. The Matrix in Figure 8.3 shows that any of the exam codes could be selected because four HPI elements is the minimum required to qualify for the highest level code (99205).

Review of Systems (ROS)

The third element of the History is the Review of Systems (ROS). In our clinical example, they are labeled as such within the clinical example, which makes it easier to identify.

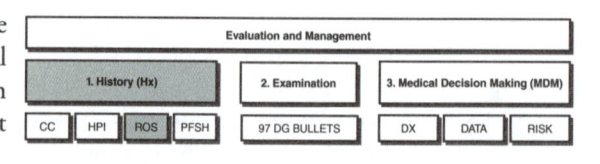

> **Note:** This is NOT the exam. It is part of the history and is generally obtained when the patient completes the Medical and Health History form (Resource 144) or provides this information verbally during the patient encounter.

According to the CPT manual, these are the 14 systems to review. Elements identified in the clinical example are listed in italics.

- Constitutional (weight loss, fatigue, etc.)
- Eyes
- Ears, nose, mouth, throat
- Cardiovascular: *present in the clinical example*
- Respiratory
- Gastrointestinal: *present in the clinical example*
- Genitourinary: *present in the clinical example*
- Musculoskeletal: *present in the clinical example but not included with the ROS. See the note below for more information.*
- Integumentary (skin and/or breast)
- Neurological: *present in the clinical example*
- Psychiatric
- Endocrine
- Hematologic/lymphatic
- Allergic/Immunologic

In the clinical example, four systems were reviewed: neurological, bowel (gastrointestinal), bladder (genitourinary), and cardiovascular. The Matrix (Figure 8.3) shows that only codes 99201, 99202 and 99203 qualify because 99204 and 99205 require at least ten elements to be reviewed.

> **Note:** The musculoskeletal system was reviewed as part of the chief complaint (CC). The CC can also count as an element of the ROS. However, HPI information cannot also be counted for ROS. There is no "double-dipping". As such, it is wise to clearly label the ROS in your documentation. The Matrix makes it clear that a 99201 is the highest code that can be selected if no ROS can be identified in the record.

Past, Family, Social History (PFSH)

The fourth element of the History is the Past, Family, Social History (PFSH). The CPT manual describes these as follows:

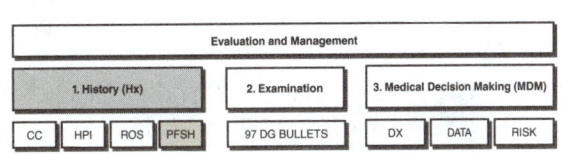

- **Past history:** A review of the patient's past experiences with illnesses, injuries, and treatments. (i.e. operations, hospitalizations, medications, allergies, dietary status)
- **Family history:** a review of medical events in the patient's family (i.e. health status of parents, children and siblings, and hereditary diseases)
- **Social history:** an age appropriate review of past and current activities (i.e. marital status, employment, drugs, alcohol, tobacco, education, sexual history)

The clinical example clearly identifies a discussion of the patient's past history (injury and surgeries), and social history (unemployed); therefore two elements are present.

> **Note:** Per the Matrix, without any PFSH, the highest level of E/M would be 99202, regardless of the other key components.

The overall history must be met or exceeded in *all* three elements. Even though the HPI and PFSH qualify for higher levels, all three components must be considered. The ROS then limits this case to a 99203 as shown in Figure 8.4.

FIGURE 8.4
History Selection Example (3 of 3)

	HPI	ROS	PFSH
99201	1-3	n/a	n/a
99202	1-3	1	n/a
99203	4+	2-9	1
99204	4+	10+	2+
99205	4+	10+	2+

2. Exam

The exam portion of an E/M encounter is defined differently in guidelines that were released in 1995 and 1997. Generally, the 1995 guidelines are best suited for a general practitioner and they essentially allow a higher code selection if more distinct body areas are examined.

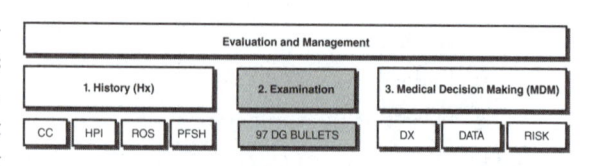

Conversely, the 1997 guidelines are generally better suited for specialists because they outline more specific elements for particular body systems, which allows for a higher level code based on a more thorough exam within a single body system. For the purposes of this example, the 1997 musculoskeletal examination guidelines have been selected, but doctors of chiropractic may find that one of the following guidelines is a closer fit to their practice model: the 1995 guidelines, the 1997 guidelines for neurological exam, or the 1997 guidelines for the multi-system exam.

> **Alert**: Providers may elect to use either the 1995 or 1997 guidelines. However, it is **not** appropriate to combine the two guidelines on a single case. The only exception allows providers to use the 1997 guidelines for an extended HPI along with other elements of the 1995 guidelines.

> See Resource 332 for the complete 1995 guidelines. See Resource 333 for the complete 1997 guidelines.

The clinical example includes the following bullets:

1. constitutional: *vital signs: blood pressure, pulse, and weight*
2. constitutional: *healthy, well-nourished, groomed*
3. cardiovascular: *no evidence of varicosities*
4. musculoskeletal: *spine: tenderness and spasm*
5. musculoskeletal: *spine: range of motion restriction*
6. musculoskeletal: *gait and station: antalgic*
7. musculoskeletal: *right lower extremity: muscle strength*
8. musculoskeletal: *left lower extremity: muscle strength*
9. skin: *right lower extremity: rashes or lesions*
10. skin: *left lower extremity: rashes or lesions*
11. gastrointestinal: *abdomen unremarkable*

12. neurological/psychiatric: *deep tendon reflexes*
13. neurological/psychiatric: *sensation and proprioception*
14. neurological/psychiatric: *alert and oriented to time and place*

According to Figure 8.3, an exam with fourteen bulleted items qualifies for 99203.

3. MEDICAL DECISION MAKING (MDM)

Medical Decision Making (MDM) is the most complex key component of Evaluation and Management coding. It assesses the management of a case by answering three questions:

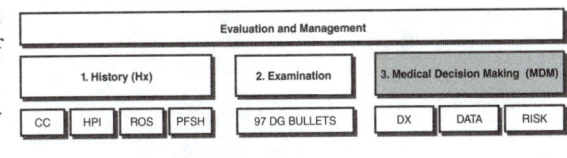

A. How many problems does the patient have? (Number of diagnoses or management options)

B. How much information needs to be reviewed to properly understand the case? (Amount and/or complexity of data to be reviewed)

C. How risky is the patient's problem? Could they lose a limb and/or die? Is this case pretty simple? (Risk of significant complications, morbidity and/or mortality)

The answer to these three questions, scored and brought together, determines the appropriate type of MDM. Note that only two of these elements must meet or exceed the level to qualify for the type of MDM selected. This is demonstrated by separately evaluating each of the three sub-components of MDM.

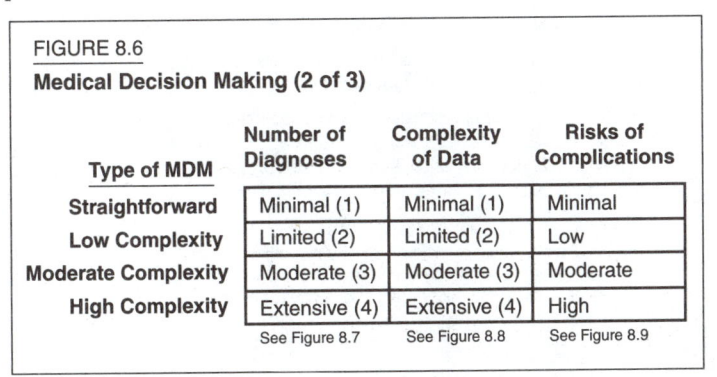

FIGURE 8.6
Medical Decision Making (2 of 3)

Type of MDM	Number of Diagnoses	Complexity of Data	Risks of Complications
Straightforward	Minimal (1)	Minimal (1)	Minimal
Low Complexity	Limited (2)	Limited (2)	Low
Moderate Complexity	Moderate (3)	Moderate (3)	Moderate
High Complexity	Extensive (4)	Extensive (4)	High
	See Figure 8.7	See Figure 8.8	See Figure 8.9

A. Number of Diagnoses and/or Management Options

Use Figure 8.7 (Number of Diagnoses/Management Options) to score the clinical example.

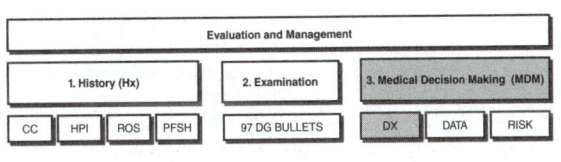

An analysis of this case reveals two problems to manage:

- The spondylolisthesis with low back pain is an established problem that is worsening (2 points).
- The radiculopathy is a new problem, and additional MRI work up is planned (4 points).

FIGURE 8.7
Number of Diagnoses and/or Management Options

Self limited or minor problem	1 Points
Established stable problem	1 Points
Established worsening problem	2 Points
New problem, no additional work up	3 Points
New problem, with additional work up	4 Points

FIGURE 8.5
Musculoskeletal Examination

System/Body Area	Elements of Examination

Constitutional	• Measurement of **any three** of the following **seven** vital signs:
	   1) sitting or standing blood pressure,
	   2) supine blood pressure,
	   3) pulse rate and regularity,
	   4) respiration,
	   5) temperature,
	   6) height,
	   7) weight (May be measured and recorded by ancillary staff)
	• General appearance of patient (eg, development, nutrition, body habitus, deformities, attention to grooming

Cardiovascular	• Examination of peripheral vascular system by observation (eg, swelling, varicosities) and palpation (eg, pulses, temperature, edema, tenderness)
Lymphatic	• Palpation of lymph nodes in neck, axillae, groin and/or other location

Musculoskeletal	• Examination of gait and station
	
	Examination of joint(s), bone(s) and muscle(s)/ tendon(s) of **four of the following six** areas: 1) head and neck; 2) spine, ribs and pelvis; 3) right upper extremity; 4) left upper extremity; 5) right lower extremity; and 6) left lower extremity. The examination of a given area includes:
	   • Inspection, percussion and/or palpation with notation of any misalignment, asymmetry, crepitation, defects, tenderness, masses or effusions
	   • Assessment of range of motion with notation of any pain (eg, straight leg raising), crepitation or contracture
	   • Assessment of stability with notation of any dislocation (luxation), subluxation or laxity
	   • Assessment of muscle strength and tone (eg, flaccid, cogwheel, spastic) with notation of any atrophy or abnormal movements
	
	NOTE: For the comprehensive level of examination, all four of the elements identified by a bullet must be performed and documented for each of four anatomic areas. For the three lower levels of examination, each element is counted separately for each body area. For example, assessing range of motion in two extremities constitutes two elements.

Extremities	[See musculoskeletal and skin]

Skin	• Inspection and/or palpation of skin and subcutaneous tissue (eg, scars, rashes, lesions, cafe-au-lait spots, ulcers) in **four of the following six** areas:
	   1) head and neck;
	   2) trunk;
	   3) right upper extremity;
	   4) left upper extremity;
	   5) right lower extremity; and
	   6) left lower extremity.
	NOTE: For the comprehensive level, the examination of all four anatomic areas must be performed and documented. For the three lower levels of examination, each body area is counted separately. For example, inspection and/or palpation of the skin and subcutaneous tissue of two extremities constitutes two elements.

Neurological/Psychiatric	• Test coordination (eg, finger/nose, heel/ knee/shin, rapid alternating movements in the upper and lower extremities, evaluation of fine motor coordination in young children) • Examination of deep tendon reflexes and/or nerve stretch test with notation of pathological reflexes (eg, Babinski) • Examination of sensation (eg, by touch, pin, vibration, proprioception) Brief assessment of mental status including: • Orientation to time, place and person • Mood and affect (eg, depression, anxiety, agitation)

This adds up to six points for number of diagnoses and/or management options. According to the MDM elements table (Figure 8.6), this qualifies for a 'high complexity' level.

> **Tip:** Consider using the same wording found in this table when documenting the patient's problems, such as "established" or "new", and "stable" or "worsening". It will make it easier for an E/M auditor to score this element the same way you do.

B. Amount and/or Complexity of Data to be Reviewed

The next element of MDM is Amount and/or Complexity of Data to be Reviewed (see Figure 8.8). If the healthcare provider needs to review records and lab tests from a dozen different providers, the case has a higher level of decision making. Alternatively, if there is very little data to consider, then the case is pretty straightforward.

Using Figure 8.8 as a guide, we see that our example only earns one point for the MRI test that was ordered. According to the MDM table (Figure 8.6), this only qualifies for a 'straightforward' level.

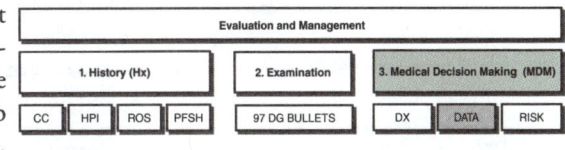

FIGURE 8.8
Amount and/or Complexity of Data Reviewed

Item	Points
Labs ordered an/or reviewed	1 Points
Test from medicine codes (90701-99199) ordered	1 Points
X-ray ordered	1 Points
Discuss results with performing physician	1 Points
Decision to obtain old records	1 Points
Review of old records	2 Points
Independent/second visualization of tests	2 Points

C. Risk of Significant Complications, Morbidity and/or Mortality

The final sub-component of MDM to review is the risk. The official 1997 table of risk (see Figure 8.9) is fairly extensive and is divided into four levels of risk. The level is selected by choosing one element from three criteria (presenting problem, diagnostic procedures ordered, and management options selected).

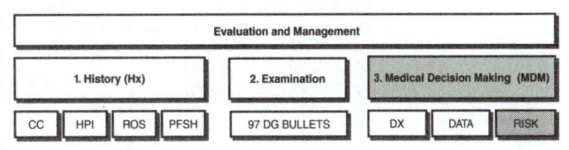

Using the Table of Risk (Figure 8.9 on the following page) as a guide, the clinical example best meets the criteria for low level of risk because there are two or more minor problems. The patient is not being sent in for surgery, is not being treated for a chronic illness, or an acute illness with systemic symptoms. These are the kinds of things that would increase the level of risk from 'low' to 'moderate.' In fact, most chiropractic cases will be considered low or minimal risk.

- See Resource 381 for a full size version of the Table of Risk.
- See Resource 391 for a chiropractic table of risk example.

FIGURE 8.9
Table of Risk

LEVEL OF RISK	PRESENTING PROBLEM(S)	DIAGNOSTIC PROCEDURE(S) ORDERED	MANAGEMENT OPTIONS SELECTED
Minimal	• One self-limited or minor problem, eg, cold, insect bite, tinea corporis	• Laboratory tests requiring venipuncture • Chest x-rays • EKG/EEG • Urinalysis • Ultrasound, eg, echocardiography • KOH prep	• Rest • Gargles • Elastic bandages • Superficial dressings
Low	• Two or more self-limited or minor problems • One stable chronic illness, eg, well controlled hypertension, non-insulin dependent diabetes, cataract, BPH • Acute uncomplicated illness or injury, eg, cystitis, allergic rhinitis, simple sprain	• Physiologic tests not under stress, eg, pulmonary function tests • Non-cardiovascular imaging studies with contrast, eg, barium enema • Superficial needle biopsies • Clinical laboratory tests requiring arterial puncture • Skin biopsies	• Over-the-counter drugs • Minor surgery with no identified risk factors • Physical therapy • Occupational therapy • IV fluids without additives
Moderate	• One or more chronic illnesses with mild exacerbation, progression, or side effects of treatment • Two or more stable chronic illnesses • Undiagnosed new problem with uncertain prognosis, eg, lump in breast • Acute illness with systemic symptoms, eg, pyelonephritis, pneumonitis, colitis • Acute complicated injury, eg, head injury with brief loss of consciousness	• Physiologic tests under stress, eg, cardiac stress test, fetal contraction stress test • Diagnostic endoscopies with no identified risk factors • Deep needle or incisional biopsy • Cardiovascular imaging studies with contrast and no identified risk factors, eg, arteriogram, cardiac catheterization • Obtain fluid from body cavity, eg lumbar puncture, thoracentesis, culdocentesis	• Minor surgery with identified risk factors • Elective major surgery (open, percutaneous or endoscopic) with no identified risk factors • Prescription drug management • Therapeutic nuclear medicine • IV fluids with additives • Closed treatment of fracture or dislocation without manipulation
High	• One or more chronic illnesses with severe exacerbation, progression, or side effects of treatment • Acute or chronic illnesses or injuries that pose a threat to life or bodily function, eg, multiple trauma, acute MI, pulmonary embolus, severe respiratory distress, progressive severe rheumatoid arthritis, psychiatric illness with potential threat to self or others, peritonitis, acute renal failure • An abrupt change in neurologic status, eg, seizure, TIA, weakness, sensory loss	• Cardiovascular imaging studies with contrast with identified risk factors • Cardiac electrophysiological tests • Diagnostic Endoscopies with identified risk factors • Discography	• Elective major surgery (open, percutaneous or endoscopic) with identified risk factors • Emergency major surgery (open, percutaneous or endoscopic) • Parenteral controlled substances • Drug therapy requiring intensive monitoring for toxicity • Decision not to resuscitate or to de-escalate care because of poor prognosis

MDM Clinical Example Summary

When comparing the results (Figure 8.10) of the three sub-components used to determine the overall level of Medical Decision Making (MDM), it is apparent that this case qualifies as 'low complexity.' *Only two* of the three criteria in the MDM table have to meet or exceed the requirements for a given level. Even though the number of diagnoses/management options was at the highest level, the amount and/or complexity of data to be reviewed is only high enough to support 'straightforward.' The risk of complications (table of risk) became the deciding factor which set the MDM type as 'low complexity.' Using the MDM table, as shown in Figure 8.10, we ignore the 'complexity of data' because the 'number of diagnoses' and 'risks of complications' meet or exceed the requirements for 'low complexity' type of MDM.

FIGURE 8.10
Medical Decision Making (2 of 3)

Type of MDM	Number of Diagnoses	Complexity of Data	Risks of Complications
Straightforward	Minimal (1)	Minimal (1)	Minimal
Low Complexity	Limited (2)	Limited (2)	Low
Moderate Complexity	Moderate (3)	Moderate (3)	Moderate
High Complexity	Extensive (4)	Extensive (4)	High

Note: Code 99205 requires a high type of MDM. This type of decision making is rare in a chiropractic office. Use this code only when warranted by medical necessity, and correctly documented.

E/M Decision Summary

Now that all three key components have been examined, they need to be compared to the requirements on the E/M Office, New Patient Matrix. Figure 8.11 demonstrates how this is done for a new patient.

FIGURE 8.11
E/M Office, New Patient Matrix (3 of 3)

	History (3 of 3)			Exam	MDM
	HPI	ROS	PFSH		
99201	1-3	n/a	n/a	1-5	straightforward
99202	1-3	1	n/a	6-11	straightforward
99203	4+	2-9	1	12+	low
99204	4+	10+	2+	all	moderate
99205	4+	10+	2+	all	high

For a new patient, all three key components have to meet or exceed the level to qualify, so in this case, the appropriate code choice would be 99203. If one component were lower, for example, the exam, then the proper code would be 99202. All three elements (History, Exam and MDM) have to meet a minimum level to qualify.

If this clinical example was for an established patient and all other factors were the same, the criteria would be different. Using the E/M Office, Established Patient Matrix (Figure 8.12), note that only two of the three key components must be met in order to qualify for a code. Therefore, the MDM component does not impact this decision. The History and Exam components meet the criteria for code 99214.

FIGURE 8.12

E/M Office, Established Patient Matrix (2 of 3)

	History (3 of 3)			Exam	MDM
	HPI	ROS	PFSH		
99211	none	none	none	none	N/A
99212	1-3	none	none	1-5	straightforward
99213	1-3	1	1	6-11	low
99214	4+	2-9	2+	12+	moderate
99215	4+	10+	2+	all	high

Code Selection by Counseling Time

E/M visit code selection is based on either the three key component areas, OR the counseling time override option when applicable. Referring back to Figure 8.1, the seventh Evaluation and Management component is Time. This component has very specific parameters which must be met in order to qualify.

E/M guidelines divide time into two categories:

1. *Pre- and post- encounter time:* Activities before and after the doctor-patient face-to-face time. This time does not count in this code selection process

2. *Intra-Service face-to-face doctor/patient time:* Doctor time performing the History, Exam, Medical Decision Making, Counseling and Coordination of Care

In a typical office visit, the three components of History, Examination and Medical Decision Making are usually the dominant components and counseling time is nominal. However, on certain occasions, time could be the overriding component. When counseling and/or coordination of care represents 50% or more of the total E/M encounter (doctor-patient face-to-face time), then time **may** become the overriding factor in code selection.

Counseling and Time

The CPT manual explains that time override is frequently used when counseling occurs during the E/M encounter. Counseling is a discussion with the patient and/or family concerning one or more of the following areas:

- Diagnostic results, impressions, and/or recommended diagnostic studies
- Prognosis
- Risks and benefits of management (treatment) options
- Instructions for management (treatment) and/or follow-up
- Importance of compliance with chosen management (treatment) options
- Risk factor reduction
- Patient and family education

Selecting the Code

When time spent in counseling and coordination of care becomes the deciding factor, match the total face-to-face time with the closest average Intra-Service Time listed in the following E/M pages. This gives you the proper code. Append modifier 25 for a significant, separately identifiable E/M service if performed on the same day as a CMT service. See Figure 8.13, *Example of Time Override Option for Established Patient.*

FIGURE 8.13
Example of Time Override Option for Established Patient

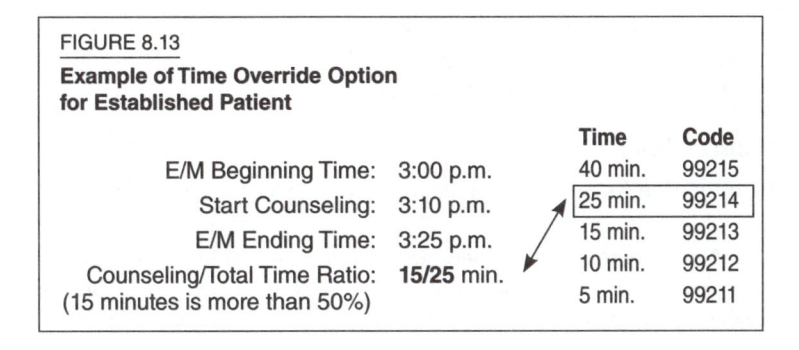

		Time	Code
E/M Beginning Time:	3:00 p.m.	40 min.	99215
Start Counseling:	3:10 p.m.	25 min.	99214
E/M Ending Time:	3:25 p.m.	15 min.	99213
Counseling/Total Time Ratio:	**15/25** min.	10 min.	99212
(15 minutes is more than 50%)		5 min.	99211

Chiropractic E/M Counseling Record

Counseling and its associated time needs to be identified and documented. This form makes it very easy to record the seven elements of counseling for a time override. It can also function as documentation for the patient encounter or be a dictation guide.

See Resource 338 for a full-size version of this form, with instructions.

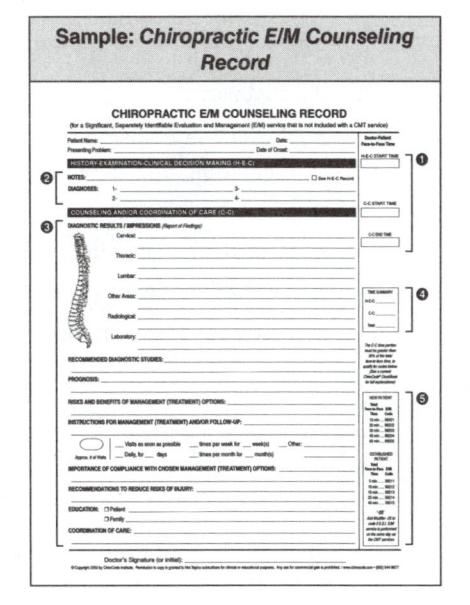

Sample: *Chiropractic E/M Counseling Record*

E/M for Chiropractic

E/M codes can be used when services are significant and separately identifiable from the routine services done within the basic Chiropractic Manipulative Treatment (CMT) code set of 98940, 98941, 98942 and 98943. This CMT code set includes a pre-manipulation patient assessment. Note the following statement regarding chiropractic services and E/M coding:

> "Chiropractic manipulative treatment (CMT) is a form of manual treatment to influence joint and neurophysiological function. This treatment may be accomplished using a variety of techniques. The chiropractic manipulative treatment codes include a pre-manipulation patient assessment. Additional Evaluation and Management services may be reported separately using modifier 25 if the patient's condition requires a significant, separately identifiable E/M service above and beyond the usual preservice and postservice work associated with the procedure." *CPT 2015*

This official CPT statement for the use of an E/M code is very clear. It eliminates any debate about the propriety of when to use E/M coding beyond CMT services, and sets the parameters for appropriate billing.

When can E/M codes be used with CMT? When significant, separately identifiable services exist; such as some of the following examples:

New patient:

- Initial evaluation
- Consultation (requested by an appropriate source. See 99241-99245)

> **Note:** According to CPT guidelines, an appropriate source includes a physician assistant, nurse practitioner, doctor of chiropractic, physical therapist, occupational therapist, speech language pathologist, psychologist, social worker, lawyer, or insurance company.
>
> If a patient requests the consultation it should be billed with the office/outpatient E/M codes, not the consultation codes.

Established patient:

- Periodic re-evaluation (e.g., a new condition, new injury, re-injury, aggravation, exacerbation, or a re-evaluation to determine if a change in treatment plan is necessary)
- Exacerbation or re-injury
- Return after lapse in care
- Counseling (using the time override)
- Release/discharge from active care.

Review: Evaluation and Management

- What is the difference between a "new patient" and an "established patient"? *H-21*
- What are the three key components of an E/M code? *H-22*
- What are the three questions addressed by Medical Decision Making? *H-27*
- When is time the deciding factor in E/M code selection? *H-32*
- Why is modifier 25 required for E/M codes when billed with a CMT code? *H-32 to H-33*

4a. CPT Procedures
Evaluation and Management Codes

The following keys apply to the tables used throughout in this Evaluation and Management chapter:

Severity of Problem

    Minor = Self-limited or minor
    Low = Low severity
    Moderate = Moderate severity
    High = High severity
    Stable = Stable, recovering or improving
    Minor Complication = Responding inadequately to therapy or has developed a minor complication
    Sig. Complic. or New = Developed a significant complication or a significant new problem
    Unst. or Sig. New = Unstable or has developed a significant new problem requiring immediate physician attention
    High, Immed. Threat = High severity and poses in immediate significant threat to life or physiologic function

History (See history table example - Figure 8.4 - on page H-26)

    Focused = Problem focused (1-3 HPI, no ROS, no PFSH)
    Expanded = Expanded problem focused (1-3 HPI, 1 ROS, no PFSH)
    Detailed, Det. = Detailed (4+ HPI, 2-9 ROS, 1 or 2 PFSH)
    Comp. = Comprehensive/IH = Interval History (4+ HPI, 10+ ROS, 2+ PFSH)

    HPI=History of Present Illness ROS=Review of Systems PFSH=Past, Family, and Social History

Exam

	97 Documentation Guidelines	95 Documentation Guidelines
Focused	1-5 bullets	1 element
Expanded	6-11 bullets	2-7 element
Detailed, Det.	12+ bullets	2-7 elements (expanded)
Comprehensive/Comp	all bullets	8+ elements

- See Resource 332 for the 1995 E/M documentation guidelines.
- See Resource 333 for the 1997 E/M documentation guidelines.

Complexity of Decision Making (See page H-27 for more on Medical Decision Making)

● = New Code for 2015 NE = Not Established ✚ = Add-on Code TC = Technical Component
▲ = Revised Code for 2015 NA = Not Applicable ⊘ = Modifier 51 Exempt 26 = Professional Component
▶◀ = New or Revised CPT Text NCCI = CCI Edits Apply -QW = CLIA Waived Test # = Resequenced Code

OFFICE OR OTHER OUTPATIENT SERVICES

The following codes are used to report evaluation and management services provided in the office or in an outpatient or other ambulatory facility. A patient is considered an outpatient until inpatient admission to a health care facility occurs.

Counseling and/or coordination of care with other physicians, other qualified health care professionals, or agencies are provided consistent with the nature of the problem(s) and the patient's and/or family's needs.

New Patient

Office or other outpatient visit for the evaluation and management of a new patient, typically face-to-face with the patient and/or family.

		Key Component Code Selection - 3 of 3			Average Intra-Service Time	
CODE	SEVERITY OF PROBLEM	HISTORY	EXAMINATION	COMPLEXITY OF DECISION MAKING	COUNSELING OVERRIDE	RVU
99201	Minor	Focused	Focused	Straightforward	10 ncci	1.22
99202	Low to Moderate	Expanded	Expanded	Straightforward	20 ncci	2.09
99203	Moderate	Detailed	Detailed	Low	30 ncci	3.03
99204	Moderate to High	Comp.	Comp.	Moderate	45 ncci	4.63
99205	Moderate to High	Comp.	Comp.	High	60 ncci	5.82

For help with codes 99201-92205 see Example #5 in Chapter 7–Clinical Examples in this *Procedure Codes* section.

Determination of Patient Status as New or Established Patient

"Solely for the purpose of distinguishing between new and established patients, **professional services** are those face-to-face services rendered by a physician and reported by a specific CPT code(s). A **new patient** is one who has not received any professional services from the physician or another physician of the **exact** same specialty and **subspecialty** who belongs to the same group practice, within the past three years.

An **established patient** is one who has received professional services from the physician or another physician of the **exact** same specialty and **subspecialty** who belongs to the same group practice, within the past three years.

When a physician/qualified health care professional is covering for another physician/qualified health care professional, the patient's encounter will be classified as it would have been by the physician/qualified health care professional who is not available. When advance practice nurses and physician assistants are working with physicians they are considered as working in the exact same specialty and exact same subspecialities as the physician."

CPT Coding Guidelines, Evaluation and Management Services Guidelines, New and Established Patients, CPT 2015

Counseling Override Option and Time

"When counseling and/or coordination of care dominates (more than 50%) the encounter with the patient and/or family encounter (face-to-face time in the office or other outpatient setting or floor/unit time in the hospital or nursing facility), then **time** shall be considered the key or controlling factor to qualify for a particular level of E/M services. This includes time spent with parties who have assumed responsibility for the care of the patient or decision making whether or not they are family members (e.g., foster parents, person acting in loco parentis, legal guardian). The extent of counseling and/or coordination of care must be documented in the medical record." -*CPT 2015.*

Established Patient

Office or other outpatient visit for the evaluation and management of an established patient, typically face-to-face with the patient and/or family.

		Key Component Code Selection - 2 of 3			Average Intra-Service Time	
CODE	SEVERITY OF PROBLEM	HISTORY	EXAMINATION	COMPLEXITY OF DECISION MAKING	COUNSELING OVERRIDE	RVU
99211	no key components are required at this coding level				5 ncci	.56
99212	Minor	Focused	Focused	Straightforward	10 ncci	1.22
99213	Low to Moderate	Expanded	Expanded	Low	15 ncci	2.05
99214	Moderate to High	Detailed	Detailed	Moderate	25 ncci	3.02
99215	Moderate to High	Comp.	Comp.	High	40 ncci	4.06

For help with codes 99211-92215 see Example #6 in Chapter 7–Clinical Examples in the *Procedure Codes* section.

Hospital Observation Services

Hospital Observation Services are not included in the *ChiroCode DeskBook*.

See Resource 362 for information about these types of services.

Consultations

A consultation is a type of evaluation and management service provided at the request of another physician or appropriate source, to either recommend care for a specific condition or problem or to determine whether to accept responsibility for ongoing management of the patient's entire care or for the care of a specific condition or problem.

A physician consultant may initiate diagnostic and/or therapeutic services at the same or subsequent visit.

A "consultation" initiated by a patient and/or family, and not requested by a physician or other appropriate source (e.g., physician assistant, nurse practitioner, doctor of chiropractic, physical therapist, occupational therapist, speech-language therapist, social worker, lawyer, or insurance company) is not reported using the consultation codes, but may be reported using the office visit, home service, or domiciliary/rest home care codes as appropriate.

The written or verbal request for a consult may be made by a physician or other appropriate source and documented in the patient's medical record by either the consulting or requesting physician or appropriate source. The consultant's opinion and any services that were ordered or performed must also be documented in the patient's medical record, and communicated by written report to the requesting physician or other appropriate source.

If a consultation is mandated (eg, by a third party payor) the modifier 32 should also be reported.

Consultation Summary

Consultation codes are different from other primary E/M services with two critical differences: 1) They must be requested by an appropriate source, and 2) there must be a written report. Appropriate sources other than physicians could include:

Physician assistant	Physical therapist	Social worker
Nurse practitioner	Occupational therapist	Lawyer
Doctor of chiropractic	Speech-language therapist	Insurance company

● = New Code for 2015   NE = Not Established   ✚ = Add-on Code   TC = Technical Component
▲ = Revised Code for 2015   NA = Not Applicable   ⊘ = Modifier 51 Exempt   26 = Professional Component
▶◀ = New or Revised CPT Text   NCCI = CCI Edits Apply   -QW = CLIA Waived Test   # = Resequenced Code

Any specifically identifiable procedure (ie, identified with a specific CPT code) performed on or subsequent to the date of the initial consultation should be reported separately.

If subsequent to the completion of a consultation the consultant assumes responsibility for management of a portion or all of the patient's condition(s), the appropriate Evaluation and Management services code for the site of service should be reported. In the office setting, the consultant should use the appropriate office or other outpatient consultation codes and then the established patient office of other outpatient service codes.

Office or Other Outpatient Consultations

New or Established Patient

The following codes are used to report consultations provided in the office or in an outpatient or other ambulatory facility, including hospital observation services, home services, domiciliary, rest home, or emergency department (see the preceding consultation definition above). Follow-up visits in the consultant's office or other outpatient facility that are initiated by the consultant or patient are reported using the appropriate codes for established patients, office visits (99211-99215), or home (99347-99350). If an additional request for an opinion or advice regarding the same or a new problem is received from another physician or other appropriate source and documented in the medical record, the office consultation codes may be used again. Services that constitute transfer of care (ie, are provided for the management of the patient's entire care or for the care of a specific condition or problem) are reported with the appropriate new or established patient codes for office or other outpatient visits, domiciliary, rest home services, or home services.

Counseling and/or coordination of care with other physicians, other qualified health care professionals, or agencies are provided consistent with the nature of the problem(s) and the patient's and/or family's needs.

Office consultation for a new or established patient, typically face-to-face with the patient and/or family.

| | | *Key Component Code Selection - 3 of 3* | | | Average Intra-Service Time | |
CODE	SEVERITY OF PROBLEM	HISTORY	EXAMINATION	COMPLEXITY OF DECISION MAKING	COUNSELING OVERRIDE	RVU
99241	Minor	Focused	Focused	Straightforward	15	1.37
99242	Low	Expanded	Expanded	Straightforward	30	2.57
99243	Moderate	Detailed	Detailed	Low	40	3.51
99244	Moderate to High	Comp.	Comp.	Moderate	60	5.19
99245	Moderate to High	Comp.	Comp.	High	80	6.35

EMERGENCY ROOM, NURSING HOME, REST HOME SERVICES

Emergency Room, Nursing Home, Rest Home Services codes are not included in the *ChiroCode DeskBook*.

See Resource 130 for information about these types of services.

HOME SERVICES

The following codes are used to report evaluation and management services provided in a private residence.

Counseling and/or coordination of care with other physicians, other qualified health care professionals, or agencies are provided consistent with the nature of the problem(s) and the patient's and/or family's needs.

New Patient

Home visit for the evaluation and management of a new patient, typically face-to-face with the patient and/or family.

		Key Component Code Selection - 3 of 3			Average Intra-Service Time	
CODE	SEVERITY OF PROBLEM	HISTORY	EXAMINATION	COMPLEXITY OF DECISION MAKING	COUNSELING OVERRIDE	RVU
99341	Low	Focused	Focused	Straightforward	20 ncci	1.55
99342	Moderate	Expanded	Expanded	Low	30 ncci	2.23
99343	Moderate to High	Detailed	Detailed	Moderate	45 ncci	3.64
99344	High	Comp.	Comp.	Moderate	60 ncci	5.11
99345	Sig. Complic. or New	Comp.	Comp.	High	75 ncci	6.18

Established Patient

Home visit for the evaluation and management of an established patient, typically face-to-face with the patient and/or family.

		Key Component Code Selection - 2 of 3			Average Intra-Service Time	
CODE	SEVERITY OF PROBLEM	HISTORY	EXAMINATION	COMPLEXITY OF DECISION MAKING	COUNSELING OVERRIDE	RVU
99347	Minor	Focused IH	Focused	Straightforward	15 ncci	1.55
99348	Low to Moderate	Expanded IH	Expanded	Low	25 ncci	2.36
99349	Moderate to High	Detailed IH	Detailed	Moderate	40 ncci	3.59
99350	Moderate to High	Comp. IH	Comp.	Moderate to High	60 ncci	4.97

IH signifies an interval history

PROLONGED SERVICES

Prolonged Service With Direct Patient Contact

Codes 99354-99357 are used when a physician or other qualified health care professional provides prolonged service involving direct (face-to-face) patient contact that is provided beyond the usual service in either the inpatient or outpatient setting. Direct patient contact is face-to-face and includes other related non-face-to-face services at that location during the same session. This service is reported in

---

Home Services

When chiropractic adjustment (CMT) services are performed in the home, use the appropriate CMT code with the place of service code '12' (home) in box 24B on the 1500 claim form. If a qualified E/M service is performed, select the appropriate E/M code for Home Services and enter the place of service code '12' on the 1500 claim form and append modifier 25.

Example

Place of Service	Type of Service	PROCEDURES, SERVICES OR SUPPLIES (Explain Unusual Circumstances) CPT/HCPCS	MODIFIER
12	1	98940	
12	1	99349	25

● = New Code for 2015 NE = Not Established ✚ = Add-on Code TC = Technical Component
▲ = Revised Code for 2015 NA = Not Applicable ⊘ = Modifier 51 Exempt 26 = Professional Component
► ◄ = New or Revised CPT Text NCCI = CCI Edits Apply -QW = CLIA Waived Test # = Resequenced Code

addition to the designated evaluation and management services at any level, and any other services provided at the same session as evaluation and management services.

See the unabridged CPT codebook for the full text of this introduction.

Example

Total Duration of Prolonged Services	Code(s)
less than 30 minutes	Not reported separately
30-74 minutes (30 minutes - 1 hr. 14 min.)	99354 X 1
75-104 minutes (1 hr. 15 min. - 1 hr. 44 min.)	99354 X 1 AND 99355 X 1
105 or more (1 hr. 45 min. or more)	99354 X 1 AND 99355 X 2 or more for each additional 30 minutes

Prolonged service in the office or other outpatient setting, requiring direct patient contact beyond the usual service;

+ 99354   first hour (List separately in addition to code for office or other outpatient Evaluation and Management service)   ncci   2.80

(Use 99354 in conjunction with codes 90837, 99201-99215, 99241-99245, 99324-99337, 99341-99350)

+ 99355   each additional 30 minutes (List separately in addition to code for prolonged service)   ncci   2.71

(Use 99355 in conjunction with code 99354)

Prolonged service in the inpatient or observation setting, requiring unit/floor time beyond the usual service;

+ 99356   first hour (List separately in addition to code for inpatient Evaluation and Management service)   ncci   2.58

(Use 99356 in conjunction with codes 90837, 99218-99220, 99221-99223, 99224-99226, 99231-99233, 99234-99236, 99251-99255, 99304-99310)

+ 99357   each additional 30 minutes (List separately in addition to code for prolonged service)   ncci   2.56

(Use 99357 in conjunction with code 99356)

Modifier Tips

Prolonged Service: Whenever the E/M service is **prolonged** or greater than the highest level, append the increased service modifier 22. Two modifiers can be used on the 1500 claim form. When using modifier 22, document the circumstances and explain in box 19 and/or attach a report.

Example

Place of Service	Type of Service	PROCEDURES, SERVICES OR SUPPLIES (Explain Unusual Circumstances) CPT/HCPCS	MODIFIER
11	1	98940	
11	1	99215	25 22

Modifier 25 for E/M Services: When E/M services are "significant and separately identifiable" they should be billed with modifier 25 appended to the appropriate E/M code. Significant, separately identifiable encounters could include new patients, periodic reevaluations, reinjury, exacerbations, counseling, releases from active care, discharges, etc.

Example

Place of Service	Type of Service	PROCEDURES, SERVICES OR SUPPLIES (Explain Unusual Circumstances) CPT/HCPCS	MODIFIER
11	1	98941	
11	1	99213	25

Note: The pre-manipulation portion of the Chiropractic Manipulative Treatment codes (9894x) does not include the necessary components of an E/M code, and should never be considered a substitution for the need for an appropriate E/M.

Prolonged Service Without Direct Patient Contact

Codes 99358 and 99359 are used when a prolonged service is provided that is neither face-to-face time in the outpatient setting, nor additional unit/floor time in the hospital or nursing facility setting during the same session of an evaluation and management service and is beyond the usual physician or other qualified health care professional service time.

This service is to be reported in relation to other physician or other qualified health care professional services, including evaluation and management services at any level. This prolonged service may be reported on a different date than the primary service to which it is related.

For complete instructions see 2015 CPT *by the American Medical Association.*

	Prolonged evaluation and management service before and/or after direct patient care;		
99358	first hour	ncci	3.07
+ 99359	each additional 30 minutes (List separately in addition to code for prolonged service)	ncci	1.48

(Use 99359 in conjunction with code 99358)

Case Management Services

Case management is a process in which a physician or another qualified health care professional is responsible for direct care of a patient and, additionally, for coordinating, managing access to, initiating, and/or supervising other health care services needed by the patient.

For complete instructions see 2015 CPT *by the American Medical Association.*

Medical Team Conferences

Medical team conferences include face-to-face participation by a minimum of three qualified health care professionals from different specialties or disciplines (each of whom provide direct care to the patient), with or without the presence of the patient, family member(s), community agencies, surrogate decision maker(s) (eg, legal guardian), and/or caregiver(s). The participants are actively involved in the development, revision, coordination, and implementation of health care services needed by the patient.

No more than one individual from the same specialty may report 99366-99368 at the same encounter.

Individuals should not report 99366-99368 when their participation in the medical team conference is part of a facility or organizational service contractually provided by the organizational or facility provider.

Medical Team Conference, Direct (Face-to-Face) Contact With Patient and/or Family

99366	Medical team conference with interdisciplinary team of health care professionals, face-to-face with patient and/or family, 30 minutes or more, participation by nonphysician qualified health care professional	ncci	1.21

(Team conference services of less than 30 minutes duration are not reported separately)

(For team conference services by a physician with patient and/or family present, see Evaluation and Management services)

Medical Team Conference, Without Direct (Face-to-Face) Contact With Patient and/or Family

99367	Medical team conference with interdisciplinary team of health care professionals, patient and/or family not present, 30 minutes or more; participation by physician	ncci	1.59
99368	participation by nonphysician qualified health care professional	ncci	1.05

(Team conference services of less than 30 minutes duration are not reported separately)

(99371-99373 have been deleted. To report telephone evaluation and management services, see 99441-99443)

PREVENTIVE MEDICINE SERVICES (WELLNESS)

This code set is also known as the **health and wellness assurance codes.** These codes are appropriate expressions of annual (initial or periodic) health and wellness encounters for infants, children, adolescents and adults. The Patient Protection and Affordable Care Act now requires many preventive services to be covered without co-payments, co-insurance or meeting deductibles.

See Resource 339 for additional information about preventive services covered by the Affordable Care Act.

Wellness-oriented practices will want to use these codes when appropriate to record the status and growth of these important health promotion services. It will provide valuable management data on the growth of true wellness services.

The extent and focus of the services will largely depend on the age of the patient.

If an abnormality is encountered or a preexisting problem is addressed in the process of performing this preventive medicine evaluation and management service, and *if the problem or abnormality is significant enough to require additional work to perform the key components of a problem-oriented E/M service,* then the appropriate Office/Outpatient code 99201-99215 should also be reported. Modifier 25 should be added to the Office/Outpatient code to indicate that a significant, separately identifiable evaluation and management service was provided on the same day as the preventive medicine service. The appropriate preventive medicine service is additionally reported.

An insignificant or trivial problem/abnormality that is encountered in the process of performing the preventive medicine evaluation and management service and which does not require additional work and the performance of the key components of a problem-oriented E/M service, should not be reported.

The "comprehensive" nature of the Preventive Medicine Services codes 99381-99397 reflects an age and gender appropriate history/exam and is **not** synonymous with the "comprehensive" examination required in Evaluation and Management codes 99201-99350.

Codes 99381-99397 include counseling/anticipatory guidance/risk factor reduction interventions which are provided at the time of the initial or periodic comprehensive preventive medicine examination. (Refer to codes 99401-99412 for reporting those counseling/anticipatory guidance/risk factor reduction interventions that are provided at an encounter **separate** from the preventive medicine examination.)

Vaccine/toxoid products, immunization administrations, ancillary studies involving laboratory, radiology, other procedures, or screening tests (eg, vision, hearing, developmental) identified with a specific CPT code are reported separately. For immunization administration and vaccine risk/benefit counseling, see 90461, 90470-90474. For vaccine/toxoid products, see 90476-90479.

ACA members may go to ACAtoday.org/UserFiles/PreventiveServicesToolkit.pdf to review their *Preventive Services Toolkit*.

RVU

New Patient

Initial comprehensive preventive medicine evaluation and management of an individual including an age and gender appropriate history, examination, counseling/anticipatory guidance/risk factor reduction interventions, and the ordering of laboratory/diagnostic procedures, new patient;

Code	Description		RVU
99381	infant (age under 1 year)	ncci	3.11
99382	early childhood (age 1 through 4 years)	ncci	3.25
99383	late childhood (age 5 through 11 years)	ncci	3.39
99384	adolescent (age 12 through 17 years)	ncci	3.82
99385	18-39 years	ncci	3.70
99386	40-64 years	ncci	4.30
99387	65 years and over	ncci	4.66

Established Patient

Periodic comprehensive preventive medicine reevaluation and management of an individual including an age and gender appropriate history, examination, counseling/anticipatory guidance/risk factor reduction interventions, and the ordering of laboratory/diagnostic procedures, established patient;

Code	Description		RVU
99391	infant (age under 1 year)	ncci	2.80
99392	early childhood (age 1 through 4 years)	ncci	2.99
99393	late childhood (age 5 through 11 years)	ncci	2.98
99394	adolescent (age 12 through 17 years)	ncci	3.26
99395	18-39 years	ncci	3.34
99396	40-64 years	ncci	3.55
99397	65 years and over	ncci	3.83

Wellness Codes and Coverage

The Wellness (Preventive Medicine Services) codes are the least understood and least used codes in most offices that are promoting health and wellness.

Sports/Athletics

Sports physicals should only be reported with a preventative medicine code if the provider performs a comprehensive history and exam. If the provider performs a brief, detailed, or extended history and exam, report the appropriate office/outpatient E/M code (99201-99215.) For Athletic Training Evaluation see 97005. See CPT Assistant, July 1996 for more information.

Use of Preventive Medicine Codes

After a patient is discharged or released for active care, these Preventive Service codes could be used. Until then, the established patient E/M code of 99211 thru 99215 would be appropriate and reported for the evaluation of outcomes, residuals and Counseling.

The intent of this Preventive Medicine code set is for services focused on periodic evaluations, re-evaluations, counseling risk factor reduction and change interventions. When the patient encounter is for such services (and not just a treatment modaltiy/adjustment) then these codes are appropriate.

● = New Code for 2015　　NE = Not Established　　✢ = Add-on Code　　TC = Technical Component
▲ = Revised Code for 2015　　NA = Not Applicable　　⊘ = Modifier 51 Exempt　　26 = Professional Component
▶◀ = New or Revised CPT Text　　NCCI = CCI Edits Apply　　-QW = CLIA Waived Test　　# = Resequenced Code

Counseling Risk Factor Reduction and Behavior Change Intervention

New or Established Patient

These codes are used to report services provided face-to-face by a physician or other qualified health care professional for the purpose of promoting health and preventing illness or injury. They are distinct from evaluation and management (E/M) services that may be reported separately when performed. Risk factor reduction services are used for persons without a specific illness for which the counseling might otherwise be used as part of treatment.

Preventive medicine counseling and risk factor reduction interventions will vary with age and should address such issues as family problems, diet and exercise, substance use, sexual practices, injury prevention, dental health, and diagnostic and laboratory test results available at the time of the encounter.

Behavior change interventions are for persons who have a behavior that is often considered an illness itself, such as tobacco use and addiction, substance abuse/misuse, or obesity. Behavior change services may be reported when performed to change the harmful behavior that has not yet resulted in illness. Any E/M services reported on the same day must be distinct, and time spent providing these services may not be used as a basis for the E/M code selection. Behavior change services involve specific validated interventions of assessing readiness for change and barriers to change, advising a change in behavior, assisting by providing specific suggested actions and motivational counseling, and arranging for services and follow-up.

For counseling groups of patients with symptoms or established illness, use 99078.

Health and Behavior Assessment/Intervention services (96150-96155) should not be reported on the same day as codes 99401-99412.

Preventive Medicine, Individual Counseling

Preventive medicine counseling and/or risk factor reduction intervention(s) provided to an individual (separate procedure);

99401	approximately 15 minutes	ncci	1.02
99402	approximately 30 minutes	ncci	1.74
99403	approximately 45 minutes	ncci	2.43
99404	approximately 60 minutes	ncci	3.15

> These code descriptions are defined as "approximately." Therefore, to select the proper code, follow the general AMA time guidelines which state that unless otherwise noted in code instructions or guidelines, "a unit of time is attained when the midpoint is passed."
>
> **Note:** Services less than 8 minutes, should not be reported because it does not reach the mid-point requirement.

For help with code 99404 see Example #21 in Chapter 7–Clinical Examples in this *Procedure Codes* section.

Behavior Change Interventions, Individual

Smoking and tobacco use cessation counseling visit;

99406	intermediate, greater than 3 minutes up to 10 minutes	ncci	.40
99407	intensive, greater than 10 minutes	ncci	.77

(Do not report 95407 in conjunction with 99406)

Alcohol and/or substance (other than tobacco) abuse structured screening (eg, AUDIT, DAST), and brief intervention (SBI) services;

			RVU
99408	15 to 30 minutes	ncci	.99
	(Do not report services of less than 15 minutes with 99408)		
99409	greater than 30 minutes	ncci	1.93
	(Do not report 95409 in conjunction with 99408)		
	(Do not report 95408, 99409 in conjunction with 99420)		
	(Use 99408, 99409 only for initial screening and brief intervention)		

Preventive Medicine, Group Counseling

Preventive medicine counseling and/or risk factor reduction intervention(s) provided to individuals in a group setting (separate procedure);

99411	approximately 30 minutes	ncci	.46
99412	approximately 60 minutes	ncci	.61

For help with codes 99411 and 99412 see Examples #22 and #23 in Chapter 7–Clinical Examples in this *Procedure Codes* section.

Other Preventive Medicine Services

99420	Administration and interpretation of health risk assessment instrument (HRA) (eg, health hazard appraisal)	ncci	.30

> Health Risk Assessments (HRA) are designed for clients with **no presenting problem.** They are ideal for screening programs and for wellness promotion. However, **if** there is a presenting problem, it would be appropriate to consider the Health and Behavior Assessment/Intervention codes (96150-96155). This code set focuses on the biopsychosocial factors important to physical health problems and treatments, and not on mental health.

99429	Unlisted preventive medicine service	ncci	NE

Non-Face-to-Face Physician Services

Telephone services are non-face-to-face evaluation and management (E/M) services provided to a patient using the telephone by a physician or other qualified health care professional, who may report evaluation and management services. These codes are used to report episodes of patient care initiated by an established patient or guardian of an established patient. If the telephone service ends with a decision to see the patient within 24 hours or next available urgent visit appointment, the code is not reported; rather the encounter is considered part of the preservice work of the subsequent E/M service, procedure, and visit. Likewise if the telephone call refers to an E/M service performed and reported by that individual within the previous seven days (either requested or unsolicited patient follow-up) or within the postoperative period of the previously completed procedure, then the service(s) are considered part of that previous E/M service or procedure. (Do not report 99441-99443 if reporting 99441-99444 performed in the previous seven days.)

> For qualified nonphysician health care providers who cannot report E/M services, see codes 98966-98968.

Telephone Services

RVU

Telephone evaluation and management service by a physician or other qualified health care professional who may report evaluation and management services provided to an established patient, parent, or guardian not originating from a related E/M service provided within the previous 7 days nor leading to an E/M service or procedure within the next 24 hours or soonest available appointment;

99441	5-10 minutes of medical discussion	ncci	.40
99442	11-20 minutes of medical discussion	ncci	.76
99443	21-30 minutes of medical discussion	ncci	1.13

For help with codes 99411 to 99443 see Examples #12 to #14 in Chapter 7–Clinical Examples in this *Procedure Codes* section.

On-Line Medical Evaluation

An on-line E/M service is a non-face-to-face encounter which must meet specific electronic requirements. It may only be used once every 7 days for the same episode of care.

For qualified non-physician health care professionals, see 98969.

For complete instructions see 2015 CPT *by the American Medical Association.*

99444	Online evaluation and management service provided by a physician or other qualified health care professional who may report an evaluation and management services provided to an established patient, or guardian, not originating from a related E/M service provided within the previous 7 days, using the Internet or similar electronic communications network	ncci	NE

For help with code 99444 see Example #15 in Chapter 7–Clinical Examples in this *Procedure Codes* section.

Interprofessional Telephone/Internet Consultations

These consultation codes are to be used in situations where the treating provider requests the opinion of another health care professional as part of their assessment and management of the patient's condition. This is done via telephone or the internet without the patient being present. For consultations which include the patient and/or family, see 99441-99444 or 98966-98969.

Typically, these are more complex or urgent situations in which face-to-face service is not feasible. They should not be used prior to an agreed upon transfer of care, however, if the decision to transfer care happens after the consultation, they may be used.

Review of data including medical records and imaging studies are included in this code and should not be reported separately. Do not report more than once every 7 days and do not report consultations which are less than 5 minutes.

For complete instructions see 2015 CPT *by the American Medical Association.*

RVU

Interprofessional telephone/Internet assessment and management service provided by a consultative physician including a verbal and written report to the patient's treating/requesting physician or other qualified health care professional;

99446	5-10 minutes of medical consultative discussion and review	ncci	NE
99447	11-20 minutes of medical consultative discussion and review	ncci	NE
99448	21-30 minutes of medical consultative discussion and review	ncci	NE
99449	31 minutes or more of medical consultative discussion and review	ncci	NE

Special Evaluation and Management Services

The following codes are used to report evaluations performed to establish baseline information prior to life or disability insurance certificates being issued. This service is performed in the office or other setting, and applies to both new and established patients. When using these codes, no active management of the problem(s) is undertaken during the encounter.

If other evaluation and management services and/or procedures are performed on the same date, the appropriate E/M or procedure code(s) should be reported in addition to these codes.

Basic Life and/or Disability Evaluation Services

99450   Basic life and/or disability examination that includes: ncci   *4.97

- measurement of height, weight and blood pressure;
- completion of a medical history following a life insurance pro forma;
- collection of blood sample and/or urinalysis complying with "chain of custody" protocols; and
- completion of necessary documentation/certificates.

Work Related or Medical Disability Evaluation Services

99455   Work related or medical disability examination by the treating physician that includes: ncci   *6.80

- completion of a medical history commensurate with the patient's condition;
- performance of an examination commensurate with the patient's condition;
- formulation of a diagnosis, assessment of capabilities and stability, and calculation of impairment;
- development of future medical treatment plan; and
- completion of necessary documentation/certificates and report.

99456   Work related or medical disability examination by other than the treating physician that includes: ncci   *7.84

- completion of a medical history commensurate with the patient's condition;
- performance of an examination commensurate with the patient's condition;
- formulation of a diagnosis, assessment of capabilities and stability, and calculation of impairment;
- development of future medical treatment plan; and
- completion of necessary documentation/certificates and report.

Other Evaluation and Management Services

99499   Unlisted evaluation and management service   NE

* = RVU gap-filled by ChiroCode Institute.

4b. CPT Procedures
Surgery Codes

Special instructions apply. See the current CPT code book or ⚙ FindACode.com for full information.

MUSCULOSKELETAL SYSTEM

Spine (Vertebral Column)

Manipulation
                                                                                                          RVU
22505   Manipulation of spine requiring anesthesia, any region   ncci   3.81

> Spinal Manipulation under Anesthesia is usually an out-patient manipulation of the posterior motor units of the spine, requiring anesthesia and designed to reduce fibroblastic proliferation, restore range of motion and visco-elasticity to the pericapsular connective tissues and paravertebral musculature to areas of spinal segmental dysfunction not amenable to in-office manipulation. When this is performed as a chiropractic procedure it requires specialized training.
>
> When two physicians work together performing distinct parts of this procedure, each should report his/her distinct operative work by appending the modifier 62 to the procedure code (example 22505-62).
>
> If the case is unusual, it would be appropriate to also append the modifier 22, and attach the report (example: 22505-62-22).
>
> See Chapter 6–Procedure Modifiers for more about modifiers 62 and 22.
>
> For CPT spinal manipulation without anesthesia, use 98940-98942.

Shoulder

Manipulation
23700   Manipulation under anesthesia, shoulder joint, including application of fixation apparatus (dislocation excluded)   ncci   5.63

Pelvis and Hip Joint
Including head and neck of femur.

Manipulation
27275   hip joint, requiring general anesthesia   ncci   5.21

Application of Casts and Strapping

These codes are for use when a cast application, strapping, or taping is used to stabilize or protect a fracture or dislocation, or to afford a patient comfort. This can be performed as an initial treatment, or as a replacement service during or after follow-up care.

Use these codes in the following situations:

- When the initial encounter involves treatment of the injury, use the codes in this section.
- When the encounter follows initial treatment performed by a different practitioner, you may still use the codes in this section.

However, do not use these codes in the following situations:

- When the initial encounter involves only strapping or casting without treatment (e.g., a sprained ankle), use the appropriate E/M and supply codes.
- When taping is used for dynamic extension, not immobilization, use the appropriate E/M and supply codes.

Note: When there is orthotic or prosthetic management and training, see codes 97760-97762.

These codes are often overlooked when performed in a chiropractic office. From a CPT coding perspective they could be used for any of the following reasons.

- Afford comfort to the patient.
- Provide initial service without restorative treatment.
- Replacement during or after follow-up care.
- Stabilize or protect fracture, injury, or dislocation.

Body and Upper Extremity

Casts

Code	Description		RVU
29035	Application of body cast, shoulder to hips;	ncci	6.37
29040	including head, Minerva type	ncci	6.28
29044	including 1 thigh	ncci	7.39
29046	including both thighs	ncci	6.76
	Application, cast;		
29049	figure-of-eight	ncci	2.10
29055	shoulder spica	ncci	6.38
29058	plaster Velpeau	ncci	3.56
29065	shoulder to hand (long arm)	ncci	2.74
29075	elbow to finger (short arm)	ncci	2.47
29085	hand and lower forearm (gauntlet)	ncci	2.72

Splints

Code	Description		RVU
29105	Application of long arm splint (shoulder to hand)	ncci	2.50
	Application of short arm splint (forearm to hand);		
29125	static	ncci	1.84
29126	dynamic	ncci	2.19
	Application of finger splint;		
29130	static	ncci	1.16
29131	dynamic	ncci	1.45

			RVU
Strapping–Any Age			
	Strapping;		
29200	thorax	ncci	1.48
29240	shoulder (eg, Velpeau)	ncci	1.61
29260	elbow or wrist	ncci	1.46
29280	hand or finger	ncci	1.44

Lower Extremity

Casts

29345	Application of long leg cast (thigh to toes);	ncci	3.90
29355	walker or ambulatory type	ncci	4.03
29358	Application of long leg cast brace	ncci	4.61
29365	Application of cylinder cast (thigh to ankle)	ncci	3.51
29405	Application of short leg cast (below knee to toes);	ncci	2.34
29425	walking or ambulatory type	ncci	2.24
29435	Application of patellar tendon bearing (PTB) cast	ncci	3.37
29440	Adding walker to previously applied cast	ncci	1.24
29445	Application of rigid total contact leg cast	ncci	3.87
29450	Application of clubfoot cast with molding or manipulation, long or short leg	ncci	4.11

Splints

29505	Application of long leg splint (thigh to ankle or toes)	ncci	2.36
29515	Application of short leg (calf to foot)	ncci	2.04

Strapping–Any Age

	Strapping;		
29520	hip	ncci	1.33
29530	knee	ncci	1.39
29540	ankle and/or foot	ncci	1.05
29550	toes	ncci	.90
29580	Unna boot	ncci	1.49
	Application of multi-layer compression system;		
29581	leg (below knee), including ankle and foot	ncci	1.77
	(Do not report 29581 in conjunction with 29540, 29580, 29582, 36475, 36476, 36478, 36479)		
29582	thigh and leg, including ankle and foot, when performed	ncci	2.01
	(Do not report 29582 in conjunction with 29540, 29580, 29581, 36475, 36476, 36478, 36479)		
29583	upper arm and forearm	ncci	1.26
	(Do not report 29583 in conjunction with 29584)		
29584	upper arm, forearm, hand, and fingers	ncci	2.01
	(Do not report 29584 in conjunction with 29583)		

Removal or Repair

Codes for cast removals should be employed only for casts applied by another individual.

29700	Removal or bivalving; gauntlet, boot or body cast	ncci	1.74
29720	Repair of spica, body cast or jacket	ncci	2.43
29730	Windowing of cast	ncci	1.83
29740	Wedging of cast (except clubfoot casts)	ncci	2.86
29750	Wedging of clubfoot cast	ncci	2.61

(To report bilateral procedure, use 29750 with modifier 50)

Other Procedures

29799	Unlisted procedure, casting or strapping	NE

CARDIOVASCULAR SYSTEM

Arteries and Veins

Vascular Injection Procedures

36415	Collection of venous blood by venipuncture	ncci	NE

NERVOUS SYSTEM

Extracranial Nerves, Peripheral Nerves, and Autonomic Nervous System

Neurostimulators (Peripheral Nerve)

64550	Application of surface (transcutaneous) neurostimulator	ncci	.45

In addition to the application code, use adjunctive codes for associated equipment and/or supplies. See associated tens codes and modifiers (rental or sales) in the supplies section.

AUDITORY SYSTEM

External Ear

Removal of Foreign Body

69210	Removal impacted cerumen requiring instrumentation, unilateral	ncci	1.39

(For bilateral procedure, report 69210 with modifier 50)

(For cerumen removal that is not impacted or does not require instrumentation, eg, by irrigation only see E/M service code, which may include new or established patient office or other outpatient services [99201-99215], hospital observation services [99217-99220, 99224-99226], hospital care [99221-99223, 99231-99233], consultations [99241-99255], emergency department services [99281-99285], nursing facility services [99304-99318], domiciliary, rest home, or custodial care services [99324-99334], home services [99341-99350])

The associated ICD-9 code is 380.4, Impacted Cerumen.

4c. CPT Procedures

Diagnostic Imaging Codes

This section includes excerpts of imaging codes that could be of interest to many primary care or Complementary and Alternative Medical (CAM) practitioners.

For complete instructions see 2015 CPT by the American Medical Association.

DIAGNOSTIC RADIOLOGY (DIAGNOSTIC IMAGING)

Head and Neck

			-TC	/-26	/Total RVU
	Radiologic examination, mandible;				
70100	partial, less than 4 views	ncci	.66	.26	.92
70110	complete, minimum of 4 views	ncci	.69	.36	1.05
	Radiologic examination, mastoids;				
70120	less than 3 views per side	ncci	.68	.26	.94
70130	complete, minimum of 3 views per side	ncci	1.04	.49	1.53
	Radiologic examination, facial bones;				
70140	less than 3 views	ncci	.53	.30	.83
70150	complete, minimum of 3 views	ncci	.77	.38	1.15
70160	Radiologic examination, nasal bones, complete, minimum of 3 views		.65	.25	.90
	Radiologic examination;				
70190	optic foramina		.66	.32	.98
70200	orbits, complete, minimum of 4 views		.77	.40	1.17

Reports: A signed, written report by the interpreting individual is considered to be part of the procedure.

Modifiers: Append the appropriate modifier when only a portion of the total service is performed. Billing without a modifier declares that **both** the technical and professional components are performed.

- TC: Append this modifier when only the technical component (TC) is performed. If it is performed by an outside source (e.g., hospital), use modifier (90)
- 26: Append this modifier when only the professional component (interpretation and report) is performed

TC Technical Component: When only the technical component is performed, it does not include the interpretation and report (professional component 26). When no modifier is used (TC or 26) it is a declaration that both components were performed.

			-TC	/-26	/Total RVU
	Radiologic examination, sinuses, paranasal;				
70210	less than 3 views	ncci	.57	.25	.82
70220	complete, minimum of 3 views	ncci	.68	.36	1.04
70240	Radiologic examination, sella turcica		.54	.29	.83
	Radiologic examination, skull;				
70250	less than 4 views	ncci	.64	.35	1.00
70260	complete, minimum of 4 views	ncci	.76	.49	1.25
	Radiologic examination, temporomandibular joint, open and closed mouth;				
70328	unilateral	ncci	.59	.27	.86
70330	bilateral	ncci	.94	.37	1.31
70336	MRI, temporomandibular joint(s)	ncci	6.85	2.09	8.94
70360	Radiologic examination; neck, soft tissue	ncci	.54	.24	.78
	CT, head or brain; (To report 3D rendering, see 76376, 76377)				
70450	without contrast material	ncci	2.04	1.22	3.26
70460	with contrast material(s)	ncci	2.94	1.61	4.55
70470	without contrast material, followed by contrast material(s) and further sections	ncci	3.61	1.81	5.42
	CT, orbit, sella, or posterior fossa or outer, middle, or inner ear; (To report 3D rendering, see 76376, 76377)				
70480	without contrast material	ncci	4.68	1.83	6.51
70481	with contrast material(s)	ncci	5.73	1.97	7.70
70482	without contrast material, followed by contrast material(s) and further sections	ncci	6.36	2.05	8.41
	CT, maxillofacial area; (To report 3D rendering, see 76376, 76377)				
70486	without contrast material	ncci	3.82	1.62	5.44
70487	with contrast material(s)	ncci	4.85	1.85	6.70
70488	without contrast material, followed by contrast material(s) and further sections	ncci	5.97	2.02	7.99
	CT, soft tissue neck; (To report 3D rendering, see 76376, 76377) (For cervical spine, see 72125, 72126)				
70490	without contrast material	ncci	3.57	1.83	5.40
70491	with contrast material(s)	ncci	4.61	1.97	6.58
70492	without contrast material followed by contrast material(s) and further sections	ncci	5.69	2.07	7.76
	MRI, orbit, face, and/or neck; (Report 70540-70543 once per imaging session)				
70540	without contrast material(s)	ncci	8.09	1.90	9.99
70542	with contrast material(s)	ncci	8.94	2.31	11.25
70543	without contrast material(s) followed by contrast material(s) and further sequences	ncci	10.70	3.05	13.75
	MRI, brain (including brain stem);				
70551	without contrast material	ncci	4.25	2.10	6.35
70552	with contrast material(s)	ncci	6.35	2.54	8.89
70553	without contrast material, followed by contrast material(s) and further sequences	ncci	7.25	3.26	10.51

● = New Code for 2015   NE = Not Established   ✚ = Add-on Code   TC = Technical Component   X-Ray = Radiologic examination
▲ = Revised Code for 2015   NA = Not Applicable   ⊘ = Modifier 51 Exempt   26 = Professional Component   CT = Computed Tomography
▶◀ = New or Revised CPT Text   NCCI = CCI Edits Apply   -QW = CLIA Waived Test   # = Resequenced Code   MRI = Magnetic Resonance Imaging

			-TC	/-26	/Total RVU
	MRI, brain, functional MRI;				
	(Do not report 70554, 70555 in conjunction with 70551-70553 unless a separate diagnostic MRI is performed)				
70554	including test selection and administration of repetitive body part movement and/or visual stimulation, not requiring physician or psychologist administration	ncci	9.53	3.03	12.56
	(Do not report 70554 in conjunction with 96020)				
70555	requiring physician or psychologist administration of entire neurofunctional testing	ncci	NE	3.69	NE
	(Do not report 70555 unless 96020 is performed)				

Chest

Code	Description		-TC	/-26	/Total RVU
71010	Radiologic examination, chest; single view, frontal	ncci	.37	.26	.63
71020	Radiologic examination, chest, 2 views, frontal and lateral;	ncci	.46	.31	.77
71021	with apical lordotic procedure	ncci	.55	.39	.94
71022	with oblique projections	ncci	.70	.47	1.17
71023	with fluoroscopy	ncci	1.22	.55	1.77
	Radiologic examination, chest,				
	(For concurrent computer-aided detection [CAD] performed in addition to codes 71010, 71020, 71021, 71022, and 71030, use 0174T. Do not report 71010, 71020, 71021, 71022, and 71030 in conjunction with 0175T for CAD performed remotely from the primary interpretation)				
71030	complete, minimum of 4 views;	ncci	.71	.45	1.16
71034	with fluoroscopy	ncci	1.68	.63	2.34
	(For separate chest fluoroscopy, use 76000)				
71035	special views (eg, lateral decubitus, Bucky studies)	ncci	.64	.26	.90
	Radiologic examination, ribs, unilateral;				
71100	2 views	ncci	.53	.32	.85
71101	including posteroanterior chest, minimum of 3 views	ncci	.62	.38	1.00
	Radiologic examination, ribs, bilateral;				
71110	3 views	ncci	.65	.39	1.04
71111	including posteroanterior chest, minimum of 4 views	ncci	.86	.46	1.32
	Radiologic examination;				
71120	sternum, minimum of 2 views		.53	.29	.82
71130	sternoclavicular joint or joints, minimum of 3 views		.67	.33	1.00
	CT, thorax;				
	(To report 3D rendering, see 76376, 76377)				
71250	without contrast material	ncci	3.58	1.46	5.04
71260	with contrast material(s)	ncci	4.63	1.78	6.41
71270	without contrast material, followed by contrast material(s) and further sections	ncci	5.72	1.96	7.68
71275	Computed tomographic angiography, chest (noncoronary), with contrast material(s) and further sections, including noncontrast images, if performed, and image postprocessing	ncci	7.02	2.74	9.76

			-TC	/-26	/Total RVU
	MRI, chest (eg, for evaluation of hilar and mediastinal lymphadenopathy);				
71550	without contrast material(s)	ncci	9.49	2.07	11.56
71551	with contrast material(s)	ncci	10.32	2.47	12.79
71552	without contrast material(s), followed by contrast material(s) and further sequences	ncci	12.95	3.21	16.16

Spine and Pelvis

72010	Radiologic examination, spine, entire, survey study, anteroposterior and lateral	ncci	1.30	.67	1.97
72020	Radiologic examination, spine, single view, specify level	ncci	.39	.22	.61

> Document the level in the patient chart and enter a note in box 19 of the 1500 claim form.
>
> Many insurance payers bundle the itemized and specific CPT codes for spinal X-rays into the single CPT code 72010 - Radiologic examination, spine, entire, survey study, anteroposterior and lateral. In response to questions, the AMA stated in the May 2002 *CPT Assistant*, "Historically, the 'Spinal Survey' accommodated the two large AP&L films for a **single study**, such as a scoliosis study to obtain measurements or to evaluate for spinal metastasis. These films are then interpreted as a single study (i.e., one interpretation of all of the films)."
>
> Subsequent to this statement by the AMA, the standard for both provider and payers is focused on clinical need and documentation. What is a single study? They cited scoliosis and metastasis. It could be appropriate to assume that "subluxation" would also be a single study. Therefore, if there are other diagnostic issues or clinical concerns it could be a **multiple study** (i.e., multiple interpretations), and it would **not** be appropriate to bundle into 72010.
>
> For the complete report see the *CPT Assistant, May 2002*.

	Radiologic examination, spine, cervical;				
72040	2 or 3 views	ncci	.60	.33	.93
72050	4 or 5 views	ncci	.80	.46	1.26
72052	6 or more views	ncci	1.03	.53	1.56
72069	Radiologic examination, spine, thoracolumbar, standing (scoliosis)	ncci	.56	.34	.90
	Radiologic examination, spine;				
72070	thoracic, 2 views	ncci	.55	.33	.88
72072	thoracic, 3 views	ncci	.65	.31	.96
72074	thoracic, minimum of 4 views	ncci	.78	.31	1.09
72080	thoracolumbar, 2 views	ncci	.60	.34	.94
72090	scoliosis study, including supine and erect studies	ncci	.76	.44	1.20
	Radiologic examination, spine, lumbosacral;				
72100	2 or 3 views	ncci	.65	.33	.98
72110	minimum of 4 views	ncci	.90	.46	1.36
72114	complete, including bending views, minimum of 6 views	ncci	1.26	.48	1.74
72120	bending views only, 2 or 3 views	ncci	.79	.34	1.13
	CT, cervical spine;				
72125	without contrast material	ncci	3.62	1.53	5.15
72126	with contrast material	ncci	4.66	1.74	6.40
72127	without contrast material, followed by contrast material(s) and further sections	ncci	5.75	1.80	7.55

				-TC / -26 / Total RVU		
	CT, thoracic spine;					
72128	without contrast material	ncci	3.61	1.42	5.03	
72129	with contrast material	ncci	4.66	1.74	6.40	
72130	without contrast material, followed by contrast material(s) and further sections	ncci	5.75	1.80	7.55	
	CT, lumbar spine;					
	(To report 3D rendering, see 76376, 76377)					
72131	without contrast material	ncci	3.58	1.42	5.00	
72132	with contrast material	ncci	4.64	1.74	6.38	
72133	without contrast material, followed by contrast material(s) and further sections	ncci	5.75	1.80	7.55	
	MRI, spinal canal and contents, cervical;					
72141	without contrast material	ncci	4.19	2.11	6.30	
72142	with contrast material(s)	ncci	6.37	2.54	8.91	
	MRI, spinal canal and contents, thoracic;					
72146	without contrast material	ncci	4.19	2.11	6.30	
72147	with contrast material(s)	ncci	6.31	2.54	8.85	
	MRI, spinal canal and contents, lumbar;					
72148	without contrast material	ncci	4.19	2.11	6.30	
72149	with contrast material(s)	ncci	6.27	2.54	8.81	
	Radiologic examination, pelvis;					
	(For a combined computed tomography [CT] or computed tomographic angiography abdomen and pelvis study, see 74174, 74176-74178)					
72170	1 or 2 views	ncci	.51	.26	.77	
72190	complete, minimum of 3 views	ncci	.74	.33	1.07	
	CT, pelvis;					
	(For a combined CT abdomen and pelvis study, see 74176-74178)					
	(To report 3D rendering, see 76376, 76377)					
72192	without contrast material	ncci	2.53	1.55	4.08	
72193	with contrast material(s)	ncci	4.65	1.66	6.31	
72194	without contrast material, followed by contrast material(s) and further sections	ncci	5.53	1.73	7.26	
	MRI, pelvis;					
72195	without contrast material(s)	ncci	8.40	2.09	10.49	
72196	with contrast material(s)	ncci	8.99	2.47	11.46	
72197	without contrast material(s), followed by contrast material(s) and further sequences	ncci	10.90	3.21	14.11	
	Radiologic examination, sacroiliac joints;					
72200	less than 3 views	ncci	.54	.25	.79	
72202	3 or more views	ncci	.64	.27	.91	
72220	Radiologic examination, sacrum and coccyx, minimum of 2 views		.53	.25	.78	
72270	Myelography, 2 or more regions (eg, lumbar/thoracic, cervical/thoracic, lumbar/cervical, lumbar/thoracic/cervical), radiological supervision and interpretation	ncci	3.23	1.91	5.14	

▶(For complete myelography of 2 or more regions via injection procedure at C1-C2, see 61055, 72270)◀

▶(72291 and 72292 have been deleted. To report, see 22510, 22511, 22512, 22513, 22514, 22515, 0200T, 0201T) ◀

-TC / -26 / Total RVU

Upper Extremities

Code	Description				
	Radiologic examination;				
73000	clavicle, complete	ncci	.53	.25	.78
73010	scapula, complete	ncci	.57	.27	.84
	Radiologic examination, shoulder;				
73020	1 view	ncci	.42	.23	.65
73030	complete, minimum of 2 views	ncci	.53	.28	.81
73040	Radiologic examination, shoulder, arthrography, radiological supervision and interpretation	ncci	2.01	.79	2.80
	Radiologic examination;				
73050	acromioclavicular joints, bilateral, with or without weighted distraction	ncci	.69	.32	1.01
73060	humerus, minimum of two views	ncci	.49	.26	.75
	Radiologic examination, elbow;				
73070	2 views	ncci	.53	.24	.77
73080	complete, minimum of 3 views	ncci	.61	.26	.87
73090	Radiologic examination; forearm, two views	ncci	.47	.24	.71
	Radiologic examination, wrist;				
73100	2 views	ncci	.57	.25	.82
73110	complete, minimum of 3 views	ncci	.73	.26	.99
	Radiologic examination, hand;				
73120	2 views	ncci	.49	.24	.73
73130	minimum of 3 views	ncci	.60	.26	.86
73140	Radiologic examination, finger(s), minimum of two views	ncci	.67	.21	.88
	CT, upper extremity;				
	(To report 3D rendering, see 76376, 76377)				
73200	without contrast material	ncci	3.57	1.42	4.99
73201	with contrast material(s)	ncci	4.56	1.65	6.21
73202	without contrast material, followed by contrast material(s) and further sections	ncci	6.02	1.73	7.75
	MRI, upper extremity, other than joint;				
73218	without contrast material(s)	ncci	8.25	1.92	10.17
73219	with contrast material(s)	ncci	8.93	2.32	11.25
73220	without contrast material(s), followed by contrast material(s) and further sequences	ncci	10.88	3.06	13.94
	MRI, any joint of upper extremity;				
73221	without contrast material(s)	ncci	4.65	1.94	6.59
73222	with contrast material(s)	ncci	8.25	2.32	10.57
73223	without contrast material(s), followed by contrast material(s) and further sequences	ncci	10.03	3.06	13.09

Lower Extremities

Code	Description				
	Radiologic examination, hip, unilateral;				
73500	1 view	ncci	.48	.26	.74
73510	complete, minimum of 2 views	ncci	.71	.32	1.03
73520	Radiologic examination, hips, bilateral, minimum of 2 views of each hip, including anteroposterior view of pelvis	ncci	.70	.40	1.10

● = New Code for 2015　NE = Not Established　✚ = Add-on Code　TC = Technical Component　X-Ray = Radiologic examination
▲ = Revised Code for 2015　NA = Not Applicable　⊘ = Modifier 51 Exempt　26 = Professional Component　CT = Computed Tomography
▶◀ = New or Revised CPT Text　NCCI = CCI Edits Apply　-QW = CLIA Waived Test　# = Resequenced Code　MRI = Magnetic Resonance Imaging

Code	Description		-TC	/-26	/Total RVU
73525	Radiologic examination, hip, arthrography, radiological supervision and interpretation	ncci	2.02	.82	2.84
73540	Radiologic examination, pelvis and hips, infant or child, minimum of 2 views	ncci	.80	.29	1.09
73550	Radiologic examination, femur, 2 views	ncci	.49	.26	.75
	Radiologic examination, knee;				
73560	1 or 2 views	ncci	.54	.27	.81
73562	3 views	ncci	.68	.28	.96
73564	complete, 4 or more views	ncci	.77	.34	1.11
73565	both knees, standing, anteroposterior	ncci	.65	.27	.92
	Radiologic examination;				
73590	tibia and fibula, 2 views	ncci	.48	.26	.74
73592	lower extremity, infant, minimum of 2 views	ncci	.52	.23	.75
	Radiologic examination, ankle;				
73600	2 views	ncci	.52	.24	.76
73610	complete, minimum of 3 views	ncci	.61	.26	.87
	Radiologic examination, foot;				
73620	2 views	ncci	.50	.22	.72
73630	complete, minimum of 3 views	ncci	.57	.24	.81
	Radiologic examination;				
73650	calcaneus [heel], minimum of 2 views	ncci	.52	.23	.75
73660	toe(s), minimum of 2 views	ncci	.59	.19	.78
	CT, lower extremity;				
73700	without contrast material	ncci	3.58	1.42	5.00
73701	with contrast material(s)	ncci	4.65	1.65	6.30
73702	without contrast material, followed by contrast material(s) and further sections	ncci	5.91	1.72	7.63
	MRI, lower extremity other than joint;				
73718	without contrast material(s)	ncci	8.26	1.92	10.18
73719	with contrast material(s)	ncci	8.97	2.30	11.27
73720	without contrast material(s), followed by contrast material(s) and further sequences	ncci	10.97	3.05	14.02
	MRI, any joint of lower extremity;				
73721	without contrast material	ncci	4.65	1.94	6.59
73722	with contrast material(s)	ncci	8.34	2.33	10.67
73723	without contrast material(s), followed by contrast material(s) and further sequences	ncci	10.08	3.05	13.13

Abdomen

Code	Description		-TC	/-26	/Total RVU
	Radiologic examination, abdomen;				
74000	single, anteroposterior view	ncci	.40	.26	.66
74010	anteroposterior and additional oblique and cone views	ncci	.64	.33	.97
74020	complete, including decubitus and/or erect views	ncci	.65	.38	1.03
74022	complete acute abdomen series, including supine, erect, and/or decubitus views, single view chest	ncci	.77	.45	1.22

CT, abdomen;

(For a combined CT abdomen and pelvis study, see 74176-74178)

(To report 3D rendering, see 76376, 76377)

Code	Description		-TC / -26 / Total RVU		
74150	without contrast material	ncci	2.49	1.69	4.18
74160	with contrast material(s)	ncci	4.63	1.82	6.45
74170	without contrast material, followed by contrast material(s) and further sections	ncci	5.33	1.99	7.32
	Computed tomography, abdomen and pelvis;				
	(Do not report 74176-74178 in conjunction with 72192-72194, 74150-74170)				
	(Report 74176, 74177, or 74178 only once per CT abdomen and pelvis examination)				
74174	with contrast material(s), including noncontrast images, if performed, and image postprocessing	ncci	8.64	3.13	11.77
74176	without contrast material	ncci	3.11	2.47	5.58
74177	with contrast material(s)	ncci	6.09	2.60	8.69
74178	without contrast material in one or both body regions, followed by contrast material(s) and further sections in one or both body regions	ncci	6.98	2.87	9.85
	MRI, abdomen;				
74181	without contrast material(s)	ncci	7.21	2.08	9.29
74182	with contrast material(s)	ncci	10.22	2.47	12.69
74183	without contrast material(s), followed by contrast material(s) and further sequences	ncci	10.93	3.22	14.15

Other Procedures

Code	Description				
76000	Fluoroscopy (separate procedure), up to 1 hour physician or other qualified health care professional time, other than 71023 or 71034 (eg, cardiac fluoroscopy)	ncci	1.07	.25	1.32
76080	Radiologic examination, abscess, fistula or sinus tract study, radiological supervision and interpretation	ncci	.79	.75	1.54
76100	Single plane body section (eg, tomography), other than with urography	ncci	1.68	.91	2.59
76120	Cineradiography/videoradiography, except where specifically included	ncci	1.98	.57	2.55
+ 76125	Cineradiography/videoradiography to complement routine examination (list separately in addition to code for primary procedure)	ncci	.NE	.42	NE

> Cineradiography/videoradiography is a motion picture view of anatomic area studied—can be either motion picture (cine) radiograph, or continuous video recording (video flourography).

76140	Consultation on X-ray examination made elsewhere, written report				NE

> **CPT code 76140** – *"Consultation on x-ray examination made elsewhere, written report"* is intended to be used when, for example, Doctor "A" from Sunnydale Hospital sends a radiograph taken at Sunnydale Hospital to Doctor "B" at Goodhope Hospital. Doctor "A" asks Doctor "B" to offer his opinion on the radiograph. Doctor "B" writes a formal report on his interpretation of the radiograph and sends a copy of this report to Doctor "A."

● = New Code for 2015   NE = Not Established   ✚ = Add-on Code   TC = Technical Component   X-Ray = Radiologic examination
▲ = Revised Code for 2015   NA = Not Applicable   ⊘ = Modifier 51 Exempt   26 = Professional Component   CT = Computed Tomography
▶◀ = New or Revised CPT Text   NCCI = CCI Edits Apply   -QW = CLIA Waived Test   # = Resequenced Code   MRI = Magnetic Resonance Imaging

This code is not intended to be used by physicians within the same institution to reread radiographs taken at that institution. Levels of Service (limited, intermediate, extended, comprehensive) include the "evaluation of appropriate diagnostic tests" which may necessitate the attending physician to personally review the radiographs taken on his patient. *-CPT Assistant, Summer 1991*

From the CPT coding perspective above, 76140 is not intended for the rereading of radiographs within the same institution or facility. Its usage is to reflect an outside second opinion (consultation) on the radiograph with a written report.

Typically, the coding for rereading would be to use the originating radiograph code and append modifiers 26 (professional component with interpretation and report) and 77 (repeat procedure by another physician. e.g., 72010-26-77).

When the initial x-ray (TC and 26) components are performed in the chiropractic office, and then sent out for a consultation opinion, the other physician should use the 76140 code.

Please note that both 76140 and modifier 26 and 77 services are for the reread and report only. It is not to be used to describe the E/M components of "Medical Decision Making" or "Counseling." The appropriate level of an E/M code includes the evaluation of appropriate diagnostic tests, and/or Counseling time with the patient. These services are on separate line items on the 1500 claim form.

Code	Description		-TC	-26	Total RVU
	3D rendering with interpretation and reporting of computed tomography, magnetic resonance imaging, ultrasound, or other tomographic modality with image postprocessing under concurrent supervision;				
	(Use 76376 & 76377 in conjunction with code[s] for base imaging procedure[s])				
76376	not requiring image postprocessing on an independent workstation	ncci	.36	.28	.64
	▶(Do not report 76376 in conjunction with 71275, 74174, 76377)◀				
76377	requiring image postprocessing on an independent workstation	ncci	1.12	.67	1.79
	▶(Do not report 76377 in conjunction with 71275, 74174, 76376)◀				
76496	Unlisted fluoroscopic procedure (eg, diagnostic, interventional)	ncci	NE	NE	NE
76497	Unlisted computed tomography procedure (eg, diagnostic, interventional)	ncci	NE	NE	NE
76498	Unlisted magnetic resonance procedure (eg, diagnostic, interventional)		NE	NE	NE
76499	Unlisted diagnostic radiographic procedure		NE	NE	NE

Diagnostic Ultrasound

Special instructions apply. See the current CPT code book or FindACode.com for full information.

> **Definitions**
>
> **B-Scan** is a diagnostic test used to produce a two-dimensional, cross-section view.
>
> **Real-time scan** is a B-scan which includes motion with time.

Head and Neck

Code	Description		-TC	-26	Total RVU
76536	Ultrasound, soft tissues of head and neck (eg, thyroid, parathyroid, parotid), real time with image documentation	ncci	2.47	.79	3.26

Non-Obstetrical

Special instructions apply. See the current CPT code book or ⌕ FindACode.com for full information.

Code	Description		-TC	-26	Total RVU
76856	Ultrasound, pelvic (nonobstetric), real time with image documentation, complete	ncci	2.38	.97	3.35

Extremities

	Ultrasound, extremity, nonvascular, real-time with image documentation;				
76881	complete	ncci	2.37	.90	3.27
76882	limited, anatomic specific	ncci	.32	.70	1.02

Other Procedures

76970	Ultrasound study follow-up (specify)	ncci	2.03	.58	2.61
76977	Ultrasound bone density measurement and interpretation, peripheral site(s), any method	ncci	.12	.08	.20
76999	Unlisted ultrasound procedure (eg, diagnostic, interventional)	ncci	NE	NE	NE

OTHER RADIOLOGIC GUIDANCE

Bone/Joint Studies

77071	Manual application of stress performed by physician or other qualified health care professional for joint radiography, including contralateral joint if indicated				1.36
77072	Bone age studies		.37	.27	.64
77073	Bone length studies (orthoroentgenogram, scanogram)	ncci	.60	.43	1.03
	Radiologic examination, osseous survey;				
77074	limited (eg, for metastases)	ncci	1.13	.65	1.78
77075	complete (axial and appendicular skeleton)	ncci	1.66	.77	2.43
77076	Radiologic examination, osseous survey, infant	ncci	1.66	1.00	2.66
77077	Joint survey, single view, 2 or more joints (specify)	ncci	.58	.48	1.06
	Computed tomography, bone mineral density study, 1 or more sites;				
77078	axial skeleton (eg, hips, pelvis, spine)	ncci	2.82	.35	3.17
	Dual-energy X-ray absorptiometry (DXA), bone density study, 1 or more sites;				
77080	axial skeleton (eg, hips, pelvis, spine)	ncci	1.10	.29	1.39
77081	appendicular skeleton (peripheral) (eg, radius, wrist, heel)	ncci	.48	.31	.79
	▶(77082 has been deleted. To report, use 77086)◀				
● 77085	axial skeleton (eg, hips, pelvis, spine), including vertebral fracture assessment		1.15	.43	1.58
● 77086	Vertebral fracture assessment via dual-energy X-ray absorptiometry (DXA)		.75	.25	1.00

> Dual-energy x-ray absorptiometry (DXA) is a non-invasive two-dimensional projection system for measuring bone mineral content and bone mineral density (BMD), using an emission of photons generated through an x-ray tube. The x-ray source produces a consistent photon flow, which leads to quality image resolution with a short scan time.

● = New Code for 2015 NE = Not Established ✚ = Add-on Code TC = Technical Component X-Ray = Radiologic examination
▲ = Revised Code for 2015 NA = Not Applicable ⊘ = Modifier 51 Exempt 26 = Professional Component CT = Computed Tomography
▶◀ = New or Revised CPT Text NCCI = CCI Edits Apply -QW = CLIA Waived Test # = Resequenced Code MRI = Magnetic Resonance Imaging

4d. CPT Procedures
Laboratory Codes

To calculate fees for these Laboratory codes, see Resource 331 to access the *ChiroCode Online Fee Calculator*. The fees produced by this calculator are taken from publically available CMS data.

Note: Annual pricing schedules are usually released by CMS in January of each year. This information is always available and current in the *ChiroCode Online Fee Calculator*.

Alert: It is essential for practices performing laboratory studies in-house to check with state and federal guidelines to ensure compliance with CLIA (Clinical Laboratory Improvement Amendments) regulations.

ORGAN OR DISEASE-ORIENTED PANELS

Note: Typically, many laboratory machines are set up to run panels, or groups of tests, to reduce costs and increase efficiency. However, these panels might not include all tests that the practitioner may require to make a proper diagnosis. This situation may require the use of additional test codes, which are separately coded. When additional tests are needed, record the individual test code as a separate item.

80048   Basic Metabolic Panel (Calcium, total)   ncci
        This panel must include the following:
        Calcium, total (82310)   Glucose (82947)
        Carbon dioxide (82374)   Potassium (84132)
        Chloride (82435)   Sodium (84295)
        Creatinine (82565)   Urea Nitrogen (BUN) (84520)
        (Do not use 80048 in addition to 80053)

80050   General Health Panel
        This panel must include the following:
        Comprehensive metabolic panel (80053)
        Blood count, complete (CBC), automated, and automated differential WBC count (85025 or 85027 and 85004)
        OR
        Blood count, complete (CBC), automated (85027) and appropriate manual differential WBC count (85007 or 85009)
        Thyroid stimulating hormone (TSH) (84443)

| 80053 | Comprehensive Metabolic Panel | ncci |

This panel must include the following:

Albumin (82040)	Potassium (84132)
Bilirubin, total (82247)	Protein, total (84155)
Calcium, total (82310)	Sodium (84295)
Carbon dioxide (bicarbonate) (82374)	Transferase, alanine amino (ALT) (SGPT) (84460)
Chloride (82435)	Transferase, aspartate amino (AST) (SGOT) (84450)
Creatinine (82565)	
Glucose (82947)	Urea Nitrogen (BUN) (84520)
Phosphatase, alkaline (84075)	

(Do not use 80053 in addition to 80048, 80076)

DRUG ▸ASSAY◂

Drug screening codes are not included in the *ChiroCode DeskBook*.

See Resource 362 for information about these types of services.

Special instructions apply. See the current CPT code book or FindACode.com for full information.

Presumptive Drug Class Screening

▶(80100, 80101, 80102, 80103, 80104 have been deleted. To report presumptive and/or definitive drug testing, see 80300, 80301, 80302, 80303, 80304)◂

4e. CPT Procedures
Medicine Codes (Chiropractic Manipulation and Therapies)

Evaluation and Management codes (99201-99499) are used to report an office visit when applicable.

Special instructions apply. See the current CPT code book or FindACode.com for full information.

BIOFEEDBACK
-TC / -26 / Total RVU

90901	Biofeedback training by any modality	ncci	1.07
90911	Biofeedback training, perineal muscles, anorectal or urethral sphincter, including EMG and/or manometry	ncci	2.38

> *Biofeedback* A training technique that enables an individual to gain some element of voluntary control over autonomic body functions; based on the learning principle that a desired response is learned when received information feedback, such as a recorded increase in skin temperature, indicates that a specific thought complex or action has produced the desired physiological response. -*Stedman's Medical Dictionary, 26th Edition*

SPECIAL OTORHINOLARYNGOLOGIC SERVICES

Vestibular Function Tests, Without Electrical Recording

92533 Caloric vestibular test, each irrigation (binaural, bithermal stimulation constitutes 4 tests)   NE

Vestibular Function Tests, With Recording (eg, ENG)

92540 Basic vestibular evaluation, includes spontaneous nystagmus test with eccentric gaze fixation nystagmus, with recording, positional nystagmus test, minimum of 4 positions, with recording, optokinetic nystagmus test, bidirectional foveal and peripheral stimulation, with recording, and oscillating tracking test, with recording   ncci   .62 2.24 2.86
▶(Do not report 92540 in conjunction with 99270, 92541, 92542, 92544, 92545)◄

			-TC	/-26	/Total RVU
92541	Spontaneous nystagmus test, including gaze and fixation nystagmus, with recording ▶(Do not report 92541 in conjunction with 92270, 92540 or the set of 92542, 92544, and 92545)◀	ncci	.28	.59	.87
92542	Positional nystagmus test, minimum of 4 positions, with recording ▶(Do not report 92542 in conjunction with 92270, 92540 or the set of 92541, 92544, and 92545)◀	ncci	.25	.48	.73
92543	Caloric vestibular test, each irrigation (binaural, bithermal stimulation constitutes 4 tests), with recording	ncci	.29	.16	.45
92544	Optokinetic nystagmus test, bidirectional, foveal or peripheral stimulation, with recording ▶(Do not report 92544 in conjunction with 92270, 92540 or the set of 92541, 92542, and 92545)◀	ncci	.27	.38	.65
92546	Sinusoidal vertical axis rotational testing	ncci	2.47	.42	2.89

Audiologic Function Tests

92550	Tympanometry and reflex threshold measurements	ncci	.59
92551	Screening test, pure tone, air only		.34
92552	Pure tone audiometry (threshold); air only	ncci	.86
92553	Pure tone audiometry (threshold); air and bone	ncci	1.02
92555	Speech audiometry threshold;	ncci	.64
92556	with speech recognition	ncci	1.03
92557	Comprehensive audiometry threshold evaluation and speech recognition (92553 and 92556 combined)	ncci	1.04
92558	Evoked otoacoustic emissions, screening (qualitative measurement of distortion product or transient evoked otoacoustic emissions), automated analysis	ncci	NE

Evaluative and Therapeutic Services

92625	Assessment of tinnitus (includes pitch, loudness matching, and masking) (For unilateral assesssment, use modifier 52)	ncci	1.96

CARDIOVASCULAR

Cardiography

	Electrocardiogram, routine ECG with at least 12 leads; (For ECG monitoring, see 99354-99360)		
93000	with interpretation and report	ncci	.48
93005	tracing only, without interpretation and report	ncci	.24
93010	interpretation and report only	ncci	.24
	Cardiovascular stress test using maximal or submaximal treadmill or bicycle exercise, continuous electrocardiographic monitoring, and/or pharmacological stress;		
93015	with supervision, interpretation and report	ncci	2.14
93017	tracing only, without interpretation and report	ncci	1.10
93018	interpretation and report only	ncci	.41

Noninvasive Physiologic Studies and Procedures

-TC / -26 / Total RVU

93740	Temperature gradient studies	.23

Other Procedures

93799	Unlisted cardiovascular service or procedure	NE NE NE

NONINVASIVE VASCULAR DIAGNOSTIC STUDIES

There are special instructions for vascular studies including supervision, interpretation, Doppler devices, duplex scans, and other non-invasive physiologic studies. See the current CPT code book or 🖱 FindACode.com for full information.

Cerebrovascular Arterial Studies

Duplex scan of extracranial arteries;

93880	complete bilateral study	ncci	4.32	.84	5.16
93882	unilateral or limited study	ncci	2.70	.56	3.26

Transcranial Doppler study of the intracranial arteries;

93886	complete study	ncci	8.46	1.37	9.83
93888	limited study	ncci	4.83	.89	5.72

Extremity Arterial Studies (Including Digits)

Special instructions apply. See the current CPT code book or 🖱 *FindACode.com for full information.*

93922	Limited bilateral noninvasive physiologic studies of upper or lower extremity arteries, (eg, for lower extremity: ankle/brachial indices at distal posterior tibial and anterior tibial/dorsalis pedis arteries plus bidirectional, Doppler waveform recording and analysis at 1-2 levels, or ankle/brachial indices at distal posterior tibial and anterior tibial/dorsalis pedis arteries plus volume plethysmography at 1-2 levels, or ankle/brachial indices at distal posterior tibial and anterior tibial/dorsalis pedis arteries with transcutaneous oxygen tension measurements at 1-2 levels)	ncci	2.17	.35	2.52

(Do not report 93922 in conjunction with 0337T)

93923	Complete bilateral noninvasive physiologic studies of upper or lower extremity arteries, 3 or more levels (eg, for lower extremity: ankle/brachial indices at distal posterior tibial and anterior tibial/dorsalis pedis arteries plus segmental blood pressure measurements with bidirectional, Doppler waveform recording and analysis, at 3 or more levels, or ankle/brachial indices at distal posterior tibial and anterior tibial/dorsalis pedis arteries plus segmental volume plethysmography at 3 or more levels, or ankle/brachial indices at distal posterior tibial and anterior tibial/dorsalis pedis arteries plus segmental transcutaneous oxygen tension measurements at 3 or more level(s), or single level study with provocative functional maneuvers (eg, measurements with postural provocative tests, or measurements with reactive hyperemia)	ncci	3.29	.63	3.92

			-TC	/-26	/Total RVU
	(Do not report 93923 in conjunction with 0337T)				
93924	Noninvasive physiologic studies of lower extremity arteries, at rest and following treadmill stress testing, (ie, bidirectional Doppler waveform or volume plethysmography recording and analysis at rest with ankle/brachial indices immediately after and at timed intervals following performance of a standardized protocol on a motorized treadmill plus recording of time of onset of claudication or other symptoms, maximal walking time, and time to recovery) complete bilateral study	ncci	4.19	.70	4.89
	(Do not report 93924 in conjunction with 93922, 93923)				

Pulmonary

Use of these pulmonary codes include both the procedure and the interpretation of test results. When a significant, separately identifiable Evaluation and Management service is performed in addition to the codes in this section, you should also use the appropriate E/M service code (99201-99350), appended with modifier 25.

Pulmonary Diagnostic Testing and Therapies

94010	Spirometry, including graphic record, total and timed vital capacity, expiratory flow rate measurement(s), with or without maximal voluntary ventilation	ncci	.77	.24	1.01
94011	Measurement of spirometric forced expiratory flows in an infant or child through 2 years of age	ncci			2.83
	Requires Moderate Sedation.				
94012	Measurement of spirometric forced expiratory flows, before and after bronchodilator, in an infant or child through 2 years of age	ncci			4.58
	Requires Moderate Sedation.				
94013	Measurement of lung volumes (ie, functional residual capacity [FRC], forced vital capacity [FVC], and expiratory reserve volume [ERV]) in an infant or child through 2 years of age	ncci			.89
	Requires Moderate Sedation.				
94060	Bronchodilation responsiveness, spirometry as in 94010, pre- and post- bronchodilator administration	ncci	1.34	.37	1.71
	(Do not report 94060 in conjunction with 94150, 94200, 94375, 94728)				
	(Report bronchodilator supply separately with 99070 or appropriate supply code)				
	(For prolonged exercise test for bronchospasm with pre- and post-spirometry, use 94620)				
94150	Vital capacity, total (separate procedure) (Do not report 94150 in conjunction with 94010, 94060, 94728. To report thoracic gas volumes, see 94726, 94727)	ncci	.60	.11	.71
94200	Maximum breathing capacity, maximal voluntary ventilation (Do not report 94200 in conjunction with 94010, 94060)	ncci	.56	.16	.72
94250	Expired gas collection, quantitative, single procedure (separate procedure)	ncci	.59	.15	.74

Code	Description		-TC / -26 / Total RVU		
94640	Pressurized or nonpressurized inhalation treatment for acute airway obstruction or for sputum induction for diagnostic purposes (eg, with an aerosol generator, nebulizer, metered dose inhaler or intermittent positive pressure breathing (IPPB) device)	ncci			.52
	(For more than 1 inhalation treatment perforemd on the same date, append modifier 76)				
	(For continuous inhalation treatment of 1 hour or more, see 94644, 94645)				
	Manipulation chest wall, such as cupping, percussing, and vibration to facilitate lung function;				
94667	initial demonstration and/or evaluation	ncci			.74
94668	subsequent	ncci			.81
94726	Plethysmography for determination of lung volumes and, when performed, airway resistance	ncci	1.13	.35	1.48
	(Do not report 94726 in conjunction with 94727)				
94727	Gas dilution or washout for determination of lung volumes and, when performed, distribution of ventilation and closing volumes	ncci	.83	.35	1.18
	(Do not report 94727 in conjunction with 94726)				
94728	Airway resistance by impulse oscillometry	ncci	.76	.36	1.12
	(Do not report 94728 in conjunction with 94010, 94060, 94070, 94375, 94726)				
+ 94729	Diffusing capacity (eg, carbon monoxide, membrane) (List separately in addition to code for primary procedure)	ncci	1.27	.26	1.53
	(Report 94729 in conjunction with 94010, 94060, 94070, 94375, 94726-94728)				
94760	Noninvasive ear or pulse oximetry for oxygen saturation; single determination	ncci			.09
	(For blood gases, see 82803-82810)				
94799	Unlisted pulmonary service or procedure		NE	NE	NE

Separate Procedure

Not understanding this term results in confusion and frustration. The helpful CPT definition is:

> "The codes designated as 'separate procedure' should not be reported in addition to the code for the total procedure or service of which it is considered an integral component.

> "However, when a procedure or service that is designated as a 'separate procedure' is carried out independently or considered to be unrelated or distinct from other procedures/services provided at that time, it may be reported by itself, or in addition to other procedures/services by appending modifier 59 to the specific 'separate procedure' code to indicate that the procedure is not considered to be a component of another procedure."

Routine muscle and range of motion testing is a component of a physical examination within the E/M service. However, in such routine examinations there could be findings that indicate a need for more definitive and quantifiable data. In such cases, these "separate procedure" codes are appropriate and accurate expressions.

NEUROLOGY AND NEUROMUSCULAR PROCEDURES

Sleep Medicine Testing

Sleep study, unattended, simultaneous recording;

			-TC	/-26	/Total RVU
95800	heart rate, oxygen saturation, respiratory analysis (eg, by airflow or peripheral arterial tone), and sleep time	ncci	3.60	1.47	5.07

(Do not report 85800 in conjunction with 93401-93227, 93228, 93229, 93268-93272, 956801, 95803, 95806)

(For unattended sleep study that measures a minimum of heart rate, oxygen saturation, and respiratory analysis, use 95801)

95801	minimum of heart rate, oxygen saturation, and respiratory analysis (eg, by airflow or peripheral arterial tone)	ncci	1.18	1.40	2.58

(Do not report 95801 in conjunction with 93401-93227, 93228, 93229, 93268-93272, 95800, 95806)

(For unattended sleep study that measures heart rate, oxygen saturation, respiratory analysis and sleep time, use 95800)

Muscle and Range of Motion Testing

Muscle testing, manual (separate procedure) with report;

95831	extremity (excluding hand) or trunk	ncci	.86
95832	hand, with or without comparison to normal side	ncci	.85
95833	total body evaluation, excluding hands	ncci	1.06
95834	total body evaluation, including hands	ncci	1.43

> "Given the subjective aspect of manual testing, the use of consistent test positions, including accurate joint placement and avoiding the use of compensatory muscle actions, must be integrated into the test in order for MMT to be utilized as an effective evaluation tool."
> -AMA CPT Assistant, August 2013
>
> See Resource 340 to review the muscle testing table by the National Institute of Environmental Health Sciences.

Range of motion measurements and report (separate procedure);

95851	each extremity (excluding hand) or each trunk section (spine)	ncci	.52
95852	hand, with or without comparison with normal side	ncci	.46

> "ROM refers to the angular distance in degrees through which the spine or a joint can be moved. This type of testing is not time based and is differentiated from strength testing."
> -AMA CPT Assistant, August 2013
>
> See Resource 341 or ACAtoday.org/coding for more information on range of motion testing, including tables.
>
> About 38% of the Relative Value Unit (RVU) is associated with the Physician Work component in these five Muscle and Range of Motion Testing codes. The amount of Work Time associated with each of these muscle and ROM procedures (16-22 minutes), confirms the fact that these tests are the brief tests normally associated with routine E/M physical examinations
>
> From a patient perspective, when these needed tests are not routine, they should be done on the same day as the E/M service.

From the CPT and RVU perspectives, when unrelated and distinct testing (beyond the normal routines within an E/M physical exam or CMT service) is performed on the same day, appending modifier 59 is appropriate. This signals the payer that a distinct procedure has occurred. Additionally, when the testing is increased, modifier 22 would also be appended. That is proper coding, even though it might be rejected by inappropriate edits that assume the code is for routine testing only.

Code	Work Time	Physician Work RVU	Malpractice RVU	Total RVU
95831	16 min.	.28	.03	.86
95832	16 min.	.29	.03	.85
95833	19 min.	.47	.01	1.06
95851	22 min.	.16	.01	.52
95852	16 min.	.11	.01	.46

Electromyography

The needle electromyographic procedures below have special instructions regarding the type of equipment used, and the interpretation of results. See the current CPT codebook or FindACode.com for full information.

Needle electromyography (EMG);

Code	Description		Work	Malpractice	Total
95860	1 extremity with or without related paraspinal areas	ncci	1.99	1.47	3.46
	(For dynamic electromyography performed during motion analysis studies, see 96002-96003)				
95861	2 extremities with or without related paraspinal areas	ncci	2.52	2.33	4.71
	(For dynamic electromyography performed during motion analysis studies, see 96002-96003)				
95863	3 extremities with or without related paraspinal areas	ncci	3.15	2.85	6.00
95864	4 extremities with or without related paraspinal areas	ncci	3.80	3.04	6.84
95865	larynx	ncci	1.67	2.37	4.04
	(Do not report modifier 50 in conjunction with 95865)				
	(For unilateral procedure, report modifier 52 in conjunction with 95865)				
95866	hemidiaphragm	ncci	1.83	1.92	3.75
95867	cranial nerve supplied muscle(s), unilateral	ncci	1.44	1.19	2.63
95868	cranial nerve supplied muscles, bilateral	ncci	1.93	1.79	3.72
95869	thoracic paraspinal muscles (excluding T1 or T12)	ncci	1.73	.57	2.30
95870	limited study of muscles in 1 extremity or non-limb (axial) muscles (unilateral or bilateral), other than thoracic paraspinal, cranial nerve supplied muscles, or sphincters	ncci	1.92	.55	2.47
	(To report a complete study of the extremities, see 95860-95864)				
95872	Needle electromyography using single fiber electrode, with quantitative measurement of jitter, blocking and/or fiber density, any/all sites of each muscle studied	ncci	1.40	4.39	5.79

			-TC / -26 / Total RVU		
	Needle electromyography, each extremity, with related paraspinal areas, when performed, done with nerve conduction, amplitude and latency/velocity study;				
	(Use 95885, 95886 in conjunction with 95907-95913)				
	(Do not report 95885, 95886 in conjunction with 95860-95864, 95870, 95905)				
+ 95885	limited (List separately in addition to code for primary procedure)	ncci	1.11	.54	1.65
+ 95886	complete, five or more muscles studied, innervated by three or more nerves or four or more spinal levels (List separately in addition to code for primary procedure)	ncci	1.26	1.32	2.58
+ 95887	Needle electromyography, non-extremity (cranial nerve supplied or axial) muscle(s) done with nerve conduction, amplitude and latency/velocity study (List separately in addition to code for primary procedure)	ncci	1.22	1.08	2.30
	(Use 95887 in conjunction with 95907-95913)				
	(Do not report 95887 in conjunction with 95867-95870, 95905)				

From a CPT coding perspective it is not appropriate to use needle EMG for static or dynamic surface EMG procedures. For **static** surface EMG or postural analysis use S3900 or 95999 and attach a report. For **dynamic** surface EMG see 96002.

Guidance for Chemodenervation and Ischemic Muscle Testing

95875	Ischemic limb exercise test with serial specimen(s) acquisition for muscle(s) metabolite(s)	ncci	1.73	1.66	3.39

Nerve Conduction Tests

95905	Motor and/or sensory nerve conduction, using preconfigured electrode array(s), amplitude and latency/velocity study, each limb, includes F-wave study when performed, with interpretation and report	ncci	1.93	.08	2.01
	(Report 95905 only once per limb studied)				
	(Do not report 95905 in conjunction with 95885, 95886, 95907-95913)				
	Nerve conduction studies;				
95907	1-2 studies	ncci	1.22	1.53	2.75
95908	3-4 studies	ncci	1.60	1.91	3.51
95909	5-6 studies	ncci	1.88	2.28	4.16
95910	7-8 studies	ncci	2.47	3.04	5.51
95911	9-10 studies	ncci	2.77	3.80	6.57
95912	11-12 studies	ncci	2.82	4.50	7.32
95913	13 or more studies	ncci	2.99	5.32	8.31

Autonomic Function Tests

Special instructions apply. See the current CPT code book or FindACode.com for full information.

-TC / -26 / Total RVU

Code	Description				
95922	Testing of autonomic nervous system function; vasomotor adrenergic innervation (sympathetic adrenergic function), including beat-to-beat blood pressure and R-R interval changes during Valsalva maneuver and at least 5 minutes of passive tilt	ncci	1.45	1.37	2.82
95924	Testing of autonomic nervous system function; combined parasympathetic and sympathetic adrenergic function testing with at least 5 minutes of passive tilt	ncci	1.80	2.53	4.33
	(Do not report 95924 in conjunction with 95921 or 95922)				
95943	Simultaneous, independent, quantitative measures of both parasympathetic function and sympathetic function, based on time-frequency analysis of heart rate variability concurrent with time-frequency analysis of continuous respiratory activity, with mean heart rate and blood pressure measures, during rest, paced (deep) breathing, Valsalva maneuvers, and head-up postural change	ncci	NE	NE	NE
	(Do not report 95943 in conjunction with 93040, 95921, 95922, 95924)				

Evoked Potentials and Reflex Tests

Code	Description				
	Short-latency somatosensory evoked potential study, stimulation of any/all peripheral nerves or skin sites, recording from the central nervous system;				
95925	in upper limbs (Do not report 95925 in conjunction with 95926)	ncci	3.62	.80	4.42
95926	in lower limbs (Do not report 95926 in conjunction with 95925)	ncci	3.28	.79	4.07
95938	in upper and lower limbs (Do not report 95938 in conjunction with 95925, 95926)	ncci	8.28	1.29	9.57
95927	in the trunk or head (To report a unilateral study, use modifier 52)	ncci	3.50	.78	4.28

How Long is 15 Minutes?

Historically, for decades "15 minutes" was accepted as up-to 15 minutes. However, in recent years more definitive approaches have been taken by payers. In 2000, in an effort to control fraud and abuse of costs, CMS adopted a policy of rounding to the nearest 15 minutes. It is a logical and simple concept. Accordingly, 8 through 22 minutes of hands-on care would be considered as one 15 minute unit of care, 23 through 37 minutes would be 2 units, etc. When more than one service code is performed the time is bundled, and the total units can not exceed the total hands-on time rule. Other policies might vary, but this CMS approach is inherently reasonable. Be aware of individual payer policies.

According to the *CPT Assistant*, March 2014, it is not appropriate to append modifier 52, Reduced Services to codes 97110-97546.

- See Resource 345 for the Medicare definition of timed codes with examples.
- See ACAtoday.org/coding for information on coding time.

				RVU	
	Central motor evoked potential study (transcranial motor stimulation); in upper and lower limbs				
95928	upper limbs	ncci	5.04	2.28	7.32
	(Do not report 95928 in conjunction with 95929)				
95929	lower limbs	ncci	5.05	2.22	7.27
	(Do not report 95929 in conjunction with 95928)				
95939	in upper and lower limbs	ncci	10.69	3.44	14.13
	(Do not report 95939 in conjunction with 95928, 95929)				
	(95934, 95936 have been deleted. To report H-reflex testing, see 95907-95913)				
95937	Neuromuscular junction testing (repetitive stimulation, paired stimuli), each nerve, any 1 method	ncci	1.35	.99	2.34
95938	Code is out of numerical sequence. See 95925-95939				
95939	Code is out of numerical sequence. See 95925-95939				
95943	Code is out of numerical sequence. See 95925-95939				

Other Procedures

95990	Refilling and maintenance of implantable pump or reservoir for drug delivery, spinal (intrathecal, epidural) or brain (intraventricular), includes electronic analysis of pump, when performed;	ncci	2.54
95991	requiring skill of a physician or other qualified health care professional	ncci	3.41
95999	Unlisted neurological or neuromuscular diagnostic procedure		NE

> Remember to attach a report.

Motion Analysis

> These procedures (96000-96004) should be performed in a dedicated motion analysis laboratory. Special instructions for computerized 3-D kinematics, 3-D kinetics, and dynamic electromyography can be found in the current CPT codebook or 🖱 FindaCode.com.
>
> Use 95860-95872 for performance of needle electromyography procedures, and 97116 for gait training.

96000	Comprehensive computer-based motion analysis by video-taping and 3D kinematics;	ncci	2.69
96001	with dynamic plantar pressure measurements during walking	ncci	2.86
96002	Dynamic surface electromyography, during walking or other functional activities, 1-12 muscles	ncci	.62
96003	Dynamic fine wire electromyography, during walking or other functional activities, 1 muscle	ncci	.55
	(Do not report 96002, 96003 in conjunction with 95860-95866, 95869-95872, 95885-95887)		
96004	Review and interpretation by physician or other qualified health care professional of comprehensive computer-based motion analysis, dynamic plantar pressure measurements, dynamic surface electromyography during walking or other functional activities, and dynamic fine wire electromyography, with written report	ncci	3.33

HEALTH AND BEHAVIOR ASSESSMENT/INTERVENTION

These codes should be used for patients with a presenting physical illness or injury, and not for the purpose of screening. Neither can these codes to be used with or as a replacement for psychiatric services (90801-90899). According to the AMA, these codes are not to be used to "identify the psychological, behavioral, emotional, cognitive, and social factors important to the prevention, treatment, or management of physical health problems." The focus of these assessment codes is not on mental health, but on "biopsychosocial factors important to physical health problems and treatments" (such as patients who are inclined to decline treatment based on fear of the protocol, such as a cancer patient who is afraid of radiation treatments, or a diabetic patient who is afraid of insulin shots).

Do not use Preventive Medicine, Individual Counseling codes (99401-99404), or Group Counseling codes (99411-99412) on the same day.

See the current CPT codebook or FindaCode.com for full information.

Alert: These codes are only for use by qualified health care professionals who are **not** eligible to report E/M services. See page H-85 for additional information on other qualified healthcare professionals.

(For health and behavior assessment and/or intervention performed by a physician or other qualified health care professional who may report evaluation and management services, see Evaluation and Management or Preventive Medicine services codes.)

Health and behavior assessment (eg, health-focused clinical interview, behavioral observations, psychophysiological monitoring, health-oriented questionnaires), each 15 minutes face-to-face with the patient;

96150	initial assessment	ncci	.61
96151	re-assessment	ncci	.58

Codes 96150 - 96151 are for face-to-face encounters with patients. It is interesting to note that these codes are for health and behavior assessments. They were created and placed in this special CPT section to accommodate the patient's biopsychosocial assessment needs. It avoids them being categorized with a mental health disorder within the CPT code set for Psychiatry services (90785-90899).

PHYSICAL MEDICINE AND REHABILITATION

Codes 97001-97755 should be used to report each distinct procedure performed. Do not append modifier 51 to 97001-97755.

If the scope of practice in your state license includes "physio therapy" or "physical therapy," it would generally be appropriate for a doctor of chiropractic to use the Physical Medicine code set of 97001-97799. Although some of these codes may have been introduced into the CPT coding system through the efforts of the American Physical Therapy Association or other associations, once they are in the CPT system they are not designated or owned by any specialty.

Licensing is critical. "Only those individuals licensed by a particular state to perform the services should use the codes to report services." -*CPT Assistant,* February 2000

Note that some states may require a type of secondary licensing and require specific training in order for doctors of chiropractic to provide these types of services.

See also Chapter 3-Commonly Used Codes in this *Procedure Codes* section for more information on 97010, 97012, 97014, 97032, 97035, 97110, 97112, 97124, 97140, S8948.

97001	Physical therapy evaluation	ncci	2.11
97002	Physical therapy re-evaluation	ncci	1.18

97001-Physical therapy evaluation and 97002-Physical therapy re-evaluation are both used to identify dynamic processes in which clinical judgments are made based on the data gathered. These evaluations result in the development of a plan for management of a patient's problems as they relate to his or her disease/disability.

Code 97001 identifies the initial assessment of the problem or difficulty which is used to determine the appropriate therapy, the increments, frequency, duration, and other factors necessary to enhance healing.

Code 97002 identifies subsequent assessments of the injury/disability to determine the progress/success of the treatment(s) given. Re-evaluations are usually performed during a treatment course. If a new problem/abnormality is encountered, then initial assessment of the new difficulty may be necessary to determine what course of action (if any) would best afford rehabilitation of the injured/disabled body area, using code 97001 to identify the new initial assessment. *-CPT Assistant, September 2001*

97003	Occupational therapy evaluation	ncci	2.39
97004	Occupational therapy re-evaluation	ncci	1.48
97005	Athletic training evaluation		NE
97006	Athletic training re-evaluation		NE

Modalities

Modality focuses on the methods of delivery. A modality consists of applying physical agents to produce therapeutic changes to tissue. These agents can include, but are not limited to thermal, acoustic, light, mechanical, or electric energy.

There are two types of modalities: 1) Supervised Modalities that do not require direct one-on-one patient contact. 2) Constant Attendance Modalities that require direct one-on-one patient contact. Some State licensing boards permit delegation to a chiropractic assistant.

Supervised

Modalities that do not require direct (one-on-one) patient contact by the provider.

Application of a modality to 1 or more areas;

97010	hot or cold packs		.17

See Chapter 3-Commonly Used Codes for more information.

97012	traction, mechanical (1 or more areas)	ncci	.45

See Chapter 3-Commonly Used Codes for more information.

97014	electrical stimulation (unattended) (1 or more areas)		.45

See Chapter 3-Commonly Used Codes for more information.

(For acupuncture with electrical stimulation, see 97813, 97814)

Alert: Don't use 97014 on Medicare claims. This general CPT electrical stimulation code has been replaced by three specific HCPCS procedure codes: G0281, G0282 and G0283. G0281 and G0282 are for wound care. Non-wound care is assigned to G0283. Do not use these "G" codes for non-Medicare claims unless required by the payer(s) (such as United Health Care in 2007). Watch payment reports for others who might follow.

Code	Description		RVU
G0283	Electrical stimulation, (unattended), to one or more areas; for indication(s) other than wound care, as part of a therapy plan of care	ncci	.39

Alert: If billing G0283 with 97032, according to NCCI edits, 97032 will not be paid unless billed with an allowed modifier.

Application of a modality to 1 or more areas;

97016	vasopneumatic devices (1 or more areas)	ncci	.54

[THESE DEVICES PROVIDE AN EXTERNAL PUMPING FORCE TO THE SOFT TISSUES OF THE LOWER OR UPPER EXTREMITIES. A SLEEVE CONTAINING SEPARATE CHAMBERS IS APPLIED TO THE EXTREMITY AND CAN BE PROGRESSIVELY INFLATED, THEREBY PROVIDING A PUMPING ACTION REQUIRED TO FACILITATE REMOVAL OF EDEMA. THE JOBST PUMP IS ONE EXAMPLE OF A VASOPNEUMATIC DEVICE. IT IS NO LONGER APPROPRIATE TO USE CODE 97016 FOR VIBROMASSAGE THERAPY.]

97018	paraffin bath (1 or more areas)	ncci	.31

[WAX TREATMENT USED TO APPLY SUPERFICIAL HEAT THAT HAS LONGER DURATION FOR THE EFFECTS ON UNDERLYING TISSUES. FOR MOST CLINICAL APPLICATIONS, PARAFFIN IS APPLIED AT TEMPERATURES BETWEEN 118 DEGREES TO 126 DEGREES FAHRENHEIT. THIS MODALITY, ALSO CALLED HOT WAX TREATMENT, IS USUALLY USED WITH THE HANDS AND FEET AND IS ESPECIALLY USEFUL FOR PAIN RELIEF IN CHRONIC ORTHOPEDIC PROBLEMS.]

97022	whirlpool (1 or more areas)	ncci	.66

[USE OF HOT OR COLD WATER AGITATED BY MOTORS WITH CURRENT BEING DIRECTED AT OR AWAY FROM THE INVOLVED BODY PART TO ACHIEVE THE DESIRED AFFECT. USEFUL IN PROMOTING MUSCLE RELAXATION (HEAT), OR REDUCTION OF MUSCLE SPASM OR SPASTICITY (COLD), AND IMPROVING CIRCULATION AND MOVEMENT.]

97024	diathermy (eg, microwave) (1 or more areas)	ncci	.18

[CREATES HEAT IN THE SOFT TISSUES, DUE TO THE RESISTANCE OFFERED BY THE TISSUES, BY THE PASSAGE OF HIGH FREQUENCY ELECTRICAL CURRENTS. THE OBJECTIVE OF THIS TREATMENT IS TO CAUSE VASODILATATION AND/OR MUSCLE RELAXATION, WITH SUBSEQUENT PAIN RELIEF. DIATHERMY ENERGY CAN CAUSE A GREATER RISE IN DEEP TISSUE TEMPERATURE THAN ANY FORM OF INFRARED ENERGY.]

97026	infrared (1 or more areas)	ncci	.17

[MODALITY WHICH USES LIGHT AND HEAT TO RAISE THE TISSUE TEMPERATURE 5 TO 10 DEGREES CENTIGRADE IN THE AREA OF APPLICATION.]

| 97028 | ultraviolet (1 or more areas) | ncci | .21 |

[MODALITY USED TO STIMULATE A VARIETY OF CHEMICAL REACTIONS IN THE SKIN AND MUCOUS MEMBRANES. USED IN CASES OF PSORIASIS, AND OTHER SKIN CONDITIONS, AND IN ASSISTING THE HEALING PROCESS OF OPEN WOUNDS. THIS ULTRAVIOLET TREATMENT IS NOT THE SAME AS PHOTOCHEMOTHERAPY TREATMENT, COMMONLY CALLED GOECKERMAN OR PUVA (PETROLATUM AND ULTRAVIOLET A).]

Constant Attendance

Constant attendance requires direct (one-on-one) patient contact by the physician or other qualified health care professional. According to the AMA, "Constant attendance involves visual, verbal, and/or manual contact with patient during provision of the service." *AMA CPT Assistant, July 2004*

Application of a modality to 1 or more areas;
(For transcutaneous electrical modulation pain reprocessing [TEMPR/scarmbler therapy], use 0278T)

| 97032 | electrical stimulation (manual), each 15 minutes (1 or more areas) | ncci | .54 |

[MODALITY USED TO APPLY ELECTRICAL CURRENT TO A SPECIFIC AREA. ATTENDED ELECTRICAL STIMULATION IS ALSO REFERRED TO AS MANUAL STIMULATION. ATTENDED STIMULATION CALLS FOR THE APPLICATION OF STIMULATION FOR SHORTER OR MORE SPECIFIC TIME FRAMES AND AT VARYING DEGREES OF CURRENT.]

| 97033 | iontophoresis, each 15 minutes (1 or more areas) | ncci | .92 |

[THE INTRODUCTION OF IONS OF SOLUBLE SALTS INTO THE BODY BY AN ELECTRIC CURRENT.]

| 97034 | contrast baths, each 15 minutes (1 or more areas) | ncci | .51 |

[ALTERNATE IMMERSION OF A BODY PART IN HOT WATER (98-112 DEGREES FAHRENHEIT) AND COLD WATER (60-75 DEGREES FAHRENHEIT).]

| 97035 | ultrasound, each 15 minutes (1 or more areas) | ncci | .36 |

See Chapter 3-Commonly Used Codes for more information.

| 97036 | Hubbard tank, each 15 minutes (1 or more areas) | ncci | .94 |

[A TANK DESIGNED FOR FULL IMMERSION OF THE BODY FOR HYDROTHERAPY. A NARROW SECTION AT THE MIDDLE OF THE TANK ALLOWS THE PROVIDER TO REACH THE PATIENT, AND A WIDER SECTION AT EACH END PERMITS FULL ABDUCTION OF THE PATIENT'S LEGS AND ARMS. THE TANK IS FITTED WITH AN AERATOR THAT AGITATES THE WATER AND PROVIDES GENTLE MASSAGE AND DEBRIDEMENT OF WOUNDS. USEFUL IN THE TREATMENT OF BURNS AND CHRONIC MULTIPLE JOINT DISORDERS.]

| 97039 | Unlisted modality (specify type and time if constant attendance) | ncci | NE |

If there is no accurate code for your modality, use 97039.

Therapeutic Procedures

The purpose of these codes is an "attempt to improve function" by direct (one-on-one) patient-practitioner contact. Most of these codes have time elements affixed to them by the AMA.

Direct one-on-one contact is required for all therapeutic procedures EXCEPT 97150.

Therapeutic procedure, 1 or more areas, each 15 minutes;

Code	Description		RVU
97110	therapeutic exercises to develop strength and endurance, range of motion and flexibility, 1 or more areas, each 15 minutes	ncci	.91

See Chapter 3–Commonly Used Codes for more information.

97112	neuromuscular reeducation of movement, balance, coordination, kinesthetic sense, posture, and/or proprioception for sitting and/or standing activities, 1 or more areas, each 15 minutes	ncci	.95

See Chapter 3–Commonly Used Codes for more information.

97113	aquatic therapy with therapeutic exercises, 1 or more areas, each 15 minutes	ncci	1.21

[ANY TYPE OF EXERCISE PERFORMED IN A WATER ENVIRONMENT. DO NOT CODE THE WATER MODALITY (EG, HUBBARD TANK, WHIRLPOOL) AND THE TYPE OF THERAPEUTIC EXERCISE (EG, NEUROMUSCULAR REEDUCATION) SEPARATELY. CODE ONLY THE AQUATIC THERAPY WITH THERAPEUTIC EXERCISE, 97113.]

97116	gait training (includes stair climbing), 1 or more areas, each 15 minutes	ncci	.80

(Use 96000-96003 to report comprehensive gait and motion analysis procedures)

[TRAINING OF THE MANNER OR STYLE OF WALKING, INCLUDING RHYTHM AND SPEED. THREE PHASES OF GAIT INCLUDE THE STANCE PHASE, THE SWING PHASE, AND THE DOUBLE SUPPORT PHASE.]

97124	massage, including effleurage, petrissage and/or tapotement (stroking, compression, percussion), 1 or more areas, each 15 minutes	ncci	.75

(For myofascial release, use 97140)

For help with code 97124 see Examples #7 and #11 in Chapter 7–Clinical Examples in this *Procedure Codes* section.

> **Caution:** When using the 97124 code on the same day as a CMT service, it may be necessary to append modifier 59 (Distinct Procedure). See page H-104 for more information.
>
> **Who can legally perform a massage?** This is determined by local or state law. Practitioners will usually find it defined within the "scope of practice" for their license. However, insurance and third party payers will reimburse according to their contracts and policies.

97139	Unlisted therapeutic procedure (specify)	ncci	NE
97140	Manual therapy techniques (eg, mobilization/manipulation, manual lymphatic drainage, manual traction), 1 or more regions, each 15 minutes	ncci	.85

For help with code 97140 see Examples #8 and #9 in Chapter 7–Clinical Examples in this *Procedure Codes* section

The CPT guidelines state that 97140 services are mutually exclusive to the CMT codes (98940-98942) when performed on the same spinal region. Also, Medicare NCCI edits categorize 97140 similarly, unless a modifier (e.g., 59) is used for a different region(s). However, Medicare law prohibits coverage and payment for non-CMT services when performed by a doctor of chiropractic. Thus, if 97140 is bundled into CMT, it would be a violation of Medicare law. Furthermore, the Medicare relative value units (RVU) do not include any non-spinal services (e.g., 97140, 97112, 97124, etc.).

Documentation Tips: When using a physical medicine procedure such as 97140, there are three things that should be documented: 1) Technique (manual traction, myofascial release, mobilization, etc.), 2) Location (cervical, thoracic, lumbar, extraspinal, etc.) and 3) Time.

97150 Therapeutic procedure(s), group (2 or more individuals)   ncci   .49

[GROUP THERAPEUTIC PROCEDURES INCLUDE CPT CODES 97110-97139. IF ANY OF THESE PROCEDURES ARE PERFORMED WITH TWO OR MORE INDIVIDUALS, THEN ONLY 97150 IS REPORTED. DO NOT CODE THE SPECIFIC TYPE OF THERAPY IN ADDITION TO THE GROUP THERAPY CODE.]

(Report 97150 for each member of group)

(Group therapy procedures involve constant attendance of the physician or other qualified health care professional [ie, therapist], but by definition do not require one-on-one patient contact by the same physician or other qualified health care professional.)

(For manipulation under general anesthesia, see appropriate anatomic section in Musculoskeletal System)

(For osteopathic manipulative treatment [OMT], see 98925-98929)

97530 Therapeutic activities, direct (one-on-one) patient contact (use of dynamic activities to improve functional performance), each 15 minutes   ncci   .99

[DYNAMIC ACTIVITIES INCLUDE THE USE OF MULTIPLE PARAMETERS, SUCH AS BALANCE, STRENGTH AND RANGE OF MOTION, FOR A FUNCTIONAL ACTIVITY. EXAMPLES INCLUDE LIFTING STATIONS, CLOSED KINETIC CHAIN ACTIVITY, HAND ASSEMBLY ACTIVITY, TRANSFERS (CHAIR TO BED, LYING TO SITTING, ETC.), AND THROWING, CATCHING, OR SWINGING.]

97532 Development of cognitive skills to improve attention, memory, problem solving, (includes compensatory training), direct (one-on-one) patient contact, each 15 minutes   ncci   .76

97533 Sensory integrative techniques to enhance sensory processing and promote adaptive responses to environmental demands, direct (one-on-one) patient contact, each 15 minutes   ncci   .82

97535 Self-care/home management training (eg, activities of daily living (ADL) and compensatory training, meal preparation, safety procedures, and instructions in use of assistive technology devices/adaptive equipment) direct one-on-one contact, each 15 minutes   ncci   .98

97537 Community/work reintegration training (eg, shopping, transportation, money management, avocational activities and/or work environment/modification analysis, work task analysis, use of assistive technology device/adaptive equipment), direct one-on-one contact, each 15 minutes   ncci   .85

97542 Wheelchair management(eg, assessment, fitting, training), each 15 minutes   ncci   .86

			RVU
97545	Work hardening/conditioning; initial 2 hours	ncci	NE
+ 97546	each additional hour (List separately in addition to code for primary procedure)	ncci	NE
	(Use 97546 in conjunction with code 97545)		

Tests and Measurements

These codes require direct one-on-one patient contact.

(For muscle testing, manual or electrical, joint range of motion, electromyography or nerve velocity determination, see 95831-95857, 95860-95872, 95885-95887, 95907-95913)

97750	Physical performance test or measurement (eg, musculoskeletal, functional capacity), with written report, each 15 minutes	ncci	.93
97755	Assistive technology assessment (eg, to restore, augment or compensate for existing function, optimize functional tasks and/or maximize environmental accessibility), direct one-on-one contact, with written report, each 15 minutes	ncci	1.01

Orthotic Management and Prosthetic Management

97760	Orthotic(s) management and training (including assessment and fitting when not otherwise reported), upper extremity(s), lower extremity(s) and/or trunk, each 15 minutes	ncci	1.08
	(Code 97760 should not be reported with 97116 for the same extremity)		
97761	Prosthetic training, upper and/or lower extremity(s), each 15 minutes	ncci	.93
97762	Checkout for orthotic/prosthetic use, established patient, each 15 minutes	ncci	1.34

Other Procedures

(For extracorporeal shock wave musculoskeletal therapy, see Category III codes 0019T, 0101T, 0102T)

97799	**Unlisted physical medicine/rehabilitation** service or procedure		NE

MEDICAL NUTRITION THERAPY

Medical Nutrition Therapy (MNT) (97802-97804) for dietary counseling provided in an outpatient setting by a state-licensed or certified dietitian, nutrition professional is considered **medically necessary** by many qualified payers.

When physicians provide nutrition services, E/M or preventive medicine codes should be used **instead** of these codes.

	Medical nutrition therapy;		
97802	initial assessment and intervention, individual, face-to-face with the patient, each 15 minutes	ncci	.98
97803	re-assessment and intervention, individual, face-to-face with the patient, each 15 minutes	ncci	.84
97804	group (2 or more individual(s)), each 30 minutes	ncci	.45
	(Physicians and other qualified health care professionals who may report evaluation and management services should use the appropriate Evaluation and Management codes.)		

ACUPUNCTURE

Acupuncture codes are based on 15 minutes of personal (face-to-face) patient contact, rather than the duration of acupuncture needle placement.

- Use either 97810 or 97813 for the initial 15-minute period; report only one initial code per day.
- Report only one add-on code per each additional 15-minute period.

According to CPT, "Significant separately identifiable E/M services above and beyond the usual preservice and postservice work associated with the acupuncture services" are not included. Report appropriate E/M services separately using modifier 25.

Code	Description		RVU
	Acupuncture, 1 or more needles;		
97810	**without** electrical stimulation, initial 15 minutes of personal one-on-one contact with the patient	ncci	1.03
	(Do not report 97810 in conjunction with 97813)		
+ 97811	**without** electrical stimulation, each additional 15 minutes of personal one-on-one contact with the patient, with re-insertion of needle(s) (List separately in addition to code for primary procedure)	ncci	.77
	(Use 97811 in conjunction with 97810, 97813)		
97813	**with** electrical stimulation, initial 15 minutes of personal one-on-one contact with the patient	ncci	1.10
	(Do not report 97813 in conjunction with 97810)		
+ 97814	**with** electrical stimulation, each additional 15 minutes of personal one-on-one contact with the patient, with re-insertion of needle(s) (List separately in addition to code for primary procedure) (Use 97814 in conjunction with 97810, 97813)	ncci	.88

[NON-PHYSICIAN ACUPUNCTURIST PRACTITIONERS SHOULD NOT USE ADDITIONAL E/M CODES UNLESS WITH PERMISSION FROM THE PAYER. HOWEVER, THEY COULD USE THE 97001-97002 EVALUATION CODES THAT WERE SPECIFICALLY CREATED FOR NON-PHYSICIANS USING THIS PHYSICAL MEDICINE AND REHABILITATION SECTION.]

OSTEOPATHIC MANIPULATIVE TREATMENT (OMT)

Osteopathic Manipulative Treatment (OMT) codes are typically not to be used by chiropractic physicians. However, from a correct CPT coding perspective, they could be used by any appropriately licensed physician or other qualified health care professional when the intent of the manipulation treatment procedure is to "eliminate or alleviate somatic dysfunction or related disorders."

Code	Description		RVU
	Osteopathic manipulative treatment (OMT);		
98925	1-2 body regions involved	ncci	.89
98926	3-4 body regions involved	ncci	1.29
98927	5-6 body regions involved	ncci	1.67
98928	7-8 body regions involved	ncci	2.05
98929	9-10 body regions involved	ncci	2.46

Body regions (by CPT) are:
- Head
- Cervical
- Thoracic
- Lumbar
- Sacral
- Pelvic
- Lower extremities
- Upper extremities
- Rib cage
- Abdomen
- Viscera

Chiropractic Manipulative Treatment (CMT)

Beginning in 2013, AMA guidelines for CMT specifically outline E/M codes 99201-99215, 99241-99245, 99307-99310, 99324-99337, and 99341-99350 as being appropriate for use with CMT services as long as they are billed with modifier 25 and the services are considered significant and separately identifiable.

Code	Description		RVU
	Chiropractic manipulative treatment (CMT);		
98940	spinal, 1-2 regions	ncci	.79
98941	spinal, 3-4 regions	ncci	1.15
98942	spinal, 5 regions	ncci	1.50
98943	extraspinal, 1 or more regions [NON-SPINE]	ncci	.77
S8990	Physical or manipulative therapy performed for maintenance rather than restoration		NE

For help with CMT codes see Examples #1-4, #7, #8, #10, #11 in Chapter 7–Clinical Examples in this *Procedure Codes* section.

"**Chiropractic Manipulative Treatment (CMT)** is a form of manual treatment to influence joint and neurophysiological function. This treatment may be accomplished using a variety of techniques." (AMA 2012). It is also known as the Chiropractic Adjustment, even though CMT is a more encompassing term.

Includes: pre-manipulation patient assessment, a variety of techniques, use of hand held assistive devices (per CMS guidelines but excluded by some payers), and could have the same diagnostic code(s) as concurrent E/M service.

Excludes: additional "significant, separately identifiable" E/M services beyond usual pre-service and post-service work. According to the RVU data, the usual pre-service and post-service time for 98940 is 5 minutes. Therefore, when there are such significant encounters taking more time, it makes sense that the CPT would acknowledge such events and label them as "significant, separately identifiable." Accordingly, such significant occasions could be with new patients, reevaluations, consultations, exacerbations, counseling, etc. Select the appropriate E/M code and append modifier 25 (significant, separately identifiable E/M service) to the E/M code.

Understanding CMT

CPT and ICD-9 Spinal Regions Do Not Correlate

Be aware that the CPT definitions of regions are not consistent with the definitions provided in ICD-9-CM. This may result in problems with payers attempting to link procedure codes directly to the diagnostic codes.

Various insurance payers have refused to acknowledge the existence of the five levels of spinal regions as outlined in the CPT codebook. They have claimed that five regions are not supported by the ICD-9 coding. They are right. Doctors are confused and frustrated in trying to follow both the CPT and ICD-9 guidelines.

Here is how the code descriptions compare. The words on the following page are taken from the actual CPT® descriptions (by the American Medical Association) and ICD-9 texts.

CPT (98940-98942)	ICD-9 (739 Series)	ICD-9 (839 Series)
(none)	Head region Occipitocervical region	(none)
Cervical region (includes atlanto-occipital)	Cervical Region Cervicothoracic region	Cervical vertebra
Thoracic region (includes costovertebral and costotransverse joints)	Thoracic region Thoracolumbar region	Thoracic vertebra
Lumbar region	Lumbar region Lumbosacral region	Lumbar vertebra
Sacral region	Sacral region Sacrococcygeal region Sacroiliac region	Sacrum Sacroiliac (joint)
(none)	(none)	Coccyx
Pelvic (sacroiliac joint) region	Pelvic region Hip region Pubic region	Other (Pelvis)

Note how the components in CPT and ICD-9 fail to all correlate with each other. Only the thoracic and lumbar regions are in total agreement. Because the ICD-9 does not correlate exactly with CPT at the lower end of the spine, the rationale of payers is that the ICD-9 does not support a 5th region. Neither does the CPT or the ICD-9 (739 series) support the coccyx (839) series as a stand alone code. Obviously, either the CPT or the ICD-9 is wrong. Some ICD-9 experts state that the subtitles listed under the ICD-9 codes are there only as helpful indicators, but are not absolutes. Nevertheless, this comparative chart reveals why the attempts to link CPT to ICD-9 creates problems. Hopefully, CPT and ICD will communicate and resolve this matter.

Background of Chiropractic Manipulative Treatment (CMT)

"Chiropractic is a health care discipline, which emphasizes the inherent recuperative power of the body to heal without the use of drugs or surgery. This is accomplished by focusing on the relationship between structure, primarily the spine, and function, as coordinated by the nervous system as that relationship may affect the preservation and restoration of health."

"Previously, Level II HCPCS code A2000 Manipulation of spine by Chiropractor was assigned to identify chiropractic services. The single A2000 code did not adequately represent all of the work included as part of the therapy used by chiropractic practitioners. Due to this, the four new codes included in CPT 1997 were developed to meet the need of more accurately describing the services performed." From *CPT Assistant*, Jan. 1997, by the American Medical Association.

Physician Work Involved

"Chiropractic adjustment is a therapeutic procedure that uses 1) controlled force, 2) leverage, 3) direction, 4) amplitude, and 5) velocity, which is directed at specific joints or anatomical regions. The complete CMT service requires a certain amount of preservice, intra-service and post-service work that is included as part of the service. This evaluation and management is necessary to determine not only what specific work will be necessary, but also to determine the effectiveness of the service being provided."

"**Preservice** work includes reviewing previously gathered clinical data (including an initial or interim history, reviewing the problem list, pertinent correspondence or reports, and other important findings and prior care), review of imaging and other test results, test interpretation, and care planning."

"**Intraservice** work includes an interactive patient reassessment (ie, determining the current status, determining indicators/contraindications, assessing the change in condition, evaluating any new complaints, correlating physical findings, and coordinating and modifying the current treatment plan). Also included in the intraservice work is a number of manipulation and post adjustment assessments that are necessary in order to adequately treat the ailment presented. This work is inherently included as part of the CMT service and would not be coded separately. If additional evaluation and management services are performed, then they may be reported separately, if and only if the patient's condition requires a significant separately identifiable E/M service above an beyond the usual pre-service work associated with the procedure." -From *CPT Assistant,* January 1997, by the American Medical Association

Substitution of E/M or 97140 Codes

The use of an E/M code and/or 97140 to report a Chiropractic Manipulative Treatment (CMT) could be considered as fraud and abuse. Always select a code that "accurately describes" the procedure performed. Get prior confirmation in writing!

Relative Value Unit (RVU) Analysis

Although time is not a component expressed in the CPT description, it is a key factor in determining the RVU for payment purposes by CMS. Significantly, the RVUs for CMT services do not include 15 minutes of work for other procedures such as 97110, 97112, 97124, 97140, etc.

Progress is being made in revising this edit. In 2006 the CPT did remove 97110, 97112 and 97124 from their bundling policies into the CMT. However, CMS's NCCI contractor has not yet taken corrective action to remove their edits.

CMT and Other Coding

CPT states that Significant Separately Identifiable (SSI) E/M services can and do exist for CMT. Upon such encounters, it is appropriate to document the special SSI E/M service and enter the appropriate E/M code on the claim form with modifier 25 being appended. Example 1 shows coding for a new patient at a level 4 service and a Chiropractic Adjustment/Manipulation.

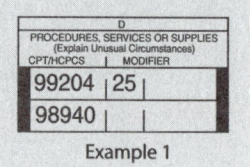

PROCEDURES, SERVICES OR SUPPLIES (Explain Unusual Circumstances)	
CPT/HCPCS	MODIFIER
99204	25
98940	

Example 1

See Resource 404 for additional information.

EDUCATION AND TRAINING FOR PATIENT SELF-MANAGEMENT

The focus of the educational and training codes is to teach the patient (including caregivers) to effectively self-manage the patient's illness or disease, as well as attempt to delay possible additional disorders or comorbidities.

According to the CPT, "the qualifications of the non-physician healthcare practitioner must be consistent with guidelines or standards established or recognized by a physician society, a non-physician healthcare professional society/association, or other appropriate source."

Some of the criteria used to establish the curriculum are as follows:

- The content must be consistent with guidelines or standards established by recognized societies as described above.
- The content must be standardized to individuals or groups of patients.
- Any modifications to the curriculum should be done only when necessary to meet the clinical needs, cultural norms, and health literacy of the patient or patients.

Typically, physician providers do not use these codes for other professionals, but rather use the appropriate Evaluation and Management codes for counseling, education and risk factor reduction intervention.

Further clarification is available in the full CPT codebook.

(For counseling and education provided by a physician to an individual, see the appropriate Evaluation and Management codes)

(For counseling and education provided by a physician to a group, use 99078)

(For counseling and/or risk factor reduction intervention provided by a physician to patient(s) without symptoms or established disease, see 99401-99412)

(For medical nutrition therapy, see 97802-97804)

(For health and behavior assessment/intervention that is not part of a standardized curriculum, see 96150-96155)

Education and training for patient self-management by a qualified, nonphysician health care professional using a standardized curriculum, face-to-face with the patient (could include caregiver/family) each 30 minutes;

Code	Description		RVU
98960	individual patient	ncci	.78
98961	2-4 patients	ncci	.38
98962	5-8 patients	ncci	.28

Non-Face-to-Face Nonphysician Services

Non-Face-to-Face Nonphysician Services codes were added in response to consumer needs and expectations for enhanced access to care. They are essential for value-based care, chronic disease management and other healthcare matters. Obviously, do not use them for the same non-face-to-face events when performed by physicians. The "qualified health care professional" status indicates a state license and is further explained on page H-84 and in the "Other Qualified Healthcare Professionals" topic below.

For physician services, see E/M codes 99441-99444.

Telephone Services

Telephone assessment and management service provided by a qualified nonphysician health care professional to an established patient, parent, or guardian not originating from a related assessment and management service provided within the previous 7 days nor leading to an assessment and management service or procedure within the next 24 hours or soonest available appointment;

Code	Description		RVU
98966	5-10 minutes of medical discussion	ncci	.40
98967	11-20 minutes of medical discussion	ncci	.76
98968	21-30 minutes of medical discussion	ncci	1.13

Other Qualified Healthcare Professionals

A qualified health care professional is a licensed health care provider who performs professional services within their state scope of practice and independently reports those services. This does not include clinical staff, such as physician assistants, who perform services under the supervision of a physician or other qualified health care professional. Physicians also meet this general definition, however, they must also satisfy additional requirements as outlined by state, federal or private payer rules and regulations.

- ● = New Code for 2015
- ▲ = Revised Code for 2015
- ►◄ = New or Revised CPT Text
- NE = Not Established
- NA = Not Applicable
- NCCI = CCI Edits Apply
- ✚ = Add-on Code
- ⊘ = Modifier 51 Exempt
- -QW = CLIA Waived Test
- TC = Technical Component
- 26 = Professional Component
- # = Resequenced Code

On-Line Medical Evaluation

RVU

98969	Online assessment and management service provided by a qualified non-physician health care professional to an established patient or guardian, not originating from a related assessment and management service provided within the previous 7 days, using the Internet or similar electronic communications network	ncci	NE

For help with code 98969 see Example #21 in Chapter 7–Clinical Examples in this *Procedure Codes* section.

SPECIAL SERVICES, PROCEDURES AND REPORTS

Codes in this section should only be used when there is not another more appropriate code that could be used. They are for use with special services that are not an integral part of the main services performed.

Codes 99050-99060 are **adjunctive** (add-on codes) in addition to the basic service provided.

Miscellaneous Services

99000	Handling and/or conveyance of specimen for transfer from the office to a laboratory	NE
99001	Handling and/or conveyance of specimen for transfer from the patient in other than an office to a laboratory (distance may be indicated)	NE
99002	Handling, conveyance, and/or any other service in connection with the implementation of an order involving devices (eg, designing, fitting, packaging, handling, delivery or mailing) when devices such as orthotics, protectives, prosthetics are fabricated by an outside laboratory or shop but which items have been designed, and are to be fitted and adjusted by the attending physician or other qualified health care professional	NE
	(For routine collection of blood, use 36415)	
99024	Postoperative follow-up visit, normally included in the surgical package, to indicate that an evaluation and management service was performed during a postoperative period for a reason(s) related to the original procedure	NE
99050	Services provided in the office at times other than regularly scheduled office hours, or days when the office is normally closed (eg, holidays, Saturday or Sunday), in addition to basic service	NE
99051	Service(s) provided in the office during regularly scheduled evening, weekend, or holiday office hours, in addition to basic service	NE
	(99052 has been deleted)	
99053	Service(s) provided between 10:00 PM and 8:00 AM at 24-hour facility, in addition to basic service	NE
	(99054 has been deleted)	
99056	Service(s) typically provided in the office, provided out of the office at request of patient, in addition to basic service	NE

List appropriate Place of Service code (POS) on the claim. See Resource 178 or 359 for POS codes.

99058	Services provided on an emergency basis in the office, which disrupts other scheduled office services, in addition to basic service	NE

			RVU
99060	Service(s) provided on an emergency basis, out of the office, which disrupts other scheduled office services, in addition to basic service		NE

> Typically, it is appropriate to use only one adjunctive code (99050-99060) on the same day.

99070	Supplies and materials (except spectacles), provided by the physician or other qualified health care professional over and above those usually included with the office visit or other services rendered (list drugs, trays, supplies, or materials provided)		NE

> 99070 is a general code. As such, it does not give most payers enough information to process your claim. Use specific HCPCS supply codes whenever possible to replace 99070. See *Section I-Supplies*.
>
> The fee for this code has not been established, because supplies vary.

99071	Educational supplies, such as books, tapes, and pamphlets for the patient's education at cost to physician or other qualified health care professional	ncci	NE
99075	Medical testimony	ncci	NE
99078	Physician or other qualified health care professional qualified by education, training, licensure/regulation (when applicable) educational services rendered to patients in a group setting (eg, prenatal, obesity, or diabetic instructions)	ncci	NE
99080	Special reports such as insurance forms, more than the information conveyed in the usual medical communications or standard reporting form	ncci	NE

(Do not report 99080 in conjunction with 99455, 99456 for the completion of Workmen's Compensation forms)

> 99080 is typically used for narrative summaries and/or reproduction costs of clinical records or x-rays made for patients or insurance companies. Some payers have set standards.

S9982	Medical records copying fee, per page		NE
99082	Unusual travel (eg, transportation and escort of patient)	ncci	NE
99090	Analysis of clinical data stored in computers (eg, ECGs, blood pressures, hematologic data)	ncci	NE

(For physician/or other qualified health care professional qualified by education, training, licensure/regulation [when applicable] collection and interpretation of physiologic data stored/transmitted by patient/caregiver, see 99091)

(Do not report 99090 if other more specific CPT codes exist, eg, 93014, 93227, 93233, 93272 for cardiographic services; 95250 for continuous glucose monitoring, 97750 for musculoskeletal function testing)

Missed Appointments

There is no CPT code for a missed appointment. It is actually a "non-service." Do not expect a third party payer to reimburse for a missed appointment. Unless the patients had prior notice of your charge policy, you shouldn't bill them either. From a risk management perspective, missed appointments need to be recorded. For example, a doctor who was sued for "patient abandonment" won the case because all "missed appointments" by the patient were recorded. It is a good practice to make sure that missed appointments are also recorded in the patient's chart.

Computer systems often permit you to make your own internal codes for such "non-service" items.

● = New Code for 2015 NE = Not Established ✚ = Add-on Code TC = Technical Component
▲ = Revised Code for 2015 NA = Not Applicable ⊘ = Modifier 51 Exempt 26 = Professional Component
►◄ = New or Revised CPT Text NCCI = CCI Edits Apply -QW = CLIA Waived Test # = Resequenced Code

			RVU
99091	Collection and interpretation of physiologic data (eg, ECG, blood pressure, glucose monitoring) digitally stored and/or transmitted by the patient and/or caregiver to the physician or other qualified health care professional, qualified by education, training, licensure/regulation (when applicable) requiring a minimum of 30 minutes of time	ncci	1.59

> Code 99091 has special usage limitations including the following:
> - May only be used once within a 30-day period
> - May not be used with certain CPT codes (eg, 93014, 93227, 93233, 93272, and 95250)
> - May not be used with an E/M service on the same day

OTHER SERVICES AND PROCEDURES

99172	Visual function screening, automated or semi-automated bilateral quantitative determination of visual acuity, ocular alignment, color vision by pseudoisochromatic plates, and field of vision (may include all or some screening of the determination(s) for contrast sensitivity, vision under glare)	ncci	NE

(This service must employ graduated visual acuity stimuli that allow a quantitative determination of visual acuity (eg, Snellen chart). This service may not be used in addition to a general ophthalmological service or an E/M service)

(Do not report 99172 in conjunction with 99173)

99173	Screening test of visual acuity, quantitative, bilateral		.09

(The screening test used must employ graduated visual acuity stimuli that allow a quantitative estimate of visual acuity (eg, Snellen chart). Other identifiable services unrelated to this screening test provided at the same time may be reported separately (eg, preventive medicine services). When acuity is measured as part of a general opthalmological service or of an E/M service of the eye, it is a diagnostic examination and not a screening test)

(Do not report 99173 in conjunction with 99172)

99175	Ipecac or similar administration for individual emesis and continued observation until stomach adequately emptied of poison (induction of vomiting)		.48
99183	Physician or other qualified health care professional attendance and supervision of hyperbaric oxygen therapy, per session	ncci	6.05
99199	Unlisted special service, procedure or report		NE

> Always include a report with a description of service when using this code or explain the service using the pink area above the service code on the 1500 claim form. Preface the explanation with "ZZ" (with no space after it).
>
> *Example:*
>
> | 24. A. DATE(S) OF SERVICE | | B. PLACE OF SERVICE | C. EMG | D. PROCEDURES, SERVICES, OR SUPPLIES (Explain Unusual Circumstances) | |
> |---|---|---|---|---|---|
> | From MM DD YY | To MM DD YY | | | CPT/HCPCS | MODIFIER |
> | ZZStatic surface EMG | | | | | |
> | 10 01 05 | 10 01 05 | 12 | | 99199 | |

99201-99499 are reserved for Evaluation and Management (E/M) codes, which begin on page H-36 in this section.

HOME HEALTH PROCEDURES/SERVICES

99600	Unlisted home visit service or procedure		NE

MEDICATION THERAPY MANAGEMENT SERVICES

Medication therapy management service(s) (MTMS) are for face-to-face patient assessment and intervention by a pharmacist, when requested by the patient. The intent is to enhance the response to medications and to manage treatment-related medication interactions or complications. MTMS includes the following documented elements: review of the pertinent patient history, medication profile (prescription and nonprescription), and recommendations for improving health outcomes and treatment compliance.

These codes represent support for consumer driven healthcare. Prudent use of drugs can be a critical concern for patients and their doctors. An alert practitioner, when performing a relevant history and/or counseling should inform their patient about this service option. There is no substitute for excellence by an experienced licensed pharmacist (who is the real drug specialist, and not just a doctor prescribing drugs or a pharmaceutical representative). Look for one or more quality pharmacists in your area. Share their contact information with your patients when appropriate.

Medication therapy management service(s) provided by a pharmacist, individual, face-to-face with patient, with assessment and intervention if provided;

99605	initial 15 minutes, new patient	ncci	NE
99606	initial 15 minutes, established patient	ncci	NE
+ 99607	each additional 15 minutes (List separately in addition to code for primary service)	ncci	NE

For additional procedures codes, see the "Category III Codes" on the following pages and Chapter 5–HCPCS Procedures Codes.

4f. CPT Procedures

Category III Codes

Category III codes are temporary codes that identify emerging technologies, services, and procedures. This allows for data gathering, payment, and research. Codes that appear in Category III may or may not eventually reach Category I status.

The full listing of the temporary Category III codes is published annually in the CPT codebook (Resource 335).

See Chapter 5–PQRS in *Section C-Medicare* for more about Category II performance measurement codes pertaining to clinical records/charts for supplemental reporting purposes.

See Resource 342 to visit the AMA website.

			RVU
0019T	Extracorporeal shock wave involving musculoskeletal system, not otherwise specified, low energy	ncci	NE
+ 0095T	Removal of total disc arthroplasty (artificial disk), anterior approach, each additional interspace, cervical (List separately in addition to code for primary procedure)	ncci	NE
0101T	Extracorporeal shock wave involving musculoskeletal system, not otherwise specified, high energy	ncci	NE
	(For application of low energy musculoskeletal system extracorporeal shock wave, use 0019T)		
	Quantitative sensory testing (QST), testing and interpretation per extremity;		
0106T	using touch pressure stimuli to assess large diameter sensation		NE
0107T	using vibration stimuli to assess large diameter fiber sensation		NE
0108T	using cooling stimuli to assess small nerve fiber sensation and hyperalgesia		NE
0109T	using heat-pain stimuli to assess small nerve fiber sensation and hyperalgesia		NE
0110T	using other stimuli to assess sensation		NE
0111T	Long-chain (C20-22) omega-3 fatty acids in red blood cell (RBC) membranes		NE
	Computer-aided detection (CAD) (computer algorithm analysis of digital image data for lesion detection) with further physician review for interpretation and report, with or without digitization of film radiographic images, chest radiograph(s),		
0174T	performed concurrent with primary interpretation (List separately in addition to code for primary procedure)		NE
	(Use 0174T in conjunction with 71010, 71020, 71021, 71022, 71030)		
0175T	performed remote from primary interpretation	ncci	NE
	(Do not report 0175T in conjunction with 71010, 71020, 71021, 71022, 71030)		

			RVU
	(0183T has been deleted. To report, use 97610)		
	(0185T has been deleted)		
	▶(0199T has been deleted)◀		
	▶(For tremor measurement with accelerometer(s) and/or gyroscope(s), use 95999)◀		
▲ 0200T	Percutaneous sacral augmentation (sacroplasty), unilateral injection(s), including the use of a balloon or mechanical device, when used, 1 or more needles, ▶includes imaging guidance and bone biopsy, when performed◀	ncci	NE
	Requires Moderate Sedation.		
▲ 0201T	Percutaneous sacral augmentation (sacroplasty), bilateral injections, including the use of a balloon or mechanical device, when used, 2 or more needles, ▶includes imaging guidance and bone biopsy, when performed◀	ncci	NE
	Requires Moderate Sedation.		
0202T	Posterior vertebral joint(s) arthroplasty (eg, facet joint[s] replacement), including facetectomy, laminectomy, foraminotomy, and vertebral column fixation, injection of bone cement, when performed, including fluoroscopy, single level, lumbar spine	ncci	NE
	Injection(s), diagnostic or therapeutic agent, paravertebral facet (zygapophyseal) joint (or nerves innervating that joint) with ultrasound guidance, cervical or thoracic;		
0213T	single level (To report bilateral procedure, use 0213T with modifier 50)	ncci	NE
+ 0214T	second level (List separately in addition to code for primary procedure) ▶(Use 0214T in conjunction with 0213T)◀ (To report bilateral procedure, use 0214T with modifier 50)	ncci	NE
+ 0215T	third and any additional level(s) (List separately in addition to code for primary procedure) (Do not report 0215T more than once per day) ▶(Use 0215T in conjunction with 0213T, 0214T)◀	ncci	NE
	Injection(s), diagnostic or therapeutic agent, paravertebral facet (zygapophyseal) joint (or nerves innervating that joint) with ultrasound guidance, lumbar or sacral;		
0216T	single level (To report bilateral procedure, use 0216T with modifier 50)	ncci	NE
+ 0217T	second level (List separately in addition to code for primary procedure) ▶(Use 0217T in conjunction with 00216T)◀ (To report bilateral procedure, use 0217T with modifier 50)	ncci	NE
+ 0218T	third and any additional level(s) (List separately in addition to code for primary procedure) (Do not report 0218T more than once per day) ▶(Use 0218T in conjunction with 0216T, 0217T)◀ (To report bilateral procedure, use 0218T with modifier 50)	ncci	NE
0278T	Transcutaneous electrical modulation pain reprocessing (eg, scrambler therapy), each treatment session (includes placement of electrodes)		NE

5. HCPCS Procedure Codes

PROCEDURES AND PROFESSIONAL SERVICES ("G" CODES)

Temporary codes listed in this section are assigned by CMS on a temporary basis. Use them with caution. Although they are current HIPAA approved code sets, not all payers are aware of or use them. Use by non-Medicare payers is optional.

Procedures and Professional Services

Code	Description		RVU
	Diabetes outpatient self-management training services;		
G0108	individual, per 30 minutes	ncci	1.48
G0109	group session (2 or more), per 30 minutes	ncci	.40
G0151	Services performed by a qualified physical therapist in the home health or hospice setting, each 15 minutes	ncci	NE
G0152	Services performed by a qualified occupational therapist in the home health hospice setting, each 15 minutes	ncci	NE
G0157	Services performed by a qualified physical therapist assistant in the home health or hospice setting, each 15 minutes	ncci	NE
G0158	Services performed by a qualified occupational therapist assistant in the health or hospice setting, each 15 minutes	ncci	NE
G0159	Services performed by a qualified physical therapist, in the home health setting, in the establishment or delivery of a safe and effective therapy maintenance program, each 15 minutes	ncci	NE
G0160	Services performed by a qualified occupational therapist, in the home health setting, in the establishment or delivery of a safe and effective therapy maintenance program, each 15 minutes	ncci	NE
G0168	Wound closure utilizing tissue adhesive(s) only	ncci	2.88
G0255	Current perception threshold/sensory nerve conduction test, (SNCT) per limb, any nerve		NE
	Medical nutrition therapy; reassessment and subsequent intervention(s) following second referral in same year for change in diagnosis, medical condition or treatment regimen (including additional hours needed for renal disease);		
G0270	individual, face to face with patient, each 15 minutes	ncci	.84
G0271	group (2 or more individuals), each 30 minutes	ncci	.45

			RVU
● G0277	Hyperbaric oxygen under pressure, full body chamber, per 30 minute interval		1.32
	Electrical stimulation, (unattended), to one or more areas;		
G0281	for chronic stage III and stage IV pressure ulcers, arterial ulcers, diabetic ulcers, and venous statsis ulcers not demonstrating measurable signs of healing after 30 days of conventional care, as part of a therapy plan of care	ncci	.39
G0282	for wound care other than described in G0281		NE
G0283	for indication(s) other than wound care, as part of a therapy plan of care	ncci	.39

> G0283 is a more specific code than the general CPT codes 97014 or 97032 for Electrical Stimulation. Failure to use this "G" code on Medicare claims will result in denials. Other payers, such as United Health Care, might also use G0283 for a therapy plan of care because it is more specific and accurate.
>
> **Alert:** If billing G0283 with 97032, according to NCCI edits, 97032 will not be paid unless billed with an allowed modifier.

G0295	Electromagnetic stimulation, to one or more areas		NE
	Complete CBC, automated (HGB, HCT, RBC, WBC,		
G0306	without platelet count) and automated WBC differential count	ncci	NE
G0307	without platelet count)	ncci	NE
G0372	Physician service required to establish and document the need for a power mobility device (use in addition to primary evaluation and management code)	ncci	.25
G0394	Blood occult test (e.g., Guaiac), feces, for single determination for colorectal neoplasm (i.e., Patient was provided three cards or single triple card for consecutive collection)		NE
G0398	Home sleep study test (HST) with type II portable monitor, unattended; minimum 7 channels: EEG, EOG, EMG, ECG/heart rate, airflow, respiratory effort and oxygen saturation	ncci	NE
G0399	Home sleep test (HST) with type III portable monitor, unattended; minimum of 4 channels: 2 respiratory movement/airflow, 1 ECG/heart rate and 1 oxygen saturation	ncci	NE
G0400	Home sleep test (HST) with type IV portable monitor, unattended; minimum of 3 channels	ncci	NE
G0402	Initial preventive physical examination; face-to-face visit, services limited to new beneficiary during the first 12 months of medicare enrollment	ncci	4.68
	Electrocardiogram, routine ECG with 12 leads;		
G0403	performed as a screening for the initial preventive physical examination with interpretation and report	ncci	.48
G0404	tracing only, without interpretation and report, performed as a screening for the initial preventive physical examination	ncci	.24
G0405	interpretation and report only, performed as a screening for the initial preventive physical examination	ncci	.24

▲ = Revised Code ● = New Code NE = Not Established

			RVU
	Follow-up inpatient consultation,		
G0406	limited, physicians typically spend 15 minutes communicating with the patient via telehealth	ncci	1.10
G0407	intermediate, physicians spend 25 minutes communicating with the patient via telehealth	ncci	2.04
G0408	complex, physicians typically spend 35 minutes or more communicating with the patient via telehealth	ncci	2.93
G0413	Percutaneous skeletal fixation of posterior pelvic bone fracture and/or dislocation, for fracture patterns which disrupt the pelvic ring, unilateral or bilateral, (includes ilium, sacroiliac joint and/or sacrum)	ncci	30.71
	Telehealth consultation, emergency department or initial patient		
G0425	typically 30 minutes communicating with the patient via telehealth	ncci	2.87
G0426	typically 50 minutes communicating with the patient via telehealth	ncci	3.86
G0427	typically 70 minutes or more communicating with the patient via telehealth	ncci	5.71
G0431	Drug screen, qualitative; multiple drug classes by high complexity test (e.g., Immunoassay, enzyme assay), per patient encounter	ncci	NE
	Smoking and tobacco cessation counseling visit for the asymptomatic patient;		
G0436	intermediate, greater than 3 minutes, up to 10 minutes	ncci	.41
G0437	intensive, greater than 10 minutes	ncci	.79
	Annual wellness visit;		
G0438	includes a personalized prevention plan of service (PPS), initial visit	ncci	4.82
G0439	includes a personalized prevention plan of service (PPS), subsequent visit	ncci	3.26
G0442	Annual alcohol misuse screening, 15 minutes	ncci	.51
G0443	Brief face-to-face behavioral counseling for alcohol misuse, 15 minutes	ncci	.73
G0444	Annual depression screening, 15 minutes	ncci	.51
G0446	Intensive behavioral therapy to reduce cardiovascular disease risk, individual,	ncci	.73
G0447	Face-to-face behavioral counseling for obesity, 15 minutes	ncci	.73
G0451	Development testing, with interpretation and report, per standardized	ncci	.27
● G0473	Face-to-face behavioral counseling for obesity, group (2-10), 30 minutes		.37
	(G0911, G0912 have been deleted)		
	(G9041-G9044 have been deleted)		

Rehabilitative Services ("H" Codes)

H0001	Alcohol and/or drug assessment	NE
H0031	Mental health assessment, by non-physician	NE
H0032	Mental health service plan development by non-physician	NE
H0038	Self-help/peer services, per 15 minutes	NE
H0049	Alcohol and/or drug screening	NE
H0050	Alcohol and/or drug services, brief intervention, per 15 minutes	NE
H2000	Comprehensive multidisciplinary evaluation	NE
H2001	Rehabilitation program, per 1/2 day	NE

RVU

Drugs Administered Other Than Oral Method ("J" Codes)

This "J" section is for injections. The Scope of Practice in some states permits injections by a trained Doctor of Chiropractic. These codes are listed here for convenience and reference.

J3420	Injection, vitamin B-12 cyanocobalamin, up to 1,000 mcg	NE
J3570	Laetrile, amygdalin, vitamin B-17	NE

Private Payer Codes ("S" Codes)

HCPCS "S" codes are temporary national codes initiated by private payers. Prior to using these codes on insurance claims to private payers, you should consult with the payer to confirm that "S" codes are acceptable. They are not payable by Medicare.

S0273	Physician visit at member's home, outside of a capitation arrangement	NE
	Medical home program, comprehensive care coordination and planning,	
S0280	initial plan	NE
S0281	maintenance of plan	NE
S0317	Disease management program; per diem	NE
S3005	Performance measurement, evaluation of patient self assessment, depression	NE
S3650	Saliva test, hormone level; during menopause	NE
S3853	Genetic testing for myotonic muscular dystrophy	NE
S3900	Surface electromyography (EMG)	NE
S5135	Companion care, adult (eg, Iadl/adl); per 15 minutes	NE
S5136	Companion care, adult (eg, Iadl/adl); per diem	NE
S5190	Wellness assessment, performed by non-physician	NE
S8301	Infection control supplies, not otherwise specified	NE
S8940	Equestrian/hippotherapy, per session	NE
S8948	Application of a modality (requiring constant provider attendance) to one or more areas; **low-level laser**; each 15 minutes	NE

> S8948 is more specific and accurate than the unlisted CPT 97139 code. If using the unlisted 97139 code, be sure to include a description in the pink shaded area above the code on the 1500 claim form.

S8990	Physical or manipulative therapy performed for maintenance rather than restoration	NE

> Typically, insurance payers do not cover manipulative therapy performed for maintenance, wellness or preventive care. Two possible ICD-9 coding options are: V70.0 for a "Health Checkup," or V82.89 for "Other Specified Conditions." When using such codes document them in the chart as a "maintenance" or "wellness" encounter.
>
> This is an appropriate and accurate code for maintenance care.

S9090	Vertebral axial decompression, per session	NE

> Although S9090 is a descriptive code, few payers honor it as a covered service. Mechanical traction (97012) is the basic modality for decompression results. However, there are many types of new equipment and protocols which go far beyond the old mechanical traction procedures. Consequently, many payers deny claims, using the rationale that more and better evidence is needed.

▲ = Revised Code   ● = New Code   NE = Not Established

Code	Description	RVU
S9117	Back school, per visit	NE
	Use S9117 with the V70.5 ICD-9 code.	
S9433	Medical food nutritionally complete, administered orally, providing 100% of nutritional intake	NE
S9445	Patient education, not otherwise classified, non-physician provider, individual, per session	NE
S9446	Patient education, not otherwise classified, non-physician provider, group, per session	NE
S9449	Weight management classes, non-physician provider, per session	NE
S9451	Exercise classes, non-physician provider, per session	NE
S9452	Nutrition classes, non-physician provider, per session	NE
S9453	Smoking cessation classes, non-physician provider, per session	NE
S9454	Stress management classes, non-physician provider, per session	NE
S9482	Family stabilization services, per 15 minutes	NE
S9976	Lodging, per diem, not otherwise classified	NE
S9977	Meals, per diem, not otherwise specified	NE
S9982	Medical records copying fee, per page	NE
S9988	Services provided as part of a phase I clinical trial	NE
S9999	Sales tax	NE

STATE MEDICAID AGENCY CODES

Code	Description	RVU
T1013	Sign language or oral interpretive services, per 15 minutes	NE

6. Procedure Modifiers

COMMONLY USED LEVEL I CPT MODIFIERS

22	Increased Procedural Services
25	Significant, Separately Identifiable Evaluation and Management Service by the Same Physician on the Same Day of a Procedure or Other Service
26	Professional Component (eg, interpretation and report of x-rays)
51	Multiple Procedures
52	Reduced Services
▲ 59	Distinct Procedural Service
76	Repeat Procedure By Same Physician
77	Repeat Procedure by Another Physician

The complete list of CPT modifiers begins on page H-99.

See Resource 343 for additional information about modifiers including articles and webinars.

COMMONLY USED LEVEL II HCPCS MODIFIERS

AT	Acute treatment (this modifier should be used when reporting service 98940, 98941, 98942)
GA	Waiver of liability statement on file

> This is a declaration of the "ABN on file".

GP	Services delivered under an outpatient physical therapy plan of care
GY	Item or service statutorily excluded or does not meet the definition of any Medicare benefit
GX	Notice of liability issued, voluntary under payer policy
GZ	Item or service expected to be denied as not reasonable and necessary
LT	Left side (used to identify procedures performed on the left side of the body)
RT	Right side (used to identify procedures performed on the right side of the body)
TC	Technical component

The complete list of HCPCS modifiers begins on page H-108.

Understanding Modifiers

Modifiers provide a way for the practitioner to report or indicate that a procedure or service has been performed but has been altered by some specific circumstance. The procedure or service was not changed in its definition or code. The appropriate use of modifiers enable practitioners to effectively respond to payment policy requirements to payer policies.

Modifiers are available to indicate that:

- A procedure or service has both a technical and professional component
- A procedure or service was performed in more than one location, and/or by more than one practitioner
- A procedure or service was reduced or increased
- Only a portion of a service was performed
- An adjunctive service was performed
- A bilateral service was performed
- Unusual events occurred during the procedure or service

Fee schedules have been developed on the basis of such modifiers. Some payers, such as Medicare, require physicians to use modifiers in some circumstances. Others do not recognize the use of modifiers by physicians in coding and billing. Communication with the payer groups ensures accurate coding and expedites payments.

Appending a modifier does not alter the basic description for the service, it merely qualifies the circumstances under which the service was provided.

Modifier Applications

Modifiers are essential tools in the coding process. They are used to enhance a code narrative to describe the circumstances of each procedure or service and how it individually applies to the patient. They are also essential ingredients to effectively communicate between providers and payers.

The correct use of modifiers is not difficult once a thorough understanding of their application is obtained. This section includes a review of the CPT modifiers which apply to chiropractic.

Modifiers have two different applications:

- Modifiers may be used to identify circumstances that significantly alter a service or procedure where reimbursement will be altered
- Modifiers may be informational only and have no impact on the normal reimbursement

Modifiers must be in two digits for all insurance claims. The 1500 claim form has space to report up to four modifiers.

Levels of Modifiers

There are three levels of modifiers. Two levels are approved by HIPAA.

- *Level I CPT numeric modifiers:* Two digits (eg, modifier 22 Increased Procedural Services) updated by the AMA yearly. There are 31 Level I modifiers.
- *Level II HCPCS alphabetic modifiers:* Ranges AA-VV are approved by HIPAA for all payers. They are updated annually by CMS.
- *Level III local modifiers:* Ranges WA-ZZ were deleted in 2003. However, Workers Compensation is exempt from HIPAA, and could have different modifiers and codes.

Level I CPT Modifiers

22   Increased Procedural Services

When the work required to provide a service is substantially greater than typically required, it may be identified by adding modifier 22 to the usual procedure code. Documentation must support the substantial additional work and the reason for the additional work (ie, **increased** intensity, time, technical difficulty of procedure, severity of patient's condition, physical and mental effort required). **Note:** This modifier should not be appended to an E/M service.

> Prior to 2008 this modifier was titled "Unusual Procedural Services." This editorial update supports the goal of "distinct reporting intent." It also clarifies that modifier 22 should not be used with an E/M service because E/M codes should use modifier 25.
>
> "In 2008 the title for modifier 22 was editorially revised to identify increased procedural services. The language was revised to include that substantially greater services than typically provided must be performed in order to report modifier 22. Documentation must support the substantial, additional work and the reason for the additional work." *CPT Changes 2008-An Insider's View*
>
> Reports are required to justify the use of this modifier and as such are closely reviewed by payers. This modifier describes services greater (more complex or time-consuming) than usual for the listed procedure. Because the physician expects greater payment from procedures using modifier 22, carriers closely watch its application and consistency of use.
>
> The nomenclature of the CPT codes is written to describe the normal, uncomplicated performance of specific procedures. When complications occur, modifier 22 should be added to the procedure code to modify the normal description and alert the payer to the unusual circumstances.
>
> It is appropriate to use modifier 22 under the following circumstances:
>
> - The complications cannot be identified by a separate code.
> - The procedure is lengthy and unusual, or beyond the code's description or RVU.
> - The services provided by the physician are increased because of unusual circumstances or complications. The work and effort would typically be increased by about 30-50 percent to justify using this modifier.
>
> Any report should include key words that highlight the increased difficulty and/or uniqueness of the procedure. Following are some of the key words that are often monitored by carriers. These words help document and justify the use of modifier 22:
>
> - Increased risk
> - Severe respiratory distress
> - Difficult
> - Extended
> - Complications
> - Unusual findings
> - Prolonged
> - Unusual contamination controls

Modifiers and HIPAA

Modifiers are divided into two groups or levels. All levels are updated annually (level I by the AMA and level II by CMS). Because of HIPAA, all prior level III local codes were eliminated in 2003; however, some payers have not yet reached full compliance and may still be using these old codes (e.g., WA to ZZ). Workers' Compensation state plans are exempt from HIPAA mandates and may have their own unique modifiers for their local payment policies.

The documentation should indicate specifics such as the length of time, the type of influencing circumstances, or the degree of difficulty which altered the original service. When modifier 22 is submitted, the claim is usually kicked out of the automated processing loop and sent to medical review. That is why an accurate clinical record with good documentation and descriptions are important (on paper or electronically).

Modifier 22 can also be used to substantiate a request for special considerations. An example would be when the chart supports the use of modifier 22. Commercial payers might allow an additional 20 to 30 percent of the procedure's value as additional reimbursement.

Example: *A patient presented for an adjustment of the spine at the chiropractor's office. The patient was a seventy-one year old obese diabetic patient. The chiropractor encountered difficulty in performing the manipulation on three areas of the spine due to the exceptionally large adipose deposits and extremely poor integrity of the muscle and fascia. The usually straightforward adjustment took an increased amount of time due to the difficulties encountered.*

Coding Example:

D PROCEDURES, SERVICES OR SUPPLIES (Explain Unusual Circumstances)	
CPT/HCPCS	MODIFIER
98941	22

25 Significant, Separately Identifiable Evaluation and Management Service by the Same Physician on the Same Day of a Procedure or Other Service

It may be necessary to indicate that on the day a procedure or service identified by a CPT code was performed, the patient's condition required a significant, separately identifiable E/M service above and beyond the other service provided or beyond the usual preoperative and postoperative care associated with the procedure that was performed. A significant, separately identifiable E/M service is defined or substantiated by documentation that satisfies the relevant criteria for the respective E/M service to be reported (see page H-21 for instructions on determining level of E/M service). The E/M service may be prompted by the symptom or condition for which the procedure and/or service was provided. As such, different diagnoses are not required for reporting of the E/M services on the same date. This circumstance may be reported by adding the modifier 25 to the appropriate level of E/M service. **Note:** For significant, separately identifiable non-E/M services, see modifier 59.

> The CPT introduction to the CMT (98940-98943) codes makes this official statement about E/M services: "The chiropractic manipulative treatment codes include a pre-manipulation patient assessment. Additional Evaluation and Management services may be reported separately using modifier 25, if the patient's condition requires a significant separately identifiable E/M service, above and beyond the usual preservice and postservice work associated with the procedure. The E/M service may be caused or prompted by the same symptoms or condition for which the CMT service was provided. As such, different diagnoses are not required for the reporting of the CMT and E/M service on the same date."

Modifier 25 is used when, on the day of a procedure, the patient's condition requires a separate E/M service above and beyond that provided with the routine preoperative and postoperative care. Without this E/M code modifier, the claim might automatically be denied by some payers.

A pure interpretation of this modifier would allow any physician to bill an E/M service on the day of a procedure if:

1. The E/M service is medically necessary and is a significant and separately identifiable service from the procedure being performed. Separate diagnostic codes are frequently used, **but the same diagnosis code may also be applicable.**

2. The documentation in the clinical record is sufficient to substantiate the E/M level of care billed. The only criteria is that the E/M service is beyond the routine (daily) E/M service associated and included in the CMT service.

E/M modifier 25 can be used whether the patient is new or established, or when there is one or more diagnoses. The physician's note must clearly indicate that the service provided was above and beyond the usual preoperative and postoperative care. If a separately identifiable service is rendered on the same day as a procedure (even if related), it should be paid. At the option of the payer, providers may be discounted for secondary services and may only receive a percentage of the amount billed.

Example: *A patient's **presenting problem** is a **suspicious knee** complaint and injury, in addition to their current treatment for sprain strain of neck. The physician performs a detailed history (E/M component #1) for the knee complaint and completes a thorough examination (E/M component #2) including the following test, sign, and reflex studies: Abduction stress test, external rotation-recurvatum test, knee flexion stress test, and Dreyer's sign.*

Coding Example:

PROCEDURES, SERVICES OR SUPPLIES (Explain Unusual Circumstances)	
CPT/HCPCS	MODIFIER
99214	25
98943	

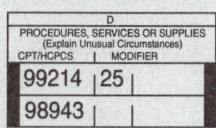

Afterward reviewing the tests and considering the treatment options (the E/M component #3), the physician performed a chiropractic adjustment of the knee to relieve pain.

Example: *An established patient is scheduled for a carpal tunnel adjustment on her wrist. When she comes to the office she reports that she is currently experiencing weakness, muscle spasms, and pain in her lower extremities. Her physician performs an adjustment to the wrist and neck for the carpal tunnel syndrome, and then spends additional time checking her general clinical condition, consisting of a detailed history and an expanded problem-focused physical with moderate to complex medical decision making due to the patient's generalized symptoms and seriousness of the origin of her pain, tingling, and muscle spasms.*

Coding Example:

PROCEDURES, SERVICES OR SUPPLIES (Explain Unusual Circumstances)	
CPT/HCPCS	MODIFIER
99214	25
98940	
98943	

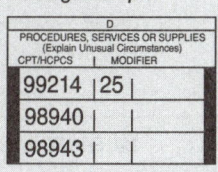

The chiropractic adjustment procedures are billed, as well as the E/M service, with modifier 25 appended to the E/M code.

Some payers might require an additional diagnosis to facilitate payment, but according to CPT guidelines this is not necessary when a separately identifiable service is furnished.

26   Professional Component

Certain procedures are a combination of a physician component and a technical component. When the physician component is reported separately, the service may be identified by adding the modifier 26 to the usual procedure number.

Modifier 26 includes the interpretation and report. Some procedures, such as x-rays, have both professional and technical components. Many of these procedures have companion codes. For example, x-rays are performed using a facility's equipment, and the technical component is billed by the facility. The physician can then bill for the professional component (reading the x-rays) using modifier 26.

Most private payers recognize the use of this modifier for those codes which have a professional and a technical component. They will pay the physician for his/her professional services and the facility for the technical component.

Coding Examples:

PROCEDURES, SERVICES OR SUPPLIES (Explain Unusual Circumstances)	
CPT/HCPCS	MODIFIER
72052	26

Physician's Office

Example: The radiologist performed a series of x-rays of the spine and billed the payer for the technical component (TC). The chiropractic physician billed for the professional component, which is the interpretation and management plan for the patient, using the modifier 26 appended to the CPT code for the specific service performed.

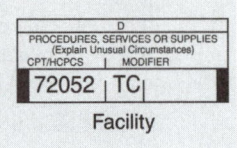

PROCEDURES, SERVICES OR SUPPLIES (Explain Unusual Circumstances)	
CPT/HCPCS	MODIFIER
72052	TC

Facility

32   Mandated Services

Services related to *mandated* consultation and/or related services (eg, third-party payer, governmental, legislative or regulatory requirement) may be identified by adding the modifier 32 to the basic procedure.

This modifier flags services required by outside sources other than the patient or the physician. If a court of law, agency, or insurance entity requires that a service be solicited, this modifier indicates such circumstances.

Depending on the payer benefit plans, reimbursement could be made at 100 percent of the allowed amount.

Example: The patient's insurance plan requires two opinions. The patient sees another practitioner for a **confirmatory consultation** *before the services were scheduled and pre-authorized. Modifier 32 signals to the insurer that the rules have been followed.*

Coding Example:

PROCEDURES, SERVICES OR SUPPLIES (Explain Unusual Circumstances)	
CPT/HCPCS	MODIFIER
99244	32

50   Bilateral Procedure

Unless otherwise identified in the listings, bilateral procedures that are performed at the same operative session, should be identified by adding the modifier 50 to the appropriate five digit code.

This modifier replaces the outdated "unilateral" and "bilateral" procedures found throughout older CPT manuals. Unless otherwise stated, procedures are considered unilateral in the codebook. In most cases, addition of the modifier 50 is the only way to report that the procedure was done on both sides. For example, when strapping is performed on the wrist on each arm, use 29260-50.

Private insurers recognize modifier 50 as long as it is used properly. In this example commercial carriers would accept billing for 29260-50. Care must be taken that the code description does not include language that describes "one or both" or "one or more" regions, which, of course, would make modifier 50 unnecessary.

In 1992, the AMA clarified in other publications the intent of the CPT guidelines for the modifier: for describing bilateral procedures as one-line entries which list the procedure code only once with modifier 50 attached. The units column would then be "1." Please note that some payers prefer having bilateral procedure codes listed twice, with modifier 50 attached to the second listing of the base procedure code.

Coding Example:

PROCEDURES, SERVICES OR SUPPLIES (Explain Unusual Circumstances)	
CPT/HCPCS	MODIFIER
29260	50

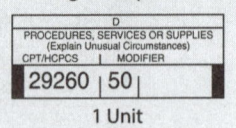

1 Unit

Some payers may prefer the reporting of the code as two line items, one with modifier RT and one with modifier LT.

Example: The patient has bilateral strapping on each side of the upper extremity (wrist or elbow).

51 Multiple Procedures

When multiple procedures, other than E/M Services, physical medicine and rehabilitation services, or provision of supplies (eg, vaccines), are performed at the same session by the same provider, the primary procedure or service may be reported as listed. The additional procedure(s) or service(s) may be identified by appending the modifier 51 to the additional procedure or service code(s). **Note:** This modifier should not be appended to designated add-on (✚) codes.

> **Alert:** According to the December 2013 issue of *CPT Assistant*, modifier 51 should **not** be appended to the CMT codes. These are separate and distinct procedures and the use of modifier 51 does not apply. However, it is possible that a payer might require the use of modifier 51 with 98943, extremity manipulation, when billed with 98940-98942. Be aware of individual payer policies which may vary from this standard.

52 Reduced Services

Under certain circumstances a service or procedure is partially reduced or eliminated at the physician's discretion. Under these circumstances the service provided can be identified by its usual procedure number and the addition of the modifier 52, signifying that the service is reduced. This provides a means of reporting reduced services without disturbing the identification of the basic service. **Note:** For hospital outpatient reporting of a previously scheduled procedure/service that is partially reduced or cancelled as a result of extenuating circumstances or those that threaten the well-being of the patient prior to or after administration of anesthesia, see modifiers 73 and 74 (see modifiers approved for ASC hospital outpatient use).

When a procedure is partially reduced, modifier 52 may be used in some situations. This alerts the payer that the service was not completed to its full extent, and provides a means of reporting reduced services without disturbing the identification of the basic service.

Coding Example:

D PROCEDURES, SERVICES OR SUPPLIES (Explain Unusual Circumstances)	
CPT/HCPCS	MODIFIER
97802	52

There are very few circumstances where this modifier applies in a chiropractic setting. Some possibilities could be the Acupuncture codes (97810-97814) or Medical Nutrition Therapy codes (97802-97804).

A cover letter describing the reduced service along with applicable documentation should accompany the claim.

Individual payer policies regarding modifier 52 may vary.

In additional to the use of modifier 52, it may also be appropriate to use a secondary or tertiary ICD code to document why the procedure was not completed. For example, V64.1 (procedure not carried out because of contraindication) or V64.3 (procedure not carried out for other reasons) may be used.

Alert: According to the March 2014 issue of *CPT Assistant*, it is not appropriate to append modifier 52 to Physical Medicine and Rehabilitation time-based codes (97110-97546). See page H-78 for more information.

| 53 | **Discontinued Procedure** |

Under certain circumstances, the physician may elect to terminate a surgical or diagnostic procedure. Due to extenuating circumstances or those that threaten the well being of the patient, it may be necessary to indicate that a surgical or diagnostic procedure was started but discontinued. This circumstance may be reported by adding the modifier 53 to the code reported by the physician for the discontinued procedure. **Note:** This modifier is not used to report the elective cancellation of a procedure prior to the patient's anesthesia induction and/or surgical preparation in the operating suite. For outpatient hospital/ambulatory surgery center (ASC) reporting of a previously scheduled procedure/service that is partially reduced or cancelled as a result of extenuating circumstances or those that threaten the well being of the patient prior to or after administration of anesthesia, see modifiers 73 and 74 (see modifiers approved for ASC hospital outpatient use).

| ▲ 59 | **Distinct Procedural Service** |

▶Under certain circumstances, it may be necessary to indicate that a procedure or service was distinct or independent from other non-E/M services performed on the same day. Modifier 59 is used to identify procedures/services, other than E/M services, that are not normally reported together, but are appropriate under the circumstances. Documentation must support a different session, different procedure or surgery, different site or organ system, separate incision/excision, separate lesion, or separate injury (or area of injury in extensive injuries) not ordinarily encountered or performed on the same day by the same individual. However, when another already established modifier is appropriate it should be used rather than modifier 59. Only if no more descriptive modifier is available, and the use of modifier 59 best explains the circumstances, should modifier 59 be used. **Note:** Modifier 59 should not be appended to an E/M service. To report a separate and distinct E/M service with a non-E/M service performed on the same date, see modifier 25.◀

Alert: Effective January 1, 2015, four new modifiers (XE, XS, XP, XU) have been created by CMS as a subset of modifier 59. While these modifiers have been created to further define Modifier 59, at the time of publication, these only apply to Medicare claims and therefore do not apply to services rendered by a doctor of chiropractic and payable by Medicare.

Check with private payers to see if they require the use of a modifier other than modifier 59 when billing timed therapy codes.

Warnings:

- Documentation in the chart/record should correctly record the parameters of treatment such as location, method of application, intensity, and time. It is fraudulent to alter documentation or billing in order to get paid.

- Simple procedures that do not require any professional clinical training, such as mechanical massage (i.e. the Genie Rub), are incidental to CMT and not billable.

Note: Some *non-government* payers do not require the use of a modifier when billing CMT with timed therapy codes.

- See Resource 392 to read more about the CMS announcement.
- See Resource 401 to read the NCCI instructions regarding modifier 59.

- See Chapter 2–Types of Insurance in *Section B–Insurance and Reimbursement* for more about benefit verification.

- See also Examples #7 and #11 in Chapter 7–Clinical Examples in this *Procedures* section for additional information.

62 Two Surgeons

When two surgeons work together as primary surgeons performing distinct part(s) of a procedure, each surgeon should report his/her distinct operative work by adding the modifier 62 to the procedure code and any associated add-on code(s) for that procedure as long as both surgeons continues to work together as primary surgeons. Each surgeon should report the co-surgery once using the same procedure code. If additional procedure(s) including add-on procedures are performed during the same surgical session, separate code(s) may also be reported with the modifier 62 added. **Note:** if a co-surgeon acts as an assistant in the performance of additional procedure(s) during the same surgical session, those services may be reported using separate procedure codes(s) with the modifier 80 or 82 added, as appropriate.

Surgeons and surgical procedures do not always mean a doctor with a knife or a knife, service (e.g., the "Application of a Cast or Strapping" is a surgical procedure from a CPT coding perspective). Accordingly, the surgical procedure code **22505–Manipulation of spine, requiring anesthesia, any region** can be done by qualified chiropractic physicians who have hospital or surgical center privileges.

Coding Example:

CPT/HCPCS	MODIFIER
22505	62 | 22

PROCEDURES, SERVICES OR SUPPLIES (Explain Unusual Circumstances)

This procedure is also known as Manipulation Under Anesthesia (MUA) in the chiropractic profession. The MUA procedure typically requires two doctors. Each doctor should bill 22505 with modifier 62. If the service is unusual, modifier 22 would also be appended with an accompanying report.

76 Repeat Procedure or Service By Same Physician

It may be necessary to indicate that a procedure or service was repeated subsequent to the original procedure or service. This circumstance may be reported by adding the modifier 76 to the repeated procedure or service.

Modifier 76 is used to report a "second" procedure which has been previously reported or performed on the same day. This may occur with interventions which must be aborted due to patient instability, or in cases where a "repeat" of the first minor procedure is necessary because the first minor procedure did not produce the desired or optimal results anticipated.

Coding Example:

CPT/HCPCS	MODIFIER
98940	76 | GA

PROCEDURES, SERVICES OR SUPPLIES (Explain Unusual Circumstances)

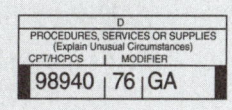

This modifier should assist in preventing denials for duplicate submission messages on EOMBs or payment reports. This modifier is usually used for radiology, laboratory, and minor surgical procedures, such as repeat blood sugar tests on the same day.

Commercial payers vary on the use of this modifier. Many do not recognize it at all, stating that they pay based on the procedure alone. Some recognize it during the global surgical period only. Others recognize it at all times when it is appropriate. In all cases the second procedure would be paid for and it would begin a new global surgical package period.

Example: A chiropractic adjustment was performed. Later that same day, no pain relief was indicated, so additional chiropractic adjustments were performed on the same date of service.

If a Medicare patient, use modifier GA and have a signed ABN form on file. Medicare will not pay for more than one CMT visit per day, and it becomes the patient's financial responsibility.

77 Repeat Procedure by Another Physician

The physician may need to indicate that a basic procedure or service performed by another physician had to be repeated. This situation may be reported by adding modifier 77 to the repeated procedure/service.

This modifier is identical to modifier 76 except that it is used when the physician repeating the procedure is **not** the same as the physician who performed the original service.

Modifiers 76 and 77 are usually not particularly reimbursement-oriented, but they are valuable in reporting the circumstances of a procedure correctly and are therefore "informational." They could "save" a claim from pending for an explanation or a denial for duplicate billing. Without this modifier the insurer could view the claim as double billing.

Coding Example:

D PROCEDURES, SERVICES OR SUPPLIES (Explain Unusual Circumstances)	
CPT/HCPCS	MODIFIER
72040	77 | 26

Additional X-ray interpretation by the DC

E/M coding by the key components includes a review and interpretation of the records and reports (x-ray, lab, etc.). However, if the x-ray report is incomplete, and a more comprehensive interpretation and report is clinically needed and performed, modifiers 26 (professional component) and 77 (repeat procedure by another physician) may be appended. In essence, your chiropractic report of the x-ray is a supplement to the initial incomplete radiologist report.

From a CPT coding perspective, it is proper to use modifier 26 for the professional component, along with modifier 77, which indicates a "repeat procedure." It would be appropriate to attach the incomplete report from the radiologist along with your comprehensive chiropractic relevancy analysis. This demonstrates to the person reviewing your claim the necessity for this "repeat" procedure.

Alert: Discussion with the patient about the x-rays is a **counseling** component within an E/M service. It is not a component of the x-ray/imaging test, interpretation and report.

80 Assistant Surgeon

Surgical assistant services may be identified by adding the modifier 80 to the usual procedure number(s).

81 Minimum Assistant Surgeon

Minimum surgical assistant services are identified by adding the modifier 81 to the usual procedure number.

90   Reference (Outside) Laboratory

When laboratory procedures are performed by a party other than the treating or reporting physician, the procedure may be identified by adding the modifier 90 to the usual procedure number.

> This modifier is used to indicate that an outside laboratory rendered the services, rather than the lab of the treating or reporting physician. This notifies the insurer that the lab services were furnished outside the physician's office and the physician is billing for the service.
>
> *Coding Example:*
>
> | PROCEDURES, SERVICES OR SUPPLIES (Explain Unusual Circumstances) | |
> |---|---|
> | CPT/HCPCS | MODIFIER |
> | 82951 | 90 |
> | 36415 | |
>
> This modifier could be used differently by non-Medicare payers. Some HMOs require that patients use specific labs with which they contract for services. In this case the physician may draw the blood (code 36415), modify the lab test by appending modifier 90 and send the specimen to the appropriate lab for testing. Other HMOs will allow the physician to bill them for the testing done in their office if they have CLIA lab certification. If a test needs to still be sent out to a reference lab the HMO may allow the physician to bill the patient for the test and then the physician will reimburse the lab later. Each carrier has their own policy regarding the use of physician labs or outside labs. In all cases payers will request information on who is actually providing the service.
>
> ***Example:*** *The patient went to the reference lab for a fasting glucose test. The laboratory and the physician's office had a billing agreement whereby the office could bill the patient (insurer) and the lab would then bill the physician's office for the service. Lab tests from the office, however, were submitted with modifier 90 (the HMO to which the patient belonged required this billing format).*
>
> **Note:** Medicare does not allow the above scenario to occur because the physician may only bill for the service that he/she actually provided. The laboratory would bill the Medicare patient and modifier 90 would not be used.

99   Multiple Modifiers

Under certain circumstances two or more modifiers may be necessary to completely delineate a service. In such situations modifier 99 should be added to the basic procedure, and other applicable modifiers may be listed as part of the description of the service.

> The paper 1500 claim form has space for up to four modifiers per procedure code. There would be very few circumstances in a chiropractic setting where there would be a need to report more than four modifiers. If such a situation arises, check with the payer to determine their preference for reporting this unique situation.

Level II HCPCS Procedure Modifiers

Modifier codes are approved jointly by the editorial panel consisting of the American Medical Association (AMA), Health Insurance Association of America (HIAA), and Blue Cross/Blue Shield (BC/BS). These two (2) digit modifier codes are appended to the basic code. Use of these national modifiers are at the option of private insurance carriers (payers). The following is a list of modifiers that might be of interest in a chiropractic office. Commonly used modifiers are in **bold type** for quick reference.

AE	Registered dietician
AF	Specialty physician
AG	Primary physician
AI	Principal physician of record
AK	Non participating physician
AM	Physician, team member service
AO	Alternate payment method declined by provider of service
AQ	Physician providing a service in an unlisted health professional shortage area (HPSA)
AR	Physician provider services in a physician scarcity area
AS	Physician assistant, nurse practitioner or clinical nurse specialist services for assistant at surgery
AT	**Acute treatment**

> Use modifier AT when reporting covered services 98940, 98941, 98942. This modifier is also known as active treatment by Medicare, which is a declaration that patients have an acute or chronic condition and active/corrective treatment is medically necessary.
>
> Consider using this quick test to determine if the AT modifier is appropriate. Is there:
> 1. A patient complaint in each area?
> 2. Objective findings to substantiate chiropractic care?
> 3. A plan to resolve the problem?
> 4. Demonstrable progress?

BO	Orally administered nutrition, not by feeding tube
CC	Procedure code change (use -CC when the procedure code submitted was changed either for administrative reasons or because an incorrect code was filed)
CG	Policy criteria applied
CH	0 percent impaired, limited or restricted
CI	At least 1 percent but less than 20 percent impaired, limited or restricted
CJ	At least 20 percent but less than 40 percent impaired, limited or restricted
CK	At least 40 percent but less than 60 percent impaired, limited or restricted
CL	At least 60 percent but less than 80 percent impaired, limited or restricted
CM	At least 80 percent but less than 100 percent impaired, limited or restricted
CN	100 percent impaired, limited or restricted
EJ	Subsequent claim for a defined course of therapy, eg EPO, sodium hyaluronate, infliximab
ET	**Emergency services**
EY	No physician or other licensed health care provider order for this item or service

F1	Left hand, second digit
F2	Left hand, third digit
F3	Left hand, fourth digit
F4	Left hand, fifth digit
F5	Right hand, thumb
F6	Right hand, second digit
F7	Right hand, third digit
F8	Right hand, fourth digit
F9	Right hand, fifth digit
FA	Left hand, thumb
GA	**Waiver of liability statement issued as required by payer policy, individual case**

> This is a declaration of the "ABN on file."

GB	Claim being resubmitted for payment because it is no longer covered under a global payment demonstration
GF	Non-physician (eg, nurse practitioner (NP), certified registered nurse anaesthetist (CRNA), certified registered nurse (CRN), clinical nurse specialist (CNS), physician assistant (PA)) services in a critical access hospital
GK	Reasonable and necessary item/service associated with GA or GZ modifier

> From a Medicare perspective, modifier GK's initial use was limited to Part A (hospitals) and DME (durable medical equipment) suppliers. It could expand to other providers because it clarifies matters. Non-Medicare payers could possibly use it, as it is an approved HIPAA code set. Accordingly, use by any payer is at their sole discretion.

GN	Services delivered under an outpatient speech language pathology plan of care
GO	Services delivered under an outpatient occupational therapy plan of care
GP	**Services delivered under an outpatient physical therapy plan of care**
GQ	Via asynchronous telecommunications system
GT	Via interactive audio and video telecommunication systems
GU	Waiver of liability statement issued as required by payer policy, routine
GW	Service not related to the hospice patient's terminal condition
GX	**Notice of liability issued, voluntary under payer policy**
GY	**Item or service statutorily excluded or, does not meet the definition of any Medicare benefit or, for non-Medicare insurers, is not a contract benefit**
GZ	**Item or service expected to be denied as not reasonable and necessary**
H9	Court-ordered
HI	Integrated mental health and intellectual disability/developmental disabilities program
HL	Intern
HN	Bachelors degree level
HO	Masters degree level
HP	Doctoral level
HQ	Group setting

HR	Family/couple with client present
HS	Family/couple without client present
HT	Multi-disciplinary team
JE	Administered via dialysate
KX	Specific required documentation on file
KZ	New coverage not implemented by managed care
LR	Laboratory round trip
LT	**Left side (used to identify procedures performed on the left side of the body)**
M2	**Medicare secondary payer (MSP)**
Q0	Investigational clinical service provided in a clinical research study that is in an approved clinical research study
Q1	Routine clinical service provided in a clinical research study that is in an approved clinical research study
Q5	Service furnished by a substitute physician under a reciprocal billing arrangement
Q6	Service furnished by a locum tenens physician
QC	Single channel monitoring
QD	Recording and storage in solid state memory by a digital recorder
QJ	Services/items provided to a prisoner or patient in state or local custody, however the state or local government, as applicable, meets the requirements in 42 CFR 411.4 (B)
QP	Documentation is on file showing that the laboratory test(s) was ordered individually or ordered as a CPT-recognized panel other than automated profile codes 80002-80019, G0058, G0059, and G0060
QT	Recording and storage on tape by an analog tape recorder
QW	CLIA waived test
	The Centers for Medicare and Medicaid Services (CMS) regulates all laboratory testing (except research) performed on humans in the U.S. due to the Clinical Laboratory Improvement Amendments (CLIA). When a simple lab test is exempt from CLIA oversight, append modifier QW.
RT	**Right side (used to identify procedures performed on the right side of the body)**
SA	Nurse practitioner rendering service in collaboration with a physician
SC	**Medically necessary service or supply**
SE	State and/or federally-funded programs/services
ST	**Related to trauma or injury**
SU	**Procedure performed in physician's office (to denote use of facility and equipment)**
SV	Pharmaceuticals delivered to patient's home but not utilized
SW	Services provided by a certified diabetic educator
SY	Persons who are in close contact with member of high-risk population (use only with codes for immunization)
T1	Left foot, second digit
T2	Left foot, third digit

T3	Left foot, fourth digit
T4	Left foot, fifth digit
T5	Right foot, great toe
T6	Right foot, second digit
T7	Right foot, third digit
T8	Right foot, fourth digit
T9	Right foot, fifth digit
TA	Left foot, great toe
TC	**Technical component**

> Under certain circumstances, a charge may be made for the technical component only. It is identified by appending modifier TC. Technical component charges are usually institutional charges and not billed by providers. Portable x-ray suppliers usually bill for the technical component with modifier TC.
>
> When only the technical component is performed, it does not include the interpretation and report (professional component 26). When no modifier is used (TC or 26) it is a declaration that both components are performed.

TF	**Intermediate level of care**
TG	**Complex/high tech level of care**
TM	Individualized education program (IEP)
TN	Rural/outside providers' customary service area
TS	**Follow-up service**
TT	Individualized service provided to more than one patient in same setting
TU	Special payment rate, overtime
TV	**Special payment rates, holidays/weekends**
UF	Services provided in the morning
UG	Services provided in the afternoon
UH	Services provided in the evening
UJ	Services provided at night
UK	Services provided on behalf of the client to someone other than the client (collateral relationship)
UN	**Two patients served**
UP	**Three patients served**
UQ	**Four patients served**
UR	**Five patients served**
US	**Six or more patients served**

7. Clinical Examples
by the ACA

These clinical examples or coding vignettes by the American Chiropractic Association (ACA) are examples of situations that could be encountered by a chiropractic office. They are **not** examples of office notes or documentation examples.

This chapter is divided into the following sections:

- Chiropractic Manipulative Treatment
- Evaluation and Management Services
- Other Related Chiropractic Services
- Telephone Services
- Online Medical Evaluations
- Preventative Medicine Services
- Preventative Medicine Counseling or Risk Factor Reductions

Guide to Clinical Examples

Code	Description	Page
97124	Massage	H-119, H-121
97140	Manual Therapy Techniques	H-118, H-120, H-121
	Chiropractic manipulative treatment, spinal,	
98940	1-2 Regions	H-114, H-119, H-120
98941	3-4 Regions	H-114, H-121
98942	5 Regions	H-115
98943	Chiropractic manipulative treatment, extraspinal, 1 or more regions	H-115
	Office or other outpatient visit,	
99201	typically 10 minutes	H-116
99202	typically 20 minutes	H-116
99203	typically 30 minutes	H-116
99204	typically 45 minutes	H-117
99205	typically 60 minutes	H-117
99211	typically 5 minutes	H-118
99212	typically 10 minutes	H-118
99213	typically 15 minutes	H-118
99214	typically 25 minutes	H-118

Physician telephone patient service,

99441	5-10 minutes of medical discussion	H-122
99442	11-20 minutes of medical discussion	H-122
99443	21-30 minutes of medical discussion	H-122
99444	Physician internet (e-mail) patient care related to patient visit within previous 7 days	H-122

Initial new patient preventive medicine evaluation,

99381	infant younger than 1 year	H-122
99382	age 1 through 4 years	H-122
99383	age 5 through 11 years	H-122
99384	age 12 through 17 years	H-122
99385	age 18-39 years	H-124
99386	age 40-64 years	H-124
99387	age 65 years and older	H-124

Established patient periodic preventive medicine examination,

99391	infant younger than 1 year	H-124
99392	age 1 through 4 years	H-124
99393	age 5 through 11 years	H-125
99394	age 12 through 17 years	H-125
99395	age 18-39 years	H-125
99396	age 40-64 years	H-125
99397	age 65 years and older	H-125

Preventive medicine counseling,

99401	approximately 15 minutes	H-126
99402	approximately 30 minutes	H-126
99403	approximately 45 minutes	H-126
99404	approximately 60 minutes	H-126

Group preventive medicine counseling,

99411	approximately 30 minutes	H-127
99412	approximately 60 minutes	H-127

Clinical Examples for CMT Codes

The following are examples of clinical situations and appropriate use of the CMT codes. They are meant only as a guide and are in no way representative of all clinical situations or manipulative technique that would require use of the CMT codes.

Example #1

98940   Chiropractic manipulative treatment, spinal, 1-2 Regions

This clinical example describes CMT service on two (2) spinal body regions of an established patient previously scheduled for this service. The previous initial examination of the patient revealed a 32-year-old female with mid-back pain, stiffness, and persistent low-back pain of two weeks' duration (2 body regions-thoracic and lumbar).

> *Description of Preservice Work*
>
> A brief evaluation of the patient reveals that chiropractic spinal manipulative treatment is clinically indicated in 2 regions: the thoracic (T5) region and the lumbar (L4) region.
>
> *Description of Intraservice Work*
>
> Diversified manipulation to T5 and to L4.
>
> *Description of Postservice Work*
>
> Chart entry and documentation, including documentation of appropriate subjective and objective assessments as well as the procedural components of this patient visit, are completed.

Example #2

98941   Chiropractic manipulative treatment, spinal, 3-4 Regions

This clinical example describes CMT service on three (3) spinal body regions of an established patient previously scheduled for this service. The previous initial examination of the patient revealed a 44-year-old man with complaints of a persistent tension-type headache noted daily for the last six months. Regular use of muscle relaxants decreased the pain temporarily, but he developed gastrointestinal irritation from the medication and is seeking a different approach to treatment. Secondarily, he described lowback pain that was noted intermittently for the past two years, but was most recently aggravated by a long bike ride. The ride aggravated his back pain to the point that he can no longer get a full night's rest due to his right-sided pelvic pain and lumbar aching (3 body regions-cervical, lumbar, pelvic).

> *Description of Preservice Work*
>
> A brief evaluation of the patient reveals that chiropractic spinal manipulative treatment is clinically indicated in 3 regions: the cervical region (C2), the lumbar region (multiple lumbar segments), and the pelvic region (right innominate).
>
> *Description of Intraservice Work*
>
> Diversified manipulation of C2; diversified right innominate adjustment of the pelvic region; and multisegmental Gonstead lumbar adjustments.

Description of Postservice Work

Chart entry and documentation, including documentation of appropriate subjective and objective assessments as well as the procedural components of this patient visit are completed. A brief telephone consultation or written summary with the patient's insurance company or referring provider to supply an update of patient progress is also conducted.

Example #3

98942   Chiropractic manipulative treatment, spinal, 5 Regions

This clinical example describes CMT on five (5) spinal body regions of an established patient previously scheduled for this service. The previous initial examination of the patient revealed a 38-year-old male who sustained injuries to multiple body parts from a fall off an extension ladder.

While trying to prevent the fall, he twisted and strained his upper and lower back and struck his head. He landed on his side on the collapsed ladder injuring his pelvis and hip. Complaints of five days' duration include neck, mid and lower back pain and stiffness, headache, and pelvic and hip pain stiffness (5 body regions-cervical, thoracic, lumbar, pelvic and sacral).

Description of Preservice Work

A brief evaluation of the patient including a review of symptoms and a focused examination of the problem and related areas reveals that chiropractic spinal manipulative treatment is clinically indicated in 5 regions: the cervical region (C5), the thoracic region (T3, T6), the lumbar region (L5), the pelvic region (left innominate), and the sacral region (sacrum).

Description of Intraservice Work

Diversified manipulation of C5; diversified manipulation of T3 and T6; Gonstead adjustment of L5; and diversified manipulation of the sacrum and left innominate.

Description of Postservice Work

Chart entry and documentation including documentation of appropriate subjective and objective assessments as well as the procedural components of this patient visit are completed. A consultation to follow up with patient's general practitioner/internist to update on patient progress.

Example #4

98943   Chiropractic manipulative treatment, extraspinal, 1 or more regions

This clinical example describes CMT on one (1) extraspinal body region on an established patient previously scheduled for this service. The previous initial examination revealed a 52-year-old patient with moderate right-sided carpal tunnel syndrome for which surgery was unsuccessful.

Besides right hand weakness and numbness, she also complains of forearm and elbow pain, which worsens as the day goes on (1 extraspinal region-upper extremities).

Description of Preservice Work (for the extraspinal portion of the service only)

A brief evaluation of the patient reveals that a chiropractic extraspinal manipulation treatment is clinically indicated in one region: the upper right extremities (elbow and hand).

Do not code from these clinical examples. Go to the procedure code pages for detailed code information.

Description of Intraservice Work

Manipulation to the right elbow; and manipulation to the right hand and wrist.

Description of Postservice Work

Chart entry and documentation, including documentation of appropriate subjective and objective assessments as well as the procedural components of this patient visit are completed.

CLINICAL EXAMPLES FOR E/M

The clinical examples included with the following are intended to illustrate clinical situations and appropriate use of the following E/M codes.

They are meant only as a guide and are in no way representative of all clinical situations that would require use of the E/M codes by chiropractic providers.

Example #5, Evaluation and Management Codes for New Patients

99201   Office or other outpatient visit, typically 10 minutes

16-year-old female high school athlete presents with severe right ankle pain and swelling after tripping yesterday.

- No history of similar problems.
- Complaints and significant findings are limited to the right ankle region.
- Treatment plan is formulated consistent with a straightforward diagnosis of right ankle strain/sprain.

99202   Office or other outpatient visit, typically 20 minutes

28-year-old male administrative assistant awoke this morning with right-sided neck pain.

- No history of trauma. Patient notes similar episode of lesser severity approximately one year ago following prolonged computer work.
- Patient appears healthy, and vital signs are normal. There is point tenderness along with restricted range of motion in the right cervical spine. There are no abnormal neurological findings.
- Treatment plan is formulated consistent with a straightforward diagnosis of acute cervical myofascitis.

99203   Office or other outpatient visit, typically 30 minutes

42-year-old mother of two bent over to pick up baby from the car seat one week ago. Patient noted immediate onset of moderate right-sided lower back pain that radiates into the right leg with numbness in the right foot.

- Diagnosed with Grade #1 spondylolisthesis at 20 years old and has experienced periodic episodes of regional low-back pain.
- Patient appears healthy, vital signs are normal, and antalgic posture is noted. No bowel or bladder impairment. Proprioception is normal. There are no signs of varicosities. There is midline tenderness and restricted range of motion in the lumbar spine. Sensory abnormalities are present in the right lower extremity; however, deep tendon reflexes and muscle strengths are normal.

- Medical decision making is focused on assessment of spondylolisthesis and radiculopathy. Plan includes lumbar spine x-rays to assess spondylolisthesis. Treatment plan is formulated consistent with noted diagnoses.

99204 Office or other outpatient visit, typically 45 minutes

57-year-old obese and hypertensive female truck driver presents with constant moderate dull burning left-sided neck pain and arm referral of insidious onset. Pain has gotten progressively worse over past 48 hours—sought urgent care yesterday.

- All body systems reviewed. Findings are negative, with the exception of insulin dependent diabetes and prior similar musculoskeletal complaints.
- Patient smokes one pack of cigarettes per day. Past history is otherwise unremarkable. Family history of heart disease and diabetes.
- Cranial nerves and EENT are normal. Respiration rate is normal. Cardiovascular examination is normal. Palpation of lymph nodes is normal, but there is point tenderness at T4-6. Examination of neck and thyroid normal.
- There is point tenderness along with restricted range of motion in the cervical spine. There is diminished sensation in the left upper extremity. Muscle strength and deep tendon reflexes are diminished. Reviewed urgent care records, including laboratory, that were faxed.
- Medical decision making is focused on ruling out myocardial infarction and assessment of cervical condition, including investigation of possible disc involvement. Plan includes cervical MRI and coordination of care for hypertension and diabetes. Treatment plan is formulated consistent with noted diagnoses.

99205 Office or other outpatient visit, typically 60 minutes

48-year-old male construction worker complains of progressive lower-back pain over past four days. Left buttock and posterior thigh pain of two days duration. Awoke this morning with marked increased low-back pain, numbness in the anal region, and a mild inability to control his bladder.

Patient brought x-rays and medical records from previous providers. All body systems reviewed. Findings are negative, with the exception of prostatic hypertrophy, lumbar spondylosis, and multiple-year history of episodic low-back and left lower extremity pain. Patient smokes three packs of cigarettes per day and drinks heavily. Past history is otherwise unremarkable.

- Family history of coronary artery disease.
- Cranial nerves and EENT are normal. Respiration rate is normal. Cardiovascular examination is normal. There are no upper motor neuron findings.
- Digital rectal examination reveals decreased sphincter tone and prostatic hypertrophy. Palpation of lymph nodes is normal. Examination of neck and thyroid are normal. There is severe muscle spasm in the left lumbar region with flexion antalgia and restricted range of motion in the lumbar spine. There is "saddle" anesthesia. Muscle strength, peripheral sensation, and deep tendon reflexes are unremarkable.
- Medical decision making is focused on confirming caudaequina diagnosis. Plan includes lumbar MRI, coordination of care with neurosurgeon, and conferencing with family to discuss diagnosis of cauda equine and risks.

Example #6, Evaluation and Management Codes for Established Patients

99211   Office or other outpatient visit, typically 5 minutes

64-year-old male, with history of mild hypertension, returns for follow-up blood pressure check.

99212   Office or other outpatient visit, typically 10 minutes

36-year-old female kindergarten teacher awoke with right scapular pain. Pain began after vacuuming.

Patient appears healthy and vital signs are normal. Point tenderness over T4-7 with active trigger points along right rhomboid. Treatment plan is formulated consistent with a straight forward diagnosis of acute right thoracic myofascitis.

99213   Office or other outpatient visit, typically 15 minutes

15-year-old male, who was seen one month ago, presents with a new injury in the right knee, which he hyperextended during a gymnastics meet.

- The pain is sharp, constant, and aggravated by weight-bearing and extension of the knee.
- The patient appears healthy, and vital signs are normal. The knee is swollen and tender with restricted range of motion. There is no sign of ligamentous instability, and muscle strength is normal. Treatment plan is formulated consistent with an acute knee sprain.

99214   Office or other outpatient, visit typically 25 minutes

A 52-year-old male presents with low-back pain after motor vehicle collision yesterday. Reported to emergency room immediately.

- History of intermittent neck pain consistent with previous diagnosis of cervical degenerative disc disease. Two years prior underwent successful left knee total joint replacement and has experienced intermittent low-back pain.
- Patient appears fit for his age, and vital signs are normal. Face is flushed, and blood pressure is slightly elevated. No sensory abnormalities; deep tendon reflexes are normal. Gait is normal. Palpation reveals tenderness of cervical and lumbar spine. Abdomen is soft and non-tender. Range of motion is restricted in both cervical and lumbar. There are no signs of ligamentous laxity. Muscle strengths are normal. All deep-tendon reflexes are within normal limits. There is normal upper- and lower- extremity peripheral sensation.
- Medical decision making is focused on assessment of acute cervical and lumbar spine injuries, including review of emergency room medical records and x-rays. Treatment plan is formulated consistent with a diagnosis of cervical and lumbar strain/sprains complicated by the presence of degenerative disc disease.

CLINICAL EXAMPLES FOR OTHER CHIROPRACTIC RELATED SERVICES

The following examples are intended to give the practitioner examples of clinical situations and appropriate use of physical medicine codes used alone and in conjunction with CMT codes. They are only meant as informational or hypothetical situations and are not intended or designed to establish a standard of clinical care or documentation. Also, these examples are not intended to be representative of all clinical situations described by a physical medicine or CMT code. All procedures should be recorded in the patient record. It is important to note that the code 97140 is reported for any number of treatment regions and is also a time-based code with units of treatment reported for each 15 minute measure of time.

Example #7

An established 39-year-old female presents to the clinic with chief complaints of cervical pain. There is a 72-hour history of the complaints, with no specific history of trauma, and the patient relates that she awoke with the complaints. She reports extreme tenderness in the cervical region, with additional reports of limited mobility. The doctor's evaluation revealed specific point tenderness, asymmetrical spasm of paracervical muscles, and an active trigger point in the belly of the left SCM muscle.

Treatment was at correcting a vertebral subluxation complex utilizing an adjustive technique. Following this procedure, post-adjustment assessment revealed increased range of motion, although there was slight limitation of motion secondary to a muscular end point restriction and expression of subjective complaints by the patient. The doctor then applied manual pressure in order to relieve the muscle spasm and utilized pressure point work, including five minutes of trigger point therapy (ischemic compression) and ten minutes of deep tissue cross friction massage in the belly of the involved muscles.

This treatment encounter would reasonably be reported as follows:

- **98940** Chiropractic manipulative treatment (CMT); spinal, one to two regions
- **97124** Massage, including effleurage, petrissage and/or tapotement (stroking, compression, percussion)

See page H-104 in Chapter 6–Procedure Modifiers for more about possible billing problems and the usage of modifer 59.

Note: In this example, 97124 is being performed at the same anatomic site as the adjustment and is thus correctly documented without Modifier 59. Be aware that the AMA and NCCI differ on the appropriateness of coding 97124 with CMT services. Although the AMA has stated that 97124 should not be bundled with CMT codes, NCCI edits state that they may not be billed together when performed to the same anatomic site. Some payer policies and edits differ from this standard and may require modifier 59 to be appended for reimbursement even when performed on the same site. As such, it is crucial to verify the insurer's policy prior to performing these procedures to the same anatomic region on the same date of service.

Example #8

An established 45-year-old male presents to the clinic with chief complaints of severe cervical and lumbosacral pain as the result of injuries incurred in a high-speed, head-on motor vehicle accident. At the time he received emergency medical treatment, with transportation to a hospital where an evaluation, diagnostic imaging and physical examination was performed. He was given a rigid cervical collar for support. Following release from the emergency room, the patient reported to his chiropractor.

History was taken and examination performed. His x-rays were requested from the emergency room and he was scheduled for care to begin the following day. He was diagnosed as having moderate soft tissue injuries in the cervical region, as well as moderate soft tissue injuries in the lumbar region. The doctor's assessment reflects that the severity of the cervical spine soft tissue injuries at present contraindicates osseous manipulation and/or adjustment. The patient's cervical spine treatment consisted of manual traction for five minutes and an additional ten minutes of postfacilitation stretch, post-isometric relaxation, and reciprocal inhibition techniques.

In the lumbar and pelvic regions, the patient receives osseous manipulative techniques. The patient tolerates the procedures well and is scheduled for a follow-up visit.

This treatment encounter would reasonably be reported as follows:

- **98940** Chiropractic manipulative treatment (CMT); spinal, one to two regions
- **97140-59** Manual therapy techniques (e.g., mobilization/manipulation, manual lymphatic drainage, manual traction), one or more regions, each 15 minutes (to describe the five minutes of manual traction and ten minutes of muscle energy techniques applied to the cervical region)

> **Note:** Modifier 59 Distinct Procedural Service-under certain circumstances, it may be necessary to indicate that a procedure or service was distinct or independent from other non-E/M services performed on the same day. Modifier 59 is used to identify procedures or services, other than E/M services, that are not normally reported together but are appropriate under the circumstances. Documentation must support a different session, different procedure or surgery, different site or organ system, separate incision or excision, separate lesion, or separate injury (or area of injury in extensive injuries) not ordinarily encountered or performed on the same day by the same individual. However, when another already established modifier is appropriate it should be used rather than modifier 59. Only if no more descriptive modifier is available, and the use of modifier 59 best explains the circumstances, should modifier 59 be used. Note: Modifier 59 should not be appended to an E/M service. To report a separate and distinct E/M service with a non-E/M service performed on the same date, see modifier 25.

See page H-104 in Chapter 6–Procedure Modifiers for more about possible billing problems and the usage of modifer 59.

Example #9

An established 45-year-old male presents to the office with exacerbation of chronic cervical pain, which flared up after sleeping two days prior. The patient's subjective complaints revealed acute cervical and thoracic regional com plaints of a non-radicular nature. Objectively, there was decreased cervical range of motion, no active extension, passive extension was reduced by 50% of normal limits, and there were active trigger points in the trapezius and sternocleidomastoid musculature. Treatment consisted of a five-minute spray and stretch procedure to the palpable trigger points in the trapezius and SCM muscles. The provider also performed, and recorded the results of, a ten-minute session of isometric contraction and relaxation techniques for the purpose of improving joint mobility in the affected ranges of motion.

This treatment encounter would reasonably be reported as follows:

- **97140** Manual therapy techniques, (e.g., mobilization/manipulation, manual lymphatic drainage, manual traction), one or more regions, each 15 minutes

Example #10

An established 45-year-old male presents for follow-up treatment of acute cervical and thoracic, non-radicular, complaints of pain. Objectively, there was decreased cervical range of motion, no active extension, with passive extension reduced by 50% and active trigger points in the trapezius and sternocleidomastoid muscles. Treatment was directed at correcting a vertebral subluxation complex of the C4 and C5 levels on the right and the C7-T1 level. Post-manipulative procedures, in the same region, included a brief session of post-isometric contraction and relaxation for the purpose of improving joint mobility.

This treatment encounter would reasonably be reported as follows:

- **98940** Chiropractic manipulative treatment (CMT); spinal, one to two regions

Example #11

An established 75-year-old woman presents for follow-up treatment of injuries incurred when she fell down a flight of steps. Subjectively, the patient complained of neck, mid-back and lower-back pain of slight to moderate severity. Objectively, spinal subluxation was identified by decreased passive range of motion, as well as significant asymmetrical paravertebral muscle spasm. There was evidence of a stable compression fracture of the T10 level, with substantial underlying degenerative joint disease and osteoporosis. Initial treatment consisted of effleurage and petrissage techniques for 15 minute interval to the thoracic and cervical areas. Treatment was directed at correcting the vertebral subluxation complex utilizing adjust ments to the cervical, lumbar and pelvic regions.

This treatment encounter would reasonably be reported as follows:

- **98941** Chiropractic manipulative treatment (CMT); spinal, three to four regions
- **97124** Massage, including effleurage, petrissage and/or tapotement

> **Note:** For traditional massage techniques, use CPT® 97124. The doctor, or therapist under the doctor's supervision, performs this service through direct contact with the patient.
>
> The July 1999 CPT Assistant reflects a question regarding manual therapy techniques, which asks to provide a description of the manual therapy techniques that may be reported with code 97140. The AMA comment is generally accurate, with the exception of inclusion of the descriptor "therapeutic massage." ACA's coding experts confirmed with AMA staff that the author's intent was to describe a form of soft tissue mobilization. The 97124 massage service includes effleurage, petrissage and/or tapotement (stroking, compression, percussion). The 97124 procedure describes a service that is different from the services that are inclusive in 97140. The services in 97140 are defined as active in nature. The 97124 services, unlike these techniques, are passive in nature and the patient does not participate in the procedure when the various massage techniques are applied to the patient.
>
> The American Physical Therapy Association coding proposal for 97140 had an accepted component indicating that massage has enough significant differences, from soft tissue mobilization, that it should be retained as a separate and distinct CPT code, as the current nomenclature described. This was accepted by the CPT Editorial Panel. However, as 97124 is a "related" service, there are many CCI coding edits that hinder the reimbursement of 97124 and 97140 on the same date of service.

> **Note:** In this example, 97124 is being performed at the same anatomic site as the adjustment and is thus correctly documented without modifier 59. Be aware that the AMA and NCCI differ on the appropriateness of coding 97124 with CMT services. Although the AMA has stated that 97124 should not be bundled with CMT codes, NCCI edits state that they may not be billed together when performed to the same anatomic site. Some payer policies and edits differ from this standard and may require modifier 59 to be appended for reimbursement even when performed on the same site. As such, it is crucial to verify the insurer's policy prior to performing these procedures to the same anatomic region on the same date of service.

CLINICAL EXAMPLES FOR TELEPHONE SERVICES

Example #12

99441   Physician telephone patient service, 5-10 minutes of medical discussion

An established patient calls with a new complaint of an injury incurred while running. The chiropractor obtains a brief history including the patient's attempt at self-treatment and the chiropractor then makes treatment recommendations, advice on bracing and home care measures and properly documents this information in the patient's clinical record. The patient is advised to call if the symptoms fail to improve.

Example #13

99442   Physician telephone patient service, 11-20 minutes of medical discussion

A patient calls the office of a chiropractor to discuss the onset of neck pain after traveling on a plane. The chiropractor obtains a brief history and makes recommendations that include advice on positions of comfort and home care measures. This interaction is recorded in the patient's clinical record. The patient is advised to call if the character of symptoms change or increase in severity. The call lasts 15 minutes and no office visit is required.

Example #14

99443   Physician telephone patient service, 21-30 minutes of medical discussion

An established geriatric patient calls to discuss onset of new episodes of pain incurred while performing at home exercises. The Chiropractor reviews the history including a review of systems, obtains a description of symptoms, and gathers information on the current exercise program. He/she makes a recommendation to change the present therapeutic exercise program and provides instruction in home care measures and spine sparing positions of comfort, which are recorded in the patient's clinical record. He/she requests follow-up in the office in one week or sooner if complaints change character or increase in severity. The call lasts 25 minutes.

CLINICAL EXAMPLES FOR ONLINE MEDICAL EVALUATIONS

Example #15

99444   Physician internet (e-mail) patient care related to patient visit within previous 7 days

An established patient emails the chiropractor to discuss a new injury incurred while weight lifting. The provider obtains a brief history and makes treatment recommendations to include home care measures and positions of comfort, as well as modification in weightlifting techniques, all of which are recorded in the patient's medical record. The patient is instructed to call if symptoms are increasing. No office visit is required.

Clinical Examples for Preventive Medicine Service Codes

Example #16, Preventive Medicine Services for New Patients

99381   Initial new patient preventive medicine evaluation infant younger than 1 year

A first time patient, male, 3-months of age, is brought in by his mother for general health evaluation. A complete family, social and medical history is taken along with a comprehensive physical examination. A complete review of systems is performed. The baby's growth and development are evaluated, including height and weight, head circumference, and hearing, as well as developmental milestones. Guidance is provided to the mother regarding appropriate use of an infant car seat; proper nutrition including continued breast-feeding; and sleep practices. Risk factors for injury or illness are discussed, along with methods to address them.

99382   Initial new patient preventive medicine evaluation, age 1 through 4 years

A healthy 3-year old girl, who is a new patient in this office, is brought in by her parents for health evaluation and supervision. A complete family, social and medical history is taken along with a comprehensive physical examination. A complete review of systems is performed.

The child's growth and development are evaluated, including height and weight and developmental milestones. Guidance is provided to the parents regarding injury prevention, including appropriate use of the car seat; nutrition; discipline and sleep practices. Risk factors are discussed and methods to address them.

99383   Initial new patient preventive medicine evaluation, age 5 through 11 years

A healthy 11-year-old male new patient is brought in by his father for health supervision and evaluation. A complete family, social and medical history is reviewed along with a review of systems. A comprehensive physical examination including height and weight, blood pressure and dental health screening is performed. Guidance is provided to the child and his father about good health habits and self care, including adequate physical activity, proper nutrition and maintenance of healthy weight.

Risk factors and methods to address them are discussed with the child and parent.

99384   Initial new patient preventive medicine evaluation, age 12 through 17 years

A female 16 year old new patient presents for health supervision and evaluation. A complete family, social and medical history is taken along with a comprehensive physical examination including height and weight, blood pressure and dental health. A complete review of systems is performed.

Scoliosis screening is done. Growth, development and behavior are assessed. Anticipatory guidance is provided regarding social habits and self care, including physical activity and good diet. Risk factors are discussed, including drug and alcohol use, tobacco use, driving responsibly and using seat belts.

99385   Initial new patient preventive medicine evaluation age 18-39 years

A new patient, 33 year old male, presents for a complete health evaluation and physical examination. He has no specific complaints or problems. A complete family, social and medical history is taken along with a comprehensive physical examination including vital signs and Body Mass Index. A complete review of systems is performed, including screening for depression. Risk factors including poor diet, tobacco use and alcohol abuse are identified. Interventions for risk factors identified are discussed. Cholesterol and blood glucose screening are recommended.

99386   Initial new patient preventive medicine evaluation age 40-64 years

A 54 year old male presents to the office for the first time for a complete health evaluation and physical examination. His complete past medical, family and social history is reviewed. Review of systems is completed. A complete age appropriate physical exam is performed including biomechanical assessment, BP, BMI and digital rectal exam. Counseling is provided regarding diet and exercise, colorectal cancer screening and smoking cessation.

99387   Initial new patient preventive medicine evaluation, age 65 years and older

A 69-year-old male, new patient, presents for a complete health evaluation and physical examination. A complete past, family and social history is taken along with a comprehensive physical examination including vital signs and Body Mass Index. A complete review of systems is performed, including screening for depression. Risk factors are identified, including weight loss, tobacco use, alcohol abuse and risk of fall. Screening is indicated for abdominal aortic aneurysm, lipids and colorectal cancer.

ESTABLISHED PATIENT

Example #17, Preventive Medicine Services for Established Patients

99391   Established patient periodic preventive medicine examination, infant younger than 1 year

An established female patient, 9-months of age, is brought in by his mother for general health evaluation. A complete family, social and medical history is taken along with a comprehensive physical examination. A complete review of systems is performed. The baby's growth and development are evaluated, including height and weight, head circumference, and hearing, as well as developmental milestones. Guidance is provided to the mother regarding injury prevention, including appropriate use of the infant car seat; hydration, nutrition; and sleep practices. Risk factors for injury or illness are discussed, along with methods to address them.

99392   Established patient periodic preventive medicine examination, age 1 through 4 years

A healthy 2-year old girl, who is an established patient in this office, is brought in by her parents for health evaluation and supervision. A complete family, social and medical history is taken along with a comprehensive physical examination. A complete review of systems is performed.

The child's growth and development are evaluated, including height and weight and developmental milestones. Guidance is provided to the parents regarding injury prevention, including appropriate use of the car seat; nutrition; discipline and sleep practices. Risk factors are discussed and methods to address them.

99393 Established patient periodic preventive medicine examination, age 5 through 11 years

A healthy 10-year-old boy who is an established patient, is brought in by his father for health supervision and evaluation. A complete family, social and medical history is taken along with a comprehensive physical examination including height and weight, blood pressure and dental health screening. A complete review of systems is performed. Guidance is provided to the child and his parent about good health habits and self care, including adequate physical activity and good diet. Risk factors are discussed and methods to address them.

99394 Established patient periodic preventive medicine examination, age 12 through 17 years

A female established patient, 15 years of age, presents for health supervision and evaluation. A complete family, social and medical history is taken along with a comprehensive physical examination including height and weight, blood pressure and dental health. A complete review of systems is performed. Scoliosis screening is done. Growth, development and behavior are assessed. Anticipatory guidance is provided regarding health habits and self care, including physical activity and good diet. Risk factors are discussed, including drug and alcohol use, tobacco use, driving responsibly, using seat belts, and safe sex.

99395 Established patient periodic preventive medicine examination age 18-39 years

A 21-year old man, established patient, presents for a complete health evaluation and physical examination. A complete family, social and medical history is taken along with a comprehensive physical examination including height, weight and Body Mass Index (BMI) and blood pressure. A complete review of systems is performed, including screening for depression.

Risk factors are identified, including poor diet, tobacco use, alcohol and drug use, injury prevention including driving responsibly and using seat belts, and risky sexual behavior. Interventions for risk factors identified are discussed. Cholesterol screening is recommended.

99396 Established patient periodic preventive medicine examination age 40-64 years

A 49-year old woman, established patient, presents for a complete health evaluation and physical examination. A complete family, social and medical history is taken along with a comprehensive physical examination including height, weight and Body Mass Index (BMI) and blood pressure. A complete review of systems is performed, including screening for depression.

Risk factors are identified, including poor diet, tobacco use, alcohol and drug use, injury prevention including using seat belts, and risky sexual behavior. Counseling for risk factors identified is provided. Cholesterol, diabetes, breast cancer and cervical cancer screening are recommended.

99397 Established patient periodic preventive medicine examination, age 65 years and older

A 75-year-old man, established patient, presents for a complete health evaluation and physical examination. A complete family, social and medical history is taken along with a comprehensive physical examination including height, weight and Body Mass Index (BMI) and blood pressure. A complete review of systems is performed, including screening for depression.

Risk factors are identified, including poor diet, tobacco use, alcohol and drug use, and injury prevention including using seat belts. Counseling for risk factors identified is provided. Aortic aneurysm, cholesterol, diabetes, and colorectal cancer screening are recommended.

Do not code from these clinical examples. Go to the procedure code pages for detailed code information.

Clinical Examples for Preventive Medicine Counseling (PMC) and/or Risk Factor Reduction for Interventions

Example #18

99401 Preventive medicine counseling, approximately 15 minutes

A 49 year old female with history of smoking one pack of cigarettes per day over the last 30 years presents to the office to assess and reinforce progress toward smoking cessation. The history of the patient notes prior attempts to quit smoking and explores possible reasons for failure.

The encounter includes reviewing the health risks of smoking and the benefits of stopping as well as the positive and negative issues regarding various options for quitting. Referral for medical management of nicotine patch or nicotine gum was offered. Handouts for smoking cessation classes were supplied and strategies for obtaining support from family and friends were offered.

Example #19

99402 Preventive medicine counseling, approximately 30 minutes

A 52 year old gentleman presents to the office with desires to select an exercise program. The discussion with the patient includes a review of the patient's current level of fitness and interest in different forms of exercise.

The interaction includes discussion regarding the risks and benefits risks of various aerobic, isotonic and isometric exercise programs. The importance of proper hydration and good nutrition support in concert with the exercise program was instructed. The patient was advised to stop any possible tobacco usage, and utilize moderation in any type of alcohol consumption.

Example #20

99403 Preventive medicine counseling, approximately 45 minutes

A 16 year old female necessitates a counseling that includes discussion of the biological aspects of conception, the benefits and risks of various contraceptive options, and the importance of consistent use of condoms for prevention of sexually transmitted diseases. Literature was provided medical referral was discussed for any potential use of pharmaceutical options.

Example #21

99404 Preventive medicine counseling, approximately 60 minutes

A 42 year old gentleman presents to the office with multiple risk factors including smoking, obesity, hypercholesterolemia, sedentary lifestyle, moderate truncal obesity and family history of cardiovascular disease.

The patient consents to discuss changes in diet and lifestyle to reduce risk of heart disease. The visit includes review with the patient any pertinent laboratory and clinical findings from the preventive visit, the risk factors that are identified and their impact on his health. Options for reducing the patient's risk factors were identified. The discussion emphasized the risk of heart disease based on the patient's current condition and family history.

There was extensive discussion of the benefits of losing weight, smoking cessation, and reducing cholesterol. We reviewed options for smoking cessation, diet change and weight loss, and assisted this gentleman in prioritizing the multiple goals.

Example #22

99411   Group preventive medicine counseling, approximately 30 minutes

Counseling session with a group of men and women to discuss early detection of breast cancer through breast self-examination and mammography and early detection of prostate cancer through appropriate screening. The counseling session about early detection of breast cancer included a discussion of the incidence and relative risk of breast cancer, instruction in breast self-examination using an anatomical model, and discussion of mammography. The male patients were advised that the effect of diet on prostate cancer risk is under study. A diet high in fat, especially animal fat, may be associated with an increased risk of prostate cancer and more studies are needed to determine if a low-fat diet with more fruits and vegetables helps prevent prostate cancer. The males were advised that studies show that a diet high in dairy products and calcium may be linked to an increased risk of prostate cancer, although the increase may be small. The men were advised that physical and laboratory evaluation were essential in screening.

Example #23

99412   Group preventive medicine counseling, approximately 60 minutes

Counseling session with a group of teenagers (13 - 15 years old) regarding substance (alcohol, drugs, tobacco) abuse. Information on selected risk factors, their impact on health and options for reducing risk is presented. We facilitated group discussion and responded to questions presented by the teenagers. The counseling session includes a discussion of the hazards of alcohol, tobacco, and drug use. We explored the reasons teenagers engage in substance abuse, and strategies for resisting peer pressure.

8. Alphabetic List

Abdomen, abdominal
   angiography 74174
   computed tomography scan 74150, 74176-74178
   magnetic resonance imaging (MRI) 74181-74183
   x-ray 74000-74022
Absorptiometry
   dual-energy x-ray 77080-77082
Acromion
   x-ray 73050
Adrenal gland
   function test 95922
Alcohol
   abuse screening 99408-99409
Allergy
   test
      food 95075
      inhalation 95075
Analysis
   vascular studies, doppler
      extremity
         arteries 93922-93923
Angiography
   computed tomographic
      abdomen
         chest 71275
Ankle
   application
      cast 29365
      splint 29505
      strapping 29540
   magnetic resonance imaging (MRI) 73721-73723
   strapping 29540
   x-ray 73600
Application
   cast
      body
         shoulder to hips 29035
      clubfoot 29450
      elbow to finger 29075
      figure of eight 29049
      hand to forearm 29085
      knee to toes 29405-29435
      rigid 29445
      shoulder 29055

      to hand 29065
      thigh
         to ankle 29365
         to toes 29345-29358
      Velpeau 29058
   compression system 29581-29584
   external fixation device
      shoulder 23700
   modality 97010-97036
   neurostimulator 64550
   splint
      calf to foot 29515
      finger 29130-29131
      forearm to hand 29125-29126
      shoulder to hand 29105
      thigh to ankle 29505
Arm
   application
      cast 29065-29075
      splint 29105-29126
   computed tomography (CT) scan 73200
   magnetic resonance imaging (MRI) 73218-73220,
      73223
   x-ray 73090
Audiometry
   comprehensive 92556
   pure tone 92551-92553
   speech 92555-92556
Auditory canal
   foreign body 69210
Autonomic Function Test 95922-95942
Biofeedback training 90875-90876, 90901-90911
Blood
   pressure
      analysis 99090-99091
      monitoring 93923, 95922
   test
      panels
         general health 80050
         metabolic 80048, 80053
Body
   cast
      removal 29700
      repair 29720

Body
  cast *cont'd*
    upper body 29035
      and head 29040
      and legs 29044-29046
  section
    x-ray 76100

Bone
  computed tomography (CT) scan
    density 77078
    facial 70486-70488
  coxa
    arthrography 73525
    manipulation 27275
    strapping 29520
    x-ray 73500-73540
  density
    appendicular skeleton 77081
    axial skeleton 77078, 77080
    ultrasound 76977
    vertebral assessment 77082
  dual energy x-ray absorptiometry 77080-77081
  facial
    fracture
      x-ray 70160
    x-ray 70100-70110, 70140-70150
  femur
    x-ray 73550
  fibula
    x-ray 73590
  humerus
    x-ray 73060
  nasal
    x-ray 70160
  scapula
    x-ray 73010
  skull
    x-ray 70250-70260
  tarsal
    x-ray 73600-73610
  tibia
    x-ray 73590-73600
  x-ray
    age study 77072
    dual energy absorptiometry 77080-77081
    facial 70100-70110, 70140-70150, 70160
    length study 77073
    osseous survey 77074-77077
    tarsal 73600-73610

Brace leg cast 29358

Brain
  computed tomography (CT) scan 70450-70470
  magnetic resonance imaging (MRI) 70551

Calcaneous
  x-ray 73650

Caloric vestibular test 92533

Canal
  auditory
    foreign body removal 69210

Cardiac
  output
    inert gas rebreathing 93799

Cardiology
  diagnostic
    electrocardiogram (ECG)
      interpretation and report 93000-93010
    stress test 93015-93018

Cardiovascular stress test 93015-93018

Care
  physician
    care plan oversight 99339-99340
      domiciliary facility 99339-99340
      home or rest home care 99339-99340
    case management 99366-99368
    online 99444
    prolonged
      direct patient contact 99354-99357
      outpatient/office 99354-99355
      without direct patient contact 99358-99359
    supervision 99339-99340
    team conference 99367
    telephone 99441-99443
  plan
    oversight 99339-99340
  therapy
    acquatic therapy
      with exercises 97113
    activities
      of daily living 97535
      therapeutic 97530
    athletic training
      evaluation 97005
      re-evaluation 97006
    check-out
      orthotic/prosthetic 97762
    cognitive skills development 97532
    community/work reintegration 97537
    contrast baths 97034
    diathermy treatment 97024
    direct, ... 97032-97039
    electric stimulation
      attended 97032
      unattended 97014
    evaluation 97001-97002
    exercises 97110
    gait training 97116
    group
      education and training 98961-98962
    group therapeutic 97150
    hot or cold pack 97010
    hydrotherapy (Hubbard tank) 97036
    individual
      home management training 97535, 98960
    infrared light treatment 97026
    iontophoresis 97033
    kinetic therapy 97530
    manual therapy 97140

Care
therapy *cont'd*
massage therapy 97124
microwave therapy 97024
neuromuscular re-education 97112
orthotics training 97760
osteopathic manipulation 98925-98929
paraffin bath 97018
physical performance test 97750T
prosthetic training 97761
sensory integration 97533
supervised procedure 97010-97028
traction 97012, 97140
ultrasound 97035
ultraviolet light 97028
vasopneumatic device 97016
wheelchair management 97542
whirlpool therapy 97022
work hardening 97545-97546
work reintegration 97537

Cast
application 29450
arm 29065, 29075
body
  upper 29035-29046
brace
  leg 29358
clubfoot 29450
cylinder 29365
finger
  splint 29130-29131
hand 29085
leg 29345-29355, 29365, 29405-29450
  brace 29358
  splint 29505, 29515
patellar tendon 29435
removal 29700
repair 29720
shoulder 29049-29058
splint
  arm 29105, 29125-29126
  finger 29130-29131
  leg 29505, 29515
wedge 29740-29750
window 29730
wrist 29085

Cerumen 69210

Cervical
disc arthroplasty
  removal 0095T
spine
  computed tomography (CT) 72125-72127
  magnetic resonance imaging (MRI) 72141-72142
  myelography 72270
  x-ray 72040-72052

Challenge
bronchial 95075

Chemotherapy administration
pump 95990-95991

Chest
angiography 71275
computed tomography (CT) scan 71250-71275
magnetic resonance imaging (MRI) 71550-71552
strapping 29200
wall
  manipulation 94667-94668
x-ray 0174T-0175T, 71010-71035, 74022

Chiropractic treatment 98940-98943

Clavicle
x-ray 73000

Clubfoot
cast 29450
  wedge 29750

Coccyx
x-ray 72220

Cognitive
skills development 97532

Cold
pack 97010

Collar bone
x-ray 73000

Compression system 29581-29584

Computed tomography
abdomen 74150
  and pelvis 74176-74178
bone density 77078
brain 70450-70470
chest 71275
ear 70480-70482
extremity
  lower 73700
  upper 73200
head 70450-70470
maxillofacial 70486-70488
neck 70490-70492
orbit 70480-70482
pelvis 72194
  with abdomen 74176-74178
plane 76100
sella 70480-70482
spine
  cervical 72125-72127
  lumbar 72131-72133
  thoracic 72128-72130
thorax 71250-71270
three dimensional 76376

Computer
analysis
  data 99090
detection
  radiograph
    chest 0174T-0175T

Consultation
interprofessional telephone/internet 99446-99449
outpatient 99241-99245
x-ray 76140

Contrast
bath 97034
radiologic study
  computed tomography (CT)
    abdomen 74160
    cervical spine 72126-72127
    chest 71275, 71551
    ear 70481-70482
    head 70460-70470
    lower extremity 73701
    lumbar spine 72132-72133
    maxillofacial 70487
    neck 70491-70492
    orbit 70481-70482
    pelvis 72193-72194
    posterior fossa 70481-70482
    sella 70481-70482
    spinal canal 72142, 72147, 72149
    thoracic spine 72129-72130
    thorax 71260-71270
    upper extremity 73201
  magnetic resonance imaging (MRI)
    abdomen 74182
    brain 70552-70553
    face 70542-70543
    lower extremity 73719-73720, 73722
    neck 70542-70543
    orbit 70542-70543
    pelvis 72196
    upper extremity 73219-73220, 73222

Costen syndrome
arthrography 70328
magnetic resonance imaging (MRI) 70336
x-ray 70328

Counseling
preventive medicine 99391-99397
  intervention 99401-99404
tobacco cessation 99406-99407

Coxa
arthrography 73525
manipulation 27275
strapping 29520
x-ray 73500-73540

Cranium
x-ray 70250-70260

Cutaneous
electrostimulation 64550

Cyst
drainage
  injection 76080

Diathermy
retina
  modality 97024

Digital
slit beam radiography 77073

Disc
arthroplasty removal 0095T

Disease
organ panel 80050

Doppler
echocardiograph
  transcranial study 93886-93923
scan
  artery 93922-93924, 93886

Drug
delivery
  refilling 95990-95991
    spinal 95990-95991
screen 80300-80304

Dual
absorptiometry
  x-ray 77080-77082

Duplex scan
artery 93880-93882

Ear
canal
  foreign body
    removal 69210
computed tomography (CT) scan 70480-70482
wax 69210

Elbow
magnetic resonance imaging (MRI) 73221
strapping 29260
x-ray 73070

Electric
application 64550
stimulation
  acupuncture 97813-97814
  modality 97014, 97032

Electro
analgesia 64550

Electrocardiography (ECG) (EKG)
monitoring
  stress test 93015-93018
routine
  interpretation and report 93000, 93010
  tracing 93005

Electromyography (EMG)
neuromuscular 95860-95872, 95885-95887
sphincter 90911
surface 96002-96004

Electronic analysis
pump 95990-95991

Encephalon
computed tomography (CT) scan 70450-70470
doppler
  transcranial 93886
magnetic resonance imaging (MRI) 70551

Evaluation
athletic training 97005-97006
body 95833-95834
occupational therapy 97003-97004
physical therapy 97001-97002

Evoked
  otoacoustic emissions 92558
  potential
    central motor 95928-95929, 95939
    somatosensory...................................95925-95928

External
  ear
    auditory canal
      removal 69210

Face
  computed tomography (CT) scan 70486-70488
  magnetic resonance imaging (MRI) 70540-70543

Facial
  bone
    fracture
      x-ray 70160
    x-ray.............................. 70100-70110, 70140-70150

Fatty acid... 0111T

Femur
  x-ray 73550

Fibula
  x-ray 73590

Finger
  x-ray 73140

Fixation
  device
    external
      shoulder 23700

Fluoroscopy 76000, 76496
  chest...71023, 71034

Foot
  cast........... 29345-29358, 29405-29445, 29505-29515
    clubfoot.. 29450
    removal.. 29700
    strapping 29540-29580
    wedging...29740-29750
    window 29730
  computed tomography (CT) scan 73700
  magnetic resonance imaging (MRI) 73723
  x-ray 73620-73660

Forearm
  cast 29075
    splint..29125-29126
  computed tomography (CT) scan 73200
  magnetic resonance imaging (MRI) 73218-73220, 73223
  ultrasound..76881-76882
  x-ray 73090

Frontal
  chest x-ray 71010-71023

Function test
  autonomic..95922-95924
  pulmonary
    airway resistance..., 94728
    capacity 94150-94200, 94729
    determination 94726, 94727
    gas
      collection 94250
      volume 94726, 94727

  inhalation... 94640
  manipulation...94667-94668
  saturation 94760
  spirometry 94010

Gait training 97116

Gland
  adrenal
    function test...95922

Group health education 98961-98962

H-reflux study...95934-95936

Hand
  cast... 29085
  magnetic resonance imaging (MRI) 73218-73223
  strapping...29280
  x-ray 73120-73130

Head
  computed tomography (CT) scan 70450-70470
  ultrasound.. 76536

Hearing
  aid
    test 92551

Heart
  output
    inert gas rebreathing 93799

Heel
  x-ray 73650

Hip
  arthrography..73525
  joint
    manipulation... 27275
  manipulation.. 27275
  strapping...29520
  x-ray 73500-73540

Home services
  established patient 99347-99350
  new patient 99341-99345

Home/house visits...................................99341-99350

Hospital services .... See FindACode.com

Hot pack treatment 97010

Hubbard tank therapy.. 97036

Humerus
  x-ray 73060

Hydrotherapy 97036

Hyperbaric oxygen pressurization/treatment.... 99183

Hypnotherapy 90880

Imaging
  3D rendering...76376-76377
  echography
    arm..76881-76882
    artery
      extracranial 93880-93882
      intracranial 93886
    follow-up 76970
    head 76536
    leg 76881-76882
    neck.. 76536
    pelvis 76856
    physical therapy 97035

Imaging cont'd
  magnetic resonance imaging (MRI)
    abdomen 74181-74183
    ankle 73721-73723
    arm 73218-73220
    brain 70551-70555
    chest 71552
    elbow 73221-73223
    face 70540-70543
    finger joint 73221-73223
    foot joint 73721-73723
    foot 73718-73720
    hand 73218-73220
    knee 73721-73723
    leg 73718-73720
    lower extremity 73718-73723
    neck 70540-70543
    orbit 70540-70543
    pelvis 72195-72197
    spine 72141
    temporomandibular joint 70336
    toe joint 73721
    unlisted 76498
    upper extremity 73218-73223
    wrist 73221-73223
  three dimensional rendering 76376-76377
  vascular studies
    arterial studies
      extracranial 93882
      extremities 93922
      intracranial 93886
    temperature gradient 93740
Infrared light treatment 97026
Infusion
  pump
    maintenance 95990-95991
Ingestion challenge test 95075
Inhalation
  treatment 94640
Injection
  paravertebral facet joint/nerve 0213T-0218T
Inner ear
  computed tomography (CT) scan 70480-70482
Insurance
  basic life/disablilty
    evaluation services 99450
    examination 99450-99456
Internal
  ear
    computed tomography (CT) scan 70480-70482
Ionization 97033
Jaw
  temporomandibular joint
    arthrography 70328
    magnetic resonance imaging (MRI) 70336
    x-ray 70328
  x-ray 70100-70110, 70328

Joint
  acromioclavicular
    arthrography 73040
  ankle
    x-ray 73600-73610
  elbow
    x-ray 73070-73080
  glenohumeral
    arthrography 73040
    manipulation 23700
    x-ray 73020-73030
  hip
    arthrography 73525
    manipulation 27275
    x-ray 73500-73520, 73540
  knee
    x-ray 73560-73565
  magnetic resonance imaging (MRI)
    lower extremity joint 73721-73723
    upper extremity joint 73221-73223
  sacroiliac
    x-ray 72200-72202
  stress application 77071
  survey 77077
  talotarsal
    magnetic resonance imaging (MRI) 73721-73723
  tarsometatarsal
    magnetic resonance imaging (MRI) 73721-73723
  temporomandibular joint
    arthrography 70328
    magnetic resonance imaging (MRI) 70336
    x-ray 70328
Kinetic therapy 97530
Knee
  magnetic resonance imaging (MRI) 73721-73723
  strapping 29530
  x-ray 73560-73565
Larynx
  electromyography 95865
Leg
  application
    brace 29358
    cast 29445-29450
      lower 29405-29435
      upper 29345-29355, 29365, 29450
      walker 29440
    splint
      lower 29515
      upper 29505
    strapping 29580
  computed tomography (CT) scan 73700
  magnetic resonance imaging (MRI) 73718-73720
  ultrasound 76881-76881
  x-ray 73592
Lumbar
  computed tomography (CT) scan 72131-72133
  magnetic resonance imaging (MRI) 72148-72149
  manipulation 22505

Lung
  pulmonology
    capacity 94150
    collection 94250
    inhalation 94640
    manipulation 94667-94668
    oximetry 94760
    spirometry 94010

Magnetic resonance
  imaging (MRI)
    abdomen 74181-74183
    ankle 73721-73723
    arm 73218-73220
    brain 70551-70555
    chest 71552
    elbow 73221-73223
    face 70540-70543
    finger joint 73221-73223
    foot joint 73721-73723
    foot 73718-73720
    hand 73218-73220
    knee 73721-73723
    leg 73718-73720
    lower extremity 73718-73723
      foot joint 73721-73723
      foot 73718-73720
      knee 73721-73723
      leg 73718-73720
      pelvis 72195-72197
      toe joint 73721
    neck 70540-70543
    orbit 70540-70543
    pelvis 72195-72197
    spine 72141
    temporomandibular joint 70336
    toe joint 73721
    unlisted 76498
    upper extremity 73218-73223
      arm 73218-73220
      elbow 73221-73223
      finger joint 73221-73223
      hand 73218-73220
      wrist 73221-73223
    wrist 73221-73223
  three dimensional rendering 76376-76377

Mandible
  x-ray 70100-70110

Manipulation
  chest wall 94667-94668
  chiropractic 98940-98943
  fracture/dislocation
    shoulder 23700
  osteopathic 98925-98929
  spine 22505

Manometry
  rectal 90911

Manual therapy 97140
Massage 97124

Mastoid(s)
  x-ray 70120-70130

Maxilla(ry)
  computed tomography (CT) scan
    70486-70488

Measurement
  lung volumes 94013
  spirometric forced expiratory flows 94011-94012

Medical
  conference 99366-99368
  evaluation, disability 99455-99456
  testimony 99075

Middle
  ear
    computed tomography (CT) scan 70480-70482

Minerva cast 29035
Motion analysis 96000, 96004

Muscle
  testing
    manual 95831-95834

Myelography
  spine 72270

Nasal
  x-ray 70160, 70210-70220

Neck
  computed tomography (CT) scan 70490-70492
  magnetic resonance imaging (MRI) 70540-70543
  ultrasound 76536
  x-ray 70360

Needle
  electromyography 95860-95872, 95885-95887

Nerve(s)
  conduction
    motor 95900-95903
    sensory 95904
  studies 95907-95913

Neural
  conduction 95900-95904

Neurology procedures
  central motor 95928-95929
  electromyography
    dynamic 96002-96004
    ischemic limb 95875
    needle 95860-95872
  evoked potentials
    central motor 95928-95929
    short latency 95925-95927
  motion analysis 96000, 96004
    range 95851-95852
  muscle test 95831-95831
    neuromuscular 95937
  nerve conduction
    motor 95900-95903
    sensory 95904
  reflex testing 95934
  somatosensory testing 95925-95927

Neuromuscular
  junction test 95937
  reduction 97112

Neurostimulators
  application 64550
New patient care
  consultation
    office/outpatient 99241-99245
    home 99341-99345
  office
    consultations 99241-99245
    initial visit 99201-99205
Non-invasive vascular studies
  extracranial 93880-93882
  extremity 93922
  intracranial 93886
Nose
  x-ray 70160, 70210-70220
Nuclear
  magnetic resonance imaging (MRI)
    abdomen 74181-74183
    ankle 73721-73723
    arm 73218-73220
    brain 70551-70555
    chest 71552
    elbow 73221-73223
    face 70540-70543
    finger joint 73221-73223
    foot joint 73721-73723
    foot 73718-73720
    hand 73218-73220
    knee 73721-73723
    leg 73718-73720
    lower extremity 73718-73723
      foot joint 73721-73723
      foot 73718-73720
      knee 73721-73723
      leg 73718-73720
      pelvis 72195-72197
      toe joint 73721
    neck 70540-70543
    orbit 70540-70543
    pelvis 72195-72197
    spine 72141
    temporomandibular joint 70336
    toe joint 73721
    unlisted 76498
    upper extremity 73218-73223
      arm 73218-73220
      elbow 73221-73223
      finger joint 73221-73223
      hand 73218-73220
      wrist 73221-73223
    wrist 73221-73223
  three dimensional rendering 76376-76377
Nutrition 97802-97804
Nystagmus test 92541-92542, 92544
Occupational therapy 97003-97004
Ocular
  orbital
    computed tomography (CT) scan 70480-70482
    magnetic resonance imaging (MRI) ... 70540-70543

Online management service
  nonphysician 98969
  physician 99444
Ophthalmology services
  screening
    computerized 99172
    visual acuity 99172-99173
    visual function 99172
  visual acuity screen 99172-99173
  visual function 99172
Optokinetic nystagmus test 92544
Orbit(al)
  computed tomography (CT) scan 70480-70482
  magnetic resonance imaging (MRI) 70540-70543
  sella turcica 70482
  x-ray 70190-70200
Organ
  panel 80050
    metabolic 80048, 80053
Orthopedic
  cast
    arm 29065, 29075
    body
      upper 29035-29046
    clubfoot 29450
    cylinder 29365
    hand 29085
    leg 29345-29355, 29365, 29405-29450
    patellar tendon 29435
    shoulder 29049-29058
    wedge 29740-29750
    window 29730
    wrist 29085
Orthoroentgenogram 77073
Orthosis 97760-97762
Osseous Survey 77074-77076
Osteopathic manipulation 98925-98929
Otorhinolaryngology services
  audiology function tests 92551
Outpatient services
  consultation 99201-99215
  established patient 99211-99215
  new patient 99201-99205
  office visit 99201-99215
  prolonged services 99354-99355
Oximetry 94760
Panel
  blood
    general health 80050
    metabolic 80048, 80053
  organ 80050
    metabolic 80048, 80053
Paraffin bath therapy 97018
Paravertebral nerve
  injection 0213T-0218T
Patella
  patellar tendon bearing (PTB) cast 29435

Pelvic
    computed tomography (CT) scan 72194, 74176-74178
    magnetic resonance imaging (MRI) 72195-72197
    ultrasound... 76856
    x-ray 72170-72190, 73540

Percutaneous
    electric nerve stimulation..................................... 64550

Performance test
    physical... 97750

Peristaltic pump
    maintenance... 95990-95991

Physical/occupational therapy
    acquatic... 97113
    activities
        daily living... 97535
        therapeutic 97530
    check-out.. 97762
    cognitive skills development 97532
    community reintegration 97537
    contrast baths 97034
    diathermy treatment 97024
    direct.. 97032-97039
    electric stimulation
        attended 97032
        unattended 97014
    evaluation 97001-97002
    exercises 97110
    group 97150
    hot or cold pack 97010
    hydrotherapy (Hubbard tank).............................. 97036
    infrared light treatment.. 97026
    iontophoresis 97033
    kinetic 97530
    manual.. 97140
    massage 97124
    microwave 97024
    neuromuscular re-education 97112
    osteopathic manipulation........................ 98925-98929
    paraffin bath 97018
    physical performance test................................... 97750
    sensory integration 97533
    supervised procedure 97010-97028
    traction 97012,97140
    training
        athletic 97005-97006
        gait 97116
        orthotics 97760
        prosthetics 97761
    ultrasound.. 97035
    ultraviolet light 97028
    vasopneumatic device 97016
    wheelchair management 97542
    whirlpool 97022
    work
        hardening 97545-97546
    work hardening... 97545-97546

Physician services
    case management.................................... 99366-99368

online 99444
prolonged
    direct patient contact 99354-99357
    outpatient/office 99354-99355
    without direct patient contact.............. 99358-99359
supervision 99339-99340
team conference 99367
telephone 99441-99443

Pinna
    computed tomography (CT) scan 70480-70482

Plantar
    pressure measurement 96001, 96004

Plethysmography
    extremities 93922-93923
    lung 94726
    total body 94726

Pneumonology
    expired gas analysis
        quantitative 94250
        therapeutic 94250
    inhalation
        treatment 94640
    manipulation of chest wall 94667-94668
    maximum breathing capacity 94200
    maximum voluntary ventilation 94200
    oximetry 94760
    spirometry
        evaluation 94010
        patient initiated with bronchospasm 94010

Positional nystagmus test 92542
Post-op visit 99024
Potential
    evoked
        motor 95928-95929
        sensory 95925-95927

Preventative medicine 99381-99397
    assessment, ... 99420
    counseling and/or risk factor reduction intervention
        behavior change 99406-99408
        group counseling 99411-99412
        individual counseling 99401-99404
    established patient 99382-99397
    new patient 99381-99387

Prolonged services 99354-99357
    without direct patient contact 99358-99359

Prosthesis
    check-out 97762
    orthotic
        checkout 97762
        training 97761
    training 97761

Psychiatric
    biofeedback training 90875-90876
    hypnotherapy 90880

Pulmonary
    function test
        airway resistance 94726, 94728
        determination of volumes 94726-94727

Pulmonary
- function tests *cont'd*
  - diffusing capacity 94729
  - expired gas analysis
    - quantitative 94250
    - therapeutic 94250
  - inhalation
    - treatment 94640
  - manipulation of chest wall 94667-94668
  - maximum breathing capacity 94200
  - maximum voluntary ventilation 94200
  - spirometry
    - evaluation 94010
    - patient initiated with bronchospasm 94010
  - thoracic gas volume 94726, 94727

Pump
- infusion
  - maintenance 95990-95991

Pure tone audiometry 92552-92553

Quantitative sensory test
- cooling 0108T
- heat-pain 0109T
- other 0110T
- touch pressure 0106T
- vibration 0107T

Radiation
- X-ray
  - abdominal 74000-74022
  - abscess 76080
  - acromioclavicular joint 73050
  - ankle 73600-73610
  - arm 73090
  - bone
    - age study 77072
    - dual energy absorptiometry 77080-77081
    - length study 77073
    - osseous survey 77074-77077
    - ultrasound 76977
  - calcaneous 73650
  - chest 71010-71035
  - clavicle 73000
  - coccyx 72220
  - consultation 76140
  - elbow 73070-73080
  - facial bones 70140-70150
  - femur 73550
  - fibula 73590
  - finger 73140
  - foot 73620-73630
  - hand 73120-73130
  - heel 73650
  - hip 73500-73540
  - humerus 73060
  - joint 77071
  - knee 73560-73564
  - leg 73592
  - mandible 70100-70110
  - mastoids 70120-70130
  - nasal bone 70160
  - neck 70360
  - orbit 70190-70200
  - pelvis 72170-72190, 73540
  - ribs 71100-71111
  - sacroiliac joint 72200-72202
  - sacrum 72220
  - scapula 73010
  - sella turcica 70240
  - shoulder 73020-73030, 73050
  - sinus tract 76080
  - skull 70250-70260
  - specimen 76098
  - spine
    - cervical 72040-72090
    - complete 72010
    - lumbosacral 72100-72120
    - standing 72069
    - thoracic 72020-72074
    - thoracolumbar 72080
  - sternum 71120-71130
  - tibia 73590
  - toe 73660
  - with contrast
    - hip 73525
    - joint 77071
    - shoulder 73040
    - spine 72270
    - tempomandibular joint 70328
    - wrist 73100-73110

Range of motion
- extremities 95851
- hand 95852

Reflex test 95936

Removal
- cast 29700
- cerumen 69210
- device
  - intervertebral disc, artificial 0095T
- ear wax 69210
- intervertebral disc, artificial
  - cervical 0095T
  - lumbar 0164T

Repair
- body cast 29720
- jacket 29720
- spica 29720

Rib
- x-ray 71100-71111

Sacroiliac joint
- x-ray 72200-72202

Sacrum
- x-ray 72220

Scan
- nuclear
  - magnetic resonance imaging (MRI)
    - abdomen 74181-74183
    - ankle 73721-73723
    - arm 73218-73220
    - brain 70551-70555

Scan
  nuclear
    MRI *cont'd*
      chest 71552
      elbow..73221-73223
      face 70540-70543
      finger joint 73221-73223
      foot joint 73721-73723
      foot 73718-73720
      hand 73218-73220
      knee 73721-73723
      leg 73718-73720
      lower extremity 73718-73723
        foot joint 73721-73723
        foot..73718-73720
        knee 73721-73723
        leg...73718-73720
        pelvis 72195-72197
        toe joint 73721
      neck 70540-70543
      orbit 70540-70543
      pelvis..72195-72197
      spine 72141
      temporomandibular joint 70336
      toe joint 73721
      unlisted...76498
      upper extremity 73218-73223
        arm 73218-73220
        elbow 73221-73223
        finger joint 73221-73223
        hand...73218-73220
        wrist 73221-73223
      wrist 73221-73223
      three dimensional rendering................76376-76377

Scanogram
  bone length studies 77073

Scapula
  x-ray..73010

Screening
  alcohol abuse 99408-99409
  audiologic function test
    pure tone, air only...92551
  drug abuse 99408-99409
  evoked otoacoustic emissions............................92558
  visual function..99172

Sella turcica.....................................70240, 70480-70482

Shock wave
  therapy
    high energy 0101T
    low energy..0019T

Shoulder
  cast..29049-29065
  fracture treatment 23700
  manipulation 23700
  strapping..29240
  x-ray..73000-73050

Sinus(es)
  x-ray...70210-70220

Skull
  x-ray..70250-70260

Sleep studies
  unattended..95800-95801

Smoking cessation....................40001F, 99406-99407

Somatosensory testing
  head 95927
  lower limbs 95926
  trunk 95927
  upper limbs...95925

Sonography
  arm 76881-76882
  arteries
    extracranial..93880-93882
    intracranial...93886
  head 76536
  leg..76881-76882
  neck 76536
  pelvis 76856

Specimen
  handling...99000-99001

Sphenoid sinus
  x-ray..70210-70220

Spica cast
  repair 29720
  shoulder..29055

Spinal
  manipulation 98940-98943

Spine
  computed tomography (CT) scan
    cervical 72125-72127
    lumbar 72131-72133
    thoracic..72128-72130
  magnetic resonance imaging (MRI)
    cervical 72141-72142
    lumbar 72148
    thoracic..72146-72147
  manipulation 22505
  myelography
    two or more regions 72270
  x-ray
    cervical 72040-72052
    lumbosacral...72100-72120
    standing..72069
    thoracic...72020-72074
    thoracolumbar 72080

Spirometry...94010

Splint
  arm
    long 29105
    short 29125-29126
  finger 29125-29131
  leg
    long 29505
    short 29515

Sternum
  x-ray..71120-71130

Stimulation
  bithermal
    caloric vestibular test.......................... 92533, 92543
  electrical
    acupuncture 97813-97814
    physical therapy 97014, 97032
  nerve
    peripheral... 95925-95927
    repetitive... 95937
  neurostimulation
    application... 64550
  transcranial
    magnetic 95939
    motor 95928-95929

Stomach
  suture
    fistula... 93880

Strapping
  ankle... 29540
  elbow.. 29260
  finger 29280
  foot 29540
  hand 29280
  hip... 29520
  knee.. 29530
  shoulder,... 29240
  thorax 29200
  toes... 29550
  Unna boot... 29580
  wrist.. 29260

Stress test
  cardiovascular 93015

Telephone
  consultation/interprofessional................. 99446-99449
  evaluation and management services.... 99441-99443

Temperature studies...93740

Tempomandibular joint
  arthrography.. 70328
  magnetic resonance imaging (MRI) 70336
  manipulation 97140
  x-ray 70328

TENS...64550, 97014, 97032

Test
  adrenal gland..95922
  allergy
    food 95075
    inhalation.. 95075
  blood
    panels
      general health 80050
      metabolic 80048, 80053
  caloric vestibular... 92533
  function
    pulmonary
      capacity... 94200
      gas
        collection.. 94250
        inhalation 94640

    manipulation 94667-94668
    saturation 94760
    spirometry 94010
  ingestion challenge...95075
  muscle
    manual 95831-95834
  neuromuscluar junction 95937
  Nystagmus 92541-92542, 92544
  optokinetic nystagmus..92544
  performance
    physical 97750
  physical performance 97750
  positional nystagmus 92542
  quantitative sensory
    cooling..0108T
    heat-pain 0109T
    other 0110T
    touch pressure..0106T
    vibration..0107T
  reflex... 95934
  somatosensory.......................................95925-95927
  stress.. 93015-93018
  torsion swing..92546

Thorax
  angiography... 71275
  computed tomography (CT) scan 71250-71275
  strapping..29200

Tibia
  x-ray 73590-73600

Tibiofibular joint
  x-ray 73590-73600

Tinnitus.. 92625

Toe
  magnetic resonance imaging (MRI)
   7372-73723
  strapping..29550
  x-ray 73660

Tomography
  3D rendering.. 76376-76377
  computed (CT) scan
    abdomen 74150
    arm.. 73200
    bone density study 77078
    brain 70450-70470
    ear.. 70480-70482
    face 70486-70488
    head 70450-70470
    leg 73700
    maxilla.. 70486-70488
    neck... 70490-70492
    orbit,.. 70480-70482
    pelvis...72194
    sella turicica 70480-70482
    spine 72125-72133
    thorax 71250-71275

Torsion swing test 92546

Toxicology screening 80300-80304

Traction therapy
   manual 97140
   mechanical 97012

Training
   biofeedback 90901-90911
   integration
      sensory 97533
   management
      home 97535
      wheelchair 97542
   orthotics 97760
   prothetics 97761
   reintegration
      community 97537
      work 97537
   self care 97535, 98960-98962
   skills, cognitive 97532

Transmittal Care Management 99495-99496

Transcranial
   doppler study 93886
   stimulation
      motor 95928-95929, 95939

Turcica
   computed tomography (CT) scan 70480-70482
   x-ray 70240

Ultrasound
   3D rendering 76376-76377
   arm 76881-76882
   artery
      extracranial 93880-93882
      intracranial 93886
   follow-up 76970
   head 76536
   leg 76881-76882
   neck 76536
   pelvis 76856
   physical therapy 97035

Unna boot 29700
   strapping 29580

Urethra
   biofeedback training 90911
   sphincter 90911

Vascular
   study
      arterial studies
         extracranial 93880-93882
         extremities 93922
         intracranial 93886
      plethysmography 94726
      temperature gradient 93740

Vasopneumatic device 97016

Velpeau cast 29058

Vestibular
   function test
      caloric 92533, 92543
      nystagmus
         otokinetic 92544
         positional 92542

         spontaneous 92541
      sinusoidal rotational testing 92546
      torsion swing test 92546

Visual
   acuity screen 99172-99173
   function screen 99172

Vital capacity measurement 94150
Wheelchair management 97542
Whirlpool therapy 97022

Whitman
   astragalectomy 97022

Work hardening 97545-97546

Wrist
   cast 29085
   magentic resonance imaging (MRI) 73221
   strapping 29260
   x-ray 73100

X-ray
   abdominal 74000-74022
   abscess 76080
   acromioclavicular joint 73050
   ankle 73600-73610
   arm 73090
   bone
      age study 77072
      dual energy absorptiometry 77080-77081
      length study 77073
      osseous survey 77074-77077
      ultrasound 76977
   calcaneous 73650
   chest 71010-71035
   clavicle 73000
   coccyx 72220
   consultation 76140
   elbow 73070-73080
   facial bones 70140-70150
   femur 73550
   fibula 73590
   finger 73140
   foot 73620-73630
   hand 73120-73130
   heel 73650
   hip 73500-73540
   humerus 73060
   joint 77071
   knee 73560-73564
   leg 73592
   mandible 70100-70110
   mastoids 70120-70130
   nasal bone 70160
   neck 70360
   orbit 70190-70200
   pelvis 72170-72190, 73540
   ribs 71100-71111
   sacroiliac joint 72200-72202
   sacrum 72220
   scapula 73010
   sella turcica 70240

Xray *cont'd*
- shoulder 73020-73030, 73050
- sinus tract 76080
- skull 70250-70260
- specimen 76098
- spine
  - cervical 72040-72090
  - complete 72010
  - lumbosacral 72100-72120
  - standing 72069
  - thoracic 72020-72074
  - thoracolumbar 72080
- sternum 71120-71130
- tibia 73590
- toe 73660
- with contrast
  - hip 73525
  - joint 77071
  - shoulder 73040
  - spine 72270
  - tempomandibular joint 70328
  - wrist 73100-73110

Notes

supplies

I SUPPLY CODES

1. Supply Coding
Page I-3

2. Commonly Used Codes
Page I-7

3. HCPCS Supply Codes
Page I-8

4. HCPCS Supply Modifiers
Page I-31

5. Alphabetic List
Page I-34

SUPPLY CODES

OBJECTIVES

Providing medical supplies to your patients, not only benefits them, but it can also contribute to practice profitability. This section helps you understand how to properly submit claims and which codes and modifiers apply.

OUTLINE

1. Supply Coding *I-3*
   - ◆ About HCPCS Supplies and Services *I-3*
   - ◆ About Durable Medical Equipment (DME) *I-4*
   - ◆ Review *I-6*

2. Commonly Used Supply Codes *I-7*
   - ◆ Commonly Used Supply Codes and Modifiers *I-7*

3. HCPCS Supply Codes *I-8*
   - ◆ Miscellaneous Services (CPT) *I-9*
   - ◆ Medical and Surgical Supplies ("A" codes) *I-9*
   - ◆ Administrative, Miscellaneous and Investigational ("A" codes) *I-13*
   - ◆ Dental Procedures ("D" codes) *I-13*
   - ◆ Durable Medical Equipment ("E" codes) *I-13*
   - ◆ Drugs Administered Other Than Oral Method ("J" codes) *I-18*
   - ◆ Temporary Codes For DMERCs' Use ("K" codes) *I-18*
   - ◆ Orthotic Procedures ("L" codes) *I-19*
   - ◆ Temporary Codes ("Q" codes) *I-30*
   - ◆ State Medicaid Agency Codes ("T" codes) *I-30*

4. HCPCS Supply Modifiers *I-31*
   - ◆ Level II Supply Modifiers (-AA to -VV) *I-32*

5. Alphabetic List *I-34*

1. Supply Coding

About HCPCS Supplies and Services

HCPCS (pronounced "hick-picks") is the Healthcare Common Procedure Coding System, maintained by the Centers for Medicare & Medicaid Services (CMS), formerly the Health Care Finance Administration (HCFA). HCPCS is a 5-digit coding system that describes physician and non-physician services and supplies.

It is the national standard for government programs administered by the CMS (i.e., Medicare, Medicaid). It is also the standard used by most insurance companies.

Technically, HCPCS is comprised of three levels or divisions:

1. **Level I - CPT Numeric Codes (00000-99999)**

   This CPT (Current Procedural Terminology) portion is maintained by the American Medical Association (AMA).

2. **Level II - CMS Alpha-numeric Codes (A0000-V9999)**

   This non-CPT portion is maintained by CMS. Codes from the non-CPT portion are easily identifiable. There is a single letter followed by 4 numbers (e.g., A9300, exercise equipment). These codes supplement the CPT codes. They exist because there is a need to more fully identify supplies and services that are not in the CPT book.

   These are national codes, and are in the public domain. Decisions regarding additions, revisions and deletions to codes or descriptors are made annually by a panel comprised of the Health Insurance Association of America (HIAA), the Blue Cross/Blue Shield Association of America, and CMS.

   There are three exceptions to panel decisions: temporary codes beginning with "H," "K" and "Q," which are reserved for exclusive use by CMS, and "S" codes which are reserved for private use by Blue Cross/Blue Shield. These temporary codes are being used while being further evaluated for full implementation into other categories or code sets.

3. **Level III - Local and State Alpha-numeric Codes (W0000-Z9999)**

   These codes were formerly reserved for state and local use. With the advent of the Health Insurance Portability and Accountability Act (HIPAA), local codes will no longer be permitted. If used, it is a HIPAA violation. However, Workers Compensation is exempt from HIPAA, and could have different modifiers and codes.

   See Resource 347 for additional information, articles and webinars about supplies.

The abridgement that follows contains HCPCS codes that could be of interest and value for chiropractic offices.

> **Note:** The existence of a code does not imply coverage by third party payers.

Why You Should Use HCPCS

Mandated Use: The use of HCPCS codes is mandated by CMS on Medicare claims, and many state Medicaid offices also require them.

Improved Communication: A provider can more clearly communicate services and supplies correctly, without the need to use narrative descriptors.

Reduced Claim Resubmissions: Inaccurate codes or incomplete narrative descriptors cause costly time delays. The claim's adjudicator must assign a code or return the claim, and the payer's reassignment of the code may be incorrect.

Quick and Efficient: Using up-to-date HCPCS codes on office forms allows office staff to assign fees quickly and easily. This saves time and money.

Faster Processing: Your coding system will be compatible with most insurance companies, speeding up claims processing.

Avoid Audits: Consistent submission of accurate claims will reduce the probability of being targeted for an audit by your carrier.

Accurate Reimbursements: Use HCPCS for accurate and complete reimbursements.
Example: Supplies billed as "over and above those usually included with the office visit" (CPT code 99070) will generally not be reimbursed unless identified with Level II or III HCPCS codes.

Code Changes

Requests for new codes are considered by CMS. See Resource 349 for more about requesting a code change.

See Resource 350 for the complete 2015 HCPCS codes.

ABOUT DURABLE MEDICAL EQUIPMENT (DME)

Within the Health Care Common Procedure Coding System (HCPCS) Level II codes set for supplies, there are many items that are classified as Durable Medical Equipment (DME). Generally, such equipment items need to meet all the following requirements:

1. Can be used repeatedly.
2. Primarily used for a medical purpose.
3. Not useful in the absence of an illness/injury.
4. Appropriate for home use.

DME and Chiropractic

Although Medicare law and regulations only pay on the three basic Chiropractic Manipulative Treatment (CMT) service codes (98940-98942), Medicare may also pay for DME codes. Here are the official instructions from the Medicare Claims Processing Manual, Chapter 12 (Resource 352):

> **220 Chiropractic Services**
> B3-4118
> **B. Durable Medical Equipment Regional Carriers Processing Claims When a Chiropractor is the Supplier**
> Effective July 1, 1999, except for restrictions to chiropractor services as stipulated in §§1861(s)(2)(A) of the Social Security Act, chiropractors (specialty 35) can bill for durable medical equipment, prosthetics, orthotics and supplies if, as the supplier, they have a valid supplier number assigned by the National Supplier Clearinghouse. In order to process claims, the Common Working File has been changed to allow specialty 35 to bill for services furnished as a supplier.

DME Application Process

The National Supplier Clearinghouse (NSC) is the national entity contracted by the Centers for Medicare & Medicaid Services (CMS) that issues Medicare DMEPOS supplier authorization numbers. The NSC provides DMEPOS supplier applications, verifies application information, and administers file activity.

- See Resource 354 for information by NSC including webinars.
- See Resource 353 for the offical CMS DME website.

Billing Process for DME Items

Once the practitioner or clinic obtains a DMEPOS supplier number, billing commences. However, the billing does not go to the usual Part B MAC. It goes to the Durable Medical Equipment Medicare Administrative Contractors (DME-MAC) in your jurisdiction.

> Note: All DME billing for Medicare is entered on a separate claim form and then transmitted to one of four designated regional DME carriers/contractors.

DME Claim Filing Centers

All DME claims are filed according to jurisdiction into one of four regions (see Resource 355):

Jurisdiction A: National Heritage Insurance Company (NHIC)

Connecticut, Delaware, District of Columbia, Maine, Maryland, Massachusetts, New Hampshire, New Jersey, New York, Pennsylvania, Rhode Island, and Vermont.

www.medicarenhic.com/dme/default.aspx

Jurisdiction B: National Government Services

Illinois, Indiana, Kentucky, Michigan, Minnesota, Ohio, and Wisconsin.

www.ngsmedicare.com/wps/portal/ngsmedicare/home

Jurisdiction C: CGS Administrators, LLC

Alabama, Arkansas, Colorado, Florida, Georgia, Louisiana, Mississippi, New Mexico, North Carolina, Oklahoma, Puerto Rico, South Carolina, Tennessee, Texas, U.S. Virgin Islands, Virginia, and West Virginia.

www.cgsmedicare.com/jc/index.html

Jurisdiction D: Noridian Administrative Services (NAS)

Alaska, American Samoa, Arizona, California, Guam, Hawaii, Idaho, Iowa, Kansas, Missouri, Montana, Nebraska, Nevada, North Dakota, Northern Mariana Islands, Oregon, South Dakota, Utah, Washington, and Wyoming.

🖱 www.noridianmedicare.com/dme/

Review: Supply Coding
■ What is HCPCS? *I-3*
■ What are the three levels of HCPCS codes? *I-3*
■ Just because a code exists, will it be covered by a third-party payer? *I-3*
■ How can using HCPCS avoid audits? *I-4*
■ What is DME? *I-5*

2. Commonly Used Supply Codes

COMMONLY USED SUPPLY CODES AND MODIFIERS

Listed below is a quick reference of commonly used supply codes and modifiers. These codes are repeated here from their respective alpha-numeric listings in this HCPCS section.

Code	Description
99070	Supplies
	This general CPT code for any supply could be used by some payers in lieu of the specific HCPCS codes
A4556	Electrodes, (eg, apnea monitor), per pair
A4557	Lead wires, (eg, apnea monitor), per pair
A4595	TENS supplies, two lead, per month
A4630	TENS replacement batteries, owned by patient
A9150	Drugs, non-prescription
	(ie, over the counter (OTC) botanicals, or nutraceuticals.)
A9152	Single vitamin/mineral/trace element, oral, per dose, not otherwise specified
A9153	Multiple vitamins, with or without minerals and trace elements, oral, per dose, not otherwise specified
A9273	Hot water bottle, ice cap or collar, heat and/or cold wrap, any type
A9300	Exercise equipment
A9999	Miscellaneous DME supply or accessory, not otherwise specified
E0100	Cane, includes canes of all materials, adjustable or fixed, with tip
E0105	Cane, quad or three prong, includes canes of all materials, adjustable or fixed, with tips
E0190	Positioning cushion/pillow/wedge, any shape or size, includes components and accessories
	(ie, cervical, lumbar, etc.)
E0210	Electric heat pad, standard
E0215	Electric heat pad, moist
	(E0238 and E0238 have been deleted. To report use A9273)
E0720	TENS, two lead, localized stimulation
E0730	TENS, four or more leads, for multiple nerve stimulation
E0850	Traction stand, free standing, cervical traction
E0942	Cervical head harness/halter
E1399	Miscellaneous durable medical equipment (DME)
E1800	Dynamic adjustable **elbow** extension/flexion device, includes soft interface material
E1805	Dynamic adjustable **wrist** extension/flexion device, includes soft interface material
E1810	Dynamic adjustable **knee** extension/flexion device, includes soft interface material
E1815	Dynamic adjustable **ankle** extension/flexion device, includes soft interface material
-NU	New equipment
-UE	Used durable medical equipment
-RR	Rental of DME (monthly)
-KR	Rental item, billing (partial month)

3. HCPCS Supply Codes

This chapter contains a numeric listing of supply codes most relevant to chiropractic offices. Pay close attention to the fees and proper usage of modifiers for some codes.

Headings

Headings are provided as a means of grouping similar or closely related items. The placement of a code under a heading does not indicate additional meaning of classification, nor does it relate to any health insurance coverage categories. This is unlike the conventions used in CPT and ICD-9/10 where section headings do relate to codes in that functional grouping.

Fees

Annual CMS pricing schedules are usually released by January of each year. This information is always available and current in the *ChiroCode Fee Calculator Worksheet* (Resource 172).

Other payers and/or states may define what is considered to be reasonable fees above the manufacturers list price for the rental and/or sale of supplies. Be aware of payer and local guidelines.

See Resource 347 for additional fee information.

Non-Supply Services

See *Section H–Procedures* for the following HCPCS (non-supply) services:

- Procedures and Professional Services
- Rehabilitative Services
- Drugs Administered Other Than Oral Method
- Private Payer Codes
- State Medicaid Agency Codes

Level I Codes

Miscellaneous Services (CPT)

Specific codes for supplies are maintained by the Centers for Medicare & Medicaid Services (CMS). The CPT retains only one general supply code, which is 99070. Some insurance companies use this code for all supplies. However, more and more payers are requesting a higher specificity of coding by use of the HCPCS supply codes.

99070 Supplies and materials provided by the physician over and above those usually included with the office visit or other services rendered (list drugs, trays, supplies, or other materials provided).

> The fee for this code has not been established because supplies vary.

Level II Codes

Medical and Surgical Supplies

A4265 Paraffin, per pound
A4290 Sacral nerve stimulation test lead, each

Incontinence Appliances and Care Supplies

A4322 Irrigation syringe, bulb or piston, each

Supplies

      Tape;
A4450   non-waterproof, per 18 square inches
A4452   waterproof, per 18 square inches
A4455 Adhesive remover or solvent (for tape, cement or other adhesive), per ounce
A4456 Adhesive remover, wipes, any type, each
A4465 Non-elastic binder for extremity
A4466 Garment, belt, sleeve or other covering, elastic or similar stretchable material, any type, each
A4480 Vabra aspirator
      Surgical stockings;
A4490   above knee length, each
A4495   thigh length, each
A4500   below knee length, each
A4510   full length, each
A4554 Disposable underpads, all sizes,
A4556 Electrodes, (eg, apnea monitor), per pair
A4557 Lead wires, (eg, apnea monitor), per pair
A4558 Conductive paste or gel, for use with electrical device (e.g., TENS, NMES), per oz.
A4559 Coupling gel or paste, for use with ultrasound device, per oz
A4565 Slings
A4566 Shoulder sling or vest design, abduction restrainer, with or without swathe control, prefabricated, includes fitting and adjustment
A4570 Splint

▲ = Revised Code   ● = New Code

A4580   Cast supplies (eg, plaster)
A4590   Special casting material (eg, fiberglass)
A4595   Electrical stimulator supplies, 2 lead, per month, (eg TENS, NMES)

Supplies for Oxygen and Related Respiratory Equipment

▲ A4601   Lithium ion battery, rechargeable, for non-prosthetic use, replacement
A4604   Tubing with integrated heating element for use with positive airway pressure device
A4606   Oxygen probe for use with oximeter device, replacement
A4615   Cannula, nasal
A4616   Tubing (oxygen), per foot
A4617   Mouth piece
A4620   Variable concentration mask

Supplies for Other Durable Medical Equipment

A4630   Replacement batteries, medically necessary, TENS, owned by patient
A4633   Replacement bulb/lamp for ultraviolet light therapy system, each
A4634   Replacement bulb for therapeutic light box, tabletop model
A4635   Underarm pad, crutch, replacement, each
A4636   Replacement, handgrip, cane, crutch, or walker, each
A4637   Replacement, tip, cane, crutch, walker, each
A4639   Replacement pad for infrared heating pad system, each

Supplies for ESRD

      Gloves;
A4927   non-sterile, per 100
A4930   sterile, per pair
A4931   Oral thermometer, reusable, any type, each
A4932   Rectal thermometer, reusable, any type, each

Supplies for Either Incontinence or Ostomy Appliance

A5120   Skin barrier, wipes or swabs, each

Shoe Supplies for Diabetics

      For diabetics only,
A5501   fitting (including follow-up), custom preparation and supply of shoe molded from cast(s) of patient's foot (custom molded shoe), per shoe
A5503   modification (including fitting) of off-the-shelf depth-inlay shoe or custom-molded shoe with roller or rigid rocker bottom, per shoe
A5504   modification (including fitting) of off-the-shelf depth-inlay shoe or custom-molded shoe with wedge(s), per shoe
A5505   modification (including fitting) of off-the-shelf depth-inlay shoe or custom-molded shoe with metatarsal bar, per shoe
A5506   modification (including fitting) of off-the-shelf depth-inlay shoe or custom-molded shoe with off-set heel(s), per shoe

A5507	not otherwise specified modification (including fitting) of off-the-shelf depth-inlay shoe or custom-molded shoe, per shoe
A5508	deluxe feature of off-the-shelf depth-inlay shoe or custom-molded shoe, per shoe

Wound Dressings

	Collagen dressing, sterile,
A6021	size 16 sq. in. or less, each
A6022	size more than 16 sq. in. but less than or equal to 48 sq. in, each
A6023	size more than 48 sq. in., each
A6024	Collagen dressing wound filler, sterile, per 6 inches
A6025	Gel sheet for dermal or epidermal application, (eg, silicone, hydrogel, other), each
	Alginate or other fiber gelling dressing;
A6196	wound cover, sterile, pad size 16 sq. in. or less, each dressing
A6199	wound filler, sterile, per 6 inches
	Composite dressing, sterile,
A6203	pad size 16 sq. in. or less, with any size adhesive border, each dressing
A6204	pad size more than 16 sq. in. but less than or equal to 48 sq. in., with any size adhesive border, each dressing
	Contact layer, sterile,
A6206	16 sq. in. or less, each dressing
A6207	more than 16 sq. in. but less than or equal to 48 sq. in., each dressing
	Foam dressing, wound cover, sterile,
A6209	pad size 16 sq. in. or less, without adhesive border, each dressing
A6210	pad size more than 16 sq. in. but less than or equal to 48 sq. in., without adhesive border, each dressing
A6212	pad size 16 sq. in. or less, with any size adhesive border, each dressing
A6213	pad size more than 16 sq. in. but less than or equal to 48 sq. in., with any size adhesive border, each dressing
A6215	Foam dressing, wound filler, sterile, per gram
	Gauze, non-impregnated, non-sterile;
A6216	pad size 16 sq. in. or less, without adhesive border, each dressing
A6217	pad size more than 16 sq. in. but less than or equal to 48 sq. in., without adhesive border, each dressing
	Gauze, non-impregnated, sterile,
A6219	pad size 16 sq. in. or less, with any size adhesive border, each dressing
A6220	pad size more than 16 sq. in. but less than or equal to 48 sq. in., with any size adhesive border, each dressing
	Gauze, impregnated with other than water, normal saline, or hydrogel, sterile,
A6222	pad size 16 sq. in. or less, without adhesive border, each dressing
A6223	pad size more than 16 sq. in., but less than or equal to 48 sq. in., without adhesive border, each dressing
	Gauze, impregnated, water or normal saline, sterile,
A6228	pad size 16 sq. in. or less, without adhesive border, each dressing
A6229	pad size more than 16 sq. in. but less than or equal to 48 sq. in., without adhesive border, each dressing
	Gauze, impregnated, hydrogel, for direct wound contact, sterile,
A6231	pad size 16 sq. in. or less, each dressing
A6232	pad size greater than 16 sq. in., but less than or equal to 48 sq. in., each dressing
A6233	pad size more than 48 sq. in., each dressing

▲ = Revised Code   ● = New Code

Hydrocolloid dressing, wound cover, sterile,
A6234   pad size 16 sq. in. or less, without adhesive border, each dressing
A6235   pad size more than 16 sq. in. but less than or equal to 48 sq. in., without adhesive border, each dressing
A6236   pad size more than 48 sq. in., without adhesive border, each dressing
A6237   pad size 16 sq. in. or less, with any size adhesive border, each dressing
A6239   pad size more than 48 sq. in., with any size adhesive border, each dressing

Hydrocolloid dressing, wound filler;
A6240   paste, sterile, per fluid ounce
A6241   dry form, sterile, per gram

Hydrogel dressing, wound cover, sterile,
A6242   pad size 16 sq. in. or less, without adhesive border, each dressing
A6244   pad size more than 48 sq. in., without adhesive border, each dressing
A6245   pad size 16 sq. in. or less, with any size adhesive border, each dressing

A6248   Hydrogel dressing, wound filler, gel, per fluid ounce

Specialty absorptive dressing, wound cover, sterile,
A6251   pad size 16 sq. in or less, without adhesive border, each dressing
A6253   pad size more than 48 sq. in., without adhesive border, each dressing
A6254   pad size 16 sq. in. or less, with any size adhesive border, each dressing
A6256   pad size more than 48 sq. in., with any size adhesive border, each dressing

Transparent film, sterile,
A6257   16 sq. in. or less, each dressing
A6259   more than 48 sq. in., each dressing

A6260   Wound cleansers, any type, any size

Wound filler;
A6261   gel/paste, per fluid ounce, not otherwise specified
A6262   dry form, per gram, not otherwise specified

A6407   Packing strips, non-impregnated, sterile, up to 2 inches in width, per linear yard

A6413   Adhesive bandage, first-aid type, any size, each

Light compression bandage,
A6448   elastic, knitted/woven, width less than three inches, per yard
A6449   elastic, knitted/woven, width greater than or equal to three inches and less than five inches, per yard
A6450   elastic, knitted/woven, width greater than or equal to five inches, per yard

A6451   Moderate compression bandage, elastic, knitted/woven, load resistance of 1.25 to 1.34 foot pounds at 50% maximum stretch, width greater than or equal to three inches and less than five inches, per yard

A6452   High compression bandage, elastic, knitted/woven, load resistance greater than or equal to 1.35 foot pounds at 50% maximum stretch, width greater than or equal to three inches and less than five inches, per yard

Self-adherent bandage, elastic, non-knitted/non-woven,
A6453   width less than three inches, per yard
A6454   width greater than or equal to three inches and less than five inches, per yard
A6455   width greater than or equal to five inches, per yard

A6457   Tubular dressing with or without elastic, any width, per linear yard

A6545   Gradient compression wrap, non-elastic, below knee, 30-50 mm hg, each

A6549	Gradient compression stocking/sleeve, not otherwise specified
	Helmet, protective,
A8000	soft, prefabricated, includes all components and accessories
A8001	hard, prefabricated, includes all components and accessories
A8002	soft, custom fabricated, includes all components and accessories
A8003	hard, custom fabricated, includes all components and accessories
A8004	Soft interface for helmet, replacement only

ADMINISTRATIVE, MISCELLANEOUS AND INVESTIGATIONAL

Miscellaneous and Experimental

A9150	Non-prescription drugs
	Over the counter (OTC) botanicals or nutraceuticals
A9152	**Single vitamin**/mineral/trace element, oral, per dose, not otherwise specified
A9153	**Multiple vitamins,** with or without minerals and trace elements, oral, per dose, not otherwise specified
A9270	Non-covered item or service
A9273	Hot water bottle, ice cap or collar, heat and/or cold wrap, any type
A9275	Home glucose disposable monitor, includes test strips
A9283	Foot pressure off loading/supportive device, any type, each
A9300	Exercise equipment
A9900	Miscellaneous DME **supply, accessory**, and/or service component of another HCPCS code
A9901	DME delivery, set up, and/or dispensing service component of another HCPCS code
A9999	Miscellaneous DME supply or accessory, not otherwise specified

DENTAL PROCEDURES

Miscellaneous Services

D9940	Occlusal guard, by report
	TMJ splint

DURABLE MEDICAL EQUIPMENT (DME)

Note: Rental fees are monthly unless otherwise specified. If the rental period is less than one month, append modifier -KR (rental item, partial month)

Canes

	Cane;
E0100	includes canes of all materials, adjustable or fixed, with tip
E0105	quad or three prong, includes canes of all materials, adjustable or fixed, with tips

▲ = Revised Code ● = New Code

Crutches

E0112	Crutches underarm, wood, adjustable or fixed, pair, with pads, tips and handgrips
E0114	Crutches underarm, other than wood, adjustable or fixed, pair, with pads, and handgrips
E0117	Crutch, underarm, articulating, spring assisted, each
E0118	Crutch substitute, lower leg platform, with or without wheels, each

Walkers

Walker,
E0140	with trunk support, adjustable or fixed height, any type
E0148	heavy duty, without wheels, rigid or folding, any type, each
E0149	heavy duty, wheeled, rigid or folding, any type

Commodes

Sitz type bath or equipment, portable; used with or without commode,
E0160	used with or without commode
E0161	with faucet attachments
E0162	Sitz bath chair

Commode chair with integrated seat lift mechanism, any type
E0170	electric
E0171	non-electric
E0172	Seat lift mechanism placed over or on top of toilet, any type

Decubitus Care Equipment

E0181	Powered pressure reducing mattress overlay/pad, alternating, with pump, includes heavy duty
E0182	Pump for alternating pressure pad, for replacement only
E0184	Dry pressure mattress
E0185	Gel or gel-like pressure pad for mattress, standard mattress length and width
E0186	Air pressure mattress
E0187	Water pressure mattress
E0188	Synthetic sheepskin pad
E0189	Lambswool sheepskin pad, any size
E0190	Positioning cushion/pillow/wedge, any shape or size, includes components and accessories (ie, cervical, lumbar, etc.)
E0191	Heel or elbow protector, each
E0193	Powered air floatation bed (low air loss therapy)
E0198	Water pressure pad for mattress, standard mattress length and width
E0199	Dry pressure pad for mattress, standard mattress length and width

Heat/Cold Application

E0200	Heat lamp, without stand (table model), includes bulb, or infrared element
E0202	Phototherapy (bilirubin) light with photometer
E0203	Therapeutic lightbox, minimum 10,000 lux, table top model

E0205	Heat lamp, with stand, includes bulb, or infrared element
	Electric heat pad;
E0210	standard
E0215	moist
E0217	Water circulating heat pad with pump
E0218	Water circulating cold pad with pump
E0221	Infrared heating pad system
E0225	Hydrocollator unit, includes pads
E0235	Paraffin bath unit, portable (see medical supply code A4265 for paraffin)
E0236	Pump for water circulating pad
	(E0220, E0230 and E0238 have been deleted. To report see A9273.)
E0239	Hydrocollator unit, portable

Hospital Beds and Accessories

E0272   Mattress, foam rubber

Hospital Bed Accessories

E0315   Bed accessory: board, table, or support device, any type

Oxygen and Related Respiratory Equipment

E0445	Oximeter device for measuring blood oxygen levels non-invasively
E0446	Topical oxygen delivery system, not otherwise specified, includes all and accessories
E0480	Percussor, electric or pneumatic home model
	Oral device/appliance used to reduce upper airway collapsibility, adjustable or non-adjustable, includes fitting and adjustment
E0485	prefabricated
E0486	custom fabricated

Monitoring Equipment

E0607   Home blood glucose monitor

Pacemaker Monitor

	Apnea monitor;
E0618	without recording feature
E0619	with recording feature

Patient Lifts

	Standing frame/table system,
E0641	multi-position (eg, three-way stander), any size including pediatric, with or without wheels
E0642	mobile (dynamic stander), any size including pediatric

Restraints

E0705   Transfer device, any type, each

▲ = Revised Code   ● = New Code

Transcutaneous and/or Neuromuscular Electrical Nerve Stimulators-TENS

	Transcutaneous electrical nerve stimulation (TENS) device,
E0720	two lead, localized stimulation
E0730	four or more leads, for multiple nerve stimulation
E0731	Form fitting conductive garment for delivery of TENS or NMES (with conductive fibers separated from the patient's skin by layers of fabric)
E0744	Neuromuscular stimulator for scoliosis
E0745	Neuromuscular stimulator, electronic shock unit
E0746	Electromyography (EMG), biofeedback device
	Osteogenesis stimulator, electrical, non-invasive;
E0747	other than spinal applications
E0748	spinal applications
E0761	Non-thermal pulsed high frequency radiowaves, high peak power electromagnetic energy treatment device
E0762	Transcutaneous electrical joint stimulation device system, includes all accessories
E0764	Functional neuromuscular stimulator, transcutaneous stimulation of muscles of ambulation with computer control, used for walking by spinal cord injured, entire system, after completion of training program
E0765	FDA approved nerve stimulator with replaceable batteries for treatment of nausea and vomiting
E0769	Electrical stimulation or electromagnetic wound treatment device, not otherwise classified
E0770	Functional electrical stimulator, transcutaneous stimulation of nerve and/or muscle groups, any type, complete system, not otherwise specified

Traction Equipment

Cervical

E0830	Ambulatory traction device, all types, each
E0840	Traction frame, attached to headboard, cervical traction
E0849	Traction equipment, cervical, free-standing stand/frame, pneumatic, applying traction force to other than mandible
E0850	Traction stand, free standing, cervical traction
E0855	Cervical traction equipment not requiring additional stand or frame
▲ E0856	Cervical traction device, with inflatable air bladder(s)

Overdoor

E0860	Traction equipment, overdoor, cervical

Extremity

E0870	Traction frame, attached to footboard, extremity traction (eg, Buck's)
E0880	Traction stand, free standing, extremity traction (eg, Buck's)

Pelvic

E0890	Traction frame, attached to footboard, pelvic traction
E0900	Traction stand, free standing, pelvic traction (eg, Buck's)

Trapeze Equipment, Fracture Frame and Other Orthopedic Devices

E0910   Trapeze bars, A/K/A patient helper, attached to bed, with grab bar

Trapeze bar, heavy duty, for patient weight capacity greater than 250 pounds,
E0911   attached to bed, with grab bar
E0912   free standing, complete with grab bar

E0935   Continuous passive motion exercise device for use on knee only

E0940   Trapeze bar, free standing, complete with grab bar

E0941   Gravity assisted traction device, any type

E0942   Cervical head harness/halter
(E0943 has been deleted. Use E0190 for cervical pillow)

E0944   Pelvic belt/harness/boot

E0945   Extremity belt/harness

E0948   Fracture frame; attachments for complex cervical traction

Wheelchair Accessories

E0992   Manual wheelchair accessory, solid seat insert

Additional Oxygen Related Supplies and Equipment

E1399   Durable medical equipment, miscellaneous

Orthotic Devices

E1800   Dynamic adjustable **elbow** extension/flexion device, includes soft interface material

E1801   Static progressive stretch **elbow** device, extension and/or flexion, with or without range of motion adjustment, includes all components and accessories

E1802   Dynamic adjustable **forearm** pronation/supination device, includes soft interface material

E1805   Dynamic adjustable **wrist** extension/flexion device, includes soft interface material

E1806   Static progressive stretch **wrist** device, flexion and/or extension, with or without range of motion adjustment, includes all components and accessories

E1810   Dynamic adjustable **knee** extension/flexion device, includes soft interface material

E1812   Dynamic knee, extension/flexion device with active resistance control
E1815   Dynamic adjustable **ankle** extension/flexion device, includes soft interface material

E1825   Dynamic adjustable **finger** extension/flexion device, includes soft interface material

E1830   Dynamic adjustable **toe** extension/flexion device, includes soft interface material

E1831   Static progressive stretch toe device, extension and/or flexion, with or without range of motion adjustment, includes all components and accessories

E1841   Static progressive stretch **shoulder** device, with or without range of motion adjustment, includes all components and accessories

---

TENS Unit Rentals

When billing a rental, use code E0720 and append modifier -RR to indicate that this is a rental only. As a rule, rental fees are usually monthly. If the rental period is less than one month, use modifier -KR instead.

▲ = Revised Code   ● = New Code

Gait Training

Gait trainer, pediatric size,

E8000	**posterior** support, includes all accessories and components
E8001	**upright** support, includes all accessories and components
E8002	**anterior** support, includes all accessories and components

Procedures and Professional Services

See *Section H–Procedures* for these "G" codes.

Rehabilitative Services

See *Section H–Procedures* for these "H" codes.

Drugs Administered Other Than Oral Method

This J code section is for injections. The Scope of Practice in some states permits injections by a trained Doctor of Chiropractic. Once you have established that this is within your scope of practice, you should also contact the insurer to determine if the injection is a covered service when performed by a DC. These codes are listed for convenience and reference.

Drugs Administered Other Than Oral Method

J3420	Injection, vitamin B-12 cyanocobalamin, up to 1,000 mcg
J3570	Laetrile, amygdalin, vitamin B-17

Temporary Codes For DMERCs' Use

This K section contains national codes assigned by CMS on a temporary basis and are for the primary use of the Durable Medical Equipment Regional Carriers (DMERC). Orthotic supply devices are listed in the "L" code series.

Supplies

K0462	Temporary replacement for patient owned equipment being repaired, any type
K0672	Addition to lower extremity orthosis, removable soft interface, all components, replacement only, each
K0739	Repair or nonroutine service for durable medical equipment other than oxygen equipment requiring the skill of a technician, labor component, per 15 minutes

(Code K0627 has been deleted. Use E0849)
(Codes K0630-K0649 have been deleted. Use L0621-L0640)

K0900	Customized durable medical equipment, other than wheelchair

Knee orthosis (ko),

- ● K0901   single upright, thigh and calf, with adjustable flexion and extension joint (unicentric or polycentric), medial-lateral and rotation control, with or without varus/valgus adjustment, prefabricated, off-the-shelf
- ● K0902   double upright, thigh and calf, with adjustable flexion and extension joint (unicentric or polycentric), medial-lateral and rotation control, with or without varus/valgus adjustment, prefabricated, off-the-shelf

ORTHOTIC PROCEDURES

Orthotic Devices

Spinal: Cervical

Cranial cervical orthosis,

L0112	congenital torticollis type, with or without soft-interface material, adjustable range of motion joint, custom fabricated
L0113	torticollis type, with or without joint, with or without soft interface material, prefabricated, includes fitting and adjustment

Cervical, flexible;

▲ L0120	non-adjustable, prefabricated, off-the-shelf (foam collar)
L0130	thermoplastic collar, molded to patient

Cervical, semi-rigid;

L0140	adjustable (plastic collar)
L0150	adjustable molded chin cup (plastic collar with mandibular/occipital piece)
▲ L0160	wire frame occipital/mandibular support, prefabricated, off-the-shelf

Cervical, collar;

L0170	molded to patient model
▲ L0172	semi-rigid, thermoplastic foam, two piece, prefabricated, off-the-shelf
▲ L0174	semi-rigid, thermoplastic foam, two piece with thoracic extension, prefabricated, off-the-shelf

Cervical, multiple post collar, occipital/mandibular supports;

L0180	adjustable
L0190	adjustable cervical bars (Somi, Guilford, Taylor types)
L0200	adjustable cervical bars, and thoracic extension

Spinal: Thoracic

L0220   Thoracic, rib belt; custom fabricated

Spinal: Thoracic-Lumbar-Sacral

(Code L0430 has been deleted.)

TLSO, flexible, provides trunk support, **upper thoracic region**, produces intracavitary pressure to reduce load on the intervertebral disks with rigid stays or panel(s), includes shoulder straps and closures,

L0450	prefabricated, off-the-shelf
L0452	custom fabricated

TLSO flexible, provides trunk support, **extends from sacrococcygeal junction to above T-9 vertebra**, restricts gross trunk motion in the sagittal plane, produces intracavitary pressure to reduce load on the intervertebral disks with rigid stays or panel(s), includes shoulder straps and closures,

L0454   prefabricated item that has been trimmed, bent, molded, assembled, or otherwise customized to fit a specific patient by an individual with expertise

L0455   prefabricated, off-the-shelf

TLSO, flexible, provides trunk support, **thoracic region, rigid posterior panel and soft anterior apron**, extends from the sacrococcygeal junction and terminates just inferior to the scapular spine, restricts gross trunk motion in the sagittal plane, produces intracavitary pressure to reduce load on the intervertebral disks, includes straps and closures,

L0456   prefabricated item that has been trimmed, bent, molded, assembled, or otherwise customized to fit a specific patient by an individual with expertise

L0457   prefabricated, off-the-shelf

TLSO, sagittal-coronal control, modular segmented spinal system,

L0491   **two rigid plastic shells,** posterior extends from the sacrococcygeal junction and terminates just inferior to the scapular spine, anterior extends from the symphysis pubis to the xiphoid, soft liner, restricts gross trunk motion in the sagittal and coronal planes, lateral strength is provided by overlapping plastic and stabilizing closures, includes straps and closures, prefabricated, includes fitting and adjustment

L0492   **three rigid plastic shells,** posterior extends from the sacrococcygeal junction and terminates just inferior to the scapular spine, anterior extends from the symphysis pubis to the xiphoid, soft liner, restricts gross trunk motion in the sagittal and coronal planes, lateral strength is provided by overlapping plastic and stabilizing closures, includes straps and closures, prefabricated, includes fitting and adjustment

Spinal: Sacroiliac

Sacroiliac orthosis,

flexible, provides pelvic-sacral support, reduces motion about the sacroiliac joint, includes straps, closures, may include pendulous abdomen design,

L0621   prefabricated, off the shelf

L0622   custom fabricated

provides pelvic-sacral support, with rigid or semi-rigid panels over the sacrum and abdomen, reduces motion about the sacroiliac joint, includes straps, closures, may include pendulous abdomen design,

L0623   prefabricated, off the shelf

L0624   custom fabricated

Spinal: Lumbar

Lumbar orthosis,

L0625   **flexible, provides lumbar support,** posterior extends from L-1 to below L-5 vertebra, produces intracavitary pressure to reduce load on the intervertebral discs, includes straps, closures, may include pendulous abdomen design, shoulder straps, stays, prefabricated, off the shelf

Lumbar orthosis, sagittal control,

▲ L0626   **with rigid posterior panel(s),** posterior extends from L-1 to below L-5 vertebra, produces intracavitary pressure to reduce load on the intervertebral discs, includes straps, closures, may include padding, stays, shoulder straps, pendulous abdomen design, prefabricated item that has been trimmed, bent, molded, assembled, or otherwise customized to fit a specific patient by an individual with expertise

| L0627 | **with rigid anterior and posterior panels,** posterior extends from L-1 to below L-5 vertebra, produces intracavitary pressure to reduce load on the intervertebral discs, includes straps, closures, may include padding, shoulder straps, pendulous abdomen design, prefabricated item that has been trimmed, bent, molded, assembled, or otherwise customized to fit a specific patient by an individual with expertise |

Spinal: Lumbar-Sacral

Lumbar-sacral orthosis,
flexible, provides lumbo-sacral support, posterior extends from sacrococcygeal junction to T-9 vertebra, produces intracavitary pressure to reduce load on the intervertebral discs, includes straps, closures, may include stays, shoulder straps, pendulous abdomen design,

| L0628 | prefabricated, off the shelf |
| L0629 | custom fabricated |

Lumbar-sacral orthosis, sagittal control,

L0630	**with rigid posterior panel**(s), posterior extends from sacrococcygeal junction to T-9 vertebra, produces intracavitary pressure to reduce load on the intervertebral discs, includes straps, closures, may include padding, stays, shoulder straps, pendulous abdomen design, prefabricated item that has been trimmed, bent, molded, assembled, or otherwise customized to fit a specific patient by an individual with expertise
▲ L0631	**with rigid anterior and posterior panels,** posterior extends from sacrococcygeal junction to T-9 vertebra, produces intracavitary pressure to reduce load on the intervertebral discs, includes straps, closures, may include padding, shoulder straps, pendulous abdomen design, prefabricated item that has been trimmed, bent, molded, assembled, or otherwise customized to fit a specific patient by an individual with expertise
L0632	**with rigid anterior and posterior panels,** posterior extends from sacrococcygeal junction to T-9 vertebra, produces intracavitary pressure to reduce load on the intervertebral discs, includes straps, closures, may include padding, shoulder straps, pendulous abdomen design, custom fabricated

Lumbar-sacral orthosis, sagittal-coronal control,
with rigid posterior frame/panel(s), posterior extends from sacrococcygeal junction to T-9 vertebra, lateral strength provided by rigid lateral frame/panels, produces intracavitary pressure to reduce load on intervertebral discs, includes straps, closures, may include padding, stays, shoulder straps, pendulous abdomen design,

| L0633 | prefabricated item that has been trimmed, bent, molded, assembled, or otherwise customized to fit a specific patient by an individual with expertise |
| L0634 | custom fabricated |

Lumbar-sacral orthosis, sagittal-coronal control,
lumbar flexion, rigid posterior frame/panel(s), lateral articulating design to flex the lumbar spine, posterior extends from sacrococcygeal junction to T-9 vertebra, lateral strength provided by rigid lateral frame/panel(s), produces intracavitary pressure to reduce load on intervertebral discs, includes straps, closures, may include padding, anterior panel, pendulous abdomen design,

| L0635 | prefabricated, includes fitting and adjustment |
| L0636 | custom fabricated |

Lumbar-sacral orthosis, sagittal-coronal control,
with rigid anterior and posterior frame/panels, posterior extends from sacrococcygeal junction to T-9 vertebra, lateral strength provided by rigid lateral frame/panels, produces intracavitary pressure to reduce load on intervertebral discs, includes straps, closures, may include padding, shoulder straps, pendulous abdomen design,

| L0637 | prefabricated item that has been trimmed, bent, molded, assembled, or otherwise customized to fit a specific patient by an individual with expertise |
| L0638 | custom fabricated |

▲ = Revised Code   ● = New Code

Lumbar-sacral orthosis, sagittal-coronal control,
> **rigid shell(s)/panel(s),** posterior extends from sacrococcygeal junction to T-9 vertebra, anterior extends from symphysis pubis to xyphoid, produces intracavitary pressure to reduce load on the intervertebral discs, overall strength is provided by overlapping rigid material and stabilizing closures, includes straps, closures, may include soft interface, pendulous abdomen design,

Code	Description
L0639	prefabricated item that has been trimmed, bent, molded, assembled, or otherwise customized to fit a specific patient by an individual with expertise
L0640	custom fabricated

Lumbar orthosis, sagittal control,

Code	Description
L0641	with rigid posterior panel(s), posterior extends from l-1 to below l-5 vertebra, produces intracavitary pressure to reduce load on the intervertebral discs, includes straps, closures, may include padding, stays, shoulder straps, pendulous abdomen design, prefabricated, off-the-shelf
L0642	with rigid anterior and posterior panels, posterior extends from l-1 to below l-5 vertebra, produces intracavitary pressure to reduce load on the intervertebral discs, includes straps, closures, may include padding, shoulder straps, pendulous abdomen design, prefabricated, off-the-shelf

Lumbar-sacral orthosis, sagittal control,

Code	Description
L0643	with rigid posterior panel(s), posterior extends from sacrococcygeal junction to t-9 vertebra, produces intracavitary pressure to reduce load on the intervertebral discs, includes straps, closures, may include padding, stays, shoulder straps, pendulous abdomen design, prefabricated, off-the-shelf
L0648	with rigid anterior and posterior panels, posterior extends from sacrococcygeal junction to t-9 vertebra, produces intracavitary pressure to reduce load on the intervertebral discs, includes straps, closures, may include padding, shoulder straps, pendulous abdomen design, prefabricated, off-the-shelf

Lumbar-sacral orthosis, sagittal-coronal control,

Code	Description
L0649	with rigid posterior frame/panel(s), posterior extends from sacrococcygeal junction to t-9 vertebra, lateral strength provided by rigid lateral frame/panels, produces intracavitary pressure to reduce load on intervertebral discs, includes straps, closures, may include padding, stays, shoulder straps, pendulous abdomen design, prefabricated, off-the-shelf
L0650	with rigid anterior and posterior frame/panel(s), posterior extends from sacrococcygeal junction to t-9 vertebra, lateral strength provided by rigid lateral frame/panel(s), produces intracavitary pressure to reduce load on intervertebral discs, includes straps, closures, may include padding, shoulder straps, pendulous abdomen design, prefabricated, off-the-shelf
L0651	rigid shell(s)/panel(s), posterior extends from sacrococcygeal junction to t-9 vertebra, anterior extends from symphysis pubis to xyphoid, produces intracavitary pressure to reduce load on the intervertebral discs, overall strength is provided by overlapping rigid material and stabilizing closures, includes straps, closures, may include soft interface, pendulous abdomen design, prefabricated, off-the-shelf

---

Definitions

Orthotics, The science concerned with the making and fitting of orthopedic appliances.

Orthosis, pl. **orthoses** An external orthopaedic appliance, as a brace or splint, that prevents or assists movement of the spine or the limbs.

Orthopaedics, or orthopedics The medical specialty concerned with the preservation, restoration, and development of form and function of the musculoskeletal system, extremities, spine, and associated structures by medical, surgical, and physical methods *(from Stedman's Medical Dictionary, 26th Edition).*

Spinal: Cervical-Thoracic-Lumbar-Sacral

L0700 Cervical-thoracic-lumbar-sacral-orthoses (CTLSO), anterior-posterior-lateral control, molded to patient model; (Minerva type)
L0710   with interface material, (Minerva type)

Scoliosis Procedures

Note: The orthotic care of scoliosis differs from other orthotic care in that the treatment is more dynamic in nature and utilizes ongoing, continual modification of the orthosis to the patient's changing condition. This coding structure uses the proper names or eponyms of the procedures because they have historic and universal acceptance in the profession. It should be recognized that variations to the basic procedures described by the founders/developers are accepted in various medical and orthotic practices throughout the country. All procedures include model of patient when indicated.

Cervical-Thoracic-Lumbar-Sacral (Milwaukee)

L1000 Cervical-thoracic-lumbar-sacral orthosis (CTLSO) (Milwaukee), inclusive of furnishing initial orthosis, including model
L1001 Cervical-thoracic-lumbar-sacral-orthosis (CTLSO), immobilizer, infant size, prefabricated, includes fitting and adjustment

Correction Pads

    Addition to CTLSO or scoliosis orthosis;
L1010   axilla sling
L1020   kyphosis pad
L1025   kyphosis pad, floating
L1030   lumbar bolster pad
L1040   lumbar or lumbar rib pad
L1050   sternal pad
L1060   thoracic pad
L1070   trapezius sling
L1080   outrigger
L1085   outrigger, bilateral with vertical extensions
L1090   lumbar sling
L1100   ring flange, plastic or leather
L1110   ring flange, plastic or leather, molded to patient model
L1120   cover for upright, each

Thoracic-Lumbar-Sacral (Low Profile)

L1200 Thoracic-lumbar-sacral-orthosis (TLSO), inclusive of furnishing initial orthosis only

    Addition to TLSO, (low profile);
L1210   lateral thoracic extension
L1220   anterior thoracic extension
L1230   Milwaukee type superstructure
L1240   lumbar derotation pad
L1250   anterior asis pad
L1260   anterior thoracic derotation pad
L1270   abdominal pad
L1280   rib gusset (elastic), each
L1290   lateral trochanteric pad

▲ = Revised Code   ● = New Code

Other Scoliosis Procedures

L1499   Spinal orthosis, not otherwise specified

Lower Limb
Knee

See also E1810–adjustable knee extension/flexion device.

Knee orthosis (KO);

L1810	elastic with joints, prefabricated item that has been trimmed, bent, molded, assembled, or otherwise customized to fit a specific patient by an individual with expertise
L1820	elastic with condylar pads and joints, prefabricated, includes fitting and adjustment
L1830	immobilizer, canvas longitudinal, prefabricated, off-the-shelf
L1831	locking knee joint(s), positional orthosis, prefabricated, includes fitting and adjustment
L1832	adjustable knee joints (unicentric or polycentric), positional orthosis, rigid support, prefabricated item that has been trimmed, bent, molded, assembled, or otherwise customized to fit a specific patient by an individual with expertise
L1834	without knee joint, rigid, custom fabricated
L1836	rigid, without joint(s), includes soft interface material, prefabricated, off-the-shelf

Ankle-Foot

See also E1815–adjustable ankle extension/flexion device.

Ankle foot orthosis (AFO);

L1900	spring wire, dorsiflexion assist calf band, custom fabricated
L1902	ankle gauntlet, prefabricated, off-the-shelf
L1904	Ankle orthosis, ankle gauntlet, custom-fabricated
L1906	Ankle foot orthosis, multiligamentus ankle support, prefabricated, off-theshelf
L1907	Ankle orthosis, supramalleolar with straps, with or without interface/pads, custom fabricated
L1910	Ankle foot orthosis, posterior, single bar, clasp attachment to shoe prefabricated, includes fitting and adjustment

Ankle foot orthosis (AFO);

L1930	plastic or other material, prefabricated, includes fitting and adjustment
L1932	rigid anterior tibial section, total carbon fiber or equal material, prefabricated, includes fitting and adjustment
L1940	plastic or other material, custom fabricated
L1945	plastic, rigid anterior tibial section (floor reaction), custom fabricated
L1951	spiral, (Institute of Rehabilitative Medicine type), plastic or other material, prefabricated, includes fitting and adjustment
L1971	plastic or other material with ankle joint, prefabricated, includes fitting and adjustment

Hip-Knee-Ankle-Foot (or Any Combination)

L2005	Knee ankle foot orthosis, any material, single or double upright, stance control, automatic lock and swing phase release, any type activation, includes ankle joint, any type, custom fabricated
L2034	Knee ankle foot orthosis, full plastic, single upright, with or without free motion knee, medial lateral rotation control, with or without free motion ankle, custom fabricated

L2035 Knee ankle foot orthosis, full plastic, static (pediatric size), without free motion ankle, prefabricated, includes fitting and adjustment

Additions to Lower Extremity Orthosis

Shoe-Ankle-Shin-Knee

L2232 Addition to lower extremity orthosis, rocker bottom for total contact ankle foot orthosis, for custom fabricated orthosis only

L2387 Addition to lower extremity, polycentric knee joint, for custom fabricated knee ankle foot orthosis, each joint

Foot, Orthopedic Shoes, Shoe Modifications, Transfers

See codes A5501-A5508 for diabetic shoe inserts.

Insert, Removable, Molded to Patient Model

Foot, insert, removable, molded to patient model;
L3000 "UCB" type, Berkeley Shell, each
L3001 Spenco, each
L3002 plastazote or equal, each
L3003 silicone gel, each
L3010 longitudinal arch support, each
L3020 longitudinal/metatarsal support, each

L3030 Foot, insert, removable, formed to patient foot [e.g. vasyli], each

L3031 Foot, insert/plate, removable, addition to lower extremity orthosis, high strength, lightweight material, all hybrid lamination/prepreg composite, each

Arch Support, Removable, Premolded

Foot, arch support, removable, premolded;
L3040 longitudinal, each
L3050 metatarsal, each
L3060 longitudinal/metatarsal, each
Ortho heel

Arch Support, Nonremovable, Attached to Shoe

Foot, arch support, non-removable attached to shoe;
L3070 longitudinal, each
L3080 metatarsal, each
L3090 longitudinal/metatarsal, each
L3100 Hallus-valgus night dynamic splint, prefabricated, off-the-shelf

Abduction and Rotation Bars

Foot;
L3160 adjustable shoe-styled positioning device
L3170 plastic, silicone or equal, heel stabilizer, prafabricated, off-the-shelf, each

Orthopedic Footwear

Orthopedic shoe, oxford with supinator or pronator;
L3201	infant
L3202	child
L3203	junior

Orthopedic shoe, hightop with supinator or pronator,
L3204	infant
L3206	child
L3207	junior
L3216	Orthopedic footwear, ladies shoe, depth inlay, each
L3219	Orthopedic footwear, mens shoe; oxford, each
L3221	depth inlay, each
L3222	hightop, depth inlay, each

Shoe Modification

Lift, elevation;
L3300	Heel, tapered to metatarsals, per inch
L3310	Heel and sole, neoprene, per inch
L3320	Heel and sole, cork, per inch
L3330	metal extension (skate)
L3332	inside shoe, tapered, up to one-half inch
L3334	heel, per inch
L3340	Heel wedge, sach
L3350	Heel wedge

Sole wedge;
L3360	outside sole
L3370	between sole
L3380	Clubfoot wedge
L3390	Outflare wedge

Heel;
L3430	counter, plastic reinforced
L3480	pad and depression for spur
L3485	pad, removable for spur

Shoe Inserts

Codes L3020 and L3030 for shoe inserts are probably the most commonly used codes in a typical chiropractic office. One code is for "molded" and the other is "formed." Ask your supplier which code best describes their orthotic supply.

In addition to any orthotic supply, don't forget the associated codes, such as an appropriate E/M, handling and conveyance (99002), and foot x-rays, if needed. Follow-up care could include orthotic management and training (97760), strapping support for foot/ankle (29540), and any therapies as clinically indicated and necessary.

See codes A5501-A5508 for diabetic shoe inserts.

Orthopedic Shoe Additions

Orthopedic shoe addition;
- L3500   insole, leather
- L3510   insole, rubber
- L3520   insole, felt covered with leather
- L3530   sole, half
- L3540   sole, full

Transfer or Replacement

- L3649   Orthopedic shoe, modification, addition or transfer, not otherwise specified

Upper Limb

Shoulder

Shoulder orthosis, (SO);
- L3650   figure of eight design abduction restrainer, prefabricated, off-the-shelf
- L3671   shoulder joint design, without joints, may include soft interface, straps, custom fabricated, includes fitting and adjustment
- L3674   abduction positioning (airplane design), thoracic and support bar, with or without nontorsion joint/turnbuckle, may include interface, straps, custom fabricated, includes fitting and adjustment
- L3677   shoulder joint design, without joints, may include soft interface, straps, prefabricated item that has been trimmed, bent, molded, assembled, or otherwise customized to fit a specific patient by an individual with expertise

Elbow

> See also E1800–adjustable elbow extension/flexion device.

Elbow orthosis (EO);
- L3702   without joints, may include soft interface, straps, custom fabricated, includes fitting and adjustment
- L3710   elastic with metal joints, prefabricated, off-the-shelf
- L3720   double upright with forearm/arm cuffs, free motion, custom fabricated
- L3730   double upright with forearm/arm cuffs, extension/flexion assist, custom fabricated
- L3740   double upright with forearm/arm cuffs, adjustable position lock with active control, custom-fabricated
- L3760   with adjustable position locking joint(s), prefabricated, includes fitting and adjustments, any type
- L3762   rigid, without joints, includes soft interface material, prefabricated, off-the-shelf

Elbow-Wrist-Hand

Elbow-wrist-hand orthoses,
- L3763   rigid, without joints, may include soft interface, straps, custom fabricated, includes fitting and adjustment
- L3764   includes one or more nontorsion joints, elastic bands, turnbuckles, may include soft interface, straps, custom fabricated, includes fitting and adjustment

Elbow-Wrist-Hand-Finger

Elbow wrist hand finger orthosis,

L3765 rigid, without joints, may include soft interface, straps, custom fabricated, includes fitting and adjustment

L3766 includes one or more nontorsion joints, elastic bands, turnbuckles, may include soft interface, straps, custom fabricated, includes fitting and adjustment

Wrist-Hand-Finger

See also E1805–adjustable wrist extension/flexion device.

Wrist-hand-finger-orthoses (WHFO);

L3806 includes one or more nontorsion joint(s), elastic bands/springs, turnbuckles, may include soft interface material, straps, custom fabricated, includes fitting and adjustment

L3807 without joint(s), prefabricated item that has been trimmed, bent, molded, assembled, or otherwise customized to fit a specific patient by an individual with expertise

L3808 rigid without joints, may include soft interface material; straps, custom fabricated, includes fitting and adjustment

Other Wrist-Hand-Finger Orthoses – Custom Fitted

Wrist hand orthosis,

L3905 includes one or more nontorsion joints, elastic bands, turnbuckles, may include soft interface, straps, custom fabricated, includes fitting and adjustment

L3908 wrist extension control cock-up, non molded, prefabricated, off-the-shelf

L3913 Hand finger orthosis, without joints, may include soft interface, straps, custom fabricated, includes fitting and adjustment

L3915 Wrist hand orthosis, includes one or more nontorsion joint(s), elastic bands, turnbuckles, may include soft interface, straps, prefabricated item that has been trimmed, bent, molded, assembled, or otherwise customized to fit a specific patient by an individual with expertise

Hand orthosis,

L3917 metacarpal fracture orthosis, prefabricated item that has been trimmed, bent, molded, assembled, or otherwise customized to fit a specific patient by an individual with expertise

L3919 without joints, may include soft interface, straps, custom fabricated, includes fitting and adjustment

Hand finger orthosis,

L3921 includes one or more nontorsion joints, elastic bands, turnbuckles, may include soft interface, straps, custom fabricated, includes fitting and adjustment

L3923 without joints, may include soft interface, straps, prefabricated item that has been trimmed, bent, molded, assembled, or otherwise customized to fit a specific patient by an individual with expertise

Finger orthosis, proximal interphalangeal (pip)/distal interphalangeal (dip),

L3925 non torsion joint/spring, extension/flexion, may include soft interface material, prefabricated, off-the-shelf

L3927 without joint/spring, extension/flexion (e.g. static or ring type), may include soft interface material, prefabricated, off-the-shelf

L3929	Hand finger orthosis, includes one or more nontorsion joint(s), turnbuckles, elastic bands/springs, may include soft interface material, straps, prefabricated item that has been trimmed, bent, molded, assembled, or otherwise customized to fit a specific patient by an individual with expertise
L3931	Wrist hand finger orthosis, includes one or more nontorsion joint(s), turnbuckles, elastic bands/springs, may include soft interface material, straps, prefabricated, includes fitting and adjustment

Finger orthosis,

L3933	without joints, may include soft interface, custom fabricated, includes fitting and adjustment
L3935	nontorsion joint, may include soft interface, custom fabricated, includes fitting and adjustment

Shoulder-Elbow-Wrist-Hand

Shoulder-elbow-wrist-hand orthosis,

L3961	shoulder cap design, without joints, may include soft interface, straps, custom fabricated, includes fitting and adjustment
L3967	abduction positioning (airplane design), thoracic component and support bar, without joints, may include soft interface, straps, custom fabricated, includes fitting and adjustment
L3971	shoulder cap design, includes one or more nontorsion joints, elastic bands, turnbuckles, may include soft interface, straps, custom fabricated, includes fitting and adjustment
L3973	abduction positioning (airplane design), thoracic component and support bar, includes one or more nontorsion joints, elastic bands, turnbuckles, may include soft interface, straps, custom fabricated, includes fitting and adjustment

Shoulder-Elbow-Wrist-Hand-Finger

Shoulder elbow wrist hand finger orthosis,

L3975	shoulder cap design, without joints, may include soft interface, straps, custom fabricated, includes fitting and adjustment
L3976	abduction positioning (airplane design), thoracic component and support bar, without joints, may include soft interface, straps, custom fabricated, includes fitting and adjustment
L3977	shoulder cap design, includes one or more nontorsion joints, elastic bands, turnbuckles, may include soft interface, straps, custom fabricated, includes fitting and adjustment
L3978	abduction positioning (airplane design), thoracic component and support bar, includes one or more nontorsion joints, elastic bands, turnbuckles, may include soft interface, straps, custom fabricated, includes fitting and adjustment

Fracture Orthoses

L3984	Upper extremity fracture orthosis; wrist, prefabricated, includes fitting and adjustment
L3999	Upper limb orthosis, not otherwise specified

Repairs

L4002	Replacement strap, any orthosis, includes all components, any length, any type

Repair of orthotic device;

L4205	labor component, per 15 minutes
L4210	repair or replace minor parts

Ancillary Orthotic Services

- L4350 Ankle control orthosis, stirrup style, rigid, includes any type interface (e.g., pneumatic, gel), prefabricated, off-the-shelf
- L4360 Walking boot, pneumatic and/or vacuum, with or without joints, with or without interface material, prefabricated item that has been trimmed, bent, molded, assembled, or otherwise customized to fit a specific patient by an individual with expertise
- L4370 Pneumatic full leg splint, prefabricated, off-the-shelf
- L4386 Walking boot, non-pneumatic, with or without joints, with or without interface material, prefabricated item that has been trimmed, bent, molded, assembled, or otherwise customized to fit a specific patient by an individual with expertise

  Replacement, soft interface material;
- L4392   static afo
- L4394   foot drop splint
- L4396 Static or dynamic ankle foot orthosis, including soft interface material, adjustable for fit, for positioning, may be used for minimal ambulation, prefabricated item that has been trimmed, bent, molded, assembled, or otherwise customized to fit a specific patient by an individual with expertise
- L4398 Foot drop splint, recumbent positioning device, prefabricated, off-the-shelf
- L4631 Ankle foot orthosis, walking boot type, varus/valgus correction, rocker anterior tibial shell, soft interface, custom arch support, plastic or other material, includes straps and closures, custom fabricated

TEMPORARY CODES

- Q4049 Finger splint, static
- Q4050 Cast supplies, for unlisted types and materials of casts
- Q4051 Splint supplies, miscellaneous (includes thermoplastics, strapping, fasteners, padding and other supplies)
- Q4082 Drug or biological, not otherwise classified, part B drug competitive acquisition program (cap)

PRIVATE PAYER PROCEDURE CODES

See *Section H–Procedures* for "S" codes.

STATE MEDICAID AGENCY CODES

- T5001 Positioning seat for persons with special orthopedic needs, for use in vehicles
- T5999 Supply, not otherwise specified

4. HCPCS Supply Modifiers

This section contains the HCPCS supply code modifiers for 2015.

A modifier provides the means by which the reporting physician or provider can indicate that a service or procedure that is being performed has been altered by some specific circumstance, but not changed in its definition or code. The judicious application of modifiers obviates the necessity for separate reports to describe the circumstance. Modifiers may be used to indicate to the recipient of a report or insurance claim that a service or supply code has been increased, decreased, adjunctive service was performed, or unusual events occurred, etc.

National Modifiers - Level I (CPT -11 to -99)

Modifiers and descriptors at the first level are by CPT-4, maintained by the AMA. These(2) position numeric codes are in the *Procedures* section. Examples are: -22 (unusual service), -52 (reduced service), -59 (distinct procedure), etc.

National Modifiers - Level II (HCPCS -AA to -VV)

These modifier codes are approved by CMS but recommended jointly by the alpha-numeric editorial panel consisting of the American Medical Association (AMA), Health Insurance Association of America (HIAA), and Blue Cross/Blue Shield (BC/BS). These two (2) position alpha-numeric modifier codes are appended to the basic code. The following is a list of all current Level II modifiers. Commonly used modifiers that might be of interest in a chiropractic office are bolded for quick reference. Modifiers for supplies are listed in this section.

Procedure modifiers are listed in the *Section H–Procedures*.

State or Local Modifiers - Level III (-WA to -WZ) [deleted by HIPAA]

HCPCS Level III modifiers (-WA to -ZZ) were formerly for local use. They have been eliminated by HIPAA mandate. Payers or providers who need modifiers must apply to the appropriate organizations (e.g., to CMS for HCPCS modifiers at level II, or to the AMA for CPT modifier codes.) However, Workers Compensation is exempt from HIPAA, and could have different modifiers and codes.

Level II Supply Modifiers (-AA to -VV)

- **-AO** Alternate payment method declined by provider of service
- **-AV** Item furnished in conjunction with a prosthetic device, prosthetic or orthotic
- **-AW** Item furnished in conjunction with a surgical dressing
- **-AX** Item furnished in conjunction with dialysis services
- **-BO** Orally administered nutrition, not by feeding tube
- **-BP** The beneficiary has been informed of the purchase and rental options and has elected to **purchase** the item
- **-BR** The beneficiary has been informed of the purchase and rental options and has elected to **rent** the item
- **-BU** The beneficiary has been informed of the purchase and after 30 days has not informed the supplier of his/her -decision
- **-CG** Policy criteria applied
- **-GA** Waiver of liability statement issued as required by payer policy, individual case
- **-GK** Reasonable and necessary item/service associated with -GA or -GZ modifier
- **-GL** Medically unnecessary upgrade provided instead of non-upgraded item, no charge, no advance beneficiary notice (ABN)

> Primarily used with Medicare

- **-GU** Waiver of liability statement issued as required by payer policy, routine notice
- **-GX** **Notice of liability issued, voluntary under payer policy**
- **-GY** **Item or service statutorily excluded or, does not meet the definition of any Medicare benefit or, for non-Medicare insurers, is not a contract benefit**
- **-GZ** **Item or service expected to be denied as not reasonable and necessary**

> No Medicare ABN form was signed by the patient.

- **-K0** Lower extremity prosthesis functional level 0: Does not have the ability or potential to ambulate or transfer safely with or without assistance and a prosthesis does not enhance their quality of life or mobility.
- **-K1** Lower extremity prosthesis functional level 1: Has the ability or potential to use a prosthesis for transfers or ambulation on level surfaces at fixed cadence. Typical of the limited and unlimited household ambulator.
- **-K2** Lower extremity prosthesis functional level 2: Has the ability or potential for ambulation with the ability to traverse low level environmental barriers such as burbs, stairs or uneven surfaces. Typical of the limited community ambulator.
- **-K3** Lower extremity prosthesis functional level 3: Has the ability or potential for ambulation with variable cadence. Typical of the community ambulator who has the ability to transverse most environmental barriers and may have vocational, therapeutic, or exercise activity that demands prosthetic utilization beyond simple locomotion.
- **-K4** Lower extremity prosthesis functional level 4: Has the ability or potential for prosthetic ambulation that exceeds the basic ambulation skills, exhibiting high impact, stress, or energy levels, typical of the prosthetic demands of the child, active adult, or athlete.
- **-KA** Add on option/accessory for wheelchair
- **-KD** Drug or biological infused through DME

-KF	**Item designated by FDA as class III device**	

If your device is an FDA Class III device, append modifier -KF to ensure higher payment.

-KR **Rental item, billing for partial month**

See -RR for a full month.

-KS Glucose monitor supply for diabetic beneficiary not treated with insulin

-LL Lease/rental (use the -LL modifier when DME equipment rental is to be applied against the purchase price)

-LT **Left side (used to identify procedures performed on the left side of the body)**

-MS Six month maintenance and servicing fee for reasonable and necessary parts and labor which are not covered under any manufacturer or supplier warranty

-NR New when rented (use the -NR modifier when DME which was new at the time of rental is subsequently purchased)

-NU **New equipment**

-RA Replacement of a DME, orthotic or prosthetic item

-RB Replacement of a part of DME, orthotic or prosthetic item furnished as part of a repair

-RD Drug provided to beneficiary, but not administered incident-to

-RR **Rental (use the -RR modifier when DME (Durable Medical Equipment) is to be rented)**

-RR is usually for one month. See -KR for partial month.

-RT **Right side (used to identify procedures performed on the right side of the body)**

-SC **Medically necessary service or supply**

-TW Back-up equipment

-UE **Used durable medical equipment**

5. Alphabetic List

Abdomen
    pad, low profile L1270
Abduction rotation bar, foot L3170
Absorption dressing A6251-A6256
Adhesive
    bandage A6413
    remover A4455
Administrative, Miscellaneous and Investigational.................. A9999
AFO E1815, E1830, L1900, L4392, L4396
Air pressure pad/mattress E0186
Alginate dressing A6196-A6199
Alternating pressure mattress/pad E0181
Ambulation device......................E0100
Amygdalin J3570
Ankle-foot orthosis (AFO)..........L1900, L4392, L4396
Anterior-posterior-lateral orthosis L0700, L0710
Arch support L3040-L3100
Back supports........................... L0621
Battery
    replacement for TENS............. A4630
Belt
    extremity.................................. E0945
    pelvic, ... E0944
Bilirubin (phototherapy) light .. E0202
Binder A4465
Biofeedback device E0746
Blood
    glucose monitor....................... E0607
Boot
    pelvic E0944
Cane............................... E0100, E0105
    accessory...................A4636, A4637
Cannula, nasal A4615
Cast
    materials, special A4590
    supplies A4580, A4590, Q4051
Cervical
    head harness/halter E0942
    orthosis L0200
    traction E0855, E0856

Cervical-thoracic-lumbar-sacral orthosis (CTLSO)..L0700, L0710
Chair
    sitz bath....................... E0160-E0162
Chin cup, cervical L0150
Cleanser, wound A6260
Clubfoot wedge.......................... L3380
Collagen
    wound dressing A6024
Collar, cervical
    multiple post L0180-L0200
    nonadjust (foam) L0120
Commode E0160
    chair........................ E0170-E0171
    lift E0172
Compressed gas system E0480
Compression stockings A6549
Contact layer.............................. A6206
Cover, wound
    alginate dressing A6196
    foam dressing......................... A6209
    hydrogel dressing A6242-A6248
    specialty absorptive dressing.............. A6251-A6256
Crutches E0118
    accessories A4635-A4637
CTLSO L1000-L1120, L0700, L0710
Decubitus care equipment........E0199
Delivery/set-up/dispensing...... A9901
Dialysis
    supplies................................... A4927
Dressing (see also Bandage)
    alginate.......................A6196-A6199
    collagen.................................. A6024
    contact layer A6206
    foam A6209-A6215
    gauze A6216
    hydrocolloid A6234-A6241
    hydrogel......................A6242-A6248
    specialty absorptive A6251-A6256
    transparent film A6257-A6259
    tubular A6457
Dry pressure pad/mattress..............E0184, E0199

Durable medical equipment (DME).......... E0100-E1830, K Codes
Eggcrate dry pressure pad/mattress..............E0184, E0199
Elbow
    orthosis (EO)...E1800, L3740, L3760
    protector E0191
Electrodes, per pair A4556
EMG E0746
Exercise equipment.................. A9300
Extremity belt/harness E0945
Filler, wound
    alginate dressing A6199
    foam dressing......................... A6215
    hydrocolloid dressing, A6240, A6241
    hydrogel dressing A6248
    not elsewhere classified A6261,A6262
Film, transparent (for dressing)......... ....A6257-A6259
Foam dressing A6209-A6215
Footdrop splint L4398
Footplate..................................... L3031
Footwear, orthopedic L3201
Fracture
    frame E0948
Gait trainer E8000-E8002
Gauze (see also Bandage)
    impregnated, ... A6222-A6233
Gel
    conductive A4558
    pressure pad E0185
Gloves.. A4927
Grab bar, trapeze E0910, E0940
Gravity traction device E0941
Hallus-Valgus dynamic splint...L3100
Halter, cervical head E0942
Hand finger orthosis, prefabricated... .... L3923
Hand restoration
    orthosis (WHFO) E1805, E1825
Handgrip (cane, crutch, walker).......... A4636
Harness E0942, E0944, E0945

Heat
   application...................E0200-E0239
   infrared heating pad
      system...............A4639, E0221
   lamp..................... E0200, E0205
   pad E0210, E0215
Heel
   protector E0191
   shoe L3430-L3485
   stabilizer..................................L3170
Helmet, head A8000-A8004
Hexalite A4590
Hydrocollator E0225, E0239
Hydrocolloid dressing...A6234-A6241
Hydrogel dressing A6242-A6248,
                        A6231-A6233
Impregnated gauze dressing... A6222
Irrigation supplies A4322
Kidney
   ESRD supply......................... A4927
Knee
   orthosis (KO)... E1810, K0901-K0902
Kyphosis pad L1020, L1025
Laetrile....................................J3570
Lead wires, per pair A4557
Lift
   shoe L3300-L3334
LSO L0621-L0640
Lumbar-sacral orthosis
   (LSO) L0621-L0640
Mask
   oxygen..................................... A4620
Mattress
   air pressure E0186
   dry pressure E0184
   hospital bed...........................E0272
   water pressure........................E0187
Monitor
   blood glucose E0607
Mouthpiece (for respiratory
   equipment) A4617
Multi-Podus type AFO L4396
Multiple post collar,
   cervical.......................L0180-L0200
Nerve stimulator with batteries E0765
Neuromuscular stimulator E0745
Noncovered services................ A9270
Nonimpregnated gauze
   dressing A6216
Nonprescription drug A9150
Occipital/mandibular support,
   cervical L0160
Oral device/appliance....E0485-E0486
Orthopedic shoes
   arch support................ L3040-L3100
   footwear L3201
   insert L3000-L3030
   lift L3300-L3334
   miscellaneous additions.......... L3500

   positioning device....................L3170
   transfer L3649
   wedge L3340
Orthotic additions
   scoliosis .L1010-L1120, L1210-L1290
   shoe...................... L3300, L3649
Orthotic devices
   ankle-foot (AFO;
      see also Orthopedic shoes).....
      ......E1815, E1830, L1900, L3160
   anterior-posterior-lateral ....
      ....L0700, L0710
   cervical.............................. L0200
   cervical-thoracic-lumbar-sacral
      (CTLSO)...............L0700, L0710
   elbow (EO) E1800, E1801, L3740
   hand, (WHFO) E1805, E1825, L3807
   hand, finger, prefabricated L3923
   knee (KO)................................ E1810
   multiple post collar L0180-L0200
   not otherwise specifiedL1499, L3999
   pneumatic splint L4350
   repair or replacement..............L4210
   replace soft interface material L4394
   scoliosis L1000 L1499
   shoulder (SO)............. L3650-L3677
   shoulder-elbow-wrist-hand
      (SEWHO) L3978
   spinal, cervical L0200
   toe E1830
   wrist-hand-finger
      (WHFO).E1805, E1806, E1825
Osteogenesis stimulator.......... E0747
Oxygen
   mask A4620
   respiratory
      equipment/supplies E0480
   tubing A4616
Pad
   gel pressure E0185
   heat E0210, E0215, E0217
   sheepskin...................E0188, E0189
   water circulating cold with
      pump E0218
   water circulating heat with
      pump E0217
Paraffin bath unit E0235
Paraffin....................................A4265
Paste, conductive A4558
Pelvic belt/harness/boot E0944
Percussor E0480
Phototherapy light.................... E0202
Plastazote................................. L3002
Pneumatic
   appliance................................. L4350
   splint L4350
Positioning seat........................T5001

Pressure
   pad E0199
Protector, heel or elbow E0191
Pump
   alternating pressure pad E0182
   water circulating pad, ... E0236
Quad cane E0105
Replacement
   battery A4630
   tip for cane, crutches, walker.. A4637
   underarm pad for crutches..... A4635
Rib belt, thoracic...................... L0220
Sacral nerve stimulation test
   lead....................................... A4290
Scoliosis.........................L1000 L1499
   additions..L1010-L1120, L1210-L1290
Seat
   insert, wheelchair................... E0992
Sheepskin pad E0188, E0189
Shoes
   arch support................ L3040-L3100
   for diabetics............................ A5508
   insert L3000-L3030
   lift L3300-L3334
   miscellaneous additions.......... L3500
   orthopedic L3201
   positioning device....................L3170
   transfer L3649
   wedge L3340-L3485
Shoulder
   orthosis (SO).......................... L3650
   spinal, cervical L0200
Sitz bath......................... E0160-E0162
Skin
   barrier, ostomy A5120
Sling.. A4565
Specialty absorptive
   dressing A6251-A6256
Spinal orthosis
   cervical................................... L0200
   cervical-thoracic-lumbar-sacral
      (CTLSO)...............L0700, L0710
   multiple post collar, ... L0180-L0200
   scoliosis L1000-L1499
Splint.................. A4570, L3100, L4350
   ankle L4398
   dynamic......... E1800, E1805, E1810,
                E1815, E1825, E1830
   footdrop L4398
Static progressive
   stretch E1801, E1806
Stimulators
   neuromuscular E0744, E0745
   osteogenesis, electrical.......... E0747
Supply/accessory/service........ A9900
Support
   arch........................L3040-L3090
   cervical................................... L0200

Surgical
   dressing A6196
   stocking A4490-A4510
Tables, bed E0315
TENS A4595, E0720
Therapeutic lightbox .. A4634, E0203
Thermometer A4931-A4932
Thoracic-lumbar-sacral orthosis (TLSO)
   scoliosis L1200-L1290
   spinal L0450-L0492
Tip (cane, crutch, walker)
   replacement A4637
TLSO L0450-L0492, L1200-L1290
Traction device, ambulatory ... E0830
Traction equipment E0840-E0948
Transcutaneous electrical nerve stimulator (TENS) E0720
Transparent film
   (for dressing) A6257-A6259
Trapeze bar E0910-E0912, E0940

Tube/Tubing
   oxygen A4616
Ultraviolet light therapy
   system A4633
Upper extremity fracture
   orthosis L3999
Ureterostomy supplies A4590
Vabra aspirator A4480
Vitamin B-12 cyanocobalamin J3420
Walker E0149
   accessories A4636, A4637
Walking splint L4386
Water
   pressure pad/mattress E0187, E0198
Wedges, shoe L3340
Wheelchair
   transfer board or device E0705
WHFO with inflatable air
   chamber L3807
Wound cleanser A6260

Wound cover
   alginate dressing A6196
   collagen dressing A6024
   foam dressing A6209
   hydrocolloid dressing. A6234-A6239
   hydrogel dressing A6242
   specialty absorptive
      dressing A6251-A6256
Wound filler
   alginate dressing A6199
   foam dressing A6215
   hydrocolloid dressing A6240, A6241
   hydrogel dressing A6248
   not elsewhere
      classified A6261, A6262
Wrist
   hand/finger orthosis
      (WHFO) E1805, E1825

ACA Template Letters

This section includes several template letters which were created by the American Chiropractic Association to assist doctors of chiropractic with specific reimbursement issues. The have been reprinted here by permission. Non-ACA members my retype the template letters and make changes as needed to fit their situation. The electronic versions of these documents are available to all ACA members through the following link:

ACA members may go to ACAtoday.org/appeals and log in to their account to access these downloadable forms.

Letters in this Section:
1. Acupuncture and Electrical Stimulation .... A - 2
2. CCI Edits .... A - 3
3. CMT Level Authorized .... A - 4
4. CPT Strapping Codes 29200-29280 and 29520-29590 .... A - 5
5. Denial of Pediatric Chiropractic Care .... A - 6
6. E/M with CMT .... A - 11
7. Hot and Cold Packs .... A - 12
8. Level of E/M Authorized .... A - 13
9. Manual Therapy .... A - 14
10. Massage .... A - 15
11. Medical Necessity .... A - 16
12. Model Provider Assignment Form Under ERISA .... A - 17
13. Physical Medicine .... A - 18

ACUPUNCTURE AND ELECTRICAL STIMULATION

<NAME OF PRACTICE>
<ADDRESS>
<PHONE/FAX>

<DATE>
<ADDRESS OF PAYER>

Re: Insurer: <INSURER>
Patient Name: <PATIENT NAME>
Date of Service: <DATE OF SERVICE>
Claim #: <CLAIM #>
Policy #: <PATIENT'S POLICY #>
Group #: <PATIENT'S GROUP #>

Thank you for your letter/EOB regarding the above referenced patient for services on <DATE OF SERVICE>. I appreciate your communication but respectfully disagree and object to your position that CPT® code #97810 and CPT code #97014 are mutually exclusive or are considered a global procedure.

According to CPT guidelines there is a specific CPT code (#97813) for acupuncture with electrical stimulation, when the electrical stimulation is applied to the needles directly as part of the acupuncture treatment. The CPT code #97810 is used when needle acupuncture is performed without electrical stimulation being applied directly to any one of the needles. The CPT code #97014 is a code used for electrical stimulation that has nothing to do with acupuncture. Your decision that these codes are mutually exclusive when performed on the same date of service is not in accordance with code usage and descriptions included in the CPT manual.

In the case of my patient referenced above, acupuncture was applied to <INSERT REGION> while electric muscle stimulation was applied to <INSERT REGION>. In my clinical opinion this was medically necessary because: <INSERT CASE SPECIFIC INFORMATION SUPPORTING TREATMENT>

Also, if your policy regarding these codes is derived from the National Correct Coding Initiative [CCI] system, it has no authority in third-party reimbursement. In a letter dated April 17, 2000, from Niles R. Rosen, MD, medical director for the National Correct Coding Initiative [CCI], to James A. Mertz, DC, president of the American Chiropractic Association, he states:

"CCI was not developed with the intent that it be used by other third party payors to process their claims."

Please correct your software or manual edit on these codes and provide reimbursement as soon as possible.

<TREATING PROVIDER'S FULL NAME>, D.C.

CC: AMERICAN CHIROPRACTIC ASSOCIATION
CPT is a registered trademark of the AMA

CCI EDITS

<NAME OF PRACTICE>
<ADDRESS>
<PHONE/FAX>

<DATE>
<ADDRESS OF PAYER>

Re: Insurer: <INSURER>
Patient Name: <PATIENT NAME>
Date of Service: <DATE OF SERVICE>
Claim #: <CLAIM #>
Policy #: <PATIENT'S POLICY #>
Group #: <PATIENT'S GROUP #>

To whom it may concern:

I have reviewed your letter on the above patient and have serious concerns about your coding and reimbursement policy, as it is not consistent with the American Medical Association's (AMA) Current Procedural Terminology (CPT) coding guidelines.

I am aware that your coding policy reflects the National Correct Coding Initiative (NCCI) edits and feel it necessary to advise you these edits are not intended for use by third-party payers. In fact, the Medical Director for NCCI, Dr. Niles Rosen, wrote in a letter to the American Chiropractic Association (ACA), dated April 17, 2000, "NCCI was not developed with the intent that it be used by third party payers to process their claims."

Since you may not be aware of this determination, I would appreciate your review and reconsideration of my claim(s) and request a revision of your reimbursement policy. Continued use of incorrect coding policy will be viewed as an unfair claim practice.

I hope to hear from you within 30 days and appreciate your immediate action on these reimbursement and policy changes.

Sincerely,

<TREATING PROVIDER'S FULL NAME>, D.C.

CC: AMERICAN CHIROPRACTIC ASSOCIATION
CPT is a registered trademark of the AMA

CMT LEVEL AUTHORIZED

<NAME OF PRACTICE>
<ADDRESS>
<PHONE/FAX>

<DATE>
<ADDRESS OF PAYER>

Re: Insurer: <INSURER>
      Patient Name: <PATIENT NAME>
      Date of Service: <DATE OF SERVICE>
      Claim #: <CLAIM #>
      Policy #: <PATIENT'S POLICY #>
      Group #: <PATIENT'S GROUP #>

To whom it may concern:

Thank you for your response to the documentation submitted regarding care for my patient, <INSERT PATIENT NAME>. I appreciate your communication, but respectfully disagree with your decision that Chiropractic Manipulative Treatment (CMT) CPT® code <ENTER CODE NUMBER> is inappropriate for my patient. I indicated that CMT CPT®code <ENTER CODE NUMBER> was necessary because: <INSERT INFORMATION WHICH SUPPORTS THE LEVEL OF CMT REQUESTED (E.G., FINDINGS FROM PHYSICAL EXAM OR X-RAY, PATIENT COMPLAINTS)>.

As you are aware, when determining which level of CMT is appropriate to treat the patient, providers must take into consideration the patient's complaints, physical findings, and many other factors. As the treating provider, I feel that my analysis of the patient, and determinations regarding care needed, are far more accurate than a determination based simply on the limited paperwork you require <ATTACH ANY FORMS INITIALLY SUBMITTED TO THE INSURER ALONG WITH ALL PERTINENT CHART NOTES, EXAM FORMS, ETC.>.

Based on the attached, I would appreciate a reconsideration of your decision in regard to the CMT level most appropriate for my patient.

Sincerely,

<TREATING PROVIDER'S FULL NAME>, D.C.

CC: AMERICAN CHIROPRACTIC ASSOCIATION
CPT is a registered trademark of the AMA

CPT STRAPPING CODES 29200-29280 AND 29520-29590

<NAME OF PRACTICE>
<ADDRESS>
<PHONE/FAX>

<DATE>
<ADDRESS OF PAYER>

Re: Insurer: <INSURER>
Patient Name: <PATIENT NAME>
Date of Service: <DATE OF SERVICE>
Claim #: <CLAIM #>
Policy #: <PATIENT'S POLICY #>
Group #: <PATIENT'S GROUP #>

To whom it may concern:

Thank you for your (select one) letter/EOB on the above mentioned patient for care provided on <INSERT DATE OF SERVICE>. I appreciate your communication, but respectfully disagree with your decision that CPT® codes 29200-29280 and 29520-29590 are not billable by doctors of chiropractic because they are considered "surgery codes."

The CPT® 2014 Professional Edition explicitly indicates that "it is important to recognize that the listing of a service or procedure and its code number in a specific section of [CPT 2014] does not restrict its use to a specific specialty group. Any procedure or service in any section of [CPT 2014] may be used to designate the services rendered by any qualified physician or other qualified health care professional or entity."

In <INSERT STATE>, the use of the strapping codes are within the scope of practice for doctors of chiropractic. A complete description of the scope of practice for doctors of chiropractic in <INSERT STATE> is accessible at: <INSERT WEB ADDRESS FOR STATE SCOPE OF PRACTICE. ABBREVIATED VERSIONS OF STATES SCOPES OF PRACTICE ARE AVAILABLE AT WWW.FCLB.ORG.>

In the case of <INSERT PATIENT'S NAME>, strapping was performed for the purpose of <INSERT STATEMENT OF MEDICAL NECESSITY>. In the attached documentation, I have clearly presented the reason these services were warranted.

If this denial is due to pre-set software edits, I urge you to consider the AMA's Current Procedural Terminology (CPT) policy regarding the classification of codes within the CPT manual. Software edits that routinely deny codes based on categorization, without consideration of state scope of practice and medical necessity, are incorrect.

I hope this nationally recognized coding source will allow you to reassess your position and provide payment within 30 days.

Sincerely,

<TREATING PROVIDER'S FULL NAME>, D.C.

Attached: <ATTACH DOCUMENTATION>
cc: American Chiropractic Association (ACA)
CPT is a registered trademark of the AMA

DENIAL OF PEDIATRIC CHIROPRACTIC CARE

<NAME OF PRACTICE>
<ADDRESS>
<PHONE/FAX>

<DATE>
<ADDRESS OF PAYER>

Re: Insurer: <INSURER>
       Patient Name: <PATIENT NAME>
       Date of Service: <DATE OF SERVICE>
       Claim #: <CLAIM #>
       Policy #: <PATIENT'S POLICY #>
       Group #: <PATIENT'S GROUP #>

To whom it may concern:

Thank you for your (select one) letter/EOB regarding the above-referenced patient for services rendered on <DATE(S) OF SERVICE>. I appreciate the time you took to communicate with me, but disagree with your determination to deny coverage for chiropractic care for children. There are a number of concerns surrounding the blanket denial of chiropractic care for children. Please consider the following issues.

Scope of Practice

Doctors of chiropractic are considered physicians by Medicare, Federal Workers' Compensation, and in the vast majority of states. Additionally, the treatment of children and adolescents has long been within the scope of practice for doctors of chiropractic. Treatment by doctors of chiropractic includes not only spinal manipulation and other forms of manual care, but also active and passive therapeutic modalities, evaluation and management services, instruction on lifestyle modifications, diet and exercise, as well as postural and nutritional advice. When treating children, doctors of chiropractic provide care for many of the same ailments as other healthcare practitioners, including respiratory problems, ear, nose, and throat problems, and general preventive care. In addition, doctors of chiropractic treat a variety of pediatric conditions including otitis media, asthma, allergies, infantile colic, and enuresis.[1] A recent report from the Centers for Disease Control (CDC) found that chiropractic/osteopathy was the most common doctor-directed CAM (Complementary and Alternative Medicine) therapy used by children.[2] A second study, published in the journal Pediatrics, found that "…chiropractors were the most common CAM providers visited by children and adolescents," estimating that 14% of all chiropractic visits were for pediatric patients. Clearly, chiropractors have become a standard part of the healthcare team for many children.[3]

Research

Effectiveness of any intervention needs to be evaluated on an individual basis, both regarding specific conditions and specific patients. Within that context, recent research has demonstrated the efficacy of chiropractic care for many non-musculoskeletal pediatric conditions. A recent systematic review of chiropractic literature found that the evidence was promising for the potential benefit of manual procedures for children with otitis media. The review also found that evidence supports that the entire chiropractic clinical encounter has a benefit to patients with asthma, cervicogenic vertigo, and

DENIAL OF PEDIATRIC CHIROPRACTIC CARE - *CONT*

infantile colic.[4] Additionally, a randomized controlled trial found that spinal manipulation had a positive short-term effect on infants with colic.[5] There is also a large body of descriptive studies supporting the effectiveness of chiropractic care for a wide variety of pediatric conditions including nursing dysfunction, headache, plagiocephaly, torticollis, constipation, and reflux.[6, 7, 8, 9, 10, 11, 12, 13, 14, 15, 16]

Research also has shown the need for pediatric treatment of back pain and other musculoskeletal conditions. A number of studies have demonstrated that children experience significant back pain and, because of the prevalence of back pain in children and adolescents, studies have been done to determine the efficacy of chiropractic management of pediatric patients. Many children are also affected by carrying heavy backpacks for school. In a study of 1,122 backpack users, 74.4 percent were classified as having back pain, validated by significantly poorer general health, more limited physical functioning, and more bodily pain.[17] Additionally, many researchers are concerned that heavy backpacks, carried by adolescents, contribute to the development of back pain. Another study, completed in 2003, found that pediatric patients with low back pain responded favorably to chiropractic management, with no complications reported.[18]

For the treatment of back pain, there are many recognized guidelines which support the use of spinal manipulation in addition to other therapies.[19] A 2007 study, published in the *Annals of Internal Medicine*, stated: "Recommendation 7: For patients who do not improve with self-care options, clinicians should consider the addition of nonpharmacologic therapy with proven benefits—for acute low back pain, *spinal manipulation* [emphasis added]; for chronic or subacute low back pain, intensive interdisciplinary rehabilitation, exercise therapy, acupuncture, massage therapy, spinal manipulation [emphasis added], yoga, cognitive behavioral therapy, or progressive relaxation."[20] Because many patients do not want to use prescription drugs to manage pain, especially when parents are considering care for their children, other passive and active interventions such as spinal manipulation should be made available to them.

A study, published in 2000 found that, "Patients with chronic low-back pain treated by chiropractors showed greater improvement and satisfaction at one month than patients treated by family physicians. Satisfaction scores were higher for chiropractic patients. A higher proportion of chiropractic patients (56 percent vs. 13 percent) reported that their low-back pain was better or much better, whereas nearly one-third of medical patients reported their low-back pain was worse or much worse."[21] Additionally, a study published in the *British Medical Journal* comparing manual therapy to physiotherapy (mainly exercise) and general practitioner care (counseling, education and drugs), found that "manual therapy resulted in faster recovery than physiotherapy and general practitioner care. Moreover, total costs of the manual therapy-treated patients were about one-third of the costs of physiotherapy or general practitioner care."[22] Given the efficacy and cost-effectiveness of spinal manipulation, this treatment option should be made available to all of your company's beneficiaries.

Clinical skills, financial impact, and patient safety

Chiropractic physicians possess more education and clinical skills in the area of musculoskeletal diagnosis and treatment compared to general medical physicians and physical therapists. A 2005 study, which sought to determine the adequacy of education in musculoskeletal medicine, concluded that "training in musculoskeletal medicine is inadequate in both medical school and non-orthopedic residency training programs,"[23]

DENIAL OF PEDIATRIC CHIROPRACTIC CARE - *CONT*

while an earlier study found that medical students "spend little time studying the neuro-musculoskeletal system and its health related problems."[24] It is confusing that your company will not allow the providers who are best suited to evaluate and treat neuro-musculoskeletal conditions to provide treatment to your younger beneficiaries. To prohibit doctors of chiropractic from treating children will not result in cost savings. Traditional care inherently has higher costs for treatment and diagnostics and the risks associated with prescriptions and invasive procedures can be high as is evidenced by a multitude of cost-effectiveness studies.

Recent studies have pointed to the safety of chiropractic care for children. A 2007 systematic review of adverse events following spinal manipulation in children found only nine serious adverse events over a 110-year period.[25] Miller et al found no adverse events following chiropractic care of 781 pediatric patients (75% under 4 months of age) involved in over 5000 chiropractic treatments from 2002-2004.[26]

Discriminatory policy/standards

As already mentioned, chiropractic care is a broad-based form of healthcare including, but not limited to, manual therapies, physiotherapies, nutritional advice, exercise prescription, and lifestyle advice. Please advise as to whether you are refusing to cover any of these services for children or if you are denying reimbursement only to those families who chose to receive those services from a doctor of chiropractic.

In addition, please help us understand whether your company denies payment to medical and osteopathic physicians, as well as physical therapists, for treatment of children and adolescents due to a lack of evidence. As the FDA did not permit research on children until 2005, most pediatric dosages have been prescribed on a hypothetical, by-weight basis because of this restriction. Policies that deny chiropractic care for children due to a lack of research hold chiropractic physicians to a different set of standards than other covered providers. I would like to request a review of your company's policies regarding care for children to ensure that there is consistency in the basis for policy determinations between clinical disciplines.

I hope that policy makers in your organization will take the time to consider these factors and review the research cited in this correspondence. Upon review of this evidence, I would like to request a review of the denial issued for care provided to a <INSERT CHILD'S AGE> child. In the case of <INSERT PATIENT'S NAME>, chiropractic care was provided for <INSERT DIAGNOSIS>. The goal of this treatment was to <INSERT TREATMENT GOALS>. A blind denial of treatment provided to this patient, without taking into consideration the benefits of chiropractic care or at least allowing a trial of care, may be a great disservice to your beneficiaries and to your company.

I look forward to hearing back from you in the next thirty days, with your responses to the questions posed and evidence presented.

Sincerely,
<TREATING PROVIDER'S FULL NAME>, D.C.
Enclosure: <INSERT CLINICAL RECORD>
cc: American Chiropractic Association

DENIAL OF PEDIATRIC CHIROPRACTIC CARE, REFERENCES

References

[1] Lee, A., Li, H., Kemper, K. Chiropractic Care for Children. Archives of Pediatric Adolescent Medicine. 2000;154:401-407.

[2] Barnes PM, Bloom B, Nahin R. Complementary and Alternative Medicine Use Among Adults and Children: United States, 2007. National Center for Complementary and Alternative Medicine, National Institutes of Health. 2008.

[3] Kemper KJ, Vohra S, Walls R, The Task Force on Complementary and Alternative Medicine the Provisional Section on Complementary, Holistic, and Integrative. Pediatrics Medicine 2008; 122(6): 1374-1386.

[4] Hawk C, Khorsan R, Lisi AJ, Ferrance RJ, Evans MW. Chiropractic care for nonmusculoskeletal conditions: a systematic review with implications for whole systems research. Journal of Alternative and Complementary Medicine 2007 Jun;13(5):491-512.

[5] Wiberg J, Nordsteen J., Nillson N. The Short-term Effect of Spinal Manipulation in the Treatment of Infantile Colic: A Randomized Controlled Clinical Trial with a Blinded Observer. Journal of Manipulative & Physiological Therapeutics; Oct99, Vol. 22 Issue 8, p517, 6p

[6] Vallone S. Chiropractic evaluation and treatment of musculoskeletal dysfunction in infants demonstrating difficulty breastfeeding. J Clin Chiro Pediatrics. 2004;6(1):349-368.

[7] Hewitt EG. Chiropractic care for infants with dysfunctional nursing: a case series. J Clin Chiropr Pediatr 1999;4(1):241-4.

[8] Lisi AJ, Dabrowski Y. Chiropractic spinal manipulation for cervicogenic headache in an 8 year old. JNMS 2002;10(3):98-103. headache--cervicogenic

[9] Hewitt EG. Chiropractic care of a 13 year old with headache and neck pain – a case report. J Can Chiro Assoc 1994;38(3):160-162.headache/neck pain

[10] Davies NJ. Chiropractic management of deformational plagiocephaly in infants: an alternative to device-dependent therapy. Chiro J Austral 2002;32(2):52-5. plagiocephaly

[11] Quezada D. Chiropractic Care of an Infant with Plagiocephaly JCCP 2004;5(1)

[12] Aker, Peter S. Cassidy, J. David. Torticollis in infants and children: a report of three cases. Journal of the Canadian Chiropractic Association 1990;34(1):13-19. torticollis

[13] Bolton PS, Bolton SP. Acute Cervical Torticollis and Palmer Upper Cervical Specific Technique: A Report of Three Cases. Chiropr J Aust 1996;263:89-93.torticollis

[14] Quist DM, Duray SM. Resolution of symptoms of chronic constipation in an 8-year-old male after chiropractic treatment. Jour Manipulative Physiol Therapeutics 2007;30(1):65-68.

[15]Hewitt EG. Chiropractic treatment of a 7 month old with chronic constipation – a

[16]Alcantara J, Anderson R. Chiropractic care of a pediatric patient with symptoms associated with Gastroesophageal reflux disease. J Chiropr Educ 2005;19(1):43.

[17]Association of Backpack Use and Back Pain in Adolescents, Spine, Posted 06/03/2003 Geraldine I. Sheir-Neiss, PhD, Richard W. Kruse, DO, Tariq Rahman, PhD, Lisa P. Jacobson, ScD, Jennifer A. Pelli, MS

[18]Evaluation of chiropractic management of pediatric patients with low back pain: a prospective cohort study. JMPT 2003 Jan;26(1):1-8

[19]AHCPR guideline 1994, URAC guidelines

[20]Annals of Internal Medicine Clinical Guidelines Diagnosis and Treatment of Low Back Pain: A Joint Clinical Practice Guideline from the American College of Physicians and the American Pain Society 2 October 2007 | Volume 147 Issue 7 | Pages 478-491

[21]Nyiendo J, Haas M, Goodwin P. Patient characteristics, practice activities, and one-month outcomes for chronic, recurrent low-back pain treated by chiropractors and family medicine physicians: a practice-based feasibility study. Journal of Manipulative and Physiological Therapeutics 2000; 23: 239-45.

[22]Primary Care - Cost Effectiveness of Physiotherapy, Manual Therapy And General Practitioner Care For Neck Pain: Economic Evaluation Alongside A Randomized Controlled Trial. Korthals-de Bos I, Hoving J, Van Tulder M, Van Molken R, Ader H, De Vet H, Koes B, et al. British Medical Journal 2003; 326: 911.

[23]Matzkin E, Smith EL, Freccero D, Richardson AB. Adequacy of education in musculoskeletal medicine. Journal of Bone and Joint Surgery February 2005;87(2):310-314.

[24]Coulter I, Adams A, Coggan P, Wilkes M, Gonyea M. A Comparative Study of Chiropractic and Medical Education. Alternative Therapies. 1998 (Sep); 4 (5): 64–75

[25]Vohra S, Johnston BC, Cramer K, Humphreys K. Adverse events associated with pediatric spinal manipulation: a systematic review. Pediatrics. 2007;119:275-283

[26]Miller JE, Benfield K. Adverse effects of spinal manipulation therapy in children younger than 3 years: a retrospective study in a chiropractic teaching clinic. Jour Manip Physiol Ther 2008;31(6):419-422.

E/M WITH CMT

<NAME OF PRACTICE>
<ADDRESS>
<PHONE/FAX>

<DATE>
<ADDRESS OF PAYER>

Re: Insurer: <INSURER>
     Patient Name: <PATIENT NAME>
     Date of Service: <DATE OF SERVICE>
     Claim #: <CLAIM #>
     Policy #: <PATIENT'S POLICY #>
     Group #: <PATIENT'S GROUP #>

To whom it may concern:

Thank you for your (select one) letter/EOB regarding <PATIENT NAME> patient for services rendered on [insert dates of service]. I appreciate the time you took to communicate with me, but disagree and object to your determination that the E/M CPT® code (E/M) is a mutually exclusive procedure when billed with a chiropractic manipulative treatment (CMT) CPT code (98940-98942).

As outlined in the American Medical Association's (AMA) Current Procedural Terminology (CPT), there are instances when it is appropriate to bill a CMT code with an E/M code on the same date of service.

The physician work component of the CMT codes includes a brief pre-manipulation patient assessment. Additional evaluation and management services may be reported separately using the modifier –25 if the patient's condition requires a significant separately identifiable E/M service, above and beyond the usual pre-service and post-service work associated with the procedure.

The E/M service may be prompted by the symptom or condition for which the procedure and/ or service was provided. On any given visit, if the patient presents more than one specific area of complaint that necessitates separate and distinct clinical evaluations, use of an E/M service code should be the service that most accurately reflects the cumulative level of all services provided during the visit. As such, different diagnoses are not required for the reporting of the E/M service on the same day.

Some specific examples of when it is appropriate to bill for both a CMT and E/M code on the same date of service are:

   New patient visit
   Established patient with new condition, new injury, aggravation, or exacerbation
   Periodic re-evaluation to assess if a treatment change is needed

For the above noted claim, the reason the E/M service was billed in addition to the CMT service was <INSERT STATEMENT OF CLINICAL NECESSITY>. I have attached documentation which supports the need for the E/M service on this date. In light of the above, please reconsider and accurately reprocess the above patient's claim within 30 days.

Sincerely,

<TREATING PROVIDER'S FULL NAME>, D.C.

Attachment: <ATTACH CLINICAL RECORD>
Cc: American Chiropractic Association
CPT is a registered trademark of the AMA

HOT AND COLD PACKS

<NAME OF PRACTICE>
<ADDRESS>
<PHONE/FAX>

<DATE>
<ADDRESS OF PAYER>

Re: Insurer: <INSURER>
       Patient Name: <PATIENT NAME>
       Date of Service: <DATE OF SERVICE>
       Claim #: <CLAIM #>
       Policy #: <PATIENT'S POLICY #>
       Group #: <PATIENT'S GROUP #>

To whom it may concern:

I received your (select one) letter/EOB regarding the services rendered for <INSERT PATIENTS NAME> on <INSERT DATE OF SERVICE>. I appreciate your communication but respectfully disagree with your findings on CPT® code 97010, hot or cold packs therapy, being denied as an integral part of the Chiropractic Manipulative Treatment (CMT) <OR INSERT EXACT DENIAL RATIONALE PROVIDED BY INSURER>.

The American Chiropractic Association (ACA) has a scientifically based policy that supports the use of hot/cold packs in cases of patient medical necessity. The policy states:

"It is the position of the American Chiropractic Association (ACA) that the work of hot/cold packs as described by CPT code 97010 is not included in the CMT CPT codes 98940-98942 in instances when moist heat or cryotherapy is medically necessary in order to achieve a specific physiological effect that is thought to be beneficial to the patient."

Indications for the application of moist heat include, but are not limited to, relaxation of muscle spasticity, induction of local analgesia and general sedation, promotion of vasodilatation, and increase of lymph flow to the area. Indications for the application of cryotherapy include, but are not limited to, relaxation of muscle spasticity, local analgesia, localized vasoconstriction, and decrease of exudates. [1]

In the case of <INSERT PATIENT NAME>, <INSERT "HOT" OR "COLD"> packs were applied to the <INSERT REGION> for the purpose of <INSERT STATEMENT ON CLINICAL NECESSITY>. In the attached documentation, I have clearly stated how the use of this therapy exceeds the preparatory stage for CMT, and the reason both distinct services were warranted. I am requesting your decision be reversed and payment made within 30 days.

Sincerely,

<TREATING PROVIDER'S FULL NAME>, D.C.

Enc: <TITLE OF DOCUMENTATION PROVIDED>
cc: American Chiropractic Association (ACA)
CPT is a registered trademark of the AMA

---

[1] Jaskoviak PA, Schafer RC. Applied Physiotherapy: Practical Clinical Applications. 2nd ed. Arlington, Va: American Chiropractic Association; 1997

LEVEL OF E/M AUTHORIZED

<NAME OF PRACTICE>
<ADDRESS>
<PHONE/FAX>

<DATE>
<ADDRESS OF PAYER>

Re: Insurer: <INSURER>
       Patient Name: <PATIENT NAME>
       Date of Service: <DATE OF SERVICE>
       Claim #: <CLAIM #>
       Policy #: <PATIENT'S POLICY #>
       Group #: <PATIENT'S GROUP #>

To whom it may concern:

Thank you for your response to the documentation submitted regarding care for the above named patient. I appreciate your communication, but respectfully disagree with your decision that Evaluation and Management (E/M) CPT® code <INSERT CODE NUMBER> is inappropriate for my patient. The reason I indicated that E/M CPT® code <INSERT CODE NUMBER> was necessary is that: <INSERT INFORMATION WHICH SUPPORTS THE LEVEL OF E/M REQUESTED (E.G., NEW PATIENT, PATIENT WITH MULTIPLE AREAS OF INJURY/EXACERBATION)>.

As you are aware, when determining which E/M code to bill, providers must take into consideration the level of history, examination, and clinical decision making involved in evaluating the patient. As the treating provider, I feel that my analysis of the complexity of the patient's case is far more accurate than a determination based simply on the limited paperwork you require. <ATTACH ANY FORMS INITIALLY SUBMITTED TO THE INSURER ALONG WITH YOUR CLINICAL NOTES, EXAM FORMS, ETC.>

Based on the attached information, I would appreciate a reconsideration of your decision in regard to the E/M level most appropriate for my patient.

Sincerely,

<TREATING PROVIDER'S FULL NAME>, D.C.

cc: American Chiropractic Association
CPT is a registered trademark of the AMA

MANUAL THERAPY

<NAME OF PRACTICE>
<ADDRESS>
<PHONE/FAX>

<DATE>
<ADDRESS OF PAYER>

Re: Insurer: <INSURER>
       Patient Name: <PATIENT NAME>
       Date of Service: <DATE OF SERVICE>
       Claim #: <CLAIM #>
       Policy #: <PATIENT'S POLICY #>
       Group #: <PATIENT'S GROUP #>

To whom it may concern:

I reviewed your correspondence regarding the above named patients' treatment on <INSERT DATE OF SERVICE>. The EOB explains that payment for CPT® code 97140, manual therapy techniques, is not available because it is considered a mutually exclusive procedure with Chiropractic Manipulative Treatment (CMT) CPT code <INSERT APPROPRIATE CMT CODE>.

The American Chiropractic Association (ACA), the largest professional association representing doctors of chiropractic (DCs) in the country, currently has two members that represent the field of chiropractic on advisory committees established by the American Medical Association (AMA) for the purpose of developing, valuing, and maintaining CPT codes. One ACA member serves on the Current Procedural Terminology/Health Care Professionals Advisory Committee (CPT/HCPAC Advisory Committee), while the other serves on the Relative Value Scale Update Committee/ Health Care Professionals Advisory Committee (RUC/HCPAC), and both are intimately involved and regularly consulted when the definition or intent of a code is in question. Based on their knowledge of the development and valuation process for CPT codes 97140 and <INSERT APPROPRIATE CMT CODE>, it is their understanding that CPT code 97140 is not a mutually exclusive procedure when provided to a different body region separate from the CMT procedure described by CPT code <INSERT APPROPRIATE CMT CODE>. When these procedures are billed together the modifier "-59" is used to delineate independent procedures were performed.

With this information in mind, I have attached a copy of my clinical record for the date(s) of service in question, and they clearly indicate that these services were provided to a separate body region. The documentation also supports that these services were clinically necessary because <insert statement of clinical necessity>.

Certain coding edits imply that CMT and CPT code 97140 can never be performed on the same date of service, even if provided to separate body regions. Please note that this is not correct CPT coding policy and has been specifically re-clarified by the AMA. For a copy of AMA CPT's position on this topic, please contact the ACA's Insurance Relations Department at insinfo@acatoday.org or call (703) 276-8800. Furthermore, if you should require additional information specific to this patient or claims appeal, please feel free to contact me at <INSERT CONTACT INFORMATION>, otherwise please forward payment for the <INSERT "DENIED" OR "REDUCED"> SERVICES WITHIN 30 DAYS.

Sincerely,

<TREATING PROVIDER'S FULL NAME>, D.C.
Attached: <CLINICAL RECORDS>
cc: American Chiropractic Association

CPT is a registered trademark of the AMA

MASSAGE

<NAME OF PRACTICE>
<ADDRESS>
<PHONE/FAX>

<DATE>
<ADDRESS OF PAYER>

Re: Insurer: <INSURER>
Patient Name: <PATIENT NAME>
Date of Service: <DATE OF SERVICE>
Claim #: <CLAIM #>
Policy #: <PATIENT'S POLICY #>
Group #: <PATIENT'S GROUP #>

To whom it may concern:

Thank you for your (select one) letter/EOB for care provided on <insert date>. I appreciate your communication, but respectfully disagree with your decision that CPT® code 97124, massage therapy, is an integral part of the Chiropractic Manipulative Treatment (CMT) (CPT codes 98940-98943).

In the March 2006 issue of the CPT Assistant Newsletter, the American Medical Association (AMA) clarified that,

"the physical medicine codes 97110-97124 represent distinctly separate and unrelated procedures not considered inclusive of the CMT described by codes 98940-98943. Therefore, when clinically relevant, it would be appropriate to report codes 97110-97124 in addition to the CMT when performed at the same anatomic site (ie, separate body regions are not required)."

CPT code 97124 describes the work inherent in massage, which is a separate and distinct service from CMT codes 98940-98942. CPT code 97124 includes procedures such as effleurage, petrissage, and/or tapotement (stroking, compression, percussion), and is billed in increments of time. Massage is applied to a large area, often crossing over several types and areas of soft tissue, and is used primarily for its restorative effects. In some cases, massage may be used for stimulating soft tissue (tapotement).

The expected outcomes of massage are also more general in nature and may, in fact, be what the patient can tolerate at the more acute stage of their treatment plan. This would include such goals as increasing circulation, decreasing muscle soreness, and decreasing muscle spasm.

In the case of this patient, massage was performed for the purpose of <INSERT STATEMENT OF MEDICAL NECESSITY>. In the attached documentation, I have clearly presented the reason both distinct services were warranted.

If this denial is due to pre-set software edits, I urge you to consider the AMA's Current Procedural Terminology (CPT®) coding policy indicates that these services may be provided on the same date of service when there is a clinical indication for each procedure. Software edits that routinely deny the service without consideration of medical necessity are incorrect. I hope this nationally recognized coding source will allow you to reassess your position and provide payment within 30 days.

Sincerely,

<Treating Provider's Full Name>, D.C.

Enc: <Title of Documentation Provided>
cc: American Chiropractic Association
CPT is a registered trademark of the AMA

MEDICAL NECESSITY

<NAME OF PRACTICE>
<ADDRESS>
<PHONE/FAX>

<DATE>
<ADDRESS OF PAYER>

Re: Patient Name: <PATIENT NAME>
      Date of Service: <DATE OF SERVICE>
      Claim #: <CLAIM #>
      Policy #: <PATIENT'S POLICY #>
      Group #: <PATIENT'S GROUP #>

To whom it may concern:

I received your recent correspondence on my patient denying care on <INSERT DATES OF SERVICE> as not being medically necessary. While I understand the need to contain healthcare costs, it should not be at the expense of patients and their need to obtain quality care.

My clinical documentation is clear and demonstrates medical necessity. It is consistent with patient care protocols taught in accredited chiropractic colleges and clearly falls under the scope of practice within this state. This patient experienced <INSERT APPROPRIATE TERM (EG., A NEW INJURY, AN EXACERBATION, RELAPSE ETC.)> that required more intensive treatment and care. The patient's condition is demonstrated by the following objective findings: <INSERT FINDINGS>. If this additional information does not allow an independent chiropractic review and/or reconsideration and full reimbursement, I would then like answers to the following:

1. What is the company's definition of medical necessity?
2. What care definitions exist for the chiropractic healthcare model for medical necessity, both acute and chronic care?
3. Are the guidelines applied to chiropractic claims developed with input from a doctor of chiropractic?
4. Are chiropractic claims reviewed by a doctor of chiropractic (DC) who is licensed in the state of <INSERT STATE> and who is, or has been, in private clinical practice at least 50 percent of the time?
5. What scientific sources and/or literature were used to support the decision on this claim? Please provide citations for the sources consulted.

Your fiduciary responsibility to the patient is to provide reasonable, fair and necessary care under the terms of the policy. Your personal attention in reviewing this situation, as well as, your company's internal medical review practices impacting the chiropractic profession, is appreciated. I have acted in good faith to provide this care and to provide you with this information and, in turn, I request that you will consider this information and provide a response within the next 30 days.

Sincerely,

<TREATING PROVIDER'S FULL NAME>, D.C.
cc: American Chiropractic Association (ACA)

CPT is a registered trademark of the AMA

MODEL PROVIDER ASSIGNMENT FORM UNDER ERISA

ASSIGNMENT OF BENEFITS / ERISA AUTHORIZED REPRESENTATIVE FORM

Financial Responsibility

I have requested professional services from _____ ("Provider") on behalf of myself and/or my dependents, and understand that by making this request, I am responsible for all charges incurred during the course of said services. I understand that all fees for said services are due and payable on the date services are rendered and agree to pay all such charges incurred in full immediately upon presentation of the appropriate statement unless other arrangements have been made in advance.

Assignment of Insurance Benefits

I hereby assign all applicable health insurance benefits to which I and/or my dependents are entitled to Provider. I certify that the health insurance information that I provided to Provider is accurate as of the date set forth below and that I am responsible for keeping it updated.

I hereby authorize Provider to submit claims, on my and/or my dependent's behalf, to the benefit plan (or its administrator) listed on the current insurance card I provided to Provider, in good faith. I also hereby instruct my benefit plan (or its administrator) to pay Provider directly for services rendered to me or my dependents. To the extent that my current policy prohibits direct payment to Provider, I hereby instruct and direct my benefit plan (or its administrator) to provide documentation stating such non-assignment to myself and Provider upon request. Upon proof of such non-assignment, I instruct my benefit plan (or its administrator) to make out the check to me and mail it directly to Provider.

I am fully aware that having health insurance does not absolve me of my responsibility to ensure that my bills for professional services from Provider are paid in full. I also understand that I am responsible for all amounts not covered by my health insurance, including co-payments, co-insurance, and deductibles.

Authorization to Release Information

I hereby authorize Provider to: (1) release any information necessary to my health benefit plan (or its administrator) regarding my illness and treatments; (2) process insurance claims generated in the course of examination or treatment; and (3) allow a photocopy of my signature to be used to process insurance claims. This order will remain in effect until revoked by me in writing.

ERISA Authorization

I hereby designate, authorize, and convey to Provider to the full extent permissible under law and under any applicable insurance policy and/or employee health care benefit plan, as my Authorized Representative: (1) the right and ability to act on my behalf in connection with any claim, right, or cause in action that I may have under such insurance policy and/or benefit plan; and (2) the right and ability to act on my behalf to pursue such claim, right, or cause of action in connection with said insurance policy and/or benefit plan (including but not limited to, the right to act on my behalf in respect to a benefit plan governed by the provisions of ERISA as provided in 29 C.F.R. §2560.5031(b)(4)) with respect to any healthcare expense incurred as a result of the services I received from Provider and, to the extent permissible under the law, to claim on my behalf, such benefits, claims, or reimbursement, and any other applicable remedy, including fines.

A photocopy of this Assignment/Authorization shall be as effective and valid as the original.

_____   _____
Patient   Date

_____   _____
Policyholder/Insured   Date

PHYSICAL MEDICINE

<NAME OF PRACTICE>
<ADDRESS>
<PHONE/FAX>

<DATE>
<ADDRESS OF PAYER>

Re: Insurer: <INSURER>
      Patient Name: <PATIENT NAME>
      Date of Service: <DATE OF SERVICE>
      Claim #: <CLAIM #>
      Policy #: <PATIENT'S POLICY #>
      Group #: <PATIENT'S GROUP #>

To whom it may concern:

I reviewed your correspondence regarding the above named patients' services rendered on <INSERT DATE(S) OF SERVICE>. I appreciate your communication but respectfully disagree and object to your findings that doctors of chiropractic (DCs) are not qualified to perform CPT® codes 97001-97799, physical medicine and rehabilitation services; therefore, I am requesting an immediate appeal of the above named denied claim.

The American Chiropractic Association (ACA), the largest professional association representing DCs in the country, has addressed this topic and they disagree with your findings. For your review, I have attached a letter from ACA member, Craig S. Little, DC, who serves on the American Medical Association's (AMA) Current Procedural Terminology Health Care Professionals Advisory Committee (CPT/HCPAC), as a representative for the ACA and the chiropractic profession. The enclosed document addresses the CPT's position on this topic, and is supported by the ACA.

With this in mind, appropriate retrospective authorization of medically necessary and reasonable services is requested. If you should require further discussion regarding the contents the enclosed letter, please contact the ACA's Insurance Relations Department at (703) 276-8800. Furthermore, additional information specific to this patient or claims appeal can be acquired by contacting me at <INSERT CONTACT INFORMATION>, otherwise please reconsider and accurately reprocess the above patient's claim within 30 days

Sincerely,
<TREATING PROVIDER'S FULL NAME>, D.C.

cc: American Chiropractic Association

CPT is a registered trademark of the AMA

Glossary

Please Note: In some instances, for the sake of brevity, the more generally accepted meanings for these terms are used as opposed to "formal" definitions.

1500 Health Insurance Claim Form The industry standard used by healthcare professionals and suppliers to submit claims for reimbursement.

abdomen The front part of the body that lies between the chest and pelvis (stomach).

ABN Advanced Beneficiary Notice of Noncoverage.

abuse Billing third-party carries such as Medicare for services that are not covered or are not correctly coded.

accept assignment A provider agrees to having the insurance payment come directly to the office instead of the patient. Generally, preferred (contracted) providers are required to accept assignment.

accreditation Process by which an organization recognizes a program of study or an institution as meeting predetermined standards.

acquired Produced by influences outside an organism, not genetic.

active care Modes of treatment requiring "active" involvement, participation, and responsibility on the part of the patient.

Activities of Daily Living (ADLs) Daily habits such as bathing, dressing and eating. ADLs are often used as an assessment tool to determine an individual's ability to function at home or in a less restricted environment of care.

actual charge A provider's usual fee for a service as indicated on a 1500 claim form. This is **not** the charge billed to the patient, which may be limited by contract with that payer.

acupuncture A practice in which needles are inserted into specific acupoints and manipulated for induction of anesthesia, relief of pain and other various conditions.

acute Refers to the condition that is the primary reason for the current encounter. Of short duration and relatively severe.

acute condition Conditions are considered "acute" within the first 4-8 weeks post-injury/illness.

add-on code Describes additional intra-service work associated with the primary procedure.

addenda Official updates to HIPAA approved code sets.

adjustment A manipulation of the spine or other articulations of the body to normalize function.

adverse Any response to a drug that is noxious, unintended, and occurs with proper dosage.

afferent Carrying impulses towards a center; when sensory nerve impulses are sent toward the brain.

aftercare An encounter for something planned in advance, for example, cast removal.

aggravation Worsening of a preexisting impairment in such a way that the degree of permanent impairment is increased.

-algia A suffix meaning "pain," as in neuralgia.

alignment Establishing a straight line between structures.

allowed (approved) amount The amount a third-party payer determines is their fee for a procedure or service. It may be less than the provider's actual charge.

anesthesia Loss of sensation caused by administration of a drug or other medical intervention.

ankylosis Stiffening or consolidation of a joint due to surgery, injury or disease.

antalgic position An abnormal position of the body, resulting from the body's attempt to minimize pain.

anterior Toward the front of the body.

anteroposterior Concerned with axis from anterior to posterior.

appeals process Legal means by which a provider may dispute reimbursements or determinations made by a third-party payer.

apportionment Distribution or allocation of causation among multiple factors that caused or significantly contributed to the injury or disease and existing impairment.

ARRA American Recovery and Reinvestment Act of 2009 is the legislation which created HITECH and added funding for many other programs, including incentives for adopting health information technology.

arthro- A prefix meaning "joint," as in arthroscope.

arthropathy The disease of a joint.

articulation The connection of bones; a joint.

assessment An evaluation or appraisal.

atlas The uppermost and most freely movable bone of the spine, located under the skull.

atrophy A decrease or shrinkage in the size of a normally developed tissue or organ.

Automobile Medical Expense Insurance (Med-Pay) Component of automobile insurance that provides compensation for health care services rendered for injuries to the driver and passengers of the subscriber's automobile, or to the subscriber if injured in another party's automobile.

autonomic nervous system The part of the nervous system that regulates involuntary action, e.g., the intestines, heart, and glands; comprised of the sympathetic and parasympathetic nervous systems.

av Atrioventricular.

balance billing Procedure of billing a patient for the remaining amount, after the payer has completed payment and any required/appropriate write-offs have been taken.

bilateral Pertaining to both sides of the body or structure.

biofeedback A training technique that enables an individual to gain some element of voluntary control over autonomic body functions.

biomechanics The application of mechanical laws to living structures.

brace An orthopedic device used to align or hold parts of the body in place.

brain stem The "primitive" (oldest) area of the brain that extends down into the cervical area of the spinal cord.

bundling (CPT Codes) process in which the submitted CPT Code is incorporated by the payer into another submitted CPT code.

bursitis Inflammation of a bursa, which is a fluid-filled sac situated where friction would otherwise develop.

capitation Reimbursement system where a payer reimburses a provider a predetermined list of services to an insured for a specified number of days.

carrier Insurer that underwrites or administers life, health, or other insurance programs.

case management Method designed to monitor and coordinate specific health services of an insured to achieve the desired health outcome in a cost-effective manner.

cast An artificial reproduction of a body part; a rigid dressing.

category Refers to ICD-9-CM diagnosis codes listed within a specific three-digit category, for example, category 250, Diabetes Mellitus.

cause That which brings about any condition or produces any effect.

central nervous system The brain and spinal cord.

cerebellum The "hind" brain.

Centers for Medicare and Medicaid Services (CMS) The federal agency which administers Medicare, Medicaid, and the Children's Health Insurance Program.

CERT Comprehensive Error Rate Testing. Helps determine the national error rate for Medicare Fee-For-Service programs.

cervical spine The vertebrae of the neck, usually seven bones.

cervicobrachial syndrome Neuropathy of brachial plexus.

Cervicocranial syndrome This syndrome comes with a variety of neurological type symptoms such as vertigo, facial pain or sinus pain. Often seems to come from misalignments of cranial bones. Sometimes referred to as Barre-Lieou syndrome.

CHAMPUS and CHAMPVA The Civilian Health and Medical Program of the Uniformed Services, and the Medical Program of the Veteran Services.

charge Price of a service provided by a practitioner.

chief complaint A concise statement describing the symptom, problem, condition, diagnosis or other factor that is reason for the encounter.

chronic Continuing over a long period of time or recurring frequently.

chronic condition Conditions are considered "chronic" after the first 12-16 weeks post-injury/illness.

-cide A suffix meaning "death," as in homicide.

claim denial management Managing the appeal process when a claim is denied.

claim review Payer process in which a claim is reviewed to validate the patient and provider identification, correct codes, and medical necessity of the provided services.

claims submission mandate By law, all claims must be submitted to Medicare by both PAR and NON-PAR providers. Patients may not submit claims.

claims processing Describes the action of submitting claims to the payer and the resulting determination.

clinical decision making see medical decision making.

clinical documentation Recording of patient health care services in an acceptable format that allows for future reference by the provider, other providers, or external entities.

closed dislocation A dislocation without an open wound.

closed fracture A fracture not accompanied by an open wound in the skin.

closed panel Designation indicating a payer is currently not accepting new providers to participate in a payer network.

closed reduction The manipulative reduction of a fracture or dislocation without incision.

closed treatment Realignment of a dislocation or fracture without incision.

CMS Centers for Medicare and Medicaid Services.

coccyx A series of small bones at the end of the sacrum.

coding The process of transferring written or verbal descriptions of diseases, injuries and procedures into numeric and/or alphanumeric designations.

co-insurance Health care cost that the insured is responsible for paying; typically based on a percentage of the charge.

column 1/column 2 Previously known as Comprehensive/Component Edits. This identifies code pairs that should not be billed together, according to the NCCI.

combination A code that combines a diagnosis with an associated secondary process or complication.

compensation reaction A new problem that results from the body's attempt to respond or adapt to a problem elsewhere in the body (e.g., the spine).

compliance program Helps prevent fraudulent or erroneous claims.

compliance regulations Conforming to billing regulations. Most are based off of the False Claims Act.

complication The occurrence of two or more diseases in the same patient at the same time.

component procedures Those services that are part of a comprehensive family of codes.

compressive lesion A malfunctioning spinal joint that puts direct pressure on a spinal nerve, resulting in nerve malfunction (a "pinched" nerve).

concurrent care The provision of similar services, e.g., hospital visits to the same patient by more than one physician on the same day.

congenital Existing at, or dating before birth.

conservative care Care that is designed to preserve health, restore function, and repair structures by nonradical methods.

consultation A type of service provided by a physician whose opinion or advice regarding evaluation and/or management of a specific problem is requested by another physician or other appropriate source.

Consumer Directed Health Care (CDHC) When a consumer uses private accounts to pay for medical expenses. Often these include Health Savings Accounts (HSA) or Health Reimbursement Accounts (HRA).

contusion An injury with hemorrhage and without a break in the skin.

conventions Refers to the use of certain abbreviations, punctuation, symbols, type faces, and other instructions that must be clearly understood in order to use a code set.

coordination of benefits When a beneficiary is covered by more than one type of insurance that covers the same health care services, one pays its benefits in full as the primary payer and the other pays a reduced benefit as a secondary or even possibly a tertiary (third) payer. When the primary payer doesn't cover a particular service but the secondary payer does, the secondary payer will pay up to its benefit limit as if it were the primary payer.

coordination of care Interaction with other health care professionals for the management of patient care.

counseling A face-to-face service between the doctor and patient.

co-payment The portion that an insurance policy designates as the amount for which the patient is responsible. New legislation waives co-pays for some preventive services.

CPT Current Procedural Terminology (CPT) is the HIPAA-approved coding system developed by the American Medical Association.

credentialing Payer review procedure where an applying, or participating provider must meet payer network participation standards in order to begin, or continue participation, in the payer network.

cryo- A prefix meaning "low temperature," as in cryotherapy.

CT Scan Computed Tomography, formerly known as CAT Scan or Computer Aided Tomography, which uses pencil-thin X-ray beams and a computer to create a type of three-dimensional X-ray.

Date of Service (DOS) Date a health care service was rendered by the provider to an insured.

deductible The amount that the beneficiary is responsible for during each calendar year before health insurance benefits begin. This applies only to services and supplies covered by the health insurance policy approved amounts–not actual charges.

Department of Defense (DOD). The federal agency which administers the healthcare programs for the military and their families. This includes both active duty military and dependents (DOD and TriCare), and retirees or detached service persons who need help or who have service-related issues (Department of Veterans Affairs Hospitals and programs for dependants).

Department of Veterans Affairs (VA) The federal agency that provides patient care and federal benefits to veterans and their dependents.

derma- A prefix meaning "skin," as in dermatome.

dermatomes Areas of skin sensitivity that reflect the function of specific nerves distributed from the spinal cord.

detailed An extended history or examination of the affected body area(s) and other symptomatic or related organ system(s).

diagnosis An expert opinion identifying the nature and cause of a patient's concern or complaint, and/or abnormal finding(s).

diathermy The therapeutic use of high frequency electrical current to create a heat response within an area of the body.

differential diagnosis The determination of which of two or more disorders with similar symptoms is the one from which the patient is suffering, by a systematic comparison and contrasting of the clinical findings.

disability Alternation of an individual's capacity to meet personal, social, or occupational demands or statutory or regulatory requirements because of an impairment.

disc A cartilage (cushion/pad) that connects and separates spinal vertebrae, absorbs shocks to the spine, protects the nervous system, and assists in creating the four spinal curves.

disc herniation Extreme bulging of the soft nucleus pulposus into a defective or weakened area of fibrous disc exterior.

disease Any deviation from or interruption of the normal structure or function of any part, organ, or system of the body that is manifested by a characteristic set of symptoms whose prognosis may be known or unknown.

dislocation The displacement of a bone.

dislocation, developmental A bone or joint displacement which is either congenital or acquired. Also known as dysplasia.

documentation The recording or pertinent facts and observations about a patient's health history and physical examination of the system(s) applicable to the current encounter.

DOD See Department of Defense.

dorsal Pertaining to the back; the twelve thoracic vertebrae are also referred to as dorsal vertebrae.

downcoding The process whereby insurance carriers reduce the value of a procedure and the resulting reimbursement, due to either 1) a mismatch of CPT code and description or 2) ICD-9-CM code does not justify the procedure or level of service.

dys- A prefix meaning "abnormal," as in dysfunction.

"E" codes Specific ICD-9-CM codes used to identify the external cause of injury, poisoning and other adverse effects.

-ectomy A suffix meaning "cutting out," as in hysterectomy.

edema A condition in which fluid fills a damaged joint area with excessive fluid, causing swelling, similar to that of a sprained ankle.

efferent Carrying away from a central organ; nerve impulses leaving the brain to peripheral tissues.

Electronic Data Interchange (EDI) Automated exchange of data and documents in a standardized format. In health care, some common uses of this technology include claims submission and payment, eligibility, and referral authorization.

Electronic Health Record (EHR) An electronic record of health-related information for an individual that conforms to national standards for interoperability, which can be created, managed, and consulted by authorized clinicians and staff across more than one health care organization.

Electronic Medical Record (EMR) An electronic record of health-related information for an individual, which can be created, gathered, managed, and consulted by authorized clinicians and staff within one health care organization. The data does not need to conform to any standards.

ePHI Electronic Protected Health Information means any electronic version of protected health information as defined by HIPAA/HITECH regulations. See also PHI.

EMG Electromyograph; a device used to measure muscle contraction resulting from electrical stimulation.

employer liability Employers can be held liable for their own actions or any actions committed by their employees that are within the scope of employment.

EMS Electro-Muscle Stimulation; a form of electrical stimulation designed to help reduce swelling and inflammation.

eponyms Medical procedures or conditions named after a person or place.

ERISA The Employee Retirement Income Security Act covers federal requirements for employer sponsored benefits such as pension and health plans.

ERISA appeals The process for appealing incorrectly adjudicated claims for employee sponsored health plans.

established patient One who has received professional services from the physician or another physician of the same specialty who belongs to the same group practice, within the past three years.

ethical behavior boundaries Fulfilling responsibilities with integrity and honesty.

etiology The cause(s) or origin of a disease.

Evaluation and Management (E/M) A category of service in the CPT to express various patient encounters.

exacerbation An exacerbation is a temporary, marked deterioration of the patient's condition because of an acute flare-up of the condition being treated.

examination The process of inspecting and testing the body and its systems to determine the presence or absence of disease or injury.

Explanation of Benefits (EOB) Statement from the payer sent to a provider and an insured explaining services provided, services denied, amount billed, amount owed by the insured, amount not paid, amount paid by the insurer, denial reasons, etc.

extension To stretch out or to spread to its fullest length or reach.

external appeal An appeal made to request the right of an independent review of a patient's case.

extraspinal Also known as nonspinal, refers to the following five regions: head (including temporomandibular joint, excluding atlanto-occipital); lower extremities; upper extremities; rib cage (excluding costotransverse and costovertebral joints); and abdomen.

facet The actual joint surface of a spinal bone, facing the adjacent bone above or below.

facilitative lesion A twisting, stretching, or irritation of nerve tissue due to a malfunctioning joint.

False Claims Act (FCA) Helps prevent persons and companies from defrauding government programs.

Federal Bureau of Investigation (FBI) The FBI investigates violations of federal criminal law and provides law enforcement assistance to federal, state, local, and international agencies. The FBI has investigated practitioners for fraud and abuse.

Federal Trade Commission (FTC) This commission deals with both consumer protection and competition jurisdiction in broad sectors of the economy. The FTC pursues vigorous and effective law enforcement, and shares its expertise with other federal and state agencies, such as HHS.

Fee for Service (FFS) Specific payment amounts for specific services rendered/received.

fee schedule List of established fees, or maximum amounts allowed, for specified health care services.

fixation Being held in a fixed position. An area of the spine, or a specific joint with restricted movement.

flexion To bend to the side or forward.

foramen A small opening, as where a nerve leaves a bone.

fracture A break or rupture in a bone.

fraud The intentional deception or misrepresentation that the individual knows to be false or does not believe to be true, perpetrated to gain some unauthorized benefit.

frontal Pertaining to the front.

functional limitation Inability to completely perform a task due to an impairment.

gatekeeper Entity responsible for overseeing and coordinating all aspects of an insured's health care including preauthorizing a referral to a specialist.

global fee Comprehensive reimbursement, for one or more related services, rendered on a date of service.

-graph A suffix meaning "record," as in radiograph.

grievance procedure Formal appeal process by which an insured or provider can voice a complaint and seek a remedy.

HCPCS Healthcare Common Procedure Coding System is the HIPAA-approved code set for specified supplies and services.

health A state of optimal physical, mental, and social well-being and not merely the absence of disease and infirmity.

Health Information Exchange (HIE) The electronic movement of health-related information among organizations according to nationally recognized standards.

Health Information Organization (HIO) An organization that oversees and governs health information exchange among organizations, according to nationally recognized standards.

Health Insurance Portability and Accountability Act of 1996 Comprised of two sections. The first title protects workers' health insurance coverage when they change or lose their job. The second title establishes national standards for electronic health transactions.

HHS Department of Health and Human Services

hierarchy A system that ranks items one above another.

HIPAA Health Insurance Portability and Accountability Act.

HIPPA title I Protects workers' and families insurance when they change or lose their job.

HIPPA title II Sets standards for electronic health care transactions for providers, health insurance plans, and employers.

history of present illness A chronological description of the development of the patient's present illness from the first sign and/or symptom to the present.

HITECH Enforcement Rule A section of the ARRA that contains breach notification provisions and increases fines and penalties for all HIPAA violations.

homeostasis A state of physiological equilibrium produced by a balance of functions and chemical composition within an organism.

hyper- A prefix meaning "over," as in hypertension.

hypermobility Excess movement of an area.

hypo- A prefix meaning "under," as in hypoglycemic.

hypomobility Restricted movement of an area.

ICD-10-CM International Classification of Diseases, 10th Revision, Clinical Modification. Use of ICD-10-CM codes begins on Oct 1, 2015.

ICD-9-CM International Classification of Diseases, 9th Revision, Clinical Modification (ICD-9-CM) is the current HIPAA approved code set for diagnoses which ends on September 30, 2015.

ilium One of the bones of each half of the pelvis. The hip.

imaging Radiological production of a clinical image using X-rays, ultrasound, computed tomography, magnetic resonance, radionuclide scanning, thermography, etc.

immobilization The process of holding a joint or bone in place with a device such as splint, cast, or brace in order to prevent an injured area from moving while it heals.

impairment An impairment is considered permanent when it has reached maximum medical improvement. Loss, loss of use, or derangement of any body part, organ system, or organ function.

indemnity insurance Health care insurance that relies on fee-for-service reimbursement and defines the maximum amounts reimbursed for covered services.

Independent Medical Examination (IME) Evaluation performed by an independent examiner, who evaluates but does not provide care for the individual.

Independent Practice Association (IPA) or Organization (IPO) Delivery model in which an insurer contracts with a physician organization, which in turn contracts with individual physicians. The IPA physicians practice in their own offices and continue to also see their FFS patients. The insurer reimburses the IPA on a capitated basis; however, the IPA may reimburse the physicians on an FFS or capitated basis.

inferior Lower in position.

inflammation A reaction of soft tissue due to injury that may include malfunction, discomfort, rise in temperature, swelling, and increased blood supply.

Indian Health Service (IHS) The federal agency which administers the healthcare programs for American Indians and Alaska Natives. It is a division of the Department of Health and Human Services (HHS).

initial intensive care A type of chiropractic care characterized by frequent visits for the purpose of eliminating or reducing the patient's major complaint.

inpatient Care Care given a registered bed patient in a hospital, nursing home, or other medical institution.

insurance reform A term broadly used to encompass legislative discussions and laws intended to improved the health care system in the U.S.

insurance reimbursement The process by which providers request compensation from insurance companies.

insurance verification Process by which you determine if the patient has insurance coverage before providing any services.

insurer Underwrites or administers life, health or other insurance programs.

inter- A prefix meaning "between," as in intersegmental.

interference Damage or deficit to the nervous system.

International Classification of Diseases, Ninth Revision, Clinical Modification (ICD-9-CM) Universal classification of disease, injury, illness, and mortality.

intervertebral In between two adjoining vertebrae.

intervertebral disc Fibrocartilage padding between vertebral bodies that acts as a shock absorber, with a pulpy center that acts as a ball-bearing. (See disc).

intervertebral foramina The lateral (side) opening through which spinal nerve roots exit the spinal column.

iontophoresis The process of using a small electric charge to deliver medicine through the skin.

-itis a suffix meaning "inflammation," as in arthritis.

joint Junction between two or more bones.

kyphosis From the side, a backward curve of the spine, aka hunchback, humpback.

late effect A residual effect (condition produced) after the acute phase of an illness or injury has ended.

lateral The side view of the body.

leins and assignment Legal process by which providers receive reimbursement for treatment provided to a patient.

letters of appeal Letter which contains a compelling case for medical necessity, and thus payment of a claim.

limiting charge A cap on how much Non-Participating physicians may bill Medicare patients.

lipping The development of a bony outgrowth.

listing A system used to describe the motion or position of vertebral segments in relation to adjacent vertebral segments.

lordosis A forward curve of the spine when seen from the side, aka hollow back, saddle back, swayback.

lumbar spine The vertebrae of the lower back, usually five bones.

maintenance care This therapy includes services that seek to prevent disease, promote health and prolong and enhance the quality of life, or maintain or prevent deterioration of a chronic condition.

managed care Techniques intended to reduce unnecessary health costs.

manifestation Characteristic signs or symptoms of an illness.

manipulation In CPT terminology, the attempted reduction or restoration of a fracture or joint dislocation to its normal anatomic alignment by the application of manually applied forces.

manual therapy Procedure by which the hands directly contact the body to treat articulations and/or soft tissues.

massage Methodical pressure, friction and kneading of the body upon bare skin.

Maximum Medical Improvement (MMI) Condition or state that is well stabilized and unlikely to change substantially in the next year, with or without treatment.

Maximum Therapeutic Benefit (MTB) Return to pre-injury/illness status or failure to improve beyond a certain level of symptomatology or disability, whatever the treatment/care approach.

Medicaid Health insurance program that provides financial medical assistance to those who can't afford to pay for coverage according to state specified levels of poverty.

medical decision making (MDM) A term by the American Medical Association for Clinical Decision Making to describe the process of establishing a diagnosis and/or selecting one of four different management option levels of service.

medical ethics Moral principles that apply to practicing medicine.

medical necessity Related to activities which may be justified as reasonable treatment for a given condition.

Medical Payments Coverage (Med-Pay) Component of automobile insurance that provides compensation for health care services rendered for injuries as defined by policy.

medical record Also known as health record. The documentation of a patient's medical history, care and treatment by a provider.

Medicare The federal health insurance program for people over the age of 65 and other individuals with disabilities due to specific diseases.

Medicare Administrative Contractor (MAC) Formerly known as "carriers," they produce Local Coverage Determinations (LCDs) for the jurisdictions they serve.

Medicare Non-Par fee allowance Medicare non-participating provider allowance. This is 95% of the Par Fee Allowance.

Medicare Par Fee allowance Medicare participating provider allowance.

Medicare Supplemental Insurance (MediGap)/Supplement Health insurance sold by private insurance companies to fill the "gaps" in Original Medicare Plan coverage. Medigap policies help pay some of the health care costs that the Original Medicare Plan doesn't cover – normally, this would be the deductible and coinsurance for covered services. Medigap policies must follow Federal and state laws and the front of a Medigap policy must clearly identify it as "Medicare Supplement Insurance".

Medigap A supplemental private insurance policy for extra benefits not covered or not fully covered by Medicare.

modifiers Codes that modify a procedure code without changing the actual code.

mobilization Movement applied singularly or repetitively within or at the physiological range of joint motion, without imparting a thrust or impulse, with the goal of restoring joint mobility.

MRI Magnetic Resonance Imaging. The use of strong magnets and radio waves to create an image of the internal structures of the body.

multiple Refers to the need to use more than one ICD-9-CM code to fully identify and code a condition.

mutually exclusive edits Identifies code pairs that are unlikely to be performed on a patient on the same day, according to the NCCI.

myelopathy A term used to describe any disease or disorder of the spinal cord itself.

myo- A prefix meaning "muscle," as in myofascitis.

NA Not applicable.

National Committee for Quality Assurance (NCQA) Non-profit managed care organization accreditation agency created to improve patient care quality and health plan performance in partnership with managed care plans, purchasers, consumers, and the public sector.

National Correcting Coding Initiative (NCCI) Rules provided by CMS to control improper coding that leads to incorrect payment on Part B insurance claims.

National Practitioner Data Bank (NPDB) Computerized data bank maintained by the Federal Government that compiles information on providers against whom malpractice claims have been paid or certain disciplinary actions have been taken.

NE Not Established.

NEC Not Elsewhere Classified.

neural canal The opening in the spine through which the spinal cord passes.

neuritis The inflammation of a nerve.

neuro- A prefix meaning "nerve," as in neurocanal.

neurological Pertaining to the nervous system.

neuromuscular reeducation A hands-on technique/approach for the evaluation and functional treatment of soft tissue injuries that occur via trauma, repetitive motion, or chronic postural fatigue.

new patient One who has not received any professional services from the physician or another physician of the same specialty who belongs to the same group practice, within the past three years (this does not apply in all situations, such as an emergency department revisit).

no-fault insurance Automobile insurance that provides coverage under the subscriber's policy regardless of who was at fault in an automobile accident.

non-participating provider A provider who chooses not to sign the Medicare Participation agreement. These providers can choose to accept assignment on a case-by-case basis; however, services that are unassigned are subject to the "limiting charge" restriction.

nonspinal See extraspinal.

NOS Not Otherwise Specified.

NPI National Provider Identifier. A 10-digit number that is required for all electronic HIPAA transactions.

NUCC National Uniform Claim Committee.

nucleus pulposus The gelatinous mass in the center of the intervertebral disc.

objective findings What the doctor finds by examination and evaluation.

oblique Slanting; diagonal.

occipital Pertaining to the lower, posterior (back) portion of the head or skull.

Office of Audit Services (OAS) The federal agency responsible for overseeing auditing services designed to examine the performance of HHS programs in order to reduce waste, abuse, mismanagement, and to promote HHS economy and efficiency.

Office of Civil Rights (OCR) The federal agency responsible for enforcing the HIPAA Privacy and Security Rules.

Office of Counsel to the Inspector General (OCIG) The federal agency responsible for providing general legal services (including fraud and abuse cases) to the OIG.

Office of Evaluation and Inspections (OEI) Conducts national evaluations to provide information and recommendations to prevent fraud, waste, or abuse, and to promote the economy, efficiency, and effectiveness of federal programs.

Office of Investigations (OI) Conducts criminal, civil, and administrative investigations of fraud and misconduct related to HHS programs. OI investigative efforts often lead to criminal convictions, administrative sanctions, and/or civil monetary penalties.

Office of Inspector General (OIG) The federal agency responsible for protecting the integrity of HHS programs by eliminating waste and fraud in these programs.

offset The recovery by Medicare of a non-Medicare debt by reducing present or future Medicare payments and applying the amount withheld to the debt incurred.

-ology A suffix meaning "study of," as in biology.

open panel Designation indicating a payer is currently accepting new providers to participate in a payer network.

opt out An official designation for a provider who agrees to operate outside the Medicare system. When a provider opts out of Medicare, he or she opts out of all Medicare programs and plans for a two year period. This option is currently not available to Doctors of Chiropractic.

osteo- A prefix meaning "bone," as in osteoarthritis.

out-of-area benefits Health care benefits available to an insured while the insured is outside the payer network geographic service area.

out-of-network benefits Health care benefits available to an insured while the insured is in the payer's geographic service area and receives service from a non-participating provider.

out-of-network provider Health care provider who is not participating in a payer network.

outcomes assessment Process by which quality of health care is researched and measured.

overpayment assessment A decision that an incorrect amount of money has been paid for Medicare services and a determination of what that amount is.

palliative treatment Treatment that relieves symptoms but not the cause of the symptom.

palpation Examining the spine with your fingers; the art of feeling with the hand.

P.A.R.T Pain, Assymetry/misalignment, Range of Motion abnormality, and Tissue/tone changes.

Part A hospital insurance benefits Hospital insurance covers institutional services for in-patients that are then billed by the hospital to the Medicare contractor. Individual providers do not submit claims for Part A services.

Part B medical insurance benefits (fee for service) Medical insurance coverage which helps to pay for all physician services that are medically necessary, outpatient hospital care and some other medical services that Part A does not cover.

Part C (Medicare Advantage) Medicare Part C is the combination of Part A and Part B. The main difference in Part C is that it is provided through private insurance companies approved by Medicare. With this program, there could be lower costs and extra benefits.

participating provider A provider who agrees to "accept assignment" for all services provided to all Medicare patients for the following year. The provider signs a Participation agreement and accepts the Participating provider fee schedule.

passive care Application of treatment procedures by the caregiver to the patient who "passively" submits to and receives care.

patho- A prefix meaning "disease," as in pathology.

pathological dislocation A displacement of a bone caused by a disease and not by traumatic injury.

pathology Structural and functional manifestations of disease.

pathophysiology A malfunction of the spine or body system(s).

patient liability Amount an insured is legally obligated to pay for services rendered.

payer (or payor) Insurer that underwrites or administers life, health, or other insurance programs.

pediatrics The care of infants and children and the treatment or prevention of their common health disorders.

peer review Evaluation of health care services, by health-care personnel of similar training, to evaluate quality and appropriateness (e.g., necessity, frequency, efficacy) of care provided.

Peer Review Organization (PRO) Organizations that review medical records and claims to evaluate quality and appropriateness (e.g., necessity, frequency, efficacy) of care provided.

peripheral nervous system The nervous system that connects the central nervous system with every cell, tissue, and organ of the body.

Personal Health Record (PHR) An electronic record of health-related information for an individual that conforms to national standards for interoperability, which can be managed, shared, and controlled by the individual.

Personal Injury (PI). Case involving medical conditions arising from an automobile crash or an accident occurring in a home or at a business site.

Personal Injury Protection (PIP) component of automobile insurance that provides compensation for health care services rendered for injuries as defined by policy.

PHI See Protected Health Information.

physical therapy Modalities and treatments within the Physical Medicine Rehabilitation section of the CPT.

physiology The biological science of essential and characteristic life processes, activities, and functions; the vital processes of an organism.

physiotherapy Treatment with physical and/or mechanical means, such as massage, electricity, etc.

-plegia A suffix meaning "paralysis," as in paraplegia.

Point-of-Service (POS) Health insurance benefits program in which subscribers can select between different delivery systems (i.e., HMO, PPO, and fee-for-service) at the time of accessing services rather than making the selection at time of open enrollment.

policy limits Maximum coverage allowed by a benefits policy. It usually refers to a "dollar limit" or a "visit limit" for a specific service or category of care.

POMR Problem Oriented Medical Record. Standard for all health care records.

post-examination An examination used to monitor the healing process and the patient's progress towards recovery.

posterior Toward the back of the body.

post-payment audits A way to recover overpayment of benefits in the past.

PPACA The Patient Protection and Affordable Care Act (PPACA) of 2010. Also known as the Affordable Care Act (ACA) or "Obamacare."

pre-existing condition Condition developed prior to issuance of a health insurance policy that may result in the limitation of coverage or benefits.

preventative/maintenance care Any management plan that seeks to prevent disease, prolong life, promote health and enhance the quality of life.

Primary Care Physician (PCP) Clinician who is accountable for addressing a large majority of personal health care needs, developing a sustained partnership with patients, and practicing in the context of family and community.

primary code The ICD-9-CM or ICD-10-CM code that defines the main reason for the current encounter.

primary coverage Policy that reimburses costs before any other insurance policy under coordination of benefits rules.

prior authorization Formal process requiring providers to obtain approval to provide particular services or procedures before they are provided.

private contract A contract between a Medicare beneficiary and a provider who has opted out of Medicare. The beneficiary agrees to give up all Medicare payments for services furnished by the provider and to pay the provider directly without regard to any limits that would otherwise apply to what the provider could charge. The contract must by in writing and must be signed before any service is provided.

private insurance companies Insurance companies which are funded and administered in the private sector.

problem focused A limited history or examination of the affected area or organ system.

prognosis A prediction of the probable course and outcome of a disease or the likelihood of recovery from a disease.

prone Lying horizontal with the face downward.

proximal Closer to reference point.

Protected Heath Information (PHI) Information held by a covered entity which concerns health status, provision of health care, or payment for health care that can be linked to an individual. PHI is protected by HIPAA/HITECH and may not be disclosed or used, except in specific situations.

qui tam Law that allows for an individual to bring suit for fraud committed against the federal government.

RAC Recovery Audit Contractors. Program that was created to detect and correct improper payments under the Medicare program.

radiograph A specially sensitized film that records the internal structures of the body by the passage of X-rays. An X-ray film.

radiology The scientific discipline of medical imaging using ionization radiation, radionuclides, nuclear magnetic resonance, and ultrasound waves.

Range of Motion The range, measured in degrees of a circle, through which a joint can be moved.

reconsideration See redetermination.

recoupment The recovery by Medicare of Medicare debt by reducing present or future Medicare payments and applying the amount withheld to the debt incurred.

recurrence A return of symptoms from a previously treated condition that has been quiescent for 30 or more days.

redetermination Medicare review process that is performed after the initial determination and denial.

referral Process of sending a patient from one practitioner to another for health care services. Health plans may require designated primary care providers authorize a referral for coverage of specialty services.

reflex An involuntary action resulting from stimulus.

Regional Health Information Organization (RHIO) An organization that brings together health care providers and organizations that govern health information exchange among them for the purpose of improving health care in a geographic region.

rehabilitative care A type of chiropractic care with the objective of strengthening the spine and providing optimum healing of the function of the spine, associated tissues, and organ systems.

reimbursement Financial compensation by a third-party payer such as an insurance company for a service or treatment.

relief care See Initial Intensive Care.

residual The long-term condition(s) resulting from a previous acute illness or injury.

Resource-Based Relative Value Scale (RBRVS) System whereby payments for services are determined by the resource costs needed to provide that service. The value of code is divided into three components: physician work, practice expense and professional liability insurance expense.

retrospective review Procedure that verifies and analyzes the medical necessity and appropriateness of health care services previously rendered to the insured.

risk management Prioritization of risks, used to minimize liability.

rule out Refers to a method used to indicate that a condition is probable, suspected, or questionable, but unconfirmed. ICD-9-CM has no provisions for the use of this term.

RVU Relative Value Unit or numeric expression of the probable intrinsic worth of one procedure/service to another. The RVU is converted into a fee by a dollar conversion factor.

sacroiliac Of or pertaining to the joints between the sacrum and ilium (hip).

sacrum The triangular bone at the base of the spine located between the ilium.

sciatica A pain that radiates from the lower back into the buttocks and down the back of the leg, caused by the irritation of the sciatic nerve, the largest nerve in the body.

scoliosis A sideways curve of the spine as viewed from the back.

-scope A suffix meaning "to see," as in microscope.

secondary diagnosis Code(s) listed after the primary code that further indicates the cause(s) code for the current encounter or defines the need for higher levels of care.

secondary payer When coordinating benefits, the health plan that pays benefits only after the primary payer has paid its full benefits. It will pay the lesser of a) its benefits in full, or b) an amount that when added to the benefits payable by the primary payer equals 100% of covered charges.

sections Refers to portions of the ICD-9-CM Tabular List that are organized in groups of three-digit code numbers. For example, Malignant Neoplasm of Lip, Oral Cavity and Pharynx (140-149).

self-insurance A situation where consumer pays for health care expenses on their own.

sequencing The process of listing ICD-9-CM codes in the proper order.

significant, separately identifiable service A service that is above and beyond the other service provided or beyond the usual service associated with the procedure that was performed. It is expressed with the modifier -25 for E/M services and other modifiers for other services.

signed consent form Primary purpose is to maintain legality for doctor and patient.

skin traction Traction of a body part accomplished by a device affixed to dressings on the body surface.

slipped disc An incorrect name given to the condition in which a disc becomes wedge-shaped and bulges. In extreme cases this pressure will cause a disc to tear or rupture. A disc cannot slip.

solo practice Physician who practices alone or with others but does not pool income or expenses.

spasm An abnormal or prolonged contraction of muscle tissue.

Specialty Care Provider (SCP) Providers other than a Primary Care Physician.

specificity Refers to the requirement to code to the highest number of digits possible: 3, 4 or 5, when choosing an ICD-9-CM code. In the *ChiroCode DeskBook* the highest specificity is identified in a single column.

spinous process A part of a posterior protruding spinal bone that can be seen or felt when examining the spine.

spurring A projecting body from a bone (see Lipping).

State Chiropractic Boards State agencies responsible for regulating and issuing licenses for Chiropractors. They define both the role and definition of Chiropractic care in their state.

State Departments of Labor and Industries State agencies responsible for regulating workers' compensation, workplace safety, labor and consumer protection, and licensing within their state.

stem Portion of word which gives the basic meaning.

stereoradiography Preparing a radiograph such that the depth, width and height can be viewed.

structural quality measure A measure that reflects the organizational, technological, and human resources infrastructure of a system necessary for the delivery of quality health care (such as the use of health information technology for the submission of measures).

sub- A prefix meaning "less than," as in subluxation.

subcategories Refers to groupings of ICD-9-CM four-digit codes listed under three-digit categories.

subdural hemorrhage A bleeding underneath the dural covering of the spinal cord, usually due to trauma which can produce abnormal function, aberra.

subjective complaints Problems identified by the patient, such as headaches, leg pain, etc.

subluxation A complex of functional and/or structural and/or pathological articular changes that compromise neural integrity and may influence organ system function and general health.

The chiropractic "subluxation" is also known as a "segmental dysfunction or "somatic" dysfunction" in ICD-9-CM language.

subrogation Procedure where an insurer recovers from a third party when the action resulting in medical (E.G., auto accident) was the fault of another person.

suffix Portion of word which modifies the root word.

superior Upper, or higher in position.

supine Lying horizontally on the back with the face upward.

supportive care Treatment for patients who have reached maximum therapeutic benefit from care.

symptom magnification Conscious and willful feigning or exaggeration of a disease or effect of an injury in order to obtain external gain.

Tabular List The portion of ICD-9-CM and or ICD-10-CM which list codes and definitions in numeric order. Also referred to as Volume 1 in ICD-9-CM.

technical component Section of a health care service that associates extra provisions other than the professional service.

technique A specific procedure, method, or maneuver used to correct spinal problems.

therapy Methods used to assist in the relief of pain, rehabilitation, and restoration of normal body functions.

Third Party Administrator (TPA) Independent organization that provides administrative services including claims processing and underwriting for other entities such as insurance companies or employers.

Third Party Claim Situation where insurance coverage applies to a party not listed in the policy, but may receive reimbursement due to negligence or fault of another.

thoracic spine Pertaining to the part of the spinal column from the base of the neck to about six inches above the waistline. (See dorsal).

timely filing Designated number of calendar days in which services must be billed to be eligible for reimbursement.

torticollis A contracted state of the neck muscles that produces a side bending of the neck and unnatural position of the head.

traction The act of drawing or exerting a pulling force, as along the long axis of a structure.

trans- A prefix meaning "across," as in transverse.

transverse process Lateral protrusions (wings) of bone from the vertebrae to which powerful muscles and ligaments attach.

treatment plan A written document which outlines the plan for helping the patient return to optimal health. It includes the progression of therapy and milestones of progress. It is a key element in establishing medical necessity.

trigger point An involuntarily tight band of muscle that is painful when pressed and can cause referred pain in other parts of the body.

ultrasound Inaudible high frequency sounds whose vibrations can be used to create a heat response in the internal structures of the body.

unassigned claim A claim in which the provider did not agree to accept only the allowed amount as payment for services. Generally, the third-party payment goes directly to the patient, not the provider.

unbundling Billing for a package of health care procedures on an individual basis when a single procedure could be used to describe the combined service.

United States Department of Justice (DOJ) The federal agency which prosecutes crimes against the nation, such as filing false claims.

United States Public Health Service (PHS) The federal agency which provides public health promotion and disease prevention services. Considered one of the United States uniformed services, agents are responsible for rapid and effective responses to public health situations.

Usual, Customary, and Reasonable (UCR) Provider's typical charge for, or payer's reimbursement rate of, a health care service.

utilization Use of services and/or supplies.

Utilization Review (UR) or Management (UM) Evaluation of quality and appropriateness (e.g., necessity, frequency, efficacy) of services, procedures, and facilities.

Utilization Review Accreditation Commission (URAC) Non-profit organization that establishes and applies health care industry standards to payer networks.

"V" codes Specific ICD-9-CM codes used to identify encounters for reasons other than illness or injury, for example, immunization.

vertebra Any of the 24 individual bones of the spinal column.

vertebral subluxation A misalignment of spinal bones that is less than a complete dislocation, but is sufficient to cause disruption of nerve system function.

vertebral subluxation complex Five specific kinds of pathology resulting from a Vertebral Subluxation: Spinal Kinesiopathology, Neuropathophysiology, Myopathology, Histopathology, and Pathophysiology.

vicarious liability In Latin, "Respondeat Superior", the responsibility of an employer for the acts of their employees.

Volume 1 See Numeric (Tabular) list of ICD-9-CM.

Volume 2 See Alphabetic Index of ICD-9-CM.

Volume 3 ICD-9-CM Procedure codes used only for hospital coding, and not in doctor offices. Volume 3 contains both a numeric listing and an alphabetic index.

wellness care Supportive care given to maintain optimal health and wellness after an annual (initial or periodic) health and wellness encounter, or release of a patient from active/rehabilitative care.

whiplash An injury to the spine at the junction of the 4th and 5th vertebrae, caused by an abrupt jerking motion, either backward, forward, or sideways.

Workers' Compensation Program that covers all medical costs incurred, and replaces wages lost as a result of a work related illness or injury.

x-rays Electromagnetic radiation that can penetrate many objects and reveal their internal structure by recording the shadow cast on photographic plates.

Frequently Asked Questions

by the ACA

Guide to Frequently Asked Questions

Question	Page
Flexion Distraction	FAQ-2
CMT Regions	FAQ-2
Extraspinal with spinal services	FAQ-2
Casting and Strapping	FAQ-3
Therapeutic Procedures with CMT in the Same Region	FAQ-3
Modifier -59	FAQ-3
NCCI Policy	FAQ-4
Massage with CMT	FAQ-4
Cox Flexion Distraction	FAQ-4
Anatomic Regions	FAQ-5
Manual Therapy Techniques	FAQ-5
Myofascial/soft tissue therapy with CMT	FAQ-5
Modifier -59 with Manual Therapy Techniques	FAQ-5
Neuromuscular Reeducation	FAQ-6
E/M Service on the Same Date as a Physical Medicine and Rehabilitation Service	FAQ-6
Combining Ultrasound and Electric Muscle Stimulation	FAQ-6
Therapeutic Exercises	FAQ-6
Myofascial release	FAQ-6
Time Units for Modalities	FAQ-7
Electrical Massager	FAQ-7
Microwave Therapy	FAQ-7
Vertebral Axial Decompression	FAQ-7

Infratonic Service FAQ-7

Group Therapy FAQ-8

Vertebral Axial Decompression FAQ-8

Electrodes FAQ-8

Dynamic Activities FAQ-8

Confirmatory Consultations FAQ-9

Re-Evaluations FAQ-9

Modifier –25 .... FAQ-9

Functional Capacity Examination FAQ-9

After-Hours Visits FAQ-9

Athletic Physical FAQ-9

Lumbosacral Support Belt FAQ-10

Durable Medical Equipment Rental FAQ-10

Cervical X-Rays FAQ-10

X-Ray Consultation FAQ-10

CMT

Q. FLEXION DISTRACTION: Is Flexion-Distraction technique considered part of Chiropractic Manipulative Treatment (CMT) codes?

A. Yes. Chiropractic treatment can be broadly organized into Chiropractic Manipulative Treatment (CMT), joint and soft-tissue mobilization, physiotherapy services, and other appropriate treatment services. The best description of Flexion-Distraction technique using existing CPT® 2007 language and codes would be the CMT codes, 98940, 98941, or 98942.

Q. CMT REGIONS: If I treat a patient by performing a Chiropractic Manipulative Treatment (CMT) to the pelvic region, the sacrum, and L5, is this a one-region adjustment, or three?

A. The five spinal regions referred to for spinal manipulative treatment are cervical, thoracic, lumbar, sacral, and pelvic. Therefore, in the instance noted above, it would be correct to code 98941, CMT, spinal, three to four regions. However, regardless of how many manipulations are performed in any given spinal region (cervical, lumbar, etc.), it counts as one region under the CMT codes. Therefore, in the example above, even if more than one segment was adjusted in the lumbar spinal region, it would still be counted as a three to four region adjustment.

Q. EXTRASPINAL WITH SPINAL SERVICES: Is it appropriate to use the extraspinal CMT code, 98943, in conjunction with the spinal CMT codes (98940, 41, 42)?

A. CMT code 98943 can be used either by itself or in conjunction with a spinal CMT code. 98943 can be billed only once per encounter.

Q. CASTING AND STRAPPING: How does one code for a casting or strapping procedure when it is performed on the same date as CMT?

A. There is evidence that some claims payers are not reimbursing for casting/strapping procedures (CPT 29000-29799) in conjunction with Chiropractic Manipulative Treatment (CMT) on the same date of service. Language exists in CPT® noting that "A physician who applies the initial cast, strap, or splint and also assumes all of the subsequent fracture, dislocation, or injury care cannot use the application of casts and strapping codes as an initial service, since the first cast/splint or strap application is included in the treatment of fracture and/or dislocation codes."

It is true that the work value of applying the initial cast, splint, and/or strap is included in the treatment of fracture and/or dislocation codes. However, the work value of initial casting and strapping is not included in the work value of CMT.

The work involved in applying the casts or splints and performing the strapping is not typically included in the evaluation and management codes when assessing a patient who has presented with an injury, nor does the CMT code (98940-98943) include the work or effort required to carry out these additional services. In typical clinical practice, it is not uncommon to immobilize patients following a manipulation or adjustment. Specifically, in the hand or wrist, immobilization is often performed with a removable splint that is either given to the patient or prescribed and obtained from a durable medical equipment vendor. In some instances, a more extensive period of immobilization may be prescribed, such as cast application. In those instances, a significant amount of additional work is required to apply the cast and should be coded and reimbursed appropriately.

Additionally, there can be many clinical situations wherein patients undergo a chiropractic adjustment or manipulation at a location on the body that is separate from that which is being treated with a cast. A specific clinical situation would include a patient who undergoes a spinal adjustment or manipulation but is treated with a cast on the right wrist for a sprain. Another example would include a patient who receives manipulation of a left ankle lesion but receives a splint or strapping for a right ankle sprain. In summary, it is appropriate to utilize casting/strapping procedures (CPT 29000-29799) in combination with CMT (98940-98943) when both procedures are medically necessary and performed on the same date of service.

Q. THERAPEUTIC PROCEDURES WITH CMT IN THE SAME REGION: Is it appropriate to bill CPT codes 97110-97124 when they have been performed in the same region as CMT?

A. It is absolutely appropriate to perform these services to the same region as CMT when clinically indicated and properly documented. Contrary to some interpretations, the modifier -59 is not required with these services when billed on the same date or same region as CMT.[1]

[1] *CPT Assistant.* March 2006; Vol. 16, Issue 3, Page 15.

Q. MODIFIER -59: I know the -59 modifier is required when billing 97140 with 98940-98943, but is the -59 modifier also required when billing 97112 with 98940-98943 and are there any restrictions on providing CMT and 97112 to the same region as there are with 97140?

A. Neuromuscular reeducation and CMT are considered 2 separately identifiable procedures; therefore, a -59 modifier is not mandatory when billing them on the same date of service. Additionally, there are no restrictions with regard to performing these services on the same body region (unlike 97140 and CMT). However, utilizing the -59 modifier is permissive as it clearly provides additional communication that you are providing a separate and distinct service and the modifier is recognized by most third party payers.

Q. NCCI POLICY: I was recently denied payment of massage and chiropractic manipulation treatment based on "NCCI Policy." What is NCCI policy and is this an appropriate denial?

A. "NCCI" stands for the National Correct Coding Initiative. The National Correct Coding Initiative was developed by the Centers for Medicare and Medicaid Services (CMS). CMS created these standards based on a number of resources including the American Medical Association CPT manual, and through review of coding practices and information from specialty societies. When NCCI was developed the ACA contacted the Medical Director of NCCI due to concerns ACA had with certain NCCI policies. At that time ACA was informed that "CCI was not developed with the intent that it be used by third party payers to process their claims." The ACA has a template letter for appealing denials based on CCI edits.

Q. MASSAGE WITH CMT: I'm receiving a number of insurance company denials stating that code 97124, massage, is not allowed on the same day as a Chiropractic Manipulative Treatment (CMT) code because it is a part of the CMT codes. Is this true?

A. CPT® 97124 describes the work inherent in massage, which is a separate and Distinct service from CMT codes 98940-98943. CPT 97124 describes work including effleurage, petrissage, and/or tapotement (stroking, compression, percussion), each 15 minutes.

Massage (CPT 97124) describes a service that is separate and distinct from those services described by Chiropractic Manipulative Treatment, Osteopathic Manipulative Treatment, and Manual Therapy Techniques. Massage, unlike those techniques, is totally passive in nature. The patient did not participate in the procedure and the various massage techniques are applied to the patient. Massage is applied to a large area—often crossing over several types of soft tissue and several areas of soft tissue— and is used primarily for its restorative effects. In some cases, massage may be used for stimulating soft tissue (tapotement). The expected outcomes of massage are also more general in nature and may, in fact, be what patients can tolerate at the more acute stage of their treatment plans. This would include such goals as increasing circulation, decreasing muscle soreness, and decreasing muscle spasm. The research available on massage techniques and their impact on the recovery of muscle function following exercise, as well as on any one of the physiological factors related to the recovery process, shows that these techniques have very little impact. Their greatest impact is on the broad factors mentioned above in terms of pain modulation, muscle tightness, and blood flow to the related tissues.

Q. COX FLEXION DISTRACTION: If I perform a regular high-velocity adjustment, side posture, on the low back, as well as COX distraction on the cervical region, am I to bill CMT with 97140 as well? I have heard that a doctor can bill both codes in this instance.

A. The COX technique is a very commonly used manipulative technique, and as such falls under the scope of Chiropractic Manipulative Treatment (CMT). Because it is considered a manipulative treatment, it does not qualify as a manual therapy under code 97140. It is, therefore, inappropriate to ever bill this technique as 97140.

97140

Q. ANATOMIC REGIONS: How is "separate body region" defined?

A. Separate anatomic regions are defined as the head region (includes the temperomandibular joints; excludes the atlanto-occipital joint), the cervical region (includes the atlanto-occipital joint), the thoracic region (includes costovertebral and costotransverse joints), the lumbar region, the sacral region (includes the sacro-coxygeal joint), the pelvic region (includes the sacroiliac joints), the lower extremities, the upper extremities, the ribcage (excludes costotransverse and costovertebral joints; includes costosternal joints), and the abdomen. Each region would include its respective articulations as well as soft tissues originating, inserting, or traversing in that region.

Q. MANUAL THERAPY TECHNIQUES: What procedures constitute "manual therapy techniques"?

A. Most, if not all, manual techniques, including mobilization, would be included in this category. Effleurage, petrissage, and tapotement would be excluded, as those techniques have their own code (97124, massage therapy).

Examples of manual therapy techniques would include passive testing of soft tissue extensibility, gross and segmental range of motion, capsular restrictions, level of muscle guarding; spinal and peripheral manual joint and soft tissue techniques; myofascial release, muscle energy and passive stretch; manual traction, passive intervetebral mobilization and manipulation, as well as capsular oscillations and stretch. Post-service work of this procedure includes documentation of treatment, including the components of the care provided, any changes in the patient's status and future plan of care, contact with physicians on patient's progress, contact with other health care professionals and family.

Q. MYOFASCIAL/SOFT TISSUE THERAPY WITH CMT: Why is it inappropriate to perform myofascial/soft tissue therapy in an area that is being adjusted?

A. According to *CPT Assistant*, February 1999, "it would not be appropriate to report code 97140 and the CMT code when provided to the same region." There is overlap of actual work inherent in both services being performed in the same body region.

Q. MODIFIER -59 WITH MANUAL THERAPY TECHNIQUES: Is a -59 modifier necessary when using a CMT and 97140 on the same visit?

A. According to *CPT Assistant*, March 1999, "Under certain circumstances it may be appropriate to additionally report CMT/OMT codes in addition to code 97140. For example, a patient has severe injuries from an auto accident with a neck injury that contraindicates CMT in the neck region. Therefore, the provider performs manual therapy techniques as described by code 97140 to the neck region and CMT to the lumbar region. As separate body regions are addressed, it would be appropriate in this instance to report both codes 97140 and 98940." In this example, modifier -59 should be appended to the manual therapy code to indicate that a distinct procedural service was provided.

Physical Medicine and Rehabilitation

Q. NEUROMUSCULAR REEDUCATION: Can CPT® 97112 Neuromuscular Reeducation be provided to individuals who do not have mobility deficits, such as those in wheelchairs or for neuromuscular reeducation for a post-stroke victim who has difficulty eating due to problems with balance or muscle control?

A. The language surrounding CPT 97112 does not in any way restrict the use of this service to individuals with central nervous system disorders. It is also important to note that in 2002 there were significant revisions to CPT 97112 Nomenclature revising examples for the type of work that can be performed are as follows. "Examples include, Proprioceptive Neuromuscular Facilitation (PNF), Feldenkreis, Bobath, BAP'S Boards, and desensitization techniques."

Additionally, in regard to the reporting of CPT® 97112, it is important to note that in March 2006, it was clarified in the CPT Assistant that, "the physical medicine codes 97110-97124 represent distinctly separate and unrelated procedures not considered inclusive of the CMT described by codes 98940-98943. Therefore, when clinically relevant, it would be appropriate to report codes 97110-97124 in addition to the CMT when performed at the same anatomic site."

Q. E/M SERVICE ON THE SAME DATE AS A PHYSICAL MEDICINE AND REHABILITATION SERVICE: Can a evaluation and management code be reported on the same date of service as a physical medicine and rehabilitation code when a manipulation has not been performed?

A. Yes, evaluation and management services can be reported on the same date of service as a physical medicine and rehabilitation code when a manipulation has not been performed.

Q. COMBINING ULTRASOUND AND ELECTRIC MUSCLE STIMULATION: What is the correct way to code for ultrasound and electric muscle stimulation delivered simultaneously from the same instrument?

A. There is no code currently available in CPT for a combination of ultrasound and electric muscle stimulation administered simultaneously from the same instrument. The correct coding approach is to bill for the more comprehensive service, which generally would be ultrasound. Most of the work values overlap when performing both of these codes together from the same instrument.

Q. THERAPEUTIC EXERCISES: What types of procedures are identified by code 97110, "therapeutic exercises to develop strength and endurance, range of motion, and flexibility"?

A. According to CPT, therapeutic exercise incorporates one parameter (strength, endurance, range of motion, or flexibility) to one or more areas of the body. Examples are treadmill (for endurance), isokinetic exercise (for range of motion), lumbar stabilization exercises (for flexibility), and gymnastic ball (for stretching or strengthening).

Q: MYOFASCIAL RELEASE: Is it possible to use code 97530, therapeutic activities, to describe myofascial release?

A. It is not appropriate to use code 97530 to describe myofascial release or other manual muscle therapies. Code 97140 best describes the technique known as myofascial release.

Q. TIME UNITS FOR MODALITIES: If I use two machines of the same type, plus another machine of a different type, can I bill three units? An insurer is denying one unit of payment saying our application of the same modality with two supervised modalities falls under treatment of "one or more body parts" with the same modality and is therefore excluded.

A. No, you cannot bill three units in this instance. Per CPT® language, "Time is not a factor in determining the use of the supervised modalities (i.e., they do not include a time component in the descriptor), and therefore, they are intended to be used only once during an encounter, regardless of the number of areas treated."

Q. ELECTRICAL MASSAGER: When using a "Jeanie Rub" or any other "electrical massager" on a patient, do I bill CPT Code 97124? In reading the coding specs for CPT Code 97124, I am unclear if this is direct hands-on-skin, or if an electrical massager is applicable.

A. No, it would not be appropriate to bill CPT 97124 when using an electrical massager. There is currently no CPT code that describes massage performed with an electrical massager. Providers should report CPT 97039, Unlisted Modality. When using CPT 97039, Unlisted Modality, it is necessary to report the modality type and time, if constant attendance.

Q. MICROWAVE THERAPY: Why are my billings for CPT 97020 being denied?

A. In 2006, Code 97020 was deleted due to infrequent use. Microwave therapy is a form of diathermy, a way of generating heat within an area of the body for therapeutic purposes. Therefore, CPT® 97024, Application of a modality to one or more areas; diathermy, has been revised with additional language in parentheses to note, "eg, microwave."

Q. VERTEBRAL AXIAL DECOMPRESSION: I have heard that a new code was developed for vertebral axial decompression. Is that accurate? If so, what is the code?

A. A temporary HCPCS code was developed for vertebral axial decompression. The code is S9090 and may be billed once per session. The S codes are developed by the Health Insurance Association of America and the Blue Cross/Blue Shield Association. S codes are created when no national code exists, but when one is needed in the private sector. It is advisable to check with individual insurers before billing this, or any, S code.

Q. INFRATONIC SERVICE: What is the appropriate CPT® code for Infratonic?

A. The manufacturers of Infratonic describe it as "a low frequency sound pain management system" and as "a low frequency electroacoustical therapeutic massager." There is currently no specific CPT code describing this modality. The ACA Coding and Reimbursement Committee recommends that doctors report this modality as 97039 - "unlisted modality." As with any other unlisted services or modalities, it may be necessary to submit supporting documentation – including information from the manufacturer - along with your claim to provide an accurate description of the work performed equipment needed and medical necessity.

Q. GROUP THERAPY: I recently began utilizing a therapy room in my practice. Under my supervision, I have several patients perform therapeutic procedures such as endurance training on treadmills. Is it appropriate to bill this as 97150, group therapy, or should I bill 97110, therapeutic procedures for each patient? Additionally, how many patients are needed to compose a 'group' under the 97150 code?

A. You would code this scenario as 97150, group therapy. It is important to remember that code 97150 should be reported for each member of the group. For code 97150, two or more individuals constitutes a 'group'. Services that can be coded as group therapy procedures include CPT® codes 97110-97139 - these procedures involve constant attendance by the physician or therapist but do not require one-on-one patient contact.

Q. VERTEBRAL AXIAL DECOMPRESSION: When billing for vertebral axial decompression therapy, should CPT code 64722 - Decompression, unspecified nerve(s) (specify) – be billed?

A. No. CPT code 64722, decompression, unspecified nerve(s) (specify), is a specific surgical code and should not be reported to describe the vertebral axial decompression procedure. CPT code 97012, Application of a modality to one or more areas, traction, mechanical, would be an appropriate code to report for various types of mechanical traction devices, including vertebral axial decompression. HCPCS code S9090, Vertebral Axial Decompression, per session, is also appropriate to report this procedure.

NOTE: Many payers have developed individual policies regarding reimbursement for this procedure. Be sure to ask payers for their specific reporting guidelines.

Q. ELECTRODES: Why am I unable to receive reimbursement from insurers when I bill HCPCS Code A4556 (Electrodes) when I perform electrical stimulation?

A. The relative value of electrodes is included in the relative value for performing the 97014 electrical stimulation service. As such, separate and distinct billings for the HCPCS code are not supported, considering the relative value of 97014 already contains the reimbursement for the electrodes.

Q. DYNAMIC ACTIVITIES: What is included in code 97530, therapeutic activities, use of dynamic activities to improve functional performance?

A. Dynamic activities include the use of multiple parameters, such as balance, strength, and range of motion, for a functional activity. Examples include lifting stations, closed kinetic chain activity, hand assembly activity, transfers (chair to bed, lying to sitting, etc.), and throwing, catching, or swinging.

Modifiers

Q. CONFIRMATORY CONSULTATIONS: I recently billed CPT code 99271 for a new patient confirmatory consultation, and I was denied reimbursement for this service. Is there a reason this E/M code was denied?

A. Yes, confirmatory consultation codes (CPT 99271-99275) have been deleted as of January 1, 2006.

Evaluation and Management (E/M) Exams

Q. RE-EVALUATIONS: Is it necessary to change the diagnosis or treatment frequency after a re-evaluation in order to charge for the E/M service?

A. A re-evaluation is normally performed on a patient at a certain time in the patient's care when a determination of altered treatment frequency or diagnosis is indicated. It is necessary for the doctor to perform an E/M service to reach these conclusions. The result of the E/M service is not a determining factor in the medical necessity for performing the E/M service. Therefore, if there is no diagnosis change or alteration of treatment frequency, the E/M service is still valid.

Coding FAQs

Q. MODIFIER −25: When billing for E/M and CMT on the same date of service, do I need to append the -25 modifier to the E/M code?

A. Yes. When billing a separate E/M code with CMT, you are indicating that you have gone above and beyond the usual pre-service and postservice work associated with the CMT. A -25 modifier must be reported to indicate that you have done so.

Q. FUNCTIONAL CAPACITY EXAMINATION: I thought I recalled seeing a CPT code for Functional Capacity Examination but I cannot pinpoint which code I should use. Could you tell me what code I should use for FCE and under what specific conditions?

A. You should use CPT® Code 97750 (Physical performance test or measurement [e.g., musculoskeletal, functional capacity], with written report, each 15 minutes). The procedure is reported according to the time spent performing the service; not according to the number of areas tested. Since this code is time based, there is no need to identify body areas treated or bilaterality. The time taken to perform the procedure identifies the amount of work involved.

Q. AFTER-HOURS VISITS: Is there a code to bill to insurance for after-hours office visits?

A. There is a series of codes to indicate services requested after hours. Each of these codes would be reported in addition to the basic service. For example, if a CMT or E/M code was billed for an after-hours visit, you report that code in addition to the after-hours code. The codes are:

99050: Services requested after office hours, but only up to 10:00 p.m.

99052: Services requested between 10:00 p.m. and 8:00 a.m.

99054: Services requested on Sundays and holidays

Q. ATHLETIC PHYSICAL: What is the appropriate code for an athletic physical?

A. The correct code would be an appropriate level E/M service based on key elements of history, exam, and medical decision-making. One would expect a complete neuromusculoskeletal exam; however, the history and medical decision making would be at lower levels so, as a general rule, one would not expect to use higher than a level three code such as 99203 or 99213. E/M codes specific to preventative services would not be appropriate since these services require a comprehensive history, which is typically not inherent in athletic physical evaluations.

Durable Medical Equipment

Q. DURABLE MEDICAL EQUIPMENT RENTAL: When I rent a piece of durable medical equipment (e.g., cervical traction equipment) to one of my patients, how do I bill the rental? Does time affect the billing? Is there a difference in billing monthly or weekly?

A. When renting a DME, the modifier -RR should be appended. HCPCS codes do not address the issue of time in a rental period. The practitioner must be able to support necessity and reasonableness, often by report, if questioned. As an example, if one were renting the type of cervical traction equipment that does not require an additional stand or frame, one would bill E0855-RR.

Radiology

Q. CERVICAL X-RAYS: When I x-ray a patient's cervical spine, I typically take three views: AP, LAT, and AP open mouth. How do I properly code for three cervical x-rays?

A. The proper code for three cervical x-rays is 72040. As described by CPT® 2001, 72040 is "Radiologic examination, spine, cervical, two or three views."

Q. X-RAY CONSULTATION: I was told to bill CPT code 76140 for my x-ray consultation when a patient brings in x-rays from an outside source. Is this correct?

A. CPT code 76140 is a service that is utilized by a radiologist, or other consultant, who reads an x-ray (or any diagnostic imaging study) but does not actually see the patient. When a patient brings in diagnostic studies from an outside source, the treating physician may review them and write a report of the findings. However, this would not be billed as a 76140. The relative work value of the E/M service includes the value for reviewing prior medical records and diagnostic studies. The amount and complexity of data to be reviewed are one of the elements of the medical decision-making "key components." It is not billed as a separate service.

ChiroCode DeskBook Index

A = Practice Management
B = Insurance and Reimbursement
C = Medicare
D = Documentation
E = Claims and Appeals
F = Compliance and Audit Protection
G = Diagnosis Codes
H = Procedure Codes
I = Supply Codes

1500 Health Insurance Claim
    Form E-12, E-13
    instructions E-14

A

Abbreviations D-16
Active care, transitioning from D-31
Acupuncture H-78
Administrative, miscellaneous and
    investigational I-13
Advanced Beneficiary Notice of Noncoverage
    (ABN) C-18
ABN for chiropractic maintenance care C-19
Advertising A-20
Allowed amount C-13
Alphabetic code list
    diagnoses (ICD-9-CM) G-100
    procedures H-129
    supplies I-34
Anatomic list (ICD-9-CM)
    abdomen G-20
    cervical and head G-14
    lower extremity G-19
    lumbar G-16
    sacral G-17
    thoracic G-15
    upper extremity G-18
Anatomic List (ICD-10-CM)
    Alphabetic list (other conditions) G-31
    Anatomic list G-21
    Additional Characters G-21
    Cervical and Head G-23

Guidelines and Conventions G-21
Lower Extremity (Extra-Spinal) G-30
Lumbar G-26
Other Conditions G-37
Sacral / Pelvic G-27
Thoracic G-24
Upper Extremity (Extra-Spinal) G-28
Annual and lifetime limits B-22
Anti-Kickback Statute F-8
Appeals
    ERISA .... See ERISA
    Expedited appeals E-42
    guidelines E-41
    hearings and reviews C-42
    Letters E-42
    Medicare C-37
    RAC Appeals F-34
    Response Letter 97110-97124 Denials . E-43
Appendices
    See ChiroCode DeskBook Online Tools
Appointment scheduling A-32
Assessments See Treatment plans
Auditory system H-48
Audits
    avoiding an F-50
    baseline audit F-38
    billing patterns F-51
    general audit protection F-48
    medical record self-audit form F-39
    not medically necessary F-53
    prepare for F-47
    protection F-46, F-48

Authorized Representative, ERISA E-50
Avoid collections A-20

B

baseline audit process F-38
Benefit notices B-16
Billing
    active treatment C-21
    agencies, outsourcing A-18
    maintenance care C-16
    personal injury B-31
    process flowchart B-18
Biofeedback H-61
Breach notification rules F-26
Business basics A-4
Business financial standards A-17

C

Cardiovascular H-62
Case management services H-36
Cash discount warning B-45
Cash/no insurance B-11, B-26
Casts and strapping H-45
Category III codes H-89
CDHP B-25
CHAMPUS and CHAMPVA B-36
Chief compliant D-18
ChiroCode DeskBook Online Tools
    See ChiroCode.com/onlinetools
ChiroCode Membership xiv
Chiropractic Manipulative
    Treatment (CMT) H-80
Civil Monetary Penalties Law F-9
Claim(s) E-1
    appeals E-41
    adjudication E-6
    based reporting example C-47
    clean claims E-4
    common errors to avoid E-9
    denial management .... *see Claim, unpaid*
    downcoded denials E-45
    electronic claims E-7
    followup procedures E-37
    form appendix .... *see Online Tools*
    filing
        late filing exceptions E-5
        paper claims E-7
        refiling / resumbitting E-6
        timely E-5
        tips E-8

    form .... *see 1500 Claim Form*
    guidelines for unpaid claims E-37
    paper claims E-7
    processing E-3
    overpayments E-38
    overview E-3
    tracking and review program,
        implement F-47
    unpaid claims E-37
    Response letter to
        97110-97124 Denials E-41
Clinical examples H-113
    CMT codes H-115
    E/M H-117
    established patient H-125
    other chiropractic related services H-119
    online Medical Evaluations H-123
    Preventive Medicine Counseling (PMC)
        and/or risk factor reduction for
        interventions H-127
    preventive medicine service codes H-124
    telephone services H-123
Clinical Laboratory Improvement Amendments..
    CLIA A-9
Clinical need E-4
Clinical review judgment C-41
CMT Coding Flowchart, Medicare ... C-23, C-26
Code of Ethics xv
Code selection process
    by counseling intraservice (time) H-19
    by key components H-18
Code sequence See Coding hierarchy
Coding conventions
    Coding hierarchy D-24, E-28, G-4,
    CPT H-5
    ICD-9-CM G-34
    ICD-10-CM G-7, G-21
Coding tips E-8
Collection(s)
    agencies A-19
    ways to avoid A-20
Commonly used codes H-11
    CPT modifiers H-96
    diagnosis codes (ICD-9-CM) G-12, G13,
        See Also anatomic list (ICD-9)
    diagnosis codes (ICD-10-CM) G-21, G22
        See Also anatomic list (ICD-10)
        Guidelines and Conventions G21
        Additional Characters G-21
    HCPCS modifiers H-97

procedure codes H-13
procedure modifiers H-14
supply codes I-7
supply codes and modifiers I-7
Common misconceptions about Medicare
    participation C-26
Communications and first impressions A-29
Compliance (and audit protection) F-3
    baseline audit F-38
    benchmarks, general F-49
    considerations A-9
    fraud and abuse F-7
    HIPAA A-33, F-14
    Medicare F-31
    need for compliance, the F-3
    OIG program guidance F-36
    OSHA requirements F-10
    plan, importance of F-6
    program F-6
    procedures F-40
    training and education F-41
Complicating factors D-26
Comprehensive error rate testing (CERT) F-33
Consultation H-28
Consumer directed health plans (CDHP) .. B-25
Continued Care, letters E-43
Continuing Education Units (CEUs) A-10
Corrections
    to patient records D-13
    guidelines for D-14
Counseling H-38
    E/M Counseling Record H-21
    counseling record H-21
Covered Entity Offices F-16
CPT
    modifiers, Level I H-99
    procedure codes H-23
        category III H-89
        diagnostic imaging H-49
        evaluation and management H-23
        laboratory H-59
        medicine (chiropractic and therapies) .. H-61
        surgery H-44

D

Daily policies and procedures manual A-29
Data mining E-6
Denials, reducing E-44
    downcoded denials E-45
Dermatological procedures H-70

Designation of
    Authorized Representative form E-50
    compliance officer F-40
Diagnosis code pointing E-4
Diagnosis codes G-1
    diagnosis coding G-3
Diagnostic imaging codes H-49
Direct Submission to Secondary Insurance for
    Medicare Non-Covered Services
    form C-26
Discount(s) B-45
    cash discount B-45
    financial hardship B-46
    programs, healthcare B-27
Documentation
    and treatment B-14
    computer generated notes D-14
    documentation challenge, the D-3
    errors by chiropractors D-5
    guidelines D-1
    initial visit, the D-18
    introduction to E/M Documentation .. H-15
    signatures D-12
    subsequent visits D-29
Dollar conversion factors B-41, B-43
Domiciliary, rest home or home care plan
    oversight services .... see Resource 130
Downcoding denials E-45
Drugs administered other than oral
    method ("J" Codes) H-94, I-18
Drug testing H-60
Durable medical equipment (DME) I-14

E

E codes G-91
E-Health Initiative C-4
Education and training for patient self-
    management H-83
Electronic Funds Transfer (EFT) F-19
Electronic Health Record (EHR) D-8
Electronic Remittance Advice (ERA) F-19
Electronic
    record keeping .... See Electronic Health Record
    (EHR)
    transaction and code set requirements ... F-18
Emergency department
    services .... See Resource 130
Enrollment, as Medicare provider C-4-
Equipment: A-13

ERISA E-47
    appeals E-47, E-51
    authorized representatitve E-50
    Designation of Authorized Representative
        form E-50
    ERISA law excerpts E-52
    Exceptions, self funded E-48
    Fiduciary duties/responsibilities ... E-49, E-53
    first steps E-49
    summary plan description E-49, E-53
Essential Health Benefits (EHB) B-22
Established patient, subsequent visits B-14
Establishing
    fees B-39
    Medicare eligibility C-15
Estimate of medical fees B-11
Evaluation and Management
    codes H-23
    examples of E/M Services H-16
    introduction to H-15
    selecting a level of service H-22
Evaluation of musculoskeletal/nervous system
        through physical exam D-23
Evergreen contracts A-18, E-40
Exclusions Database A-25, F-43
Expedited appeals E-42
Explanation of benefits (EOB) B-16

F

False Claims Act F-8
Family history D-21
Fax and photocopier caution F-18
Federal
    Employee insurance plans B-37
    Employee Health Benefits (FEHB) Program..
        B-38
    Truth in Lending Act A-18
    Workers' Compensation B-36
Fee calculators
    See ChiroCode DeskBook Online Tools
Fees
    conversion factors C-31
    discounts B-45
    dollar conversion factors B-41, B-43
    fee calculations B-44
    financial hardship policy B-46
    Medicare C-30
    Relative Value Units B-41
    setting fees A-17
    Usual, Customary, & Reasonable (UCR) B-40

Fee schedules B-39
    discounts B-45
    Medicare C-30
    methodologies B-40
    other fee schedules B-45
    personal injury B-31
Filing .... See Claims
Financial
    Consent Policy B-10
    Hardship Policy and Application B-10, B-46,
        B-47
    standards, business A-17
Firing A-27
First report of inury B-34
Flowcharts
    acute care algorithm D-37
    chronic care algorithm D-39
    billing process B-18
    Medicare CMT coding C-23-26
    Medicare fees decision chart C-33-35
    treatment of spine related pain D-35
Forms
    1500 Health Insurance Claim Form E-12
    ABN for Chiropractic Maintenance
        Care C-18
    Advanced Beneficiary Notice (ABN) C-17
    Chiropractic E/M Counseling Record . H-21
    Designation of Authorized
        Representative Form E-50
    Direct Submission to Secondary Insurance
        for Medicare Non-Covered Services. C-26
    Estimate of Medical Fees B-11
    Financial Hardship Policy and
        Application B-10, B-47
    Informed Consent for Chiropractic
        Treatment B-9, D-34
    Insurance Information B-8
    Letters for continued care E-43
    Letter of protection or liens B-30
    Maintenance Care Notice C-20
    Medical and health history B-8, D-22
    Medical Record Self-Audit form F-39
    Medicare reconsideration request form . C-41
    Medicare redetermination request form C-39
    Medicare status questionnaire C-15
    Notice of Medicare coverage for
        chiropractic care C-18
    P.A.R.T. Documentation D-22
    Patient Financial Responsibility Letter B-7
    Patient Information B-7

Patients' Global Impression of Change (PGIC) Scale D-45
Prompt Pay Letter E-38
Request for a Medicare Hearing by an Administrative Law Judge C-42
Request for review of administrative law judge (ALJ) Medicare decision/dismissal C-42
Response Letter to 97110-97124 Denials E-43
Response Letter to Refund Demands F-55
Rowland-Morris Low Back Pain and Disability Questionnaire................. D-44
Third-Party Refund Demand Letter....... F-55
Transfer of Appeal Rights C-39
Troubleshooting using EOMB............... C-39
Verification of Insurance Coverage........ B-12
Voluntary Refund Form E-38
Welcome Letter B-6
Forms, full-sized
   See ChiroCode DeskBook Online Tools
Fraud and abuse F-7
   six important laws F-8
Frequently Asked Questions FAQ-1

G

Gifts and other inducements A-22
Glossary .... See End of Book
Government
   compliance programs............................... A-9
   health insurance programs B-35
      Federal Employee Plans B-37, B-38
      Federal Workers' Compensation B-36
      Medicaid B-37
      Military and Veterans B-36
Group
   health plans B-21
   practice options A-6
Guidelines
   appeals.. E-41
   Chiropractor's services C-28
   documentation D-1
   Medicare C-1
   unpaid claims E-39

H

Hardship policy (discount), financial............ B-46
HCPCS
   procedure codes................................... H-91
   supply codes I-8
   supply modifiers I-31
   Why use HCPCS I-4
Health and behavior assessment/intervention H-69
Health Care Fraud Statute F-10
Healthcare reform B-21
   shared savings programs............................A-7
Health history, past D-21
Health insurance coverage B-11
Health Reimbursement Arrangement (HRA) B-26
Health Savings Accounts (HSA) B-25
Help wanted ads... A-26
Highest specificity coding............................. G-4
HIPAA compliance F-14
   breach notification........ see Breach Notification
   covered entity offices............................... F-16
   electronic transactions F-18
      EFT and ERA F-19
   HITECH enforcement requirements..... F-26
   mobile devices and breaches F-16
   national identifier requirements F-29
   Omnibus final rule F-18
   penalties F-26
   privacy requirements.............................. F-20
   safeguards F-24
   security requirements............................. F-24
HIPAA Privacy Policy Form and Acknowledgement B-9
Hiring and firing... A-25
HITECH enforcement requirements F-26
Home services .... see Resource 130
Hospital services...........................see Resource 130

I

ICD-9-CM
   alphabetic list .... See Alphabetic list (ICD-9)
   anatomic list .... See Anatomic list (ICD-9)
   numeric list .... See Numeric list (ICD-9)
ICD-9-CM and ICD-10-CM
   code map - ICD-9 to ICD-10 ....G-9
   differences G-7
ICD-10-CM
   anatomic list .... See Anatomic list (ICD-10)
   guidelines and conventions....................G-21
   numeric list .... See Numeric list (ICD-10)
   placeholders..G-22
Imaging, diagnostic H-49
Independent contractors............................. A-33

Informed Consent for Chiropractic Treatment
    Form B-9, D-34
Informed Financial Consent Policy............. B-10
Initial visit B-13
    documentation requirements D-18
Inpatient consultations H-30
Insurance and Reimbursement B-1
    annual & lifetime limits........................ B-22
    business related A-11
    consumer driven plans B-25
    cyber A-12
    disability A-12, B-12
    federal employee plans B-37
    Forms .... See Forms
    government programs B-35
    information form B-8
    malpractice A-11
    managed care B-23
    medicaid B-37
    military and veterans B-36
    personal injury B-28
    plans, types of B-21
    property A-11
    reimbursement B-3
    secondary to medicare C-9
    supplemental C-8
    traditional B-21
    Workers' Compensation A-12, B-32
Interviewing A-26

L

Laboratory codes H-59
Late filing exceptions E-5
Laws
    ERISA E-47
    Medicare benefit policy manual C-27
Leasing equipment A-13
Letter(s)
    Continued care E-43
    Letter of Protection B-30
Liability insurance B-29
Licensing, professional A-10
Liens and assignment B-30
Lifetime limits B-22
Limiting charge C-6, C-13, C-14, C-35

M

MAC (Medicare Administrative Contractors)
Mail and correspondence, handling A-31

Maintenance care
    maintenace vs. active C-16
    billing B-16, C-16
    otice C-20
Managed care (HMO, PPO, etc) B-23
Marketing your practice A-20
Maximum medical improvement B-22
Measure Applicability Validation (MAV) C-46
Medicaid B-37
Medical and health history form B-8, D-22
Medical and surgical supplies I-9
Medical Benefits Payments ("MedPay") B-29
Medical expense recovery B-28
Medical fees .... See Fees
Medical necessity D-4
Medical Record Self-Audit Form F-39
Medical Savings Accounts (MSA) B-26
Medical team conferences H-36
Medicare
    Advantage plans, (Part C) C-10
    Administrative Contractors (MAC) C-11
    allowed amount C-6, C-13-14, C-30-35
    appeals C-36
    Benefit policy manual C-27-29
    billing help C-20
    CMT coding flowchart C-23-26
    common misconceptions C-26
    compliance F-31
    coverage of chiropractic services .. C-15, C-28
        coverage and limitations C-28
        eligibility C-15
        Medicare status questionnaire C-15
    fee
        schedule C-30
        decision chart C-32-35
    forms .... See Forms
    Inusrance
        secondary C-9
        medicap (supplemental) C-9
    jurisdictions (MAC) C-12
    limiting charge C-6,
        C-8, C-9, C-13, C-14, C-30-34
    misinformation on chiropractic
        services C-7, C-8, C-16, C-19, C-26
    modifiers, ... See Modifiers
    non-participation C-8
    Part C C-10
    Par/Non-Par Comparison C-5, C-6
    participation C-6, C-32
        advantages B-24

disadvantages B-24
comparison table C-6
participation status C-32
payment C-6
PQRS *See Physician Quality Reporting System*
provider enrollment C-4
PECOS C-5
revalidation C-5
Status Questionaire form C-15
summary notice B-17
Medication therapy mgmt services H-88
Medicine codes (chiropractic manipulation and
therapies) H-61
Medigap C-9
Military and Veterans B-36
Misinformation on chiropractic
services C-7, C-8, C-16, C-19, C-26
Modalities H-71
Modifiers
level I CPT H-99, I-9, I-31
level II supply I-9, I-32
Medicare C-21
understanding modifiers H-97
Multi-DC clinics A-6
Multi-disciplinary practice (MDP) A-6
Multiple diagnoses on a claim form E-5
Multiple employer welfare arrangements
(MEWA) B-26
Musculoskeletal system H-44
Mutually Exclusive (NCCI edits) H-8

N

National Correct Coding Initiative
(NCCI) F-32, H-7
edit challenges H-8
NCCI Edits for commonly used codes .. H-9
National identifier requirements F-29
Necessity for treatment D-20
Nervous system H-47
Networking A-22
Neurology and neuromuscular procedures . H-65
New patient initial visit B-13
No-fault states B-30
No-insurance and the cash practice B-26
Non-face-to-face services
nonphysician H-84
physician H-40
Noninvasive vascular diagnostic studies H-63
Nonphysician services, non-face-to-face H-84

Notice of Medicare coverage for chiropractic
care C-18
Numeric list, ICD-9-CM (Tabular) G-33
congenital anomalies (740-759) G-66
diseases of
blood/blood-forming organs (280-289) ....
G-33
circulatory system (390-459) G-45
digestive system (520-579) G-45
genitourinary system (580-629) G-46
musculoskeletal system (710-739) .. G-46
nervous system(320-389) G-38
endocrine, nutritional metabolic diseases,
and immunity disorders (240-279) . G-35
infectious/parasitic diseases (001-139) .. G-35
injury and poisoning (800-999) G-72
maintenance/wellness care (S8990) G-90
mental disorders (290-319) G-37
supplemental classification of external
causes of injury and poisoning
(E000 to E999) G-92
supplementary classification of factors
influencing health status and contact
with health services (V01 - V91) G-85
symptoms, signs, and Ill-Defined
Conditions (780-799) G-69
Nursing facility services .... *See Resource 130*
Nutrition therapy H-78

O

Office
equipment and software A-13
policies B-13
space: own vs lease A-5
services H-24
consultations H-29
OIG Compliance .... *See Compliance, OIG*
Omnibus 2013 Final Rule F-18
On-line medical evaluation H-41, H-84
Online tools xii
Orthotic procedures I-19
Definitions I-22
OSHA A-9, F-10
Osteopathic manipulative treatment
(OMT) H-79
Oswestry low back pain questionnaire D-44
Otorhinolaryngologic services H-61
Outcomes assessment D-43
Patients' Global Impression of
Change (PGIC) Scale D-45

Revised Oswestry Low Back
    Pain Questionnaire D-45
Rowland-Morris Low Back Pain and
    Disability Questionnaire D44
Outsourcing services A-14, A-18
Overpayments C-11, E-38, F-41

P

Pain, treatment of spine related algorithm .. D-35
Panels, joining A-22
Panels, organ or disease-oriented H-59
Paperwork Segment (PWK) E-8
P.A.R.T. Documentation Form D-24
Participation
    Medicare C-6
    Panels B-24
Patient
    financial responsibilities A-18
        Patient Financial Responsibility Letter B-7
    history D-19
    information B-13
    records, quality D-10
    Welcome Packet B-6
Patient Protection & Affordable Care Act
    (PPACA) A-7, E-48
Patients' Global Impression of Change
    (PGIC) Scale Form D-45
Payers, working with A-22
Payment concerns B-16
Payment, Medicare how it works C-6
Payment offsets, fighting F-55
Payment reports B-16, E-37
PECOS C-5
Pedestrian/Bicycle,
    personal injury inurance B-29
Penalties, HITECH F-26
Penalty for failure to timely
    provide required informaiton E-55
Performance measurement codes
    for chiropractic C-47, C-48
Personal injury B-11, B-28
    liens and assignment, ... B-30
    letter of protection B-30
    Medical Benefits Payments ("MedPay") . B-29
    no fault Ssates B-30
    Personal injury protection (PIP) B-29
    Uninsured/ Underinsured Motorist (UM/
        UIM) Coverage B-29
Physical examination D-22, D-30
Physical medicine and rehabilitation H-70

Physical therapy H-70
Physician Self-Referral Law F-8
Physician Quality Reporting System
    (PQRS) C-44
Policies & Procedures Manual A-29
PPACA essential health benefits (EHBs) B-22
PQRS ....
    See Physician Quality Reporting System
Practice management A-1
    groups A-23
Pre-authorization B-12
Preventive medicine services H-37
Privacy
    program review F-28
    protections and rights F-22
    requirements F-20
Private payer codes ("S" codes) H-94
Private sector plans E-47
Problem-Oriented Medical Record D-10
Procedure
    codes/coding H-1
    modifiers H-96
    professional services ("G" codes) H-91
Prolonged services H-35
Prompt filing B-16
Prompt pay discounts (TOS) B-47
Pulmonary H-64
Purchasing equipment A-14

R

Radiologic guidance other H-58
Radiology, diagnostic H-49
RBRVS components and fees B-42
Record keeping D-7
    abbreviations D-14
    Electronic Health Record (EHR) D-8
    guidelines for corrections D-14
    organizing the chart D-7
    Problem-Oriented Medical Record D-10
    standards for proper record keeping D-7
Recovery Audit Contractors (RAC) F-33
Redetermination & Reconsideration C-39
    redetermination checklist C-40
Refund requests and demands F-54
Registration process B-13
Rehabilitative services ("H" codes) H-94
Reimbursement Life Cycle B-5, E-3, E-34
Relative Value Units B-41
    dollar conversion factor B-41, B43
    RBRVS components B-42

Remittance advice B-17
Request for
    Medicare hearing by an administrative law
        judge C-42
    review of administrative law judge (ALJ)
        Medicare decision/dismissal C-42
    treatment.. B-5
Resource icons, legend to using xvii
Response Letter
    97110-97124 denials E-40
    refund demands F-55
Revalidation C-5
Review Erisa Appeals E-55
Review questions .... See end of each chapter
Rowland-Morris Low Back Pain and Disability
    Questionnaire D-45

S

Scheduling appointments A-32
Secondary insurance C-9
Security requirements F-24
Self-disclosure protocol (SDP) F-40
Self-funded plans E-48
Self-insurance (consumer driven plans) B-25
Services and procedures, other H-87
Shared Savings Programs A-7
Signatures D-12
Social Media A-21
Software selecting A-15
Solo or group practice A-6
Special evaluation/management services H-42
Special services, procedures and reports H-84
Staffing A-25
Starting & Maintaining a Thriving Practice ... A-3
Strapping H-45
Subluxation, diagnosis/coding C-20, D-23
Subsequent visits B-13, D-29
    documentation requirements D-27
Supplemental insurance
    (Medigap) C-7, C-9, C-13
Supply codes I-1
    supply coding I-3
    commonly used I-7
Supply modifiers
    supply modifiers I-7, I-31
    level II I-32
Supportive and productive staff A-25
Surgery codes H-44

T

Taxonomy codes F-29
Telephone services H-40, H-84
    clinical examples H-123
Telephone skills and duties A-31
Temporary codes For DMERCs' use I-18
Therapeutic procedures H-74
Third-party refund demand letter F-55
Timely filing of claims E-5
Traditional Insurance (individual or group) . B-21
Training staff A-28
Transitional care management services H-43
Treatment and documentation B-14
Treatment parameters D-43
Treatment plans D-30
    See ChiroCode DeskBook Online Tools
    Medicare requirements D-42
    treatment plan components D-42
Treatment visits D-28
    treatment visit notes D-28

U

Ultrasound, diagnostic H-57
Unbundling H-7
Unpaid claims, guidelines E-37
Unprocessable claims C-36, E-38
Usual, Customary, and Reasonable (UCR) . B-40

V

V codes G-84
Value based modifier (VBM) C46
Vascular diagnostic studies, noninvasive H-63
Verification of
    PQRS Reporting Status C-48
    coverage B-33
    insurance coverage form B-12
Virtual cards F-19
Voluntary Employee Benefit Associations
    (VEBA) B-26
Voluntary Refund Form E-38

W

Welcome packet B-6
Wellness services H-37
What to do if you are audited F-49
Work plan, OIG F-43
Work-related illness or injury B-32

Workers' Compensation B-11, B-32
    federal B-36
    first report of injury B-34
    loss of work time B-34
    state guidelines and fee schedules B-34
    verification of coverage B-33
    work-related illness or injury B-32
Working with payers A-23

Other Products from ChiroCode®

ICD-10 Coding for Chiropractic

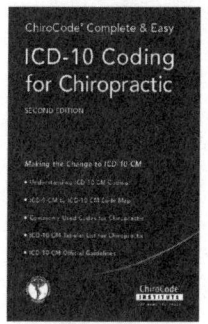

Is your office ready for ICD-10-CM? The Centers for Medicare & Medicaid Services (CMS) have set the deadline of October 1, 2015 for ICD-10-CM implementation. Your practice will benefit greatly from getting a head start on the changeover with this comprehensive resource from ChiroCode®.

Get this book NOW to avoid any interruption to your revenue stream. Written by the experts you trust, this book will be one of your most valuable tools during this industry conversion process.

Regular Price: $129
ChiroCode Member Price: $99

HIPAA Compliance - 3rd Edition

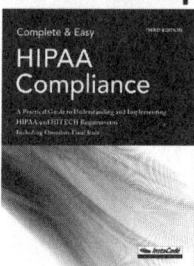

A simple and practical guide to implementing all HIPAA, HITECH and Omnibus 2013 Final Rule components. Includes all forms and policies to meet compliance requirements. This quick start manual, with essential forms, addresses all your top concerns, ensuring that you stay HIPAA compliant.

Includes customizable forms in Microsoft Word format. Not only do we tell you what needs to be in your forms, we actually have those forms available to download so you can quickly customize them for your office.

Regular Price: $149
ChiroCode Member Price: $119

How To Defeat IME Doctors Who Deny Your Claims

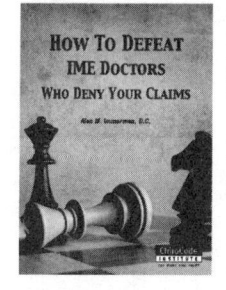

This book will give you the ammunition you need to counter reports from IME chiropractors and orthopedic surgeons. You will have arguments, key references and modern peer-reviewed literature to support the care you have rendered.

Arm yourself with this book so that you will be ready to defend your cases when assaulted by unfair IME reports. There is no other book available that provides this level of support for your personal injury practice.

Author: Dr. Alan Immerman

Regular Price: $89
ChiroCode Member Price: $79

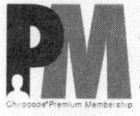

ChiroCode Premium Membership
- Discounts on most products, including coding books.
- ChiroCode Coding and Billing assistance by email.
- ChiroCode Webinars On Demand

Price: 29.99 MO / 299.99 YR

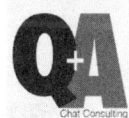

Q&A Chat Consulting
Do you need to talk with our coding, billing, or compliance experts?
We can guide you through your most difficult questions, customized to your own practice.

Price: $70 / 30 minutes

ChiroCode®

REGISTER FOR FREE CHIROCODE ALERTS

Stay Updated Throughout 2015

Register now for free *ChiroCode Alerts*. Changes can and do happen throughout the year. You'll get weekly coding and reimbursement updates and tips, as well as announcements of free *ChiroCode Webinars*. The alerts are sent by email, and are also posted on the ChiroCode.com website.

Your email privacy is assured. We will never share your information with anyone.

There are two ways to register for your ChiroCode Alerts:

1) Internet: Go to ChiroCode.com/register
2) Fax: Fill out and send this page to (602) 997-9755

Thank you for registering.

Register for ChiroCode Alerts

☐ Please register me to receive FREE ChiroCode Alerts by email.

Doctor or other name _____

Practice or other business name _____

Address _____

City/State/Zip _____

Phone _____ Fax _____

Email address _____

Signature _____

Date _____

ChiroCode INSTITUTE